"Prepare for a paradigm shift in the world of essential oil therapy. In *Aromatica Volume 2*, the dichotomy between the vitalistic and scientific/analytic philosophies which has overshadowed clinical practice for many years is finally resolved. A new way of approaching clinical practice is presented – one which integrates the diagnostic principles of traditional Chinese, Greek, Japanese Kampo and Ayurvedic medicine with empirical and scientific evidence which informs the clinical use of essential oils. This is a masterpiece, and highly recommended for all serious practitioners of essential oil therapy."

*—Jennifer Peace Rhind, author, mentor and essential oil consultant*

"In this eagerly awaited second volume, Peter Holmes applies decades of clinical experience and scholarly endeavour to a field of plant therapy in need of the very insights that inform the book. *Aromatica* blends advanced aromatherapy, Chinese medicine and clinical expertise to yield an illuminating and accessible approach to Integrative Essential Oil Therapeutics."

*—Gabriel Mojay, Founding Co-Chair of the International Federation of Professional Aromatherapists (IFPA) and author of* Aromatherapy for Healing the Spirit

"Holmes' *Energetics* has been a valuable reference in my clinical work for 30 years. Peter is one of the rare thought leaders in herbalism who understand that history, philosophy and science are all essential prerequisites for precision parsing of the materia medica into clinical practice. In *Aromatica Volume 2*, Peter extends his tried and tested approach to (his beloved) essential oils - and aromatherapy will be all the richer."

*—Jonathan Treasure, Medical Herbalist, Oregon*

"Here is the perfect book for the advanced aromatherapist who is interested in applying energetics within their aromatic practice. Holmes provides not only the introduction into aromatic energetics, but then follows up with oil energetics in the Materia Aromatica. The crowning glory is all the safety information given in methods of essential oil delivery."

*—Inga Wieser, ND, MS, APAIA, MH, President of Alliance of International Aromatherapists*

"There are a relative handful of 'must-have' books on the therapeutic use of essential oils that I keep on my main bookshelf for easy reference and study. Peter's *Aromatica Volume 1* and now *Volume 2* are definitely on this short list! Highly recommended for any practitioner truly interested in essential oil therapy.

Peter's knowledgeable blending of the physical and energetic qualities of essential oils using both Western and Eastern approaches gives a comprehensive overview of the therapeutic benefits of each essential oil covered in his profiles."

*—Ron Guba, Aromatic Medicine educator, and Director of the Center for Aromatic Medicine, Melbourne, Australia*

# AROMATICA

A Clinical Guide to Essential Oil Therapeutics

VOLUME 2: APPLICATIONS AND PROFILES

## PETER HOLMES LAc, MH

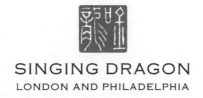

SINGING DRAGON
LONDON AND PHILADELPHIA

First published in 2019
by Singing Dragon
an imprint of Jessica Kingsley Publishers
73 Collier Street
London N1 9BE, UK
and
400 Market Street, Suite 400
Philadelphia, PA 19106, USA

*www.singingdragon.com*

**Library of Congress Cataloging in Publication Data**
A CIP catalog record for this book is available from the Library of Congress

**British Library Cataloguing in Publication Data**
A CIP catalogue record for this book is available from the British Library

ISBN 978 1 84819 303 1
eISBN 978 0 85701 257 9

Printed in the United Kingdom

*Dedicated to my students, who have provided both
the motivation to write and the encouragement
to finish this text.*

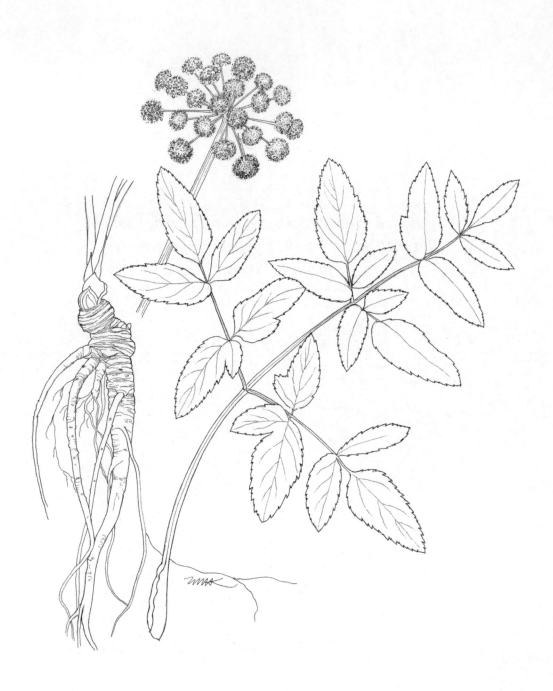

# Contents

# 1

# The Clinical Applications of Essential Oils

## A SYSTEMIC APPROACH

This chapter will attempt to do the impossible: to take a systemic approach to the therapeutic uses of essential oils with the full knowledge that the odds against being successful are unfavourable. Their clinical uses have too short a history, their applications are too varied, and the current dichotomy between clinical experience and scientific research is too great. Despite these odds, if we are to make progress to a truly integrated and effective approach to essential oil use, it becomes necessary at this time to scan all the therapeutic knowledge about the oils through the lens of basic clinical criteria. We must ask ourselves some fundamental questions: Do essential oils mainly treat the psyche or the body, or both? What is the relative influence of olfaction and absorption in any effective treatment with essential oils? What are the best forms of delivery and preparation methods for essential oils? What types of illnesses are best treated with essential oils? And what are the best treatment paradigms for the clinical applications of essential oils?

With those exploratory themes in mind, we could certainly do worse than summarize the main types of conditions that essential oils are known so far to address with remarkable success (Chabènes 1838; Gattefossé 1937; Maury 1961; Valnet 1975; Belaiche 1979; Pénoel 1990; Buckle 2003; Price and Price 2007; Franchomme 2015).

- **Symptom relief.** Regardless of the route of administration adopted, essential oils are known to provide good and often rapid relief of signs and symptoms, both acute and chronic – pain and fatigue being the most common ones relieved or reduced. The use of essential oils in most delivery forms generally tends to induce a feeling of wellbeing; this may or may not be accompanied by relief of a particular sign or symptom. The main symptoms that are indicated for selecting a particular oil are summarized in the 'Specific symptomatology' sections of this materia aromatica.

- **The treatment of psychological conditions.** Used for olfaction by mild inhalation in their vapour form, essential oils have proven highly effective for treating mental and emotional conditions, including the treatment of mood disorders and various psychological states. These include anxiety, depression, bipolar syndrome, PMS, ADHD and many other such conditions, whether formally diagnosed in Western medicine or not. Any essential oil that evokes a pleasant subjective response in the individual is a good candidate for aromatic therapy by olfaction. This includes oils with many different types of fragrance qualities, ranging from fresh-pungent to sweet-green to floral-sweet. The main symptoms and disorders that are indicated for the psychological use of an oil are summarized in the 'Psychological' sections of this materia aromatica.

- **The treatment of infections.** Since the mid-19th century, if not earlier, essential oils have been applied experimentally and clinically to treating a large variety of infectious conditions. Scientific studies in vivo and in vitro continue to confirm their efficacy, both in their gaseous and liquid phase, in inhibiting the activity and development of most microbes, including bacteria, fungi, viruses and spirochetes. Important oils commonly employed for treating a range of acute and chronic infections of various kinds include Niaouli, Cajeput, Tea tree, Thyme ct. thymol, Oregano, Palmarosa, Clove and Cinnamon. The main infectious conditions indicating use of a particular oil are summarized in the 'Antimicrobial actions' subsections of physiological functions and indications.

- **The treatment of the general terrain of the individual.** Like herbal and homeopathic remedies, essential oils also excel at regulating imbalance of the individual terrain, especially when used over time. In functional and diagnostic terms, this includes a terrain characterized by tension, weakness, heat, cold, dry, damp, and so on. In physiopathological terms, a terrain may be dominated by a particular pathology, e.g. chronic inflammation; congestion; fungal, viral or bacterial dominance; or simply be the result of certain organ or endocrine dominance, such as a hepatic terrain or an oestrogen-dominant terrain. Almost any essential oils may address the whole terrain that underlies specific symptoms, syndromes and disorders. Those least likely to be appropriate for terrain treatment are those with a single dominant fragrance note and chemical constituent, such as Lemon, Cajeput and Wintergreen. Oils for treatment may be given in many different forms of delivery, all depending on individual needs. The main terrain conditions indicating use of a particular oil are given at the start of the sections on physiological functions and indications.

## Making Systemic Differentiations among Clinical Applications

Ambiguity and conflation now plague anyone wanting to use essential oils for therapeutic purposes. Essential oils in all their varieties have been commercialized and popularized to the utmost extent of legality, and beyond – they have finally entered the cultural mainstream of the Western lifestyle. Healthcare practitioners wishing to embrace the use of essential oils as therapeutic agents clearly need to set themselves apart from popular 'aroma culture' and its profit-driven underpinnings. But herein lies the catch. In order to successfully differentiate themselves, they first need to define themselves through their therapeutic work. The task is mainly about defining clearly and accurately the many ways in which the oils may be put to therapeutic purposes. Practitioners need to clarify their treatment applications before and in order to define themselves.

Terms such as 'aromatic medicine', 'clinical aromatherapy', 'aesthetic aromatherapy' and 'psychoaromatherapy' have become increasingly common. Each term purports use in a particular healthcare setting and with particular therapeutic intentions – but at best, these definitions are ambiguous and confusing: most imply the exclusive use of oil aroma, despite that not always being the case. As discussed in Chapter 1 of the first volume, the problem with these terms is that it is arguably counterproductive today to even use the term 'aromatherapy', which logically and properly refers to a form of treatment solely based on olfaction and which clearly indicates the therapeutic use of oil aroma alone. Outworn traditional definitions such as 'aromatherapy' and 'aromatic' serve merely to conflate and obscure the true purpose and methodology of different therapeutic applications. Furthermore, these terms erode clarity among practitioners and adherents as regards their own treatment styles and methods. In so doing, they undermine essential oil therapy itself.

It would clearly be more accurate and positive to describe any clinical application of essential oils simply as a particular form of essential oil therapy – this is an important issue of terminology. Regardless, however, there is a second problem here: no truly complete and systemic explanation of the ways in which essential oils positively benefit the individual during treatment exists. The oils are extremely – and confusingly – versatile in their applications in any clinical context. Whether used in their vapour or liquid form, the pathways and processes of absorption and therapeutic effect of essential oils are numerous and polyvalent, and their physiological interactions complex (Buckle 2003; Harris and Harris 2006a; Rhind 2012). It is now well established that there are many means and mechanisms by which essential oils positively influence individual wellbeing and, in a clinical context, treat actual disorders. Most of them are not fully understood.

These means include activation of cerebral neural networks through olfaction; absorption of an essential oil vapour by the respiratory system when inhaled; absorption of the oils through the skin when applied topically; and absorption through the mucous membrane when applied in specialized delivery forms such as pessaries, suppositories and gel caps. Taken together, these pathways of essential oil absorption and influence form a highly complex web whose pharmacodynamics we are only just beginning to understand. For instance, in the case of dermal oil application, there is still no definite agreement, for any particular oil, as to the amount of essential oil actually absorbed into the body's internal environment. Lack of serious studies on this extremely basic issue is partly the cause, in addition to simplistic adherence to received assumptions. Likewise, the effect of oil inhalation itself is still not fully understood for its therapeutic implications. This is partly because of the twin simultaneous olfactory and physiological processes involved, and partly because of the numerous variables that may swing results one way or another, such as the length and depth of oil inhalation, the type of oil used, the intention and expectations of treatment shared by the client and practitioner, and so on.

At the same time, the research evidence that is available needs to be translated into a treatment context, if we are to draw meaningful conclusions for actual practice. For a practitioner to make effective and intentional choices among the many methods available for delivering essential oils to a client, the pathways and processes of oil absorption simply need to be understood for their final therapeutic effect, which in turn will indicate the types of conditions most likely to benefit from their use. The evidence of research is just a place to start. To be of any clinical use, scientific findings still need to be interpreted for their clinical significance. Interpretation is everything.

Clearly, if a practitioner is to intentionally direct essential oil treatment to a patient's particular needs, it becomes crucial to systemically clarify the pathways, gateways and processes through which the oils are taken up and absorbed. This will allow him or her to make clear distinctions among the various types of essential oil treatments and will help avoid the conflation of these pathways into a generic, nonspecific 'aromatherapy'. The result will be clearer definitions among the various possible treatments with essential oils, which will finally suggest accurate naming of these different treatments. In practice, systemic clarification allows one to make primary decisions about whether to focus on treating mind or body, and whether olfaction or absorption would be the best treatment route. This in turn will determine the choice of appropriate methods of treatment to obtain the most effective results. On a larger scale, making these systemic distinctions will in turn yield the additional benefit of bridging the gap, unfortunately still enormous, between essential oil applications based purely on theoretical evidence, and clinical practice based on the evidence of cumulative traditional empirical experience.

Table 1.1 Pathways of Essential Oil Treatment

| | Vapour | | Liquid | | | | |
|---|---|---|---|---|---|---|---|
| **Treatment pathway** | **Internal** | | | | | **External** | |
| **Absorption gateway** | **Respiratory** | **Respiratory** | **Oral** | **Rectal** | **Vaginal** | **Dermal** — **Oil based** | **Dermal** — **Water based** |
| **Organ and system tropism** | Brain and neuroendocrine system | Upper and lower respiratory system, stomach | Intestines, liver, kidneys, brain; systemic | Large intestine, lower respiratory; systemic | Female reproductive system | Soft tissue, including skin, muscles, tendons, joints | |
| **Effect and process** | **Psychological by olfaction** | **Physiological by tissue absorption** | | | | | |
| **Delivery methods** | Mild to moderate inhalation, e.g. diffusion, tissue or fingertip inhalation | Deep inhalation, e.g. steam inhalation, nebulization, medicated cotton wool | Gelatin capsules, honey, sublingual drops and tablets, lingual honey | Suppositories | Pessaries, sponges, vaginal serums | Topical lotions, liniments, creams, ointments, plasters | Topical gels, compresses |

# Pathways of Essential Oil Treatment

*The two therapeutic effects: psychological and physiological*

A primary rubric for clinical practice is to divide the various essential oil treatments into psychological versus physiological types of applications. All possible pathways of influence really boil down to either a psychological effect or a physiological one: the realm of the psyche on one hand, with its gamut of instinctive, emotional, mental and spiritual functions, and the physical body with its many functional systems on the other hand. As a result, it becomes crucial for the practitioner to differentiate any clinical application of essential oils according to the treatment intention. If an effect on the psyche is intended, then inhalation techniques of the oils in vapour form are the best (although by no means the only) choice. Applications by inhalation are indicated when mental and/or emotional issues are foremost in the patient's presentation, or simply when working with clients in the context of a counselling or psychology practice. The administration method in this case would be direct or diffuse olfactory stimulation, which could be delivered in any number of ways, such as direct gentle methods of inhalation, and ambient inhalation through diffusion of the oils into the immediate environment. However, if treating physiological conditions such as infection and inflammation, then physiological absorption of the oils in liquid form is the obvious application of choice. Physical disorders require specific targeted methods of internal delivery such as gel caps, suppositories, nebulizer inhalation and various topical preparations, largely depending on the location of the condition.

The psychological and physiological effects of an essential oil are best understood by examining the two complementary pathways that it may take to influence an individual. The psychological effect is achieved mainly through the process of olfaction, which makes use of an oil purely as olfactory information. The physiological effect is obtained primarily through the process of physical absorption of an oil as a physiochemical substance. Both types of effect clearly depend on the various gateways that facilitate them, which in turn point the way to the best forms of essential oil delivery.

*The two essential processes: olfaction and absorption*

In the most basic terms, essential oil applications rely for their effects on either the process of olfaction – using an oil in vapour form – or by application onto or absorption into the body – using an oil in liquid form. Any essential oil application should be pivoted on one of these processes.

The first type of application involves gentle inhalation of an oil's fragrance for the process of olfaction. Here the oil will deliver its benefits essentially in terms of the information that its fragrance provides to the limbic system. The end result of olfactory uptake is essentially a psychological response. This involves many dynamics, such as sense perception, memory association and mental changes in both content and type, as well as an important instinctual response in terms of liking or disliking the oil fragrance, coupled with an emotional response of some kind. Eventually, however, the neuroendocrine effect of olfaction will also end up affecting physical tissues, not least by modulating the two-way exchange of hormonal and neural peptides between the brain and intestinal microflora – the brain-gut axis. Although olfaction mainly produces a psychological effect, it also may activate the psyche's complex pathways of influence on the body itself.

The second type of clinical application involves causing a physical uptake of an oil as a medicinal substance, i.e. by judicious insertion into one of the body's orifices, or by application of the oil topically. The aim here is treatment of a physical ailment by causing tissue absorption with resultant alterations in physiological functions at every level – cellular, tissue and organ systems. The dominant effect is clearly a physiological response. Eventually, however, as this response begins to involve peptides and neuroendocrine functions – especially in the intestinal microflora and the brain – it will also end up creating a secondary psychological effect. Although tissue absorption essentially produces a physiological effect therefore, it will in turn tend to stimulate the effects of physiological functions on the psyche.

Understanding the primary and secondary systemic effects of olfactory stimulation and physical absorption on the individual is key to understanding the complementary relationship between a psychological and a physiological effect. In so doing, it clearly illuminates the difference between psychology and physical medicine, as well as their essential and complementary relationship. The two essential processes point unequivocally to the unity of mind and body.

In clinical practice, distinguishing between olfaction and absorption will suggest specific treatment strategies that are truly based on the needs of the individual condition. By offering many options beyond simplistic treatments based on a one-size-fits-all approach, this will allow the practitioner to go to the source of the individual's ailment and to provide comprehensive body-mind treatment that goes beyond symptom relief.

Making a clear distinction between an olfactory and a physiological treatment with essential oils takes into account the important consequences for those oils that exert a different effect in vapour versus liquid form. The result of conflating olfaction with absorption has been ignorance of this major difference that certain oils exhibit. In many cases, their systemic effect is simply different and, in some cases, exactly the opposite. This is generally seen in those oils whose pharmacological profile is no useful indication of their olfactory effect, and often in those posessing two or more dominant constituents. Oils high in aldehydes, such as citral and citronellal for instance – the green-lemony oils that include Lemongrass, May chang and Lemon eucalyptus – are uplifting and clarifying when gently inhaled. When deeply inhaled and absorbed, however, their physiological effect is the exact opposite: calming and relaxing. Certain other oils too exhibit a marked incongruence between their olfactory and physiological effect, including Myrrh, Laurel, Fennel, Cardamom,

Patchouli, Vetiver, Wintergreen, Helichrysum, Atlas cedarwood, Red and green mandarin, and Basil ct. methylchavicol.

In turn, this phenomenon points to the fact that an oil's pharmacological profile is not necessarily a reliable indicator of its psychological impact. It puts to question the traditional – and still staunchly upheld – tenet of understanding essential oils solely through their pharmacognosy. Once again, it suggests that understanding their fragrance profile is at least as, if not more, important than their pharmacological one. Certainly, when it comes to understanding the broad psychological effects of essential oils, knowing their fragrance type clearly becomes inescapable. Ultimately, defining oils by their fragrance is yet another way of deepening our connection with the plant kingdom, as well as of expanding our ability to access the richness of all life in general.

**Table 1.2 The Five Gateways for the Physiological Delivery of Essential Oils**

| Essential oil delivery gateway | Respiratory | Oral | Rectal | Vaginal | Dermal |
|---|---|---|---|---|---|
| Local recipients and delivery methods | Sinuses, middle ear – hot steam inhalation | Brain, sinuses – sublingual, lingual | Rectum – suppository | Vagina, cervix – vaginal serum, sponge, pessary | Skin, other soft tissues – liniment, perfusion |
| Internal organ beneficiaries and delivery methods | Upper and lower respiratory systems, brain – deep inhalation, strong nebulization | Intestines, microflora, liver – gel cap | Colon, lungs – suppository | Uterus, bladder – serum, sponge, pessary | |
| Systemic distribution | Moderate, short-lived | Good | Excellent, prolonged | None | Very poor, unpredictable |

## The Five Orifice Gateways of Essential Oil Treatment

Key to determining the choice of delivery method for any essential oil treatment is understanding the treatment gateways or openings through which an oil can be delivered to exert its psychological or physiological effect. These gateways are four of the body's main orifices – nose, mouth, rectum and vagina – plus the skin. Any essential oil treatment entails one or more of these common gateways: the respiratory, oral, rectal, vaginal and dermal gateways. They are major portals that allow essential oils to access certain internal organs and systems. Essentially, they are not the final beneficiaries of treatment in their own right, but rather facilitators of many types of treatment, systemic as well as local, internal as well as superficial. The oral gateway of treatment, for example, is an important entryway for essential oils to reach the digestive tract and, from there, the internal environment. However, although the mouth is the beginning of the digestive tract, it is clearly also possible to treat problems in the oral cavity itself. With the right choice of delivery method, oils administered through any of the major gateways can produce an internal effect. Likewise, all five orifice gateways have the potential for producing physical absorption of an oil – including respiratory oil uptake by moderate to deep, extended inhalation, and dermal application when delivered to particular reflex zones and points.

The respiratory and dermal treatment gateways in particular are unique in facilitating two very different processes. Inhalation of an essential oil is a delivery method able to achieve two different, distinct effects, psychological or physiological, depending on the intensity and length of inhalation. When an oil is inhaled mildly and briefly, olfaction is the main initial result, involving translation of gaseous oil molecules into neural impulses. However, when an oil is inhaled deeply and for a length of time, physiological absorption is the main eventual result, as it crosses the membranes and enters the circulation. Being the portal to both olfactory stimulation of the psyche and physiological absorption, the respiratory gateway by inhalation is clearly a highly versatile and effective form of essential oil treatment. In practice, it deserves careful consideration and precise use with respect to the specific treatment intention desired.

The skin, closely related to the lungs, is the other organ gateway that is able to achieve a dual effect with dermal application of an essential oil: on one hand physiological absorption by three distinct mechanisms, on the other hand a reflex effect by nerve stimulation and somatic resonance. Both these effects, like respiratory intensity and length of inhalation, are also best applied to different types of treatment.

Oil absorption engages fully when applied to topical conditions involving a limited body area, whereas reflex effects shine when used to treat internal and more systemic conditions. Marguerite Maury herself, the founder of British Aromatherapy, fully understood the complex effects of an essential oil on the skin. She realized early on that correct and effective delivery through the skin was not just about considering the issue of oil absorption, but also a matter of taking into account its reflex action on reflex zones and acupuncture points (Maury 1961, 2004).

These two effects combined, along with the minor olfactory aspect of skin applications, conspire to make the highly exposed dermal gateway not only the most versatile and easy-to-use of all gateways but, by the same token, the one most vulnerable and most fraught with dangers as well. While its versatility mirrors respiratory versatility, it requires careful, considered use in essential oil therapy.

The dynamics of the treatment gateways and the applications that they suggest are best described in the practical terms of the three basic processes involved, namely olfactory stimulation, respiratory/oral/rectal/vaginal absorption, and topical dermal application.

# 2

# Methods of Essential Oil Delivery

## GATEWAYS AND METHODS OF DELIVERY

The systemic approach to essential oil therapeutics trickles down to the very specific delivery methods chosen for treatment. Once the practitioner decides on olfaction or absorption as the fundamental form of treatment – depending on the primary concern, psychological or physiological – the next decision is about the treatment gateway to be chosen. Many factors will determine that choice: whether the patient's condition is acute or chronic, local or systemic, and so on, along with its many details. Each treatment gateway is a special entry that allows treatment of particular body systems, organs and tissues. Each has both advantages and disadvantages, and offers a variety of specific delivery methods for consideration.

### Olfactory Stimulation by Mild Inhalation

*Using the respiratory gateway*

The first use of the respiratory gateway is when an individual gently inhales an essential oil simply to obtain olfactory stimulation. Here the oil is used for the information that fragrance provides, not for its actual substance or energy. What counts here is its fragrance content, not its physical form. The result is a broad effect that, for better or for worse, may be labelled a psychological one. The oil here evokes a mental-emotional response.

In the process of olfaction, an essential oil is taken up as a fragrant vapour in the olfactory epithelium, where the dendrites, the olfactory nerves, translate its chemical structure into a neural impulse, which in turn is amplified by the olfactory bulb.

The neural information finally reaches the brain's limbic system without any step-down process of any kind – unlike the information received from all other senses, which is greatly reduced by the olfactory bulb. From the limbic system, the impulse reaches the hypothalamus and selectively various other brain centres. These then release various peptides, i.e. hormones and neurotransmitters, that evoke in the individual the mental and emotional response particular to that essential oil.

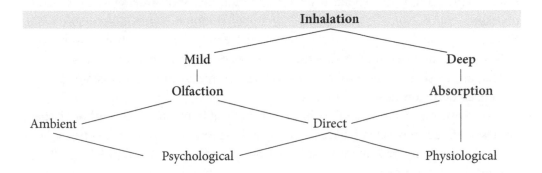

As the end result of the process of olfaction, the psychological response presents several different aspects. Firstly, it usually involves several dynamics such as cognition, sense perception, memory association and mental changes in both type and content. Secondly, olfaction usually generates a significant instinctual response in terms of liking or disliking the oil fragrance. Thirdly, it often triggers an emotional response that may affect mood and ultimately also behaviour. In addition, this psychological response may create a secondary effect on physiological functions, especially in conditions related to unproductive stress. This effect is mediated by psycho-neuroendocrine functions as a whole. Many skin, digestive and respiratory disorders, for instance, and especially when involving pain, may be beneficially influenced by the psychological effects of essential oils used purely by olfaction. In the hands of a skilled practitioner, even a formulation designed for a physiological application may be useful for its olfactory dimension. As noted in Volume 1, the majority of popular medicinal preparations in the past certainly also doubled as perfumes.

Olfactory stimulation of the upper respiratory gateway by mild inhalation of an essential oil is the safest way to use essential oils; it is the one widespread and time-tested practice for all aromatic substances in many different contexts. It represents true 'aromatic' therapy. For today's practitioner it represents a potentially powerful pathway of treatment to the extent that the majority of current disorders seen in the West arguably involve mental-emotional imbalance. This does not include frank infectious diseases and epidemics, of course. Olfactory stimulation can be seen as the most important contribution of essential oil therapy in its many forms to both prevent and treat illness in general.

## Clinical applications

The main purpose of olfaction by mild inhalation is to promote psychological balance and wellbeing, as well as to treat actual mental and emotional conditions. Selecting suitable essential oils for olfaction should be done with reference to the basic model of stimulant, relaxant and regulating oils – their three basic psychological functions. Most mood disorders may be positively influenced through olfaction, including anxiety states, depression, PMS, bipolar disorder, attention deficit disorders (ADD, ADHD), obsessive-compulsive disorder (OCD) and post-traumatic stress disorder (PTSD). Essential oils can be very effective in treating these disorders: their direct modulation of limbic and neuroendocrine functions involves primary, autonomic emotions such as fear, anger, sorrow and euphoria, as well as psychic or soul-related states such as shame, anxiety, confusion and despair.

Aromatic olfaction is also known to be beneficial in mental states, although these are less defined in psychiatric terms. They include loss of cognitive functions, poor concentration, impaired memory, distractibility, and schizoid and psychotic states. Essential oils can positively influence even minor mood changes, including those caused by a physical disorder. These include the mental-emotional symptoms involving common conditions such as insomnia, dysmenorrhoea, neurasthenia, adrenal fatigue and dysregulation, and chronic pain conditions in general.

Finally, all stress-related symptoms in general will also benefit from the use of oil olfaction because of its secondary physiological effect. They include those conditions often thought of as psychosomatic, such as psychogenic skin conditions (e.g. neurogenic eczema and seborrhoea), neurogenic asthma and heart conditions, irritable bowel syndrome (IBS) and urinary incontinence.

## Delivery methods

The delivery methods for the olfactory use of essential oils in practice divide into direct olfaction and indirect olfaction by ambient diffusion.

### DIRECT OLFACTION BY MILD INHALATION

To produce direct olfaction by inhalation, the essential oil should be inhaled gently and smelt for only one to four cycles of the breath. This may be done directly from a bottle of oil, from a few drops on a tissue or handkerchief, from a cotton-wool ball inside a ziplock bag, or from a drop placed on the forefinger and thumb held together. If smelling directly from a bottle, the orifice reducer or dropper may be removed. It is important here to keep wafting the oil slowly from one nostril to the other rather than have it pointing only to one nostril. It is always best to start at a small distance below the nose and, when the whole fragrance is perceived, slowly move the oil closer until an ideal, comfortable distance is found.

Olfaction should be discontinued if the oil is for any reason experienced as unpleasant. Ideal oils are those that are much liked, but oils that evoke only a neutral response at first are also acceptable candidates for olfactory treatment. If these are strongly indicated therapeutically, the client will often experience an increased appreciation for their odour during one or several sessions and will in turn derive increasing benefit from their use.

Direct olfaction can stand in nicely for indirect ambient olfaction when the individual is in transit, e.g. in cars, planes and trains, or when in public or semi-public spaces (often restricted) where discretion is appropriate, as in airports, public waiting rooms, classrooms and the like. Mild olfaction can refresh, uplift, energize or relax, all depending on the oils chosen – often a lifesaver in acute travel situations. Citrus oils such as Bergamot, Grapefruit and Mandarin (red, green or yellow), single or blended, are especially versatile in such situations. Most of these oils are able to uplift, creating alertness and optimism, while also balancing the mood in difficult situations that may arouse anxiety, frustration, and so on. Also, citrus oils are the most likely to be enjoyed by anyone else in close proximity. However, many green-fragrance oils also show their first-aid worth in thorny travel situations, especially unexpected and traumatic experiences; these oils include Lavander, Lavandin and, in dilution, Blue tansy, Roman camomile and Sambac jasmine absolute.

Direct olfaction is the delivery method of choice when mental emotional symptoms are acute. It can act fairly quickly, for instance, for acute anxiety, fear, agitation, panic attack, etc., but also for acute brain fog, falling into a stupor, etc. However, direct olfaction also serves chronic mood disorders quite nicely if done regularly and when the right oils are selected.

Several types of essential oils are appropriate for acute conditions:

- Rosy-sweet oils for acute anxiety and worry, including Geranium, Rose absolute, Helichrysum and Jasmine absolute

- Sweet-green oils for acute anger and frustration, including Blue tansy, German camomile, Roman camomile and Sambac jasmine absolute

- Herbaceous-green oils for acute racing mind and nervous tension, including Lavender, Clary sage, Marjoram and Hyssop

- Pungent oils for acute brain fog or stupor, including Peppermint, Niaouli, Rosemary, Ravintsara and Black spruce

- Sweet-woody oils for acute worry, obsession or compulsion, including Cedarwood (any type), Sandalwood, Siam wood, Myrrh and Patchouli

- Rooty oils for acute manic elation or dissociation, including Vetiver, Dong quai, Lovage root and Spikenard

- Lemony oils for acute discouragement or despair, including Bergamot, Grapefruit, Lemongrass, May chang and Kaffir lime petitgrain

- Pungent oils for acute grief or sadness, including Saro, Rosemary, Green myrtle and Spike lavender

It is important to be clear about which treatment is intended, olfactory or physiological, and to stick to that decision. Any inhalation over three breath cycles will definitely cause increasingly significant physiological absorption. If a combined olfactory and physiological effect is intended, such as in acute situations, it may be appropriate to go over the limit of three breath cycles and continue up to eight.

However, note again here that not all oils have the same or even similar effect in the olfactory phase as in their physiological phase. Caution is especially required in the case of the green-lemony, aldehyde-rich oils, such as Lemongrass, May chang and Coriander leaf. By olfaction these oils promote alertness, good judgement and optimism; by physiological absorption they exert a calming effect on the nervous system, causing drowsiness and systemic relaxation – the very opposite of their olfactory effect. Certain other oils also exhibit a marked difference between their olfactory and physiological effect. Helichrysum, for example, by olfaction is a rosy-sweet supporter and balancer that promotes emotional security and stability; by absorption the oil is a high-ester systemic relaxant and hypnotic. Cardamom is another example; by olfaction a sweet, spicy-pungent oil for promoting confidence and courage, the oil once absorbed will act as a nervous sedative and systemic relaxant – again very different effects. Being aware of the possible difference between the olfactory and absorptive effects of an oil will always guide the practitioner to the best oil selection. Key here is knowing an oil's fragrance profile and noting the difference from its pharmacological profile.

## INDIRECT OLFACTION BY AMBIENT DIFFUSION

Diffusing essential oils into the immediate environment by very mild, low-level continuous oil inhalation will also cause olfactory stimulation. There are several ways in which essential oils may be diffused to release their ambient scent. They all come down to two distinct processes: evaporation and nebulization. Oil evaporation, or vaporization, is created with the use of heat or cold air. Oil nebulization is produced either by ultrasound in water or with compressed air in a specialized glass nebulizer.

Note that the various devices available that diffuse essential oils by evaporation or nebulization are commercially often called 'diffusers' and 'nebulizers' without discrimination between these two very different processes. Add to this confusion mistaken concepts such as the conflation of oil evaporation and oil burning.

Ambient diffusion is the most common method available for releasing essential oil fragrance into the environment. Extremely versatile, it is employed in both domestic and therapeutic settings, including living spaces, bedrooms, daycares, homecare centres and clinics of all kinds (ranging from spas to professional practitioners' treatment rooms to hospitals). It enjoys a wide range of applications – aesthetic, psychological and mildly physiological. Ambient diffusion of the right oils has a wide range of advantages, serving mainly to:

- Create a pleasant scentscape and welcoming ambience at home and at work to enhance wellbeing

- Mask and reduce unpleasant odours

- Gently balance mental-emotional conditions

- Reduce ambient microbial load and thereby create a more sanitary space

- Prevent chronic upper and lower respiratory infections

The power of ambient diffusion, especially with use of a nebulizer (either type), should not be underestimated for any of these tasks. The types of essential oils that excel here include:

- Sweet-lemony oils for creating a welcoming scentscape in a work environment, including Bergamot, Nerolina, Red mandarin, Palmarosa and Lemongrass

- Lemon, Gapefruit, Cedarwood and Patchouli for masking bad odours

- Rosy-sweet and sweet-woody oils for promoting mental-emotional stability, including Rose absolute, Geranium, Helichrysum, Cedarwood, Siam wood and Sandalwood

- Widely antimicrobial, fresh-pungent oils high in 1,8 cineole and monoterpenes, including several Eucalyptus oils (including the blue-gum, narrow-leaf, river red gum and blue-leaf species), Niaouli, Cajeput, Ravintsara and Thyme ct. thymol for sanitizing a space by reducing its microbial load

- Antimicrobial fresh-pungent oils high in monoterpenes and 1,8 cineole with a strong tropism for respiratory functions: all of the above and Green myrtle

Studies in the last 50 years show that essential oils diffused or nebulized in healthcare environments such as clinics, nursing homes and hospitals are significantly able to prevent infections by reducing germ transmission. The surprise here is not the strong antiseptic action of essential oils, but rather the extremely limited extent to which their proven antimicrobial effect is currently engaged in communal spaces whose load of infection-producing microbes is known to be extremely high. Certainly, in the face of increasingly common nosocomial and antibiotic-resistant infections, nebulization of strong antimicrobial oils high in monoterpenes (as those listed above) in these environments has now become a sheer necessity.

To create a successful oil blend for ambient diffusion, see in, 'Perfumery status' Chapter 6 of Volume 1. In most cases, a good blend that is not fatiguing to the nose requires a good balance of head, heart and base notes or, if base-note oils are not included, at least a nice proportion of head and heart notes. If the blend is intended mainly for therapeutic purposes, then the balance of fragrance notes is not as crucial, but simply useful to ensure acceptability and a non-fatiguing effect.

- **Heat aromatic evaporation.** This common, reliable method of diffusing essential oils relies on their ability, when stimulated by a warmth source, to rapidly evaporate and release their fragrance. The majority of traditional aroma diffusers, also called aroma burners or oil burners or vaporizers, work on this principle. A small ceramic or glass bowl filled two-thirds with water or vegetable oil to which several drops of undiluted essential oil is added is gently heated from below by a tea light candle or electric coil. The greater the oil's fragrance intensity, the fewer the drops that are needed. Ensure that the water or vegetable oil does not start boiling, smoking or burning. If it dries out, a ceramic bowl may crack and a glass bowl may break. Using a vegetable oil base is especially good for creating a warm, intimate and meditative ambience, especially with balsamic resin oils such as Myrrh, Cistus, Benzoin or Frankincense.

  Both heat and cold types of aromatic ambient diffusion mainly exert an aesthetic and psychological effect; their action is too mild to sanitize interior space and prevent the spread of infection. They are ideal for living and work spaces rather than healthcare environments.

  Heat diffusers are especially useful for diffusing the fragrance of oils of a thicker consistency, such as Cedarwood, Sandalwood, Myrrh and Benzoin: these should not be used in a glass nebulizer and not in all ultrasound diffusers. Their other obvious advantage is that they are free of noise (unlike some nebulizers) and are easy to maintain – the bowl is easily cleaned after each session with detergent or rubbing alcohol. Note that, because heat rises, heat diffusers are less effective in rooms with high ceilings, where much of the aromatic vapour will be lost in the room's headspace.

- **Cold aromatic evaporation.** This less common type of ambient diffusion also causes evaporation, not with heat but with fan-driven cold air that blows through an absorbant cartridge impregnated with several drops of essential oil or oil blend. Being less efficient than heat diffusion, ambient olfaction remains very mild. The advantages of cold diffusion are many. They include diffusion for children, sensitive individuals and any family or work setting involving more than just a few people, for which an innocuous, universally acceptable fragrance is desired. Single oils or blends with a strong character that are suspected of being too intense to be really effective may also be tested first by cold diffusion.

- **Ultrasound aromatic nebulization.** Now a common form of ambient oil diffusion, ultrasound nebulizers operate by generating ultrasound waves of 100 Hz or less in a reservoir of cold water to which between 5 and 20 drops of essential oil or blend have been added. Ultrasound causes the water surface with its oils to vibrate, thereby noiselessly generating a fragrant ionizing mist. Ultrasound nebulization has the unique advantage of nicely producing not only ambient fragrance, but also ionization and humidification of the surrounding space. This makes it very useful not only in dry climates and dry living and work spaces in general (e.g. in dry air from wintertime heating), but also in environments where sanitized air is the ideal, such as spas, clinics and hospitals. The olfactory effect of ultrasound nebulization is mild to moderate, depending on the setting of the unit. Certainly, it cannot replace compressed-air nebulization for saturating a space with an oil's full molecules of fragrance, nor as a delivery method for the internal absorption of essential oils by deep inhalation (see below).

- **Compressed air aromatic nebulization.** This type of nebulization is less common and more specific to the internal use of essential oils (see below). Nevertheless, a nebulizer (sometimes called an atomizer) that operates by pumped compressed air is also a highly versatile vehicle for ambient oil diffusion. When on a low setting, the pump rheostat (volume control) acts as a diffuser of fragrance that creates only mild olfaction – like an ultrasound nebulizer but somewhat stronger, although without the extra humidification. As little as ten minutes of nebulization per hour is required to saturate an average room of 60 m$^2$, which also makes the hum of the pump motor less of an issue. The purely aesthetic result of compressed air nebulization makes its use worthwhile. No other device is able to achieve the extraordinary effect of producing a three-dimensional panorama of pure fragrance like the compressed air nebulizer.

  When the rheostat of the compressed air nebulizer is turned up, it will perform as a treatment device for absorbing oils physiologically in larger quantities through sustained inhalation (see below).

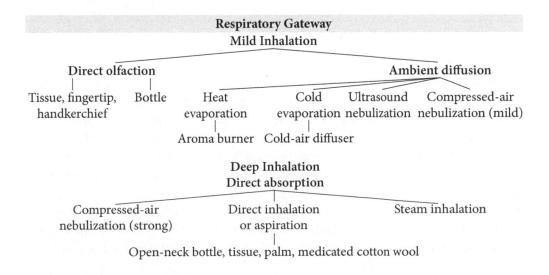

**Respiratory Gateway**
Mild Inhalation

Direct olfaction                                             Ambient diffusion

Tissue, fingertip,   Bottle        Heat            Cold         Ultrasound      Compressed-air
handkerchief                       evaporation     evaporation  nebulization    nebulization (mild)

                                   Aroma burner    Cold-air diffuser

Deep Inhalation
Direct absorption

Compressed-air                     Direct inhalation                    Steam inhalation
nebulization (strong)              or aspiration

            Open-neck bottle, tissue, palm, medicated cotton wool

# Physiological Absorption by Deep Inhalation

## Using the respiratory gateway

The second use of the respiratory gateway is deep and prolonged inhalation of an essential oil in order to obtain physiological absorption. This makes use of an oil not for its psychological effect, but purely for the substantial or physical effect that it causes. What counts here is the oil's physical substance and form rather than its fragrance or olfactory information. The result is primarily a physiological effect that evokes functional alterations in the body. In addition to modulating body functions, this effect when prolonged may eventually also cause tissue changes.

When an essential oil is deeply inhaled as a vapour, it will fairly easily penetrate the nasal and lower respiratory epithelium; condensation of the oil vapour then gets under way. Entering the bloodstream through the pulmonary alveoli, it fully condenses to a liquid state and quickly reaches the tissues of its tropism, which include various brain centres. Studies show that the quantity of oil actually absorbed with inhalation depends mainly on the intensity and length of time that its vapour is inhaled. Ultimately therefore, intense inhalation actually constitutes an internal method of oil delivery.

Apart from circulatory uptake, another factor that contributes to the absorption of a lipophilic oil on inhalation is its attraction to the lipid-rich tissues of the brain. As it diffuses across the membranes and the cribiform plate, it enters (and alters!) the cerebrospinal fluid – a significant factor to practitioners of craniosacral therapy.

The pharmacological dynamics of essential oil absorption and elimination are many and complex. The physiological actions of essential oils are fairly specific and range from mild to strong. However, their net effect is nothing less than systemic, even though different oils show a different tropism for certain tissues and body systems. Deep inhalation of essential oils, like other gateways of internal delivery, should therefore ideally be performed by practitioners trained to a level of competence in internal medicine.

## Clinical applications

Respiratory absorption by inhalation is most useful for treating upper and lower respiratory conditions, as these are the gateway tissues involved. This includes all pathologies of the mucous membrane with excessive or scanty dry sputum; all hypersensitivity disorders such as allergic sinusitis and rhinitis, and atopic asthma (with caution); all upper and lower respiratory infections with inflammation, e.g. rhinitis, pharyngitis, bronchitis and pneumonia; all tense, spasmodic conditions of the bronchi such as asthma, croup and airway reflux with chronic cough; and all chronic, weak conditions of the lungs and bronchi. Please refer to the Repertory for suggested oils.

Secondarily, other physiological conditions will also respond to prolonged inhalation, especially those associated with the organs above the diaphragm, the heart and coronary circulation. Upper digestive functions in the stomach and duodenum are also fairly easily influenced by respiratory absorption. Equally, where a psychological effect is desired at the same time with a judicious selection of oils, inhalation may well be able to address both the physiological and psychological aspects of a particular condition. In this case, however, it is again crucial to be aware of the difference between an oil's olfactory effect and its physiological effect – the two may be entirely different.

The final use for deep respiratory inhalation is to quickly help resolve acute mental-emotional states. This could be acute psychological trauma, including shock, acute grief, anger, fear and elation, especially when erupting from chronic suppression, as well as other acute distressed emotions or mental states such as panic attacks, compulsions, mania and schizoid episodes. For oil suggestions, please see 'Direct olfaction by mild inhalation' above.

## Cautions for all delivery methods of deep inhalation

- Any essential oil causing skin irritation or sensitization should not be used by deep inhalation. This especially refers to oils with aggressive constituents, such as Clove, Cinnamon, Oregano and Thyme ct. thymol. Citral-rich oils such as Lemongrass and May chang may also need to be avoided.

- Oils containing neurotoxic ketones, such as Sage, Hyssop, Cistus and many Artemisia oils listed under the Tarragon profile, are also contraindicated by deep inhalation; they may provoke passing nervous conditions.

- Oils high in monoterpenes, such as Cajeput, Rosemary, Ravintsara and Niaouli, should be used cautiously in hypersensitive patients, especially in those with multiple chemical sensitivity (MCS) syndrome.

- Deep inhalation is cautioned in clients prone to asthma and in those highly allergic or hypersensitive in general, e.g. with hyperhistamine syndrome. In these patients, other internal methods of delivery are often more appropriate. Children with asthmatic tendencies are particularly vulnerable to bronchospasm on exposure to inhaled essential oils.

- Deep inhalation is contraindicated in any room where a baby is present.

## Delivery methods

### Absorption by deep inhalation

- **Compressed air nebulizer inhalation.** The compressed air aroma nebulizer is the optimal device for achieving physiological absorption of essential oils by inhalation. A variant of the nebulizer of Western medicine, this device was specially designed in the mid-20th century for delivering undiluted essential oils internally through the respiratory pathway. An air pump feeding an upright glass funnel compresses air into a small glass funnel that contains two fine glass tubules, one emitting the compressed air, the other the essential oil. The action of the air on the oil causes the essential oil to microvibrate and release microscopic oil droplets (1–3 micrometres in size) into the air in a fine and highly aromatic mist. Nebulization is so obtained.

There is no immediate evaporation in this nebulization process, as there is with diffusers; evaporation from oxidation is extremely slow. On the contrary, the nebulizer microionizes and negatively charges the essential oil molecules, which ensures that the microionized fragrance remains actively suspended in the space even when the nose is no longer able to detect it. This process generates a deep, wide scentstage with highly concentrated olfactory surface space. This ensures that the essential oil molecules are all fully released, available and freely absorbable. Compressed air nebulization is the cleanest way to smell essential oils in their unaltered, original state. It also remains one of the most effective methods for treating conditions by respiratory absorption, both direct and ambient.

Delivery by oil nebulization is especially effective for treating respiratory conditions, including infections, upper and lower respiratory congestion, and pain and inflammation in general. Treatment consists of 10–15-minute nebulizing sessions with the nebulizer positioned several feet directly in front of the client. The glass nozzle at the top should be pointing to the client. This may be repeated several times a day in the case of acute conditions such as respiratory infections and toxic congestion from environmental pollutants such as dust, gas, smoke and chemicals.

It is important to note that only undiluted essential oils should be used for efficient nebulization. Any dilution in a vegetable oil or alcohol, or any inclusion of absolutes, will sooner rather than later cause a nebulizer to malfunction.

The aroma nebulizer is also excellent for improving ambient air quality; in this case the rheostat volume should be set low to medium. The higher the volume is turned up, the more the nebulizer's function will change from olfactory diffusion to physical absorption; these two processes increase and decrease simultaneously in an inverse gradient. Medium volume would seem ideal in larger rooms in clinics and other healthcare settings. This will produce a nice balance between promoting psychological wellbeing by producing a pleasing scentscape, and achieving a sanitary, low-microbe quality of the airspace by including highly antimicrobial oils such as Niaouli, Cajeput and Palmarosa. At medium volume, nebulizer diffusion could certainly be intermittent to prevent olfactory fatigue. At low volume, diffusion could last longer before needing to stop, if at all necessary.

Even though the aim of nebulization is physiological treatment, it is always best to create an oil blend that is also pleasant; this also will contribute hugely to prevent olfactory fatigue and client or patient acceptance.

The only inconvenience of the aroma nebulizer is possible interference from the noise of the pump motor itself – noise levels vary widely from noiseless to a noticeable hum. However, any hum may be masked by soft music, a water fountain, and so on. Regular maintenance is also important for this type of nebulizer. For optimal performance, the inside of the glass funnel should be cleaned with rubbing alcohol or a similar solvent about every two weeks.

It is important to obtain a nebulizer with a sufficiently strong air pump. At its maximum volume, the pump should have the capacity of pumping out 300 litres of air per hour. This optimum output is neccessary to obtain a smooth, homogenous and fine nebulization. Failing that, a weaker pump tends to fractionate the oil, at first easily diffusing the more pleasant volatile top notes and only later diffusing the middle and often less pleasing base notes – and then with increasing difficulty. The result over time may well be a thickened residue of oil at the funnel base. This will eventually require replacing the funnel with a new one.

- **Direct inhalation.** To achieve any significant physiological absorption from an oil directly, the essential oil should be inhaled for four to eight cycles of the breath. Each in- and out-breath should be deep. This should ideally be done from an open-necked bottle of oil, i.e. a small 2 or 4 ml vial, or a 10 ml bottle with the orifice reducer (dropper) removed. The bottle should be wafted at a short distance below both nostrils. This is also called dry inhalation, in contrast to steam or wet inhalation.

  Again, this intense form of direct inhalation can stand in for the more effective inhalation available with the use of a compressed air nebulizer. This technique may be useful when travelling and especially in public spaces.

  A milder but still effective method of direct inhalation is to put 2 drops of oil onto a tissue or handkerchief and inhale deeply. A somewhat stronger effect is produced by dropping 1 or 2 drops of oil onto the palm of the hand and gently rubbing both palms together before cupping them over the nose and mouth and inhaling. Both methods achieve a combination of olfaction and mild absorption and so may exert both a psychological and mildly physiological effect.

  One of the best methods for achieving direct inhalation for treating upper respiratory conditions is the medicated cotton wool in the form of a nasal plug. Use 2–3 drops of non-irritant oil(s) per plug, place one snugly into each nasal entrance and inhale freely. As the oils are absorbed by the upper respiratory and eustachian tube mucosa, they are able to treat various infections, relieving pain, congestion and inflammation in the process. This user-friendly technique was perfected by the Hospital for Diseases of the Throat and described in their 1872 Pharmacopoeia, where Eucalyptus, Camphor and Menthol were standard antimicrobial decongestants, alongside remedies such as alum, boric acid and tinctures of iodine and witch hazel.

A variant technique sometimes used to obtain physiological absorption into the lungs and the whole system is oral aspiration. Here the aromatic vapour of an oil is breathed in with an open mouth, not through the nose. However, oral aspiration was traditionally better performed with an inhaler device filled with hot water sprinkled with antimicrobial oils (inhaler devices were used for both oral aspiration and nasal inhalation). Aspiration of the medicated hot moist air produces especially good absorption by the eustachian tube and bronchi, and is able to treat a variety of infectious, inflammatory and congestive conditions, including those of the middle ear.

- **Steam inhalation.** Essential oil vaporizing with warm steam is a simple traditional technique for treating upper respiratory conditions. Drop 2–3 drops of oil on a basin or bowl of hot water, place a thick towel over the head to form a fairly airtight tent and gently inhale the aromatic steam for about five minutes. Repeat four times a day. Steam inhalations are indicated for sinus, middle ear and chest conditions in particular, both infectious and congestive, and especially viral infections, including influenza. Steam inhalation is often combined with other delivery methods that treat these conditions.

  An alternative for the shower or bath is to use a steaming hot washcloth. Drop 1–2 drops of oil onto the washcloth, cup over the nose and inhale. With suitable stimulating or relaxing oils, the aromatic washcloth can also act as a nice morning pick-me-up or evening unwind.

  **Caution:** Never use boiling water for a steam inhalation to prevent severe disintegration of the oil by sudden oxidation, as well as acute burning. Refrain from using more than 4 drops and from steaming longer than five minutes to prevent irritating the nasal and bronchial mucosa; this can happen rapidly in children. Those with an asthmatic tendency should be cautious with steam inhalation.

## Physiological Absorption by Other Internal Delivery Methods

*Using oral, rectal and vaginal gateways*

Using essential oils in liquid form as a type of internal medication or remedy requires careful consideration as regards the choice of three main factors:

- The gateway of delivery

- The method of delivery

- The dosage and dilution for delivery

The many ways of introducing essential oils into the body's internal evironment essentially divide into oral intake, rectal delivery and vaginal delivery – i.e. through the body's main orifices or gateways. These are the classic medical applications of essential oils that practitioners throughout Europe, and especially in France, have developed over at least 300 years. To these types of delivery may be added more popular skin application techniques using the arch of the foot, the creases of the wrist and elbow, the sublingual area, and so on.

The aim of choosing internal delivery of essential oils is to maximize transport to the internal environment in order to create a physiological effect. Essential oils possess the almost unique ability to cross the protective barriers of the mucosa and skin, enter the general circulation, and join the body's internal environment – regardless of the particular gateway chosen. The extent to which an oil is able to reach the interior depends both on the amount of tissue vascularization and the location of absorption to which they are exposed. For both reasons, absorption is greatest in all mucosa-rich areas, such as the lungs, rectum, vagina and digestive tract.

Oil quality is an important factor for all of these internal methods of delivery. For practitioner use, only oils that meet all four criteria that define a bioactive oil remedy may be considered (see Volume 1, Chapter 3). Using inferior oils for mild inhalation is an excusable error, although an aesthetic travesty; using them as internal remedies is unconscionable.

## Clinical applications

Because delivering essential oils through the gateways to the body's interior creates significant physiological effects, it is especially important when treating to consider the choice of administration or delivery method, the dosage, excipient (if any), frequency, length of treatment, and so on. The methods chosen will all vary according to the therapeutic context, the location and nature of the disorder, the functions and tropism of the particular oils used, and other miscellaneous factors. The most common types of conditions treated in this way with essential oils include pain, inflammation, infections and hypersensitivity of most kinds.

Note that the oral and rectal gateways possess the best systemic delivery effects and are especially chosen for treating these systemic conditions. Oral and rectal deliveries are also well suited for treating long-term imbalance of the individual terrain, such as functional states of weak, damp, tense, hot, cold or dry terrain. Again, for best results and for long-term improvement or cure, it is best to undertake treatment of the whole terrain based on a functional Six-Condition or other similar diagnosis (see Chapter 4 and Appendix B).

Each body gateway has particular uses, advantages and disadvantages; these should guide the practitioner to the best choice of delivery method for a particular patient. It is common for a practitioner to combine one or two delivery methods, as well as to combine internal and topical, or internal and respiratory, treatment gateways, all depending on the nature of the condition under treatment, e.g. whether acute or chronic, mild or severe, and whether other treatment methods are being used concurrently.

Currently, a small number of doctors, medical herbalists, naturopaths and aromatherapists have adopted these internal delivery methods, often in combination with herbal medicines, nutritional advice, etc. Their practice is based on some degree of professional training in internal medicine (i.e. physiological biomedicine). However, note that the therapeutic intention and efficacy of an internal treatment relies entirely on the particular model of medicine that informs them. Allopathic and vitalistic types of medicine both have their indications and applications, although used together they prove more effective. When essential oils are incorporated within a particular type of medicine, they can only be as effective as they are understood and practised in the context and terms of that system. Chapter 4 discusses some possible ways of integrating both approaches.

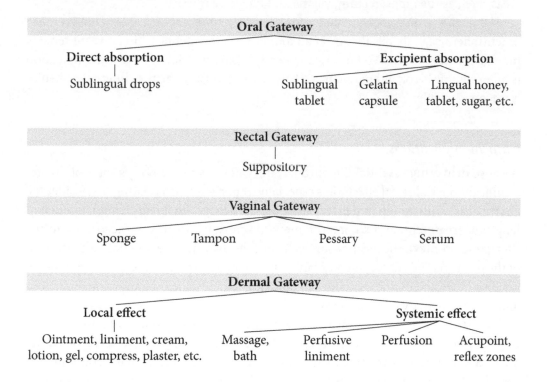

## Delivery methods

### Oral delivery

Taking an essential oil as a bioactive remedy by mouth is an important and commonly used delivery method. It is also surprisingly versatile, considering that the oil may not only be ingested, but also applied to the oral cavity itself. Oral administration generally exerts a systemic effect, although the prime target organ is the digestive tract. Most essential oils suitable for internal consumption may be considered for the appropriate oral delivery method. Certain oil applications, especially sublingual and lingual ones, are also able to treat local conditions of the oral mucosa, the gums, nose, sinuses and throat. Oral gels, for instance, may be used for mouth ulcers and gingivitis, for their antibacterial and plaque-inhibiting actions, and possibly for their balancing effect on the oral microbiota.

**Dosage considerations:** Doses of essential oils and excipients or liquid bases are given in this section both in milligrams (mg) and in drops (and in millilitres or ml for larger quantities). Doses should be counted with a standard eyedropper (vertical drop dispenser), not directly from the orifice reducer or 'dropper' in essential oil bottles, whose opening size varies enormously. Although many practitioners accustomed to drug or herbal pharmacy are experienced in working in mg and ml measurements, practical usage often favours dosing essential oils by the number of drops, especially when small quantities are being prepared.

There are many factors that create variability of the final dose; these are often overlooked. They include small variations in the density of essential oils, the drop size of the standard eyedropper, the fact that the oils commonly in use, once absorbed, do not exert a simple drug-like action, and the fact that oil doses, proportions and dilution percentages are usually rounded off when a formula is created. Given all these variables, it is hardly practical to insist on measuring all dosages by weight, i.e. milligrams, alone. However, to ensure accurate and safe prescribing, it is clearly important to know the equivalents among drops, milligrams and millilitres.

Note that all equivalents between mg and drops are approximate because, as noted, they directly depend both on the density of the oil and on the size of the dropper. With oils of higher density, such as Clove, Vetiver, Cinnamon leaf, Sandalwood and Rose absolute, less than 30 drops will make 1 g or 1 ml. As a general rule, however, these approximations apply:

- 1 drop = 30 mg of essential oil
- 30 drops of essential oil = 1 g or 1 ml

**Caution:** Most essential oils are irritating to the mucous membrane, even more so than to the skin. For oral use an essential oil should always be first administered via a gelatin capsule or prepared with a diluting agent to make a medicated oil before being swallowed. This can prevent gastrointestinal irritation and, in the case of highly irritant, caustic oils such as Oregano, Cinnamon and Thyme ct. thymol, avoid severe irritation and burns to the throat and stomach.

For oral use, the essential oil itself should first be made into a medicated oil. Whether the essential oil is to be swallowed or not, it should as a rule be first diluted in an oily excipient such as a vegetable oil (e.g. olive or coconut oil), which is able to properly disperse the essential oil. Honey is also able to disperse an essential oil. As a last resort, a non-dispersing excipient, such as some jam, syrup or even a piece of soft bread, may also serve for oral use. The traditional popular French method of putting one or two drops of oil onto a sugar cube is therefore no longer recommended. Equally, simply drinking down essential oils in water is clearly contraindicated.

Essential oils whose therapeutic status is Strong with acute toxicity should never be considered for oral or any other internal form of delivery (see Volume 1, Chapter 4). Those oils with Medium-strength status (i.e. those that possess some cumulative toxicity) should only be used under competent practitioner advice. Any oil considered for oral use should first be checked for its gelatin capsule dosage in Part II of this text, as well as for its therapeutic and pharmacological precautions. These precautions specify the various toxicities found in essential oils, such as neurotoxicity (e.g. from certain oils containing ketones), hepatotoxicity (from high-phenol oils) and photosensitivity (from oils containing coumarin). Any carcinogenic potential is also mentioned under the pharmacological precautions for each oil.

The oral intake of essential oils is generally contraindicated in children under five years, during pregnancy, and with gastric and duodenal ulcers present.

- **Gelatin capsule.** Using a gelatin capsule, herafter referred to as a gel cap, is the cleanest, safest and most effective technique for oral essential oil intake. The medicated oil is thereby delivered directly to the small intestine, from where it passes through the liver before being distributed systemically by the circulation. Gel cap delivery exerts a local effect in the gut, followed by a systemic effect. The local effect is aided by a certain amount of immediate absorption of the oil in the gut before moving on to the liver first pass. Local absorption from the gel cap into the gut is enhanced by the presence of a vegetable oil rather than any other excipient.

  Because of its local effect in the gut, gel cap delivery is the best choice for treating digestive conditions of most kinds, acute and chronic, spasmodic or congestive, infectious or non-infectious. It is also very appropriate for treating intestinal dysbiosis of the microflora (microbiome) and resultant disorders, such as intestinal hyperpermeability (leaky gut syndrome), chronic inflammation, microbial toxicosis and infection. Treating the intestinal microflora directly will in turn not only promote microbial balance of the body's whole symbiotic microflora, but also generate positive hormonal changes in general; it will especially benefit brain and neurological functions through the significant brain-gut axis of peptide communication.

  The gel cap is also an important delivery method for treating a wide range of acute and chronic systemic conditions of all organ systems. Infections, inflammations and allergies, as well as congestive conditions of the circulation, liver, uterus, lungs and other organs, all respond well to oral gel caps.

Although in theory almost any essential oil that is therapeutically safe is suitable for gel cap use, all the cautions above strictly apply. However, the best candidates are always the oils of culinary herbs and spices, both temperate and tropical, since the digestive tract has long adapted to those in the course of human evolution. They include most of the lipflower family oils, such as Basil, Thyme and Spearmint, and spice oils such as Ginger, Cardamom and Cinnamon. Edible citrus fruit oils, such as Mandarin, Grapefruit and Sweet orange, are also preferable. However, oils from medicinal plants in general, including resins (e.g. Myrrh, Cistus and Frankincense), may also be used safely.

- **Choosing the right excipient.** To maximize the bioavailability of a medicated gel cap through local absorption in the gut, it is important to prepare a vegetable oil excipient for the capsule that is mucosa-friendly – a medicated oil, in short. Ensuring good lymphatic absorption can therefore enhance the treatment of both intestinal disorders and conditions at a distance in other organ systems. Alternative excipients are hydrated silica or silica gel, and phospholipids such as phosphatidylcholine (also found in the dispersant Disper), all of which are also well assimilated in the gut. Most other excipients (such as clay, starches and herb powders), however, will not promote local absorption of the essential oil, resulting in a weaker effect.

   Size 00 or 0 gelatin capsules (40 mg and 80 mg respectively) are best for adults, 000 size for children aged 5 to 12. Using a plain vegetable oil, each capsule may be prepared individually. Or a separate batch of medicated oil can first be prepared, using the dosage guidelines below. If preparing gel caps individually, each empty capsule must be filled first with the essential oil or essential oil formula (blend) – usually just two or three drops – then topped up with a vegetable oil before shutting the cap with its top. Once a batch of capsules is made, they should be kept in a refrigerator to reduce or prevent leakage of the medicated oil. They should be used within three months, before the essential oil degrades the gelatin. Gel caps containing high-phenol oils, such as Clove and Oregano, should be used within a few days.

- **Choosing the right dosage.** Because essential oils are highly concentrated remedies, choosing the correct dose for oral use is paramount. As a general guideline, the daily oral dose of essential oil for an adult weighing 70 kg ranges from 200 to 400 mg, or 7 to 14 drops counted with a separate dropper. The lower dose of this calculation is loosely based on the conservative rule of 1 drop per 10 kg of weight. Note again that this dosage applies to a single oil or any combination of oils constituting a formula. It also applies to the intake of medicated liquids (see below).

The total number of drops of oil or formula should therefore be adjusted up or down based on the following factors:

–   The patient's weight. A 90 kg patient should receive about 9 drops of oil daily; a teenager weighing 45 kg, 4–5 drops daily; a child over 5 weighing 20 kg, only 2 drops per day.

–   The patient's age and metabolic condition. Younger and older individuals have a lowered capacity for both metabolizing and eliminating essential oils. A child's elimination functions are not fully formed until around age 12. Individuals with liver congestion and impaired phase-II detoxification should especially receive lower and more gradual doses. In addition to needing lower doses that start quite small and gradually increase, younger and older individuals with chronic conditions should, whenever possible, be treated with mild, gentle oils and with ambient oil diffusion rather than by internal oil delivery.

–   The nature of the patient's condition, especially whether acute or chronic. Acute conditions require larger and/or more frequent intake, but usually for only three or four days; chronic conditions require smaller and/or less frequent intake, but for a longer duration of up to three weeks before a break of at least two days. When treating the patient's terrain (most often a chronic condition), the functional diagnosis of tense/weak, hot/cold, dry/ damp will also help determine the right dose.

–   The therapeutic status of the oil itself. The correct, safe dosage for oils with some cumulative toxicity, such as Oregano, Sage and Wintergreen, is relatively less; the length of intake is also severely limited in this case.

–   Any other simultaneous medication, such as herbal teas, tinctures, nebulizer sessions and topical applications. The synergistic action of combined delivery methods produces a greater effect and a higher dose than each single method on its own.

•   **Dosage summary.** In chronic conditions, the most common gel cap dose for an adult is 2–3 drops (60–90 mg) per cap, taken three times a day. The total number of drops is therefore 6–9 drops (180–270 mg) per day. The usual dose for an adolescent is 2 drops twice daily; for a child over 7, 1 drop twice daily.

Acute conditions in adults usually need a stronger dose of 4–6 drops per gel cap every three or four hours, or 4–6 gel caps at regular strength daily; for children of 5–12 years, 3–5 regular gel caps daily. This intense dosing should be discontinued after two days.

A safe effect is obtained by taking one gel cap at the end of each meal. Taken between meals, the effect may be somewhat stronger but requires more accurate oil selection. Intake typically consists of a ten-day course followed by four days of abstinence; this can be repeated several times. For treating chronic conditions, five days on and two days off is another good rule of thumb.

**Caution:** Children under 5 and infants should not be given medicated gel caps, only suppositories by rectal delivery (see below). A minority of patients may experience gastric intolerance to gel caps, resulting in burping and hiccups; other delivery routes are best chosen in that case.

## Medicated liquid

Essential oils that are non-irritant to the mucous membrane may also be ingested directly with an emulsifier or dispersant to make an emulsified medicated liquid. A dispersant such as Solubol or Disper (made in France) is ideal for this purpose, although honey or maple syrup will also serve. While Disper is an alcohol-based dispersant, Solubol contains almost entirely vegetable-based ingredients. A medicated liquid is well absorbed and may replace use of a gel cap, but is overall not quite as clean and effective a technique. Various types of medicated liquid can also be prepared for making gargles, syrups, mouthwashes, and so on.

An ingestible medicated liquid that uses Solubol or Disper as a dispersant should consist of a 5–10% essential oil dilution, which is 15–30 drops of essential oil (or formula) per 10 ml of dispersant. Add 5–10 drops of this milky medicated liquid to some water and take two or three times a day. The maximum recommended daily dose is generally 30 drops divided into two or three doses.

A simpler rubric for making a single dose is to mix 3 drops of essential oil in 1 teaspoon (5 ml) of dispersant (an approximate 2% dilution) and to add the mix to half a glass of water.

Excellent gargles for treating all throat and oesophagus infections, as well for overuse of the vocal cords, can also be prepared with a medicated liquid. Use 15–30 drops of essential oil to 100 ml of the dispersant Solubol or Disper – a 0.5–1% dilution. Mix well with water, hydrosol or herb tea (Sage leaf infusion is traditional for sore throat), add a pinch of sea salt (optional) and gargle freely – once an hour in acute conditions. For children, half the essential oil dose should be used. The right hydrosol on its own is also very effective.

Medicated syrup is another convenient (although very sweet) type of medicated liquid useful for treating throat infections and other throat conditions. For adults, add 2–4% of non-irritant essential oils to a plain syrup, 2% for children and 1% for infants. To make an average 2% dilution, add 3 drops of essential oil or blend to 5 ml (1 teaspoon) of syrup, or 60 drops of oil to 100 ml of syrup.

A herbal tincture may also be reinforced with a non-irritant essential oil. One drop can be added to each 30 ml or 1 oz of tincture. The higher the alcohol content, the better the essential oil will disperse in the tincture. In France some practitioners favour a base of 50% tincture and 40–45% vegetable oil (e.g. olive or apricot kernel oil), to which 5–10% essential oils are added. The dose is 40 drops in some water twice daily.

## Sublingual application

Essential oils that are non-irritant to the mucous membrane may be given sublingually, i.e. dropped underneath the tongue. The sublingual area is rich in capillary perfusion, which allows rapid oil absorption to the brain and secondarily the throat and organ systems at a distance while avoiding the liver's first pass. Sublingual delivery is locally effective not only for throat conditions (hoarseness, dryness, irritation and infection), but also for any related coughing. The unpleasant taste of most essential oils and the irritation they cause to the sublingual mucosa are both severe limitations to this delivery technique. Preparing a medicated oil first is once more an answer, as the oil may then be retained sublingually for up to a minute. For sublingual delivery of a medicated oil, a 50:50 dilution of an essential oil (or formula) in a vegetable oil such as olive or coconut oil, or some honey, is acceptable. Another solution is to immediately swish an undiluted oil under the tongue with water as soon as it causes pain – which often occurs within seconds.

An alternative is the medicated tablet or pastille, a neutral tablet of lactose or calcium carbonate, or even a Vitamin C tablet. Drop 1 drop of essential oil (or formula) on one side and optionally another drop on the other side of the tablet. Once the oil has soaked in, allow the medicated tablet to slowly dissolve under the tongue.

Whether diluted or not, the dose of essential oil should again only be 2–3 drops for each application. Up to 5 drops may be fine if taken once only, for instance using Lavender or Marjoram oil as a sedative before bedtime in the case of severe insomnia. Again, great caution regarding the use of irritant essential oils is advisable.

## Lingual application

One drop of essential oil – preferably a small drop – may be dropped onto the tongue surface, where it will disperse into the nasal passages. Half a teaspoonful of honey serves as an excellent excipient for lingual delivery, especially thick honey. A semi-solid medicated honey will be retained longest on the tongue. This technique is particularly useful for treating nose and sinus infection and inflammation, and for relief of such symptoms as mucus congestion, runny nose and sinus pain. The choice of oils is wide, depending on the condition being treated.

If preparing a larger supply, use 25 drops of essential oil (or formula) to 50 ml of honey and mix well; this is a 1.5% dilution. For most conditions, 1 teaspoon is taken two or three times a day for eight days.

## Aromatic tisane

Essential oils can also make excellent aromatic infusions that are as pleasant to drink, inhale and smell as they are medicinal in effect. Aromatic tisanes are similar in effect to herbal tisanes or infusions, but there is a trade-off: while aromatic tisanes are definitely stronger than herbal ones, they do not include the plant's water-soluble constituents found in the latter.

Evenly mix 4 drops of essential oil (or formula) with a teaspoon of honey, maple syrup or molasses in a cup. Pour on hot (but not boiling) water. The 4 drops of oil are necessary for this preparation as about half the oil will be lost in evaporation and as deposit on the cup wall.

## Rectal delivery
### Suppository

Along with gel cap delivery and deep inhalation, rectal delivery is the other important application for producing systemic internal absorption of essential oils. Practitioners have relied on medicated suppositories introduced by rectum as a safe and highly effective technique for many centuries. As the suppository dissolves within about six minutes after insertion, the essential oils are easily absorbed by the highly permeable rectal mucosa, taken up by the haemorrhoidal veins and the inferior vena cava, and quickly reach the internal environment before being eliminated by the lungs. A significant amount of absorption by the pelvic lymphatic circulation also occurs.

If the aim is systemic absorption of the active essential oils, delivery by suppository is generally somewhat more effective than oral gel cap delivery for the simple reason that it avoids any possible enzymatic action on the oils and largely (but not entirely) bypasses the liver's first pass (phase-II detoxification) – a considerable factor with gel caps. Furthermore, relatively higher and therefore stronger doses of essential oils may be given with a suppository than with a gel cap. However, as with oral and respiratory delivery, the oils are also able to exert a local effect at the location of insertion and to target major beneficiary organs before being absorbed systemically.

The main beneficiary organs of suppositories are the colon and the lungs, as well as the pelvic organs (bladder, uterus and other reproductive structures in general). A wide range of intestinal and pelvic conditions can benefit from them and, as the oils are eliminated by the lungs, they can lower respiratory disorders such as acute bronchial and lung infections and inflammations. Suppositories can also shift chronic terrain conditions of these organs, especially congestive or damp (e.g. intestinal dysbiosis, pelvic and uterine congestion, BPH, bronchial phlegm congestion), infectious (viral, bacterial, fungal, parasitic) or inflammatory conditions (e.g. IBS, IBD, prostatitis, interstitial cystitis, bronchitis). Locally, suppositories will also treat internal and external haemorrhoids and anal fissures.

Suppositories have the unique advantage of being suited for babies, infants and young children, as these are unable to tolerate oral delivery of essential oils before the age of 5. A wide range of children's conditions will respond to suppository treatment with essential oils, including coughs, fevers, respiratory infections, emotional upsets, bedwetting, and eruptive children's diseases such as measles and chickenpox.

**Caution:** All cautions given under 'Oral delivery' (above) apply equally strongly to rectal delivery of essential oils by suppository. In addition, formulating for a suppository requires complete accuracy in terms of the choice of oils and the avoidance of other oils. Partly for local and partly for systemic protection, all possibly irritant, rubefacient and allergizing oils should strictly be avoided.

*Choosing the right excipient and dosage*

The traditional excipients for preparing a suppository are cacao or cocoa butter and shea butter; singly or combined they work well. Other excipients in use today include Witespol, which consists of hydrogenated coco glycerides.

The dose of essential oils in a suppository is calculated by 5 mg (about one-sixth of 1 drop) per kg of body weight. Depending on the type of condition being treated, especially whether acute or chronic, as a general rule the following dosage ranges apply:

- Babies aged up to 6 months: 1 g suppository with 40–75 mg (about 1.5–2.5 drops) of essential oil

- Infants aged 6 to 24 months: 1 g suppository with 60–90 mg (2–3 drops) of essential oil

- Children aged 2 to 8: 2 g suppository with 90–120 mg (3–4 drops) of essential oil

- Children aged 8 to 12: 2 g suppository with 120–150 mg (4–5 drops) of essential oil

- Adults: 3 g suppository with 120–210 mg (4–7 drops) of essential oil

First gently melt the excipient in a jar in a double boiler. Cocoa butter melts at around 35°C, whereas Witespol usually melts at 36°C, just below body temperature. Stir in and mix the essential oil formula well with the molten base excipient. Using a large pipette or turkey baster, pour the now-medicated oil into suppository moulds and set to harden in the refrigerator until ready for use.

The typical suppository treatment consists of 2–4 suppositories per day for a maximum of eight days. In the case of long-term terrain treatment, 1 suppository a day is sufficient.

VAGINAL DELIVERY

Vaginal sponges and pessaries are the main traditional preparations for essential oil delivery for treating various local conditions of the external female genitalia, vagina and genital tract. Because the essential oils are eventually absorbed into the inferior vena cava, disorders of the organs in the pelvic basin, such as the bladder, may also be treated using this method.

**Caution:** All cautions given under 'Oral delivery' (above) apply even more strictly to vaginal delivery of essential oils by suppository. Because the vaginal mucosa is highly sensitive, formulating for vaginal preparations requires complete accuracy in terms of the choice of oils and the avoidance of other oils. Partly for local and partly for systemic protection, all possibly irritant, rubefacient and allergizing oils should be strictly avoided.

## Vaginal serum and sponge

Both preparations make use of a vegetable oil that is medicated with essential oils. The medicated oil or serum is either inserted into the vagina manually or, better still, inserted with the help of a natural sea sponge that is retained for two hours. Either way, because the vaginal mucosa is highly permeable, the medicated oil allows the essential oils to be well absorbed locally and into the pelvic basin.

Courses of treatment with daily vaginal applications of a medicated serum, either direct or with a sponge, can be as short as a few days and as long as several weeks. When done on a regular basis, vaginal serums and sponges are an excellent way of maintaining vaginal and pelvic health by regulating the vaginal microbiota, helping keep its pH acid, and strengthening the vaginal mucosa. They can relieve the symptoms of vaginal dryness, itching, pain and discharge seen in infectious and inflammatory disorders such as bacterial vaginosis, yeast overgrowth, vaginitis and cervicitis. They are also directly and indirectly able to treat urinary infections, themselves sometimes the result of forms of vaginitis.

When taken in prolonged courses over weeks or months, the overall vaginal and pelvic terrain can be modified positively, regardless of its nature, bacterial or fungal. In energetic terms, sponges are mainly able to resolve conditions of dryness (e.g. from oestrogen deficiency) and damp (e.g. from infection).

The choice of essential oils used will clearly vary, depending on the type of condition being treated. However, hormonally active oils, such as Rose, Geranium and Palmarosa, often yield good results, possibly by supporting oestrogen levels and promoting a healthy glycogen- and lactobacilli-rich environment of the vaginal microbiota. When treating infections, non-irritant antimicrobial oils are chosen, such as Palmarosa, Tea tree, Niaouli, Green myrtle and Thyme ct. linalool.

### Choosing the right sponge, excipient and dilution

Natural, unbleached sea sponges are ideal for vaginal use – the kind harvested in the Greek islands, for instance, often available in art supply stores. Unbleached sponges are various shades of brown and dark orange, whereas bleached sponges are light sand coloured – these tend to fall apart after a few uses. Synthetic cosmetic sponges or regular tampons should be avoided because of the plastic fibres and chemical additives they contain. Natural, unsprayed tampons are viable but still less effective than a sponge, as they are too absorbent.

The best oily excipient is hazelnut oil, as it has almost the same pH as the healthy vagina, although other vegetable oils are perfectly fine to use as well. It is also possible to prepare a vaginal sponge using as an excipient a hydrosol, a herbal infusion or decoction, or a very dilute and low-alcohol tincture.

Sterilize or autoclave the sponge first for 20 minutes before use; several sponges may be sterilized at once for several days' supply. Briefly soak the dry sponge in the medicated oil, insert vaginally and retain for up to two hours – no longer (see caution below). This allows the oils to treat both local conditions and, as the oils permeate upward, conditions of the cervix and pelvic organs, including the bladder.

The dilution range for the medicated vaginal serums and sponges is 0.5–2% of essential oils. A 1% dilution is fine for treating chronic conditions of vaginal irritation, dryness or shrinking, and for treating a terrain imbalance of the pelvis or bladder over several weeks or months. However, up to 2% dilution is often required for treating acute infections. The dilution should also be adjusted up or down, based on the patient's body size.

To make a 1% dilution, use 30 ml or 1 oz of carrier oil and add 10 drops (300 mg) of essential oil or formula. When using highly concentrated oils such as Rose or Neroli, as little as 5 drops (150 mg) per oz are needed. To make sure that the dilution is comfortable to the vaginal tissue, do a test insertion first; then dilute further if necessary.

**Caution:** In addition to the cautions above relating to all vaginal delivery of essential oils, medicated vaginal sponges should never be retained for more than two hours to prevent development of the acute bacterial infection, toxic shock-like syndrome. For this reason, they should be inserted and removed during the day, never at night.

### Pessary

A pessary is a soft 2–3 g suppository that is inserted vaginally and dissolves at body temperature. It may be given for the same functions and indications as the vaginal serum or sponge. Like the latter, it can also be used for many weeks at a time as it does not disrupt the vaginal microflora – on the contrary, with the right choice of essential oils it will achieve the same benefits both locally and at a distance among the pelvic organs. A pessary is made of the same excipients as a suppository and requires the same dilutions and dosage ranges (see above).

## Physiological Effects by Dermal Delivery Methods

### Using the dermal gateway

Essential oils can provide a large number of both topical and systemic internal effects by dermal delivery. The skin is an important gateway for administering essential oils because of its great ability to sustain and assimilate them. The low molecular weight of most essential oils allows a certain amount of diffusion through the skin, the rate and amount of which is largely determined by the condition of its most superficial layer, the stratum corneum. At the same time, the skin, like the mucosa, is a sensitive, exposed yet protective interface that may easily be irritated or sensitized by:

- Inappropriate selection of essential oils for dermal application

- Inappropriate dilution of essential oils in a carrier oil or other excipient

- Inappropriate frequency of essential oil applications over time

Skin delivery may be highly beneficial and is certainly easy and practical – but it should be adopted with great care.

Delivery through the dermal gateway can treat both local conditions by topical application, and systemic conditions by internal delivery. It is crucial above all for the practitioner to be clear about the type of treatment intended, local or systemic, and decide on the best dermal delivery method on that basis. In order to determine the optimal choice of preparation for each particular client, the practitioner should consider two fundamental factors that determine the bioavailability – and ultimate effectiveness – of an essential oil:

- The degree of essential oil absorption through the skin that may be achieved

- The degree of reflex action in the skin through nerve endings and reflex energetic resonance

These primary considerations will directly determine the best dilution strength for, and the frequency and duration of, a particular dermal oil application for safe and effective results.

## Dermal absorption

The amount of essential oils that the skin is able to absorb, as well as the absorption rate, is a complex issue (Buckle 2003; Bensouilah and Buck 2006; Harris and Harris 2006a; Rhind 2012; Bonneval and Dubus 2014; Franchomme 2015; Guba 2017). A review of findings is that, in summary:

- The skin is generally porous to essential oils, especially those high in lipophilic compounds, but possesses extremely variable porosity or permeability. This is due to its metabolic state, e.g. whether sluggish, congested and toxin-laden, or whether efficient, active and possessing good elimination – the skin is the body's largest organ of waste elimination.

- The skin's very top layer, the stratum corneum, freely absorbs essential oils, forming a type of reservoir. Because of physical and metabolic barriers, however, only much smaller amounts and selective constituents are able to penetrate further layers of the epidermis, and finally the dermis with its capillary perfusion.

- Those constituents that are finally absorbed may have been altered by the skin's metabolism: they may still be active or have been rendered inactive.

If still active, they may also be present in quantities insufficient to produce a pharmacological effect.

- Essential oil absorption and elimination occurs at different rates. In various experiments, absorption ranged from 20 to 40 minutes (e.g. volatile, fresh-pungent, monoterpene-rich oils such as the Eucalyptus oils, Niaouli and Ravintsara) to more than 120 minutes (e.g. denser, more viscous, large-molecule oils such as Vetiver, Benzoin and Sandalwood). These rates depend as much on the oil's physical characteristics as on its particular components, as well as on the terrain of the skin's metabolism itself.

- Certain essential oil constituents are also known to be absorbed and eliminated at different rates, ranging from 20 minutes (e.g. 1,8 cineole, some monoterpenes and benzyl acetate), to 30 or 40 minutes (e.g. linalool, eugenol, linalyl acetate, geranyl acetate), to 120 minutes (e.g. citral, geraniol coumarins, methyl salicylate).

In short, the dermal absorption of essential oils is highly variable and dependent on numerous factors. Its clinical usefulness for reliable physiological intervention is questionable. Certainly, the all-too-common assumption that essential oils applied onto the skin are easily and consistently able to reach the internal environment, resulting in reliable physiological effects, is clearly an erroneous one. To put the issue in further perspective: transdermal absorption of essential oils has been shown in general to be only about one-third as effective as oral delivery in reaching the internal environment, and even less effective than rectal delivery by suppository (Franchomme 2015). Arguably, this low effectiveness and inconsistency is insufficient to warrant using dermal absorption as a gateway for delivery of essential oils to the internal environment. Regardless, if a practitioner is to obtain reliable results with dermal applications, careful consideration of these basic issues is required.

DERMAL REFLEX ACTION

The reflex action that an essential oil may cause in and just below the skin should also be considered. The first type of reflex action is stimulation of peripheral nerve endings and larger dermatomes, such as are found thoughout the body, including on the ear. Here an essential oil may cause a positive effect at a distance, reversing the pathway of somatic dysfunction from the nerve root to the area of typical pain or rash. Neural stimulation is one basis for the evident efficacy of essential oil applications to these areas for treating physiological dysfunctions at a distance.

The second type of reflex action is the energetic resonance between the area of application and physiological functions, such as is described by various systems of somatic resonance, e.g. reflexology systems on the hand, face, foot and abdomen, as well as by acupuncture and marma points. Resonance includes electromagnetic, myofascial and other phenomena that would explain reflex signalling. Although few studies of this type have been conducted with essential oils, the evidence of clinical experience fully substantiates both types of reflex action.

## Clinical applications

Considering the high variability of essential oil absorption and the fairly consistent reflex action of essential oils on certain skin zones – and lacking more extensive scientific studies – the evidence of clinical experience shows that:

- **Topical forms of dermal delivery** are generally reliable for treating local superficial conditions involving the skin itself, the joints, muscles, and so on – mainly because of the oils' effective local and superficial absorption. However, because topical applications require low dilutions, are larger than a small, precise zone or point, and produce insufficient reflex activity, they are less suited for treating systemic conditions.

   Applications for treating purely local conditions topically include medicated liniments, ointments, creams, lotions and compresses, which in herbal pharmacy may also contain herbal extracts (usually tinctures) such as Capsicum and Benzoin. Diluted essential oils, undiluted hydrosols, infused herbal oils and tinctures are all very useful ingredients for these preparations. As with systemic applications, these topical preparations can also be formulated to be very specific and able to treat a variety of local soft tissue conditions, including:

   - **Skin lesions of many kinds,** such as wounds, scars, eczema, psoriasis, acne, ulcers and bedsores, using oils with various topical actions such as vulnerary, astringent, antimicrobial, tissue regenerating (cytophylactic), anti-inflammatory, analgesic and antipruritic. Generally useful essential oils for skin lesions include Lavender, Spike lavender, Geranium, Yarrow, Patchouli, Roman camomile, Myrrh, Tea tree, Niaouli and Helichrysum.

   - **Hot, inflamed, swollen conditions of the skin, muscles, joints and tendons,** often with muscle cramps or reflex pain or itching (which may also lead to infection), using neuromuscular relaxant oils with analgesic, anti-inflammatory and spasmolytic actions. These include Yarrow, Marjoram, German camomile, Roman camomile, Blue tansy, Helichrysum, Wintergreen, Peppermint, Tarragon and Basil ct. methylchavicol.

   - **Cold, atonic conditions of the skin, muscles, joints and tendons,** often with numbness, tingling, joint stiffness, muscle cramps or pain, etc., using warming arterial and nervous stimulants, with anti-inflammatory and analgesic actions in the case of chronic inflammation and pain, and possibly capillary stimulant and rubefacient actions. Useful oils here include Ginger, Cajeput, Rosemary (all chemotypes), Clove, Pimenta berry, Juniper berry, Spike lavender, Black pepper, Nutmeg and Ravintsara.

- **Internal types of dermal delivery** are able to reliably treat systemic internal conditions. This is mainly because of the oils' good reflex actions at a distance through reflex zones and acupuncture points – and despite often poor and highly variable absorption. However, by the same token, these specialized applications are less suited for treating local conditions.

Applications for treating systemic conditions through the skin include massage, perfusive liniments, perfusions, and reflex zone and acupoint applications. Because they are able to address a wide range of systemic and internal conditions, they are useful both for treating particular disorders, especially with a marked terrain imbalance present, and for general preventive and health-maintenance purposes.

CHOOSING THE RIGHT DILUTION AND CARRIER OIL
These two factors are crucial for safety and success with all dermal applications.

The dilution range for all essential oil applications to the skin begins where the dilution to the mucosa leaves off. The best range is 5–20%, which is 45–180 drops (1.5–6 ml) of essential oil (or formula) per 30 ml or 1 oz of vegetable carrier oil. The general rules that apply are that:

- The greater the surface area of skin covered, the higher the dilution required, as a larger quantity of essential oil is applied.

- The smaller the area of skin covered, the lower the dilution required, as a smaller quantity of essential oil is applied.

- The final choice of dilution percentages should also factor in the metabolic condition of the client's skin, e.g. whether clear or congested, dull or sensitive, dry or moist.

At one end of the spectrum, a whole-body massage with a medicated carrier oil needs a 2–5% dilution, whereas at the other end a single spot or point application may be at 100%, i.e. undiluted. Although the dilution percentages for all other delivery methods fall somewhere in between these extremes, a dilution above 30% is rarely necessary for dermal application, and then only for one or two applications.

The best excipients for dermal delivery in general are vegetable oils, which provide a controlled, safe release of essential oils into the skin's layers. Preferred oils are those that allow the best absorption of essential oils by the skin – the more fluid and less dense, the better. Apricot kernel, peach kernel and hazelnut oil are said to be absorbed down to the hypodermis, while jojoba, avocado and macadamia nut oil are also well absorbed. Furthermore, each vegetable oil possesses its own therapeutic properties that should be considered when making any preparation for skin application. Each oil inherently has specific energetic and physiological characteristics that can contribute significantly to the quality of the final preparation. However, note that these qualities are only fully active when the oil is cold-pressed and unrefined. In overview:

- Apricot kernel, peach kernel, hazelnut and wheatgerm oils are optimal carrier oils for general use; they easily permeate the skin without leaving it greasy.

- Tamanu, kukui nut, evening primrose, borage seed, jojoba and olive oils are good choices for their specific treatment properties.

- Argan, hazelnut, avocado, rosehip seed, macadamia nut, camellia, almond, walnut, wheatgerm, ricebran, sesame and hemp seed oils are more often chosen for skin-care applications.

Another possible excipient is the use of silica gel, to which a small amount of vegetable oil has been stirred in. Mineral oils should never be used on the skin because they are not absorbed and may irritate the skin.

## *Cautions for all dermal methods of delivery*

- Many essential oils may cause skin irritation, skin sensitization or photo-sensitization. They should only be used on the skin with due caution, especially as regards the appropriate dilution in an excipient – often a vegetable carrier oil – the type of excipient, and the location and frequency of use. This especially refers to oils with aggressive constituents, such as the oils of Clove, Cinnamon bark, Cinnamon leaf, Oregano, Winter savoury and Thyme ct. thymol. Citral-rich oils such as Lemongrass and May chang may also need to be avoided for many applications except in very low dilutions (see the detailed section on topical safety status in Volume 1). The risk of skin irritation and sensitization is especially high in individuals who are generally hypersensitive, and in those with allergy conditions, such as atopic dermatitis (eczema). It is also high in those exposed to frequent ambient diffusion of fragrance products – especially if these are fragrance chemicals.

- If absolute extracts are incorporated in topical preparations, their exact sensitizing potential should be considered. It is higher in such absolutes as Lavender, Lavandin, Jasmine and Nutmeg.

- Topical applications on the face containing Eucalyptus or Peppermint oil are contraindicated in infants up to age 3. Babies' skin and mucosa up to 12 months are too permeable and sensitive for direct applications.

- Treating any area of traumatized or broken skin requires especially conservative selection, dilution and frequency of application of essential oils. Skin reactions should be closely watched.

*Delivery methods for treating local topical conditions*

A wide range of topical applications may be prepared for topical conditions of the skin, tendons, muscles and other soft tissues in general. These are traditionally differentiated into hot, acute versus cold, chronic conditions, and dry versus weeping or wet conditions. Pain and irritation are the main symptoms, to which any microbial involvement should also be noted.

The following represent the more important preparations that can incorporate essential oils. Further details and preparation instructions may be found in the author's *The Energetics of Western Herbs* (2007).

### LINIMENT

Also known as an embrocation, a liniment is a medicated vegetable oil rubbed or massaged into the skin and muscles. It can be prepared separately or with a herbal infused oil, with or without the addition of essential oils.

The dilution range for liniments is 5–15%, i.e. 45–135 drops (1.5–4.5 ml) of essential oil per 30 ml or 1 oz of vegetable oil.

Liniments provide excellent contact with the skin and have extremely varied applications. They are employed for all of the major indications for topical applications (above) – most skin lesions; for treating hot, inflamed, swollen surface conditions; and for cold, atonic conditions. In addition, applying a medicated liniment is also useful to:

- **Relieve local tissue trauma with pain and swelling**, such as sprains, strains, bruises, cuts, insect stings (including mite and tick bites), and all wounds without bleeding. Oils such as Geranium, Helichrysum, Myrrh, Frankincense and Roman camomile are useful for these.

- **Repel small insects** with such oils as Citronella, Lemongrass, Lemon eucalyptus, Geranium and Patchouli.

- **Treat an internal organ, bone or tissue:** see 'Perfusion and reflex zone application' and 'Acupoint application' below.

### OINTMENT

Also known as a salve, balm or unguent, an ointment is an infused herbal oil thickened with beeswax applied directly to the skin. Ointments have the advantage of providing even more extended contact with the skin than liniments, creating an excellent soothing, protective and healing layer for chronic conditions especially. Because they also help retain water, ointments are especially useful for rough, dry skin, such as on the elbows, knees and feet. Ointments also help retain body heat and are therefore highly effective for stimulating and warming a large range of cold conditions presenting as deep aches, chronic rheumatic and arthritic pain, stiffness, and so on. However, because they provide a slow, extended release of essential oils into the skin, there is also a greater chance of ointments causing skin reactions.

The dilution range for ointments is 2–5%, i.e. about 20 drops of essential oil per 30 g (1 oz) of beeswax.

A 30 g amount of beeswax is usually melted in 300 ml of vegetable oil. For a stiffer ointment, use just 200 ml of vegetable oil.

Ointments serve mainly to:

- **Warm and stimulate** in cold conditions of the skin, muscles and joints, including broken veins and capillaries, muscle pain, numbness and stiffness, and cold arthritis or rheumatism. Appropriate oils include Cajeput, Ginger, Rosemary, Spike lavender, Juniper berry and Pimenta berry.

- **Moisten and protect** dry, irritated, scaly, itching skin, as found in dry eczema, dermatosis, psoriasis, and dry, chapped skin or lips. Complementary essential oils include Benzoin, Copaiba, Patchouli, German camomile, Sandalwood, Rose absolute and Vetiver. Good infused oil bases here include those made of emollient herbs such as Marigold (Calendula) flower, Plantain leaf, Chickweed herb, Comfrey leaf and Gotu kola herb.

- **Protect and heal** wounds, cuts, sprains and contusions with such oils as Lavender, Yarrow, Geranium, Helichrysum and Patchouli in a tissue-regenerating infused oil base of Marigold flower, Arnica flower, Selfheal spike, Tansy mustard herb or Lady's mantle herb. Tissue-healing and protective ointments are also excellent for treating varicose veins and indolent varicose ulcers. For ulcers, the ointment should be pasted around the affected part and used in conjunction with an antiseptic wash or hydrosol.

## CREAM AND LOTION

A cream is a light vegetable or infused oil preparation mixed with a water-based extract, such as a hydrosol, herbal tea or tincture, and emulsified with beeswax or lanolin. While similar to an ointment, creams have the advantage of penetrating faster and promoting more rapid tissue healing. Moreover, creams allow the skin to breathe by not clogging the pores and so are excellent for warm, damp areas of the body, such as the groin.

They will quickly soothe and cool in all irritated and hot skin conditions, and can both moisten dry skin and hydrate wet, weepy skin conditions, as needed. Creams should be used sparingly and reapplied often. The essential oils used in creams are generally the same as the moistening, protecting and healing oils listed for ointments above.

The dilution range for creams is 0.5–2%, i.e. 5–20 drops of essential oil per 30 ml or 1 oz of vegetable oil. For example, 15 g, or 0.5 oz, of beeswax is first melted in 50 ml of vegetable oil, and 50 ml of hydrosol or herbal tea is then very slowly mixed in with the help of an electric food mixer. Finally, the essential oil or formula may be mixed in.

A lotion is simply a thinner, more liquid cream with a higher water content, which makes it more cooling. Lotions soak in more easily and interfere less with clothing. They are especially useful for treating delicate, sensitive skin – as in infants and children. They are excellent for cooling and soothing hot or inflamed skin rashes caused by an allergy (dermatitis), and also for sunburn or radiation burns. They should also be applied frequently. Cooling, soothing oils in low 0.5–1% dilutions are especially suited to lotions, and include Yarrow, German camomile, Roman camomile, Blue tansy and Helichrysum.

## Compress

Also known as a fomentation, a compress is water applied to the skin with a cloth at strategic places. A simple water compress is used to deliver therapeutic heating or cooling effects to the chosen area. A medicated compress is prepared by adding an essential oil or tincture to the water, or by substituting a hydrosol or herbal tea for the water. Here the medicated liquid can reinforce the heating or cooling effects of a compress. The oils or hydrosols chosen depend entirely on the condition being treated.

Fold and immerse a gauze bandage, fresh washcloth or handkerchief in cold or warm hydrosol, herb tea or water medicated with essential oil. For the latter, use 5–10 drops (45–90 mg) per 30 ml or 1 oz of water. Apply the medicated compress over the affected part and cover with a dry towel, waxed cloth, hot or cold pad, or water bottle. Leave the compress on for two to four hours, changing if necessary.

An aromatic compress can serve all treatment functions for topical forms of dermal delivery in general, using the example essential oils or hydrosols above. In general:

- **Cold compresses** are cooling and decongesting for acute hot, inflamed or congested conditions, including red, itchy rashes; burns, including from radiation; hot feet; acute injury; fever; a hot congested head; pelvic congestion; and painful liver or gallbladder congestion. For greater effectiveness, the compress can be applied both locally and at a distance, especially on the calves, feet, or nape of neck. For weeping, damp skin conditions with exudate, a judicious choice of astringent hydrosol or essential oil for a compress at room temperature is useful – including Geranium, Petitgrain, Sage, Myrrh, Green myrtle and Thyme ct. geraniol.

- **Warm compresses** are restoring and strengthening for cold, weak conditions, especially when chronic, including injuries that are two or three days old, as well as fatigue, debility or neurasthenia. They can also be relaxing and warming in tense, cold conditions presenting as aches and pains, muscle tension and spasms, neuralgia, dysmenorrhoea, cold arthritis, fibromyalgia, and so on.

*Delivery methods for treating systemic internal conditions*

AROMATIC MASSAGE

Whole-body 'aromatherapy' massage is a systemic form of treatment that combines the benefits of touch with those of essential oils in both their vapour and liquid form. Its highly positive effects on wellbeing should not be underestimated. They result from the seamless synergy of three therapeutic pathways:

- A psychological effect as the oils are gently released to olfaction

- A mild, general whole-person balancing effect as the oils blanket and non-specifically engage the body's reflex systems

- The physical manipulation of soft tissues with its combined physiological, energetic and emotional benefits

These pathways combined may generate an additional layer of pleasure to the therapeutic process that can only potentiate the latter by enhancing receptivity to treatment.

It is interesting to note that in aromatic massage the essential oils play a dual role as a liquid remedy on one hand capable of a certain amount of physiological effect, and an aromatic remedy on the other hand with a definite olfactory effect on the psyche. When these twin effects are combined with touch, a potent cocktail for general improvement of whatever kind is assured. In the hands of a skilled practitioner, aromatic massage can be both effectively therapeutic and preventive.

To the extent that the oils exert a physiological effect, the oils chosen may be functionally *relaxant*, *stimulant*, *sedative* or *restorative* (see Chapter 4).

To the extent that the oils exert a psychological effect, the oils chosen may be either stimulant, relaxant or regulating.

It is worth remembering at this point that although the common complaint among many clients is 'stress', the stress experience often arises from an internal weakness, especially from a deficiency in adrenocortical cortisol and in available thyroxine – and/or from unresolved pathogenic emotional blocks. The fundamental treatment in that case is not further use of *relaxant* oils such as Lavender, Camomile (all types), Marjoram and Clary sage, but instead *restorative* and *stimulant* oils such as Rosemary, Ravintsara and Niaouli. If a dual effect is required, regulating oils with a more complex chemistry, such as Petitgrain, Green myrtle, Laurel and Tea tree, are here the best choice.

Massage of different areas in itself will provide certain benefits, as many traditional systems of massage attest. Back massage is possibly the most fundamental treatment, and more widely acting than the more focused spinal liniment. Massage up the forearms towards the heart exerts a relaxant effect that is useful for relieving tension and anxiety, helping with insomnia, anxiety, and so on. Massage up the legs is excellent for venous stagnation in the lower limbs and also exerts a mild sedative effect.

Each procedure may be enhanced with the judicious addition of essential oils – that is, the right oil and the right dilution in a carrier oil.

## Choosing the right dilution and carrier oil

Depending on the intensity of fragrance desired, the optimal dilution range for massage is 2–4%, i.e. 20–40 drops of single essential oil or blend per 1 oz of vegetable oil. See 'Clinical applications' above for a discussion of dilutions and the best vegetable carrier oils to consider. More often than not, a blend of different vegetable oils is chosen, based on the amount of absorption required – for instance, a combination of apricot kernel and sweet almond oil.

Essential oils with a sweet or sweet-green fragrance quality should be diluted more than others as they have a greater emotional impact. When combined with the sensory-emotional aspect of massage, they have the potential for being effective catalysts for emotional release and transformation. The sweet oils in question include Geranium, Rose absolute, Rose oil, Neroli and Jasmine absolute. Typical sweet-green oils include Blue tansy, Roman camomile, German camomile, Marjoram and Sambac jasmine absolute.

### Aromatic bath

Aromatic and therapeutic bathing has been practised – and enjoyed – throughout history. Similar to aromatic massage, it is a systemic form of treatment that combines the benefits of warm water with that of essential oils in both vapour and liquid form. The aromatic bath gently combines the following two therapeutic pathways:

- A psychological effect as the hot water releases some of the oils' fragrance to olfaction

- A therapeutic effect on the whole person as the oils are mildly absorbed and gently engage the body's reflex systems

As in aromatic massage, this treatment makes full use of essential oils as aromatic remedies by olfaction, and as liquid remedies by physical contact. The key agent that facilitates both processes is the warm bath water, as it brings circulation to the body's surface, opens the pores and promotes absorption through the skin and the respiratory mucosa. This is unlike therapeutic bathing or hydrotherapy proper, which uses different water temperatures, including cold water, delivered in different ways for different durations; the short cold-water sitz bath is such a classic example.

It is important to emulsify the essential oil or blend it first with a little vegetable oil, liquid soap or shampoo to make sure that it disperses evenly throughout the water. Failing that, the oils will simply float on the water's surface before quickly evaporating. For a **whole-body aromatic bath** mix anywhere from 5 to 10 drops with the emulsifier before stirring well into the bath water. The ideal water temperature is 34–37°C (hotter than that becomes depleting). Soak for 10–20 minutes.

The choice of essential oils depends on the same therapeutic intentions as with aromatic massage, considering both the olfactory and the physiological routes of treatment. A simple rubric is to decide between stimulating versus relaxing oils and warming versus cooling ones.

However, if a simple relaxing and reviving evening bath is wanted to close the work day, 5–10 drops of essential oil are sufficient. Regulating oils would then be the top choice, such as Lavender, Lavandin, Marjoram, Bergamot, Nerolina, Green myrtle or Siberian fir; the water temperature would not be over 34°C and the soaking time would also tend to be shorter. Bath salts medicated with essential oils are another way of introducing a beneficial aromatic treatment element.

For **foot and hand aromatic baths**, use 3–10 drops of essential oil for a basin full of warm water, stir briefly and immerse the feet or hands up to the ankles or wrists for about ten minutes. The oils may be emulsified first, but in this case it is not necessary. The same treatment considerations and choice of essential oils as for the whole-body bath apply. As well as reviving and warming the body in general (especially after a long, tiring day), foot baths are particularly useful for increasing circulation in the feet, both arterial and venous.

Foot and hand aromatic baths also take advantage of the excellent innervation and diverse reflex zones found in the extremities. They have their origin in the traditional herbal foot and hand baths advocated for centuries by herbal medicine practitioners, and popularized in the 20th century by Maurice Mességué.

**Caution:** Peppermint oil should be avoided in baths because of its intensely cold sensation on the skin. Aromatic baths are contraindicated in babies under six months. Baths, as well as all topical applications, with any Peppermint or Eucalyptus oil are contraindicated in infants and toddlers up to age three. Ambient diffusion may be created for them by simply dropping 1–2 drops of a non-irritant essential oil or blend into a nearby washbasin full of hot water.

### Perfusive liniment

In this very versatile preparation, essential oils are diluted with a vegetable carrier oil to make a medicated oil that is applied topically onto a limited area – optionally with brief, gentle massage. The perfusive liniment engages essential oils for treating organs by reflex action at a distance rather than for treating local soft tissue conditions. This was a cornerstone of Marguerite Maury's (1961) treatments with essential oils.

The medicated liniment is applied on a limited area of the body and can be either gentle or vigorous. It may be repeated several times a day. If done vigorously with the intention of stimulating circulation and generating warmth, in France it is often called a friction. A perfusive liniment is also known as a simple unction, 'onction' in French medicine, and in traditional herbal pharmacy in England was simply called an 'anointing', with no religious implications attached.

The dilution range for perfusive liniments is 10–20% (3–6 ml) of essential oil in 30 ml (1 oz) of vegetable oil carrier. The higher the dilution chosen, the more it becomes important to change or alternate the area of application so as to avoid any possible skin irritation or sensitization.

The following are some examples of perfusive liniments for different areas and suitable essential oils:

- Chest: *expectorant, mucolytic* and *antimicrobial* oils for all types of respiratory conditions, e.g. Eucalyptus oils, Hyssop, Spearmint, Niaouli, Laurel, Green myrtle, Spike lavender. These are good choices for the traditional 'chest rub'

- Solar plexus zone: *relaxant nervous restorative* oils for emotional upset, e.g. Lavender, Marjoram, Clary sage, Nerolina, Petitgrain bigarade

- Abdomen: *analgesic, spasmolytic anti-inflammatory* oils for intestinal and gynaecological colic, pain or inflammation, e.g. Roman camomile, Basil ct. methylchavicol, Fennel, Nutmeg, Helichrysum

- Shoulder and neck: *muscle-relaxant* and *stimulant spasmolytic* oils, e.g. Marjoram, Fennel, Laurel, Tropical basil, Nutmeg, Cinnamon leaf, Pimenta berry

- Upper back: the same oils as the chest for respiratory conditions

- Mid-back adrenal zone: *adrenocortical restorative* oils for loss of stamina, collapse or acute allergic reaction (anaphylaxis), e.g. Rosemary ct. cineole, Scotch pine, Black spruce, Hemlock spruce, Thyme ct. thymol

- Low back: the same as for the abdomen

- Other organ zones, e.g. the liver, pancreas, kidneys, ovaries: a wide range of oils apply

A special perfusive liniment is the **spinal liniment**: here the oils act through spinal innervation and address both tense and weak conditions that require relaxant or restorative oils respectively. Because individual tension is determined by neuroendocrine functions, all neurological conditions may be treated in this way. The origin of spinal treatment remains unknown but undoubtedly goes back to ancient times; William Salmon (1691) reports the use of Laurel berry oil (*oleum baccarum Lauri*) 'being anointed on the backbone' for recurrent or intermittent agues, i.e. fevers. Interestingly, he also highlights the traditional affinity of Laurel for nervous and neuromuscular functions: 'The berries…are cephalick, comfort the nerves, cure palsies, convulsions and epilepsies, ease pains after travel…'

*Relaxant/sedative* oils for nervous system tension include Lavender, Clary sage, Petitgrain bigarade, Marjoram and Thyme ct. linalool.

*Restorative/stimulant* oils for nervous system weakness include Scotch pine, Black spruce, Niaouli, Laurel, Frankincense and Spike lavender.

Chapter 4 discusses in detail *relaxant* and *restorative* oils for the nervous system, most of which are pertinent to spinal liniments.

## Perfusion and reflex zone application

Perfusion engages rapid circulatory absorption in particular areas of the body where the skin is finer and the veins more superficial, e.g. at the inner wrist, the cubital crease, the popliteal crease, the temples and the foot arch. One drop of an undiluted non-irritant oil is gently applied to and spread over the small area, which is then occluded or covered with the fingers to prevent evaporation. Alternatively, several drops of oil diluted to 15–30% may also be used, technically making a perfusive liniment. In the case of precious oils such as Rose, Rose absolute, Helichrysum, Neroli, Jasmine absolute and Sambac jasmine absolute, a 5–10% dilution is ample for a good perfusion. Once applied to the inner wrist, the drop of oil can be spread out by circling and holding both wrists together. If used on a regular basis, however, perfusion requires some caution to prevent skin reactions. Alternating the areas of delivery from the very start is always helpful, especially to those with sensitive skin.

Perfusion can treat an extremely wide range of conditions by application to these areas, each of which also possesses its own typical effects. As suspected, in some cases a good reflex action may also be obtained at these sensitive parts of the body where reflex zones are often present. In other cases, the reflex zones are located in other places, such as the hands, feet, sacrum and face. Here the oils depend largely on an energetic reflex action at a distance rather than on simple absorption – especially on the hands and feet where physical absorption is rather poor compared to the rest of the body.

The arch of the foot is a particularly useful and versatile area of application for perfusions – the crescent between the foot sole and the medial plane. While high in vascular perfusion, unlike the thickened foot sole itself, it is also a good reflex zone – and especially to the spine in reflexology (and in that sense complementary to the spinal liniment). Another advantage of foot-arch perfusion is that it is less sensitizing than the delicate area at the body's major joints – the inner wrist, cubital crease and popliteal fossa. Apply one drop of essential oil or blend onto the foot arch area, rub in gently for a few seconds, cover with the fingers and hold for at least one minute. Repeat on the other foot or do both feet at the same time. A nice variation, once the oil has been applied to both feet, is to lock both foot arches together; this can be most comfortably done while lying down by placing one leg vertically and the other horizontally.

Furthermore, perfusion of many essential oils and absolutes – including the precious florals – can exert a nice psychological as well as physiological effect if inhaled at the same time. By olfaction they are put to especially good use in floral perfusions onto the inner wrist, effectively doing 'double duty' as a remedy for both body and soul.

ACUPOINT APPLICATION

This specialized, newly developed type of application is based on Chinese medicine pathophysiology and is similar to acupuncture and acupressure – although it also possesses notable differences with these. An essential oil is very lightly placed undiluted – in some cases diluted 10–50% in a carrier oil – onto an acupuncture point and held for at least a minute and until some kind of change is experienced. Acupoint treatment relies on triggering healing changes in the individual by engaging energetic resonance or reflex action at a distance through the body's network of energy meridians. This technique engages the combined effects of both the energy and information of an essential oil – despite the fact that no olfactory stimulation is involved. It does not engage oil absorption as a liquid substance with known pharmacological effects, as when one of the body's gateways is used to deliver the oil internally.

Once the practitioner has decided on a plan of treatment based on a Chinese medicine diagnosis, the basic aim is to choose an oil that possesses the same energetic functions as a selected acupoint. Because both oils and acupoints have several (and in some cases many) important energetic functions, the combination decided on will always engage one or two functions in particular. There is no one-to-one correlation between them. For example, a sweet-woody oil such as Atlas cedarwood placed lightly onto K-3 *taixi* will create a restorative effect on the patient's Yin and a calming, centring effect on the spirit; if placed on CV-6 *qihai* it will strengthen the Kidney and reduce urogenital discharges; if placed on LU-5 *chizi* it will resolve bronchial phlegm, decongest and promote expectoration.

Conversely, a major acupoint such as SP-6 *sanyinjiao* has many potential primary functions that may be stimulated by oils as different as Geranium (to nourish the Blood and regulate menstruation), Juniper berry (to warm and activate the Lower Warmer and promote menstruation), Rosemary (to resolve Middle Warmer damp and relieve abdominal pain), Marjoram (to calm the spirit and relieve agitated depression) and Petitgrain (to resolve damp-heat in the skin and relieve neurogenic eczema or neurodermatitis).

Clearly, acupoint application relies on knowledge of essential oils in the same context and medical terms as acupuncture theory itself. The backbone of this knowledge is the author's system of fragrance energetics – specifically the theory of how their various fragrance energies, their *xiang qi*, impact energy circulation in the individual. This is summarized in Appendix A.

Like the internal use of essential oils as liquid medicines, acupoint application too requires special training. However, because here the oils are being engaged for their energetic, not physiological, functions, the special training involves more than just knowledge of the theory of their use in Chinese medicine. Any successful acupoint application additionally calls for a willingness on the practitioner's part to develop his or her clinical skills for professional practice, such as receptive observation, greater sensitivity and loving presence.

# 3

# Using Essential Oils for Their Physiological Functions

## Two Types of Evidence

As specialized but integral preparations within herbal medicine and pharmacy, essential oils have a long history of consistent clinical use in Europe since the Middle Ages – alongside tinctures, decoctions, aromatic waters and many other herbal preparations. The physiological functions and indications of essential oils have always been embedded in the therapeutic principles and practices of herbal medicine. However, because herbal medicine itself since its earliest days has contained both currents of vitalistic and analytic paradigms, essential oils too have been employed on the basis of these two very different types of therapeutic expression (see Volume 1, Chapter 5). Developed over many centuries, both approaches have helped practitioners recognize the appropriate indications of the oils for relieving symptoms, treating disorders and addressing terrain conditions.

The modern healthcare practitioner is increasingly interested in benefiting from the strong treatment potential of essential oils in physical medicine. However, he or she is unfortunately faced with the poignant allure of these two very different but equally persuasive approaches. In the vitalistic tradition on one hand, as disorders are becoming increasingly complex and multifactorial, there is the draw to explore unorthodox and often more effective essential oil applications; conversely, however, there is also the tendency to fall back on the traditionally assumed functions of aromatic remedies. In the analytic tradition on the other hand, in the context of ubiquitous allopathic Western medicine, there is the pull of the easy rationalization of scientific pharmacology and the comfortable reassurance of research studies; conversely, however, there is also the exciting prospect of discovering new oil applications based on these studies.

It is timely then to investigate basic questions about essential oil functions from both vitalistic and analytic–scientific perspectives – questions such as those relating to the true meaning of evidence and the actual efficacy of different approaches to treatment. Continuing to engage a systemic approach here will allow us to begin reconciling the currently estranged relationship between these two different paradigms of practice. The insights it provides will help resolve the current glaring dichotomy between the medical applications of essential oils based on their traditional functions and those based on modern scientific pharmacology and research.

## The Epistemology of Essential Oil Use in Physical Medicine

The fundamental question raised by these turbulent paradigm currents concerns the exact epistemology of the therapeutic use of essential oils. How much of the information on essential oils that we have today is clinically really reliable? How much of it has been validated through scientific research? And how much of the scientific approach is useful for clinical practice? These are reasonable and weighty questions which can only be clarified by proposing general guidelines, not answered with final and definitive conclusions.

### *The evidence of clinical experience as clinical science*

There are essentially two sources of knowledge regarding an oil's functions and indications; it is important to clarify their differences. The first source is the clinical experience accumulated by generations of European herbal medicine and pharmacy practitioners in the Greek–Galenic medicine tradition making use of herbal remedies in their various preparation forms (tinctures, fluid extracts, aromatic waters, essential oils, etc.). This empirical clinical evidence goes back to herbal medicine practitioners in monasteries and nunneries during the Middle Ages, as well as to the wide assortment of herbalists, doctors, wise women and midwives who have used them ever since. This large current of clinical experience constitutes a clinical science in its own right and expresses a vitalistic paradigm. It has carried right through to the present day, as attested by countless herbals, pharmacopeias and dispensatories in all major European languages. As a clinical science it is expressed in the very core language of vitalistic remedy functions, such as *restorative, stimulant, relaxant, astringent* and *sedative*. It is also expressed in the basic functional pathology conditions that indicate their use, such as weakness, tension, heat, cold, dryness and damp.

With the development of pharmacies in the early Renaissance in Italy and then Central Europe, certain herbal practitioners increasingly experimented with alchemical preparations, essential oils among them (see Volume 1, Chapter 1). Alchemists had originally developed essential oil distillation from aromatic herbs in the 1200s, following their discovery of spirit alcohol. From the 1400s onwards, these essential oils became a special and integral part of traditional Western pharmacy and medicine. As the alchemists continuously developed and refined the technique of water-based distillation, essential oils eventually became almost as commonly available as aromatic waters, which had been the most central herbal preparation of all since prehistory. Many types of practitioners, including pharmacists, herbalists and perfumers, as well as allopathic and homeopathic doctors, all enjoyed the wide general availability of essential oils for use in their practice continuously until the early 1900s. The oils were a significant component in the wide arsenal of remedies that Western practitioners had at their disposal.

During the 19th century, for instance, highly skilled Eclectic physicians in North America made extensive use of particular essential oils, as recorded in the voluminous tomes of *King's American Dispensary*. The *US Pharmacopeia* of 1855 includes monographs on 23 officinal oils, which implies a much larger number actually being available and used in a clinical setting. Pharmacist, medical researcher and practitioner Samuel Hahnemann, who developed homeopathic medicine in the early 1800s, was completely conversant with essential oil remedies. In his texts he advises caution and even contraindication for the use of particular pungent oils such as Camphor and Peppermint in patients undergoing treatment with homeopathic remedies; he believed such oils would antidote homeopathic treatment. These statements would not have been necessary if these oils had not been in common currency at the time.

Empirical knowledge is always the primary source of knowledge, whether it eventually becomes 'scientific' or not. It is the foundation for the clinical knowledge of essential oils – one of the main contributions of the vitalistic tradition. The functions and indications of almost every essential oil in the materia aromatica are solidly based on its empirical uses in its country of origin – and regardless of the particular preparation form used. Even oils based on herbs that did not originally belong to the materia medica of Western herbal medicine, such as Niaouli, Tea tree, Lemongrass, Palmarosa and Ylang ylang, were at first still used empirically by Western practitioners on the basis of known indigenous folk uses of the whole herb. In the in-between case of essential oils that became lost to herbal medicine during the course of time, such as Helichrysum oil, these oils too rely for their modern uses on a core of traditional herbal usage. Helichrysum the herb was since earliest times a common liver decongestant and an expectorant remedy in its native Italy, being widely prepared in infusion, tincture, aromatic water and essential oil form. This is all that French practitioners in the 20th century had to go by as they began experimenting with the distilled oil: Helichrysum had never become a mainstream remedy in Western pharmacy. Had they ignored this herb's empirical information from Italy, Helichrysum would never have become the important aromatic remedy it is today and, ironically, science would never have been able to validate its clinical actions through pharmacology and research in the first place.

## The modern reduction of clinical science

The empirical evidence of clinical science is clearly significant and once again very much relevant today. Despite that, however, currently it has unfortunately found only limited recognition among practitioners of Western medical healthcare who choose to include essential oils in treatment. This is largely because chemical pharmacology, despite its obvious imperfections, still remains the ruling allopathic medical epistemology – along with the weighty modernistic paradigm or meme generally inherent in Western culture (see Volume 1, Chapter 5). The emphasis here is on the evidence demonstrated by modern scientific research regarding the use of oils, while the evidence of clinical science is minimized. It is assumed that clinical evidence alone, with its purely functional descriptions of essential oil effects and indications, is unreliable and therefore without real value. Despite this attempt at reduction, Western practitioners often find it difficult to cleanly separate research-based information from received clinical information. Whether it is realized or not, the two sources of evidence are often conflated (see below).

Moreover, the same reductionist approach exists within herbal medicine itself: when branded as phytotherapy (a newly coined term borrowed from French medicine), it attempts, again rarely with full success, to limit herb actions to those supported by both research evidence and the hindsight *a priori* logic of structure–function pharmacology (see below). However, as prominent herbal medicine practitioners have pointed out, this reductionistic approach rarely succeeds on its own (Mills and Bone 2000). It is a simple case of throwing out the baby with the bathwater – to the serious loss of modern essential oil therapy. We now know that it is largely the political rise of the synthetic pharmaceutical industry that eroded and finally watered down the 800-year-old clinical body of evidence acquired by hard-won empirical experience.

One argument for relying on scientific evidence alone as the basic epistemology for essential oil use draws its validation from noting how the functions of a herb in essential oil form differ from its functions in tincture, decoction, aromatic water and other preparations. It assumes that past practitioners and pharmacists were unaware of the therapeutic differences as well as commonalities among different preparation forms. However, a simple glance at herbal and pharmacopeia text from 1550 to the 1880s makes it clear that past practitioners were quite aware of the differences. One key example among many is Louis Jourdan's relatively modern *Pharmacopée universelle* of 1828, which is an exhaustive comparative survey of the many pharmaceutical preparation forms of the main traditional herbal and mineral remedies at that time – and it predictably includes aromatic waters and essential oils, like most other pharmacopeias before and after it. An earlier text that clearly differentiates among various herbal preparations is W.H. Ryff's *Reformierte Deutsche Apotheck* of 1573 – a wonderfully exhaustive compendium of herbal preparations (Ryff in 1545 had already devoted a separate volume to the aromatic waters distilled in his day in his landmark *Neu Gross Destillirbuch*).

While there are clearly some functional distinctions among the various preparation forms of a single herb, this does not invalidate the functions and indications they do have in common. In the case of important and well-known oils, such as Lavender and Peppermint, modern research with its pharmacological underpinnings has amply vindicated most of their empirical functions and uses in both tincture and essential oil form. The actions that may not have been scientifically validated remain secondary and do not appear to reflect their uses in different preparation forms.

As regards terminology, all of the terms that Western herbal medicine uses to describe a herb's functions and indications have always applied equally to essential oils. This includes broad actions based on functional vitalistic concepts, such as *restorative (tonic)*, *relaxant*, *stimulant* and *sedative*, as well as more specific tissue actions such as *anti-inflammatory*, *astringent*, *demulcent*, *diuretic*, *mucostatic* and *haemostatic*. In the case of oils that have no history of herbal medicine use, science alone now has often failed to recognize some of their basic functions. Geranium oil is a case in point. Based on all clinical evidence, it has a good astringent action. This important function is not spelled out today simply because an astringent action cannot be tested by modern research methods, therefore making it not even recognized. This lack of definition is not aided by the fact that Geranium oil does not contain any typically astringent constituents, such as tannins or resins, always found in astringent herbs. Nevertheless, this oil's astringency is a key aspect of its wide range of treatment actions, especially for tissue trauma and skin lesions in general…all without the help of tannins. This example underscores the importance of not relying on reductionist scientific evidence alone to obtain a complete clinical profile for an essential oil. It points once more to the major contribution that a vitalistic approach can make to obtain a complete profile of an oil's therapeutic properties.

The main functions of herbal medicines that do *not* carry over easily to essential oils are the moistening, demulcent and emollient actions. Because of their intrinsic fine, ethereal and volatile nature, oils are generally unable to perform these particular functions. Nevertheless, a few oils are indirectly able to evoke a hydrating effect on a particular tissue: Sandalwood, for instance, is well documented for relieving dry cough and also serves as a good emollient for dehydrated and irritated skin. Using a suitable preparation form for dry conditions will also help bring out the hydrating effects of certain oils – for example, steam inhalations for dry upper respiratory conditions, topical lotions for dry skin conditions, and so on.

The same danger of discarding the useful along with the useless can occur when looking through the lens of scientific evidence to compare the functions and indications of different chemotypes of a single species, as with the oils of Thyme and Rosemary. Again, evident here is the pull that convenient rationalization of chemistry-based deductive pharmacology provides. In both these oils, the common uses among their various chemotypes by far outweigh their differences. It is misleading to focus on their differences as though they were entirely different remedies – clinical and historical evidence again does not support this full-scale reductionism (Duraffourd and Lapraz 2002). It is important to recognize an oil's traditional profile of uses as a whole, integral remedy, not as a collection of separate constituents. This in turn is based on knowledge of how the remedy performs in clinical practice, not how its isolated constituents behave in the laboratory.

### The evidence of deductive pharmacology and structure–function theory

While traditional uses of essential oils closely followed the dominant theories of Greek–Galenic medicine in the vitalistic paradigm, by the 18th century, along with the rise of the analytic sciences, they saw another, different interpretation of their clinical applications. As discussed in Volume 1, Chapter 1, in tandem with the development of chemical and biological sciences, it became clear that the oils' physiochemical properties could actually be analysed and tracked. Later in the 19th century, with the discoveries of Louis Béchamp and Louis Pasteur that highlighted the involvement of microbes in disease causation and progression, essential oils aroused further interest by demonstrating *in vivo* activity against pathogenic microbes such as bacteria and fungi. The scientific overhaul of essential oil pharmacognosy and pharmacology culminated in manuals such as Gildemeister and Hoffmann's landmark *Die Aetherischen Oele* of 1899. The 19th- and 20th-century models of mechanistic biochemistry and bacteriology validating the oils' potential therapeutic effects in physical medicine remain with us to this day.

The second justification for the knowledge of the essential oil functions presented in this materia aromatica is the evidence of modern science. This knowledge is based partly on scientific studies and partly on deductive analytical pharmacology interpreted according to structure–function theory. Both fields of analytical science have yielded much of our knowledge of the mechanisms of action of essential oils on tissue functions. In so doing they have both refined known oil actions and expanded their potential uses. It is interesting as well as reassuring to know, for instance, that Bergamot, Petitgrain, Lavender and Clary sage oils contain linalyl acetate, a constituent proven to restore and protect nerve-cell functions (Faucon 2015). This specific information supports and *may* even expand these oils' traditional uses concerning neurological and mental dysfunctions.

Structure–function theory is the basis for scientific evidence still relied on today to rationalize essential oil functions. Here an oil's functions, like those of herbs, are presumed to equate the sum total of the known actions of its chemical constituents, and in direct proportion to the quantity of its constituents. The focus is not on investigating the clinically known actions of the whole oil, but on the experimentally known actions of its isolated constituents. This theory is based on the deductive *a priori* reasoning that each constituent possesses a definite, predictable action on living tissue, and that an oil's functions must therefore result from the proportional actions of all its constituents.

## The limitations of a priori deductive pharmacology

The limitations of this simplistic reductionistic interpretation of plant pharmacognosy and general approach to pharmacology are readily apparent when scientific analysis is compared to the reality of clinical results. With quite a few essential oils, a large difference between structure–function theory and practice is seen. Acute examples of theory–practice contradiction are Mandarin and Sweet orange oils. Mandarin oil contains up to 94% monoterpenes, Sweet orange oil up to 98% – constituents that are theoretically known to be stimulant and energizing in nature, as seen in Lemon, Rosemary, Ravintsara and many other oils known for their *nervous stimulant* and *restorative* actions. Yet despite their dominance in stimulant monoterpenes, both Mandarin and Sweet orange oils are used clinically for their reliable *nervous sedative* action – the exact opposite of what would be expected. Marjoram is another good example of an oil dominant in *stimulant* monoterpenes and monoterpenols, whose therapeutic effect is chiefly *systemically relaxant* and *sedative*. With many other oils, the incompatability between chemistry theory and clinical practice is not quite so glaring but still uncomfortable. That notwithstanding, the limitation of structure–function theory is often ignored for the sake of providing some semblance of scientific authority in the face of absent or limited true evidence-based research.

Still keeping to deductive reasoning, the theory of potentiation and inhibition among essential oil constituents is often cited as a modification to the basic assumptions of the structure–function theory. The effect of a constituent, major or minor in quantity, is said to be increased or inhibited by another constituent. A minor or trace constituent may therefore enhance a major constituent, thereby increasing its effect and possibly inhibiting the expression of other constituents. Or a minor constituent may directly inhibit the action of a major constituent, thereby modifying its effect and possibly allowing other constituents to become more expressive. This is the only way that the striking inconsistencies found between the clinical action of some essential oils and their structure–function explanation come deductively close to being reconciled.

Certainly, in the end it is difficult to generalize on the interaction of oil constituents, making potentiation and antagonism by definition impossible to predict. The laws governing the precise interactions and synergy among essential oil constituents remain unknown. The complexity of possible interactions often defies rationalization of their clinically known and experimentally proven actions. This is especially the case with oils of diverse and numerous constituents, such as Niaouli, Laurel and Green myrtle. The element of unpredictability seems to increase with the greater complexity of their components.

Oils with a relatively simple pharmacognosy profile tend to be more predictable. This includes those dominant in a single constituent or family of constituents, such as Lemon, Eucalyptus, Wintergreen and Roman camomile. Their chemical profile may be seen to closely match their clinical functions, based on the known and purported actions of their isolated constituents. With these oils, there is often little obvious difference between the action of the whole oil and its dominant constituent. Here the whole oil assumes a more linear, drug-like character than the complex character of an oil with a complex chemistry, or even the more complex character of a whole-herb preparation. With this type of oil the *a priori* approach still appears to work, despite its questionable logic and inherent limitations. Even so, even in oils that are overwhelmingly dominated by a single component, such as in Ravintsara, minor constituents definitely contribute to their final therapeutic functions: in this case, the highly active nature of the oxide 1,8 cineole appears to be softened and modified by monoterpenols, monoterpenes and sesquiterpenes. Juniper berry is similar, with its *stimulant* monoterpene dominance evidently balanced by *relaxant* monoterpenols and sesquiterpenols.

Regardless, it is tempting to assume that these predictably acting oils perform therapeutically in the way they do *because* of their particular profile of constituents. However, this is the *a priori* reasoning of deduction that reverses observation and assumption, and therefore may contradict the evidence of clinical experience. Moreover, the working logic of structure–function is then speculatively applied to oils with a much less predictable chemical profile – with equally less success. The topsy-turvy *a priori* approach of structure–function law is especially challenged when applied to oils of greater chemical complexity, in which unpredictability plays a stronger part – which ultimately designates *all* oils except for those few with a very simple pharmacognosy profile. And it certainly does nothing to explain the important tropism that oils exhibit for particular organ functions or types of tissue.

Explaining the clinical actions of the majority of the materia aromatica in terms of structure–function deduction alone therefore becomes virtually impossible. This is especially the case with oils containing a wide spectrum of different chemical families, such as Clove, Cistus, Hyssop, Laurel, Yarrow, Niaouli, Cardamom and Green myrtle, whose synergy of many constituents is virtually impossible to decipher. In these oils the deductive *a priori* approach simply breaks down, making it very difficult to justify their clinical functions by structure–function theory. This unfortunate (and ultimately unscientific) dichotomy between scientific theory and clinical experience clearly points to the serious limitations of current scientific pharmacology to provide theoretical evidence for the therapeutic efficacy of essential oils.

When all is said and done, it is generally conceded today that scientific knowledge of essential oils – their traditional pharmacognosy and pharmacology – is still rudimentary. At the same time, there is a growing awareness of other mechanisms at work in essential oil activity. It is admitted that there are other factors – poorly understood – that contribute to determining oil functions. For instance, little is known about how the electromagnetic properties of essential oils interact with their chemical properties; the main thing known is that the oils work as a single electrochemical unit. We still have no model to describe this unitary functioning (Faucon 2015). As a result, only so much of an oil's actions can be explained with the structure–function model of deductive pharmacology.

## *The* a posteriori *solution of inductive pharmacology*

A realistic solution to the structure–function conundrum would suggest adopting the stricter logical method of *a posteriori* reasoning of inductive logic. This logical procedure allows us to see an oil's chemistry as a *range of potential or possible actions* rather than a certain number of fixed and predictable actions. It also allows for the ever-present factor of unpredictability inherent in the synergy of its chemistry. There is a big difference between saying that Lavender oil has a calming effect *because* it contains esters that are calming – *a priori* reasoning based on deductive pharmacology theory – and saying that Lavender has a calming effect *and* we see esters in its composition that *may* contribute to its calming effect – *a posteriori* reasoning based on inductive observation.

It is always less useful to deduce the actions of an oil simply in terms of the unknown potential actions of its relative constituents. It is more accurate and logical to infer the actions of an oil's constituents based on the known clinical functions of the whole oil. (This difference incidentally also highlights the two basic types of theories, those based on speculation – endemic to the Western thought process – and those based on observation of phenomena – typical of Oriental thought.) Moreover, as Chapter 4 will argue, the *a posteriori* evidence for an oil's functions, based on the evidence of observed treatment results, is more useful in that it provides a greater context for understanding its analytical actions. It is the key that opens the possibility for integrating the vitalistic and analytic approaches – both valuable – to essential oil therapeutics.

# 4

# Integrative Essential Oil Therapeutics

## Vitalistic and Analytical Approaches to Treatment

Practitioners currently making therapeutic use of essential oil and herbal remedies now have a unique opportunity – that of benefiting from two quite distinct approaches to treatment: the vitalistic and the analytical. These approaches and their clinical modalities stem directly from the vitalistic and the scientific paradigms, both strongly present today (see Volume 1, Chapter 5). However, their true benefits will not be reaped if drawn on in eclectic fashion as separate, unconnected strands of information. Their benefits can only be obtained by using an integrated approach, such as the one proposed in the present materia aromatica. What exactly does this integrated modern solution involve, and what are the specific benefits to a clinical practice? Ultimately, the aim is clinical results.

Despite modern appearances, more medical systems originated in the vitalistic tradition than in the analytical approach. This approach is based on recognizing and utilizing the concept of a vital force in medical theory and treatment. Variously called *qi*, *prana* and *ruh* in traditional systems, this fundamental concept of a life energy inherent in all of life allows individual illness to be gauged with reference to a state of health – a reference that allopathic Western medicine lacks. Vitalism is the basis for traditional Chinese medicine, Ayurvedic medicine and traditional Greek–Galenic, or Tibb Unani, medicine – the three main extant classical medical systems that today are once again alive and well. The failing of Western medicine as a preventive and curative system now unavoidably allows for the resurgence of traditional vitalistic systems such as these. Likewise, ethnobotanists in many countries, including in Africa, East Asia and South America, use their research to document and make available medicinal plant wisdom that is on the brink of extinction.

And yet, the analytical approach is all-pervasive, largely fuelled by commercialized drug treatment of insurance-defined diseases in combination with scientific research of narrow parameters. The scientific – and scientismic – nature of Western discourse is so widespread that the lay population accepts it as a *de facto* gold standard, especially in medical discussions. As a result, in the area of essential oil therapeutics this has led to the strange alliance of analytical pharmacology, based on essential oil pharmacognosy, with holistic British aromatherapy. The alliance is a strange one because the point of scientific pharmacology is simply to clarify essential oil actions when taken internally as a medicine. However, because it aims to treat the whole person, the point of British aromatherapy is essential oil olfaction by mild inhalation, not internal ingestion.

This situation presents at worst an insufferable contradiction, at best a disconcerting paradox. Our task now is to clarify the terms and methods of each paradigm approach, so that a truly positive, universally beneficial and, above all, clinically effective integration can be achieved.

Historically, the physiological uses of essential oils were never separate from herbal medicine in the West and, for the most part, remain so to this day. Therefore, oils and herbs will be considered jointly here as remedies. Nowhere is the close relationship between herbal and essential oil prescribing more evident than in the area of therapeutics, including remedy selection and formulation.

## The vitalistic and analytical functions of remedies

There are two keys to understanding the traditional vitalistic functions of herbal and essential oil remedies. Firstly, as discussed in Chapter 3, their traditional functions are squarely based on the evidence of clinical experience rather than on the evidence of scientific research. Secondly, they are based on a pathology of physical functions rather than on a pathology of structural tissue changes. However, the term *functional medicine* itself was only coined in the early 19th century by a French physician – and it has certainly never refered to nutrition alone.

Vitalistic herbal medicine simply approaches herbal and essential oil functions based on their observed final effect on the body. *Astringents* tighten tissues, *expectorants* promote expectoration of phlegm, *carminatives* relieve indigestion, *vulneraries* treat wounds, *uterine stimulants* or *emmenagogues* promote menstruation, *decongestants* relieve congestion, *anti-infectives* treat infections, *antiallergics* treat allergies, *detoxicants* and *alteratives* treat states of toxicosis, and so on. These broad remedy actions all refer to the condition being treated rather than to the remedy itself. In turn, the conditions being treated are described here as syndromes (symptom patterns) rather than discrete disorders (diseases), and whole-terrain conditions or constitutions rather than particular tissue states and their symptoms.

By contrast, the analytical approach aims, instead of observing a remedy's final effect, to understand its specific actions, and its mechanisms of action, on physical tissues. Scientific pharmacology describes tissue conditions, not functional conditions. It relies on theory-based analytical research on the medicinal plant or oil itself (usually in the laboratory), rather than on its observed therapeutic functions in clinical practice. Practitioners of modern phytotherapy and French 'aromatic' medicine therefore feel more comfortable with tissue-based remedy actions such as *anti-inflammatory, analgesic, antiseptic, antimicrobial, antibacterial, antiviral, antifungal, antioxidant* and *oestrogenic* or *oestrogen-like*. After all, their aim is precisely to relieve tissue lesions and other states, such as infection, inflammation and pain.

Arising from different approaches, we can now usefully clarify the difference between these two types of remedy terminologies. For example, in connection with a remedy that treats wounds, a *vulnerary* function in vitalistic herbal medicine can entail several specific tissue actions, such as *analgesic, anti-inflammatory, tissue-regenerating* (*ci-catrisant* in French), *detumescent, antiseptic* and *anti-haematomal*. None of these tissue actions replace the functional action of a *vulnerary* remedy; collectively they all contribute to its *vulnerary* action. Likewise, the *cerebral sedative* function becomes a *hypnotic* or *anxiolytic* action in a science-based context. An *antiallergic* action becomes an *antihistamine* and *anti-inflammatory* action. A *neuromuscular relaxant* effect is described as being s*pasmolytic, anti-inflammatory* and *analgesic*.

Clearly, the two types of descriptions, the vitalistic and the analytical, share no equivalents – despite being connected. This lack of equivalence is especially apparent with broad functional remedy actions that have no clear corresponding tissue actions, such as *digestive stimulant, uterine restorative* and *venous decongestant*, not to mention basic terms such as *warming, cooling, drying* and *moistening*. The challenge at this interface of two very different terminologies is now to keep them clearly separate. Confusingly, numerous terms used for herb and oil actions belong to both clinical ex- perience and scientific research, thus blurring the boundary between these distinct modalities. Terms such as *stimulant, relaxant, sedative, diuretic* and *analgesic* are used both to designate clinical functions and to describe tissue effects based on research. The practitioner should be aware of this situation and interpret these terms decisively as either vitalistic or analytical, depending on the context in which they are found.

## *The tropism of herbal and essential oil remedies*

The fundamental way of thinking about how plant remedies relate to the body and its many dysfunctions is by the symptoms they relieve. This is common to all systems of herbal medicine worldwide. A characteristic particular to vitalistic therapies, however, is the notion of tropism – how remedies can positively affect major functions of particular organs and body systems. In all medical traditions, practitioners have always categorized herbal and aromatic remedies according to their ability not only to relieve major symptoms but also to treat dysfunctions of the organ that is their main focus. The tropism or affinity that they observed remedies to exhibit in practice resulted in basic designations such as *digestives* (i.e. remedies for digestive conditions), *cordials* (for heart conditions), *hepatics* (for liver conditions), *cephalics* (for brain conditions) and *respiratories* (for respiratory conditions). Sometimes these descriptions include an action, as in the vague concept of 'tonic', even though they still basically refer to the tropism of organ functions; this is the case with the terms *diuretic* and *uterine tonic*, for instance.

Knowing the tropism of an essential oil is as important for understanding how it will perform clinically as knowing its particular functions. While most oils affect the nervous system in one way or another, they intrinsically gravitate more to certain body systems than to others. For example, while Geranium and Marjoram oils both share a strong tropism for the nervous system, Geranium also has a good tropism for the organs below the diaphragm – the liver, pancreas and adrenal glands, and also the female reproductive system and the whole venous circulation. Marjoram's additional tropism, however, is for the whole neuromuscular system, from the cerebral circulation down to bladder functions. By strongly affecting neuromuscular functions, it is able to exert a widespread net of influence – unlike Geranium, which by regulating blood supply is focused on the organs in the trunk and the venous circulation.

Other pairs of essential oils share a superficial similarity of both tropism and chemical consituents, yet on closer inspection also exhibit marked differences. Laurel and Green myrtle are one such pair. Both oils share a major tropism for the nervous, respiratory, digestive and urogenital systems, and both are restorative to these organ functions. Both oils are excellent *expectorants* and *spasmolytics*. More than anything, both are clinically valued for the excellent results they obtain in many kinds of respiratory conditions. However, digging deeper, we find that Laurel has a much stronger affinity for the neuromuscular system, whereas Green myrtle exerts a stronger effect on the mucous membrane and fluid circulation. In addition, Laurel has a better tropism for the brain, for mental functions, whereas Green myrtle is especially tropic to the pelvic organs and the liver. Comparing their tropism in terms of their energy movement, it becomes clear that Laurel has a rising and dispersing effect, affecting the body's upper and exterior parts (brain, peripheral neuromuscular tissues). In contrast, Green myrtle has a good sinking and interiorizing effect that engages the lower internal organs (liver, uterus, prostate, bladder, pelvic blood and lymph circulation). Taking the next step to consider their fundamental actions, we note that Laurel is an excellent *relaxant* and *stimulant* on the organs of its tropism, whereas Green myrtle is a premier decongestant to its tropic organs. This completes the outline of their commonalities and differences in their tropism and fundamental functions.

Clearly, considering the tropism of an essential oil in relation to its fundamental broad actions yields the clearest and most memorable clinical profile. Without knowledge of this basic, systemic profile, the practitioner will simply see that both oils are *expectorant* and *spasmolytic*, and therefore largely interchangeable – as well as each possessing a long list of unrelated specific actions.

## *Treating the terrain with herbal and essential oil remedies*

Another characteristic of vitalistic systems of medicine is the notion of terrain treatment. Terrain designates the whole underlying condition that forms a larger context for symptoms, disorders and syndromes in an individual. It is the ground or energy field in which imbalance or illness is able to grow, describing a person's predispositions to imbalance. In one sense, terrain is the individual internal environment and the way it responds to stressors – physical and psychological. Different individuals will respond to the same stressor in very different ways because of major differences in their terrain. Terrain therefore includes hereditary strengths and weaknesses. A wide range of differences in dietary habits, lifestyle, emotional expression, and so on also continuously feed and modify the individual terrain. Ultimately, the individual terrain encompasses the sum total of hereditary and acquired features that a patient brings to the practitioner, even though the complaint may be a single symptom. Practitioners throughout the ages have sought to address this terrain not only to achieve a cure, but also to prevent relapse – above and beyond treating symptoms.

However, the terrain of illness is a highly malleable concept, one that various practitioners have applied to a variety of different treatment strategies. Although the word was only coined in the 19th century, it was actually a revival of the ancient concept of individual typing. Greek medicine practitioners developed the earliest recorded typologies. These rested on the Four Temperament types, the phlegmatic, choleric, sanguine and melancholic, which were also called the Four Element types or constitutions – Water, Fire, Air and Earth, respectively. They were based on the Greek medicine theory that, even in relative good health, each person possesses a particular mix (*krasis*) of the four basic body fluids (*tessera chumoi*) in quantity and quality. Knowing this mix helped the practitioner diagnose the individual's *dyskrasia*, or pathological fluid mix. (Incidentally, the word *chumoi* was mistakenly translated as 'humours' in the 16th century by Elizabethan Greek language scholars.) Regardless, the Four Temperaments are still generally known and discussed peripherally. The brilliant behavioural psychologist Eysenck, for example, was easily able to integrate their psychological attributes with two basic pairs of human character dimensions: introversion versus extroversion, and stability versus instability (Eysenck and Eysenck 1969).

With the neoplatonic revival of the Renaissance, practitioners of iatromathematics developed the Seven Planetary types. Based on the classical inner planets, this system of medical astrology discussed these planetary constitutions in detailed manuals, complete with elaborate illustrations. Herbs and formulas were assigned to treat various conditions arising in the planetary constitutions. Various treatment methods, such as cupping, phlebotomy and hydrotherapy, as well as herbal treatment, were prescribed for rebalancing and treating conditions arising from planetary terrain imbalance. Continuing the idea of treating a person's fundamental terrain, Samuel Hahnemann in the early 1800s then developed his system of homeopathy on the very basis of diagnosing by the patient's specific symptomatology – the homeopathic constitutions. This materia aromatica too carries forward the idea of specific symptomatology as an aid to essential oil selection (see Volume 1, Chapter 6). A few modern practitioners, such as P. Franchomme and D. Baudoux, have also developed interesting models of terrain treatment, for the most part based on typologies informed by essential oil pharmacognosy.

However, the concept of terrain is also used to describe the terrain of illness, without reference to a particular typology. It can serve both vitalistic descriptions of illness as well as allopathic ones, and energetic as well as physiological ones. For example, a woman presenting the common condition of pelvic congestion with systemic poor venous circulation and heavy clotted periods may be described as having an underlying congestive or damp terrain. Individuals with persistent, often inherited, allergies or autoimmune disorders may be said to present an allergic or immune-dysregulated terrain. A patient with immune impairment, chronically susceptible to viral infections and tested positive for chronic dormant viruses, could also be defined as having a viral terrain. Likewise, in the case of fungal infections such as candidiasis, a fungal terrain, and so on. These descriptions of fundamental terrain imbalance all describe a predisposition to particular conditions and symptomatologies.

The clearest examples of terrain imbalance today are endocrine–hormonal imbal- ances: these will create systemic pervasive shifts in the individual terrain that, if untreated, can dominate the whole symptomatology and persist for years. Good examples of endocrine terrain imbalance include hypothyroid syndrome (often with thyroxine resistance), hypoadrenal syndrome (or low-cortisol syndrome), oestrogen accumulation syndrome (with oestrogen dominance) and hyperhistamine syndrome. Completing the picture, these terrain syndromes may also be described in vitalistic or energetic medicine terms. Oestrogen accumulation, for example, generates a systemic condition diagnosed by the pathogenic qualities of Damp, Heat, Tension and Weakness (see Appendix B). Hypoadrenal syndrome diagnostically presents a Weak or Weak-Tense condition, and so on. These multifactorial conditions are true modern-day syndromes, not disorders or diseases, because they have either no single cause or no known cause. Chronic fatigue syndrome, fibromyalgia and multiple chemical sensitivity are further examples of latter-day syndromes. It is the chronic, systemic and pervasive nature of these endocrine syndromes that causes a marked and long-term imbalance of the terrain.

In each essential oil profile, the oil's ability to treat the terrain is referenced in two ways. Firstly, 'Specific symptomatology' at the start of the Therapeutic Functions and Indications section portrays the broadest picture of the specific whole-person terrain that the oil will treat in an individual (see Volume 1, Chapter 6 for a detailed discussion of specific symptomatology). Secondly, the indicated terrain is also described under 'Physiological' in terms of its essential diagnostic function, using as a basis Six-Condition diagnosis. Yarrow oil, for instance, is useful for treating Damp or congestive and Hot or hypersthenic terrain with its combined *stimulant* and *cooling* (*heat-clearing*) major functions.

## Using the six diagnostic conditions with herbal and essential oil remedies

The practitioner seeking to treat the terrain that is causing illness should make a systemic, holistic or whole-person diagnostic evaluation of some kind. The Six Conditions of Pathology is one such systemic diagnostic model that allows the practitioner to establish a diagnostic conclusion about the patient's condition and, on that basis, to adopt certain treatment principles. It can be used along with the conventional scientific approach to form the integrated modality that truly modern and efficacious essential oil therapy requires.

Six-Condition diagnosis is a new model of diagnosis in the vitalistic tradition that updates the diagnostic parameters of the Eight Principles from Chinese medicine and integrates them with the main diagnostic principles of traditional Greek medicine, Japanese Kampo medicine and Ayurvedic medicine (see Appendix B). Based on many years of research and practice into the principles and practices of traditional Greek and Ayurvedic medicine, it takes the best of the world's three major medical systems and integrates them into a larger dialectic diagnostic model that is more relevant to the types of terrain imbalances seen today.

The Six Conditions model consists of three pairs of opposite pathological conditions that include both physiological and psychological signs and symptoms: Tense versus Weak, Hot versus Cold, and Dry versus Damp conditions. These six conditions hinge on the three main parameters of tension, warmth and moisture. The individual patient may present one or more of these conditions in any combination, although Tension, Heat and Dryness (the three Yang conditions) are often found together (in any combination), just as Weakness, Cold and Damp (the three Yin conditions) are often seen together. In chronic conditions of terrain imbalance, however, Yang and Yin types of conditions will typically combine, as in the above example of oestrogen accumulation in women, where symptoms of pathological Damp, Heat, Tension and Weakness are often found together. This dialectic model of therapeutics makes complex conditions with their many symptoms much clearer and therefore easier to treat. When the time is right, it helps the practitioner tailor treatment to the underlying terrain rather than continue relieving symptoms or managing the particular Western disorder. This diagnostic model can provide the link in herbal and essential oil prescribing that has been missing for several centuries since the demise of Greek–Galenic medicine in the 18th century.

The treatment principle and functional remedy actions for each condition are as follows:

- Tense conditions require relaxing with the use of *relaxant* remedies.
- Weak conditions require restoring with the use of *restorative* remedies.

- Hot conditions require cooling with the use of cool *sedative* remedies.

- Cold conditions require warming with the use of *warm stimulant* remedies.

- Damp conditions require decongesting with the use of *decongestant* remedies.

- Dry conditions require moistening with the use of *demulcent* or *emollient* remedies.

The essential oil remedies that treat each of these conditions are discussed in detail below under 'The Six Functional Actions of Essential Oils'.

## An Integrated Approach to Essential Oil Therapeutics

Herbal and essential oil medicine today are clearly polarized between two very different modalities of approach, the vitalistic and the analytic–scientific. Both clearly have intrinsic value and contribute much to current healthcare in various sectors. Today's practitioner has the unique opportunity of being able to make integrated use of both vitalistic and scientific modalities. To realize this goal, however, means avoiding the classic error of throwing out the baby with the bathwater – an integration that does not breach the integrity and clinical usefulness of either approach. Moreover, it also means avoiding the common pitfall of simply placing the two modalities side by side, of making them available as alternatives – as sometimes seen in clinics that propose integrative treatment. If the goal here is to allow the practitioner to truly benefit from the positive benefits of each system without invalidating either one, a true synthesis into a larger encompassing system must be achieved. This necessarily entails establishing a new single modality, a unified approach to essential oil therapy.

Specifically, the ideal unified system would use the vitalistic modality of herbal medicine and its dialectic process as a basic general context, while using the analytic–scientific modality as discrete specific content of information. This is analogous to the relationship between form and content. The synergy of both modalities not only creates a larger picture with more information, it also allows the practitioner to modulate between both as needed. In other words, they create a bridge that allows one to focus on analytical information in one direction, and on vitalistic meaning in the other direction.

Here are some specific examples of the integrated modality applied to particular areas.

### *Pathology*

Through patient questioning and lab tests, one can determine the syndrome, specific symptomatology and terrain as the context for the specific disorder with its pathogenesis. For example, chronic fatigue syndrome (CFS) with its typical symptoms (the context) may present hypothyroid and hypoadrenal syndromes (the content). Or conversely, hypothyroid and hypoadrenal syndromes combine to create CFS.

If these endocrine syndromes were not recognized or diagnosed as underpinning the CFS, treatment would not be as targeted as it might be. Once the connection between the CFS disorder and the endocrine syndromes is made, treatment can concentrate on boosting thyroid and adrenocortical functions (e.g. with functional thyrotropic remedies such as Pimenta berry oil and cortisol inducers such as Rosemary and Black pepper) rather than simply focus on increasing cellular energy production and mitochondrial repair with monoterpene-rich oils, and so on.

## Diagnosis

By differentiating patient symptom-signs, making a Six-Condition diagnosis establishes a terrain context for a specific tissue disorder (e.g. infection, inflammation, swelling, sclerosis – the content) – for example, interstitial cystitis presenting a Damp-Hot-Tense condition.

However, in another person it may be possible to see interstitial cystitis in the larger context of a Damp-Cold-Weak condition – for instance with hypothyroid syndrome present – which would change the treatment to a large extent. Without diagnosing the terrain context (both local and systemic), interstitial cystitis would simply, and inadequately, be treated with *analgesic*, *spasmolytic* and *anti-inflammatory* oil remedies – regardless of their basic nature and tropism, i.e. whether *relaxing* or *restoring*, *warming* or *cooling*, and regardless of their affinity for certain organs, and so on. Although the use of such oils as Roman camomile, Marjoram and Basil ct. methylchavicol would certainly relieve urgent spasmodic symptoms and gain patient confidence, they may not be able to treat the underlying terrain, in this example Damp-Hot-Tense or Damp-Cold-Weak terrain. However, with a more focused selection of oils or with an individual oil formula, it would be possible to treat both the terrain and the painful inflammatory tissue condition.

## Therapeutics

The Six-Condition diagnosis leads immediately to a cogent and specific treatment strategy. For example, a Damp-Cold condition can be relaxed with oils possessing *decongestant*, *warming*, *stimulant* and *analgesic* actions.

If this condition were menstrual cramps with bearing-down pains before onset of the period, for example, this would establish congestive dysmenorrhoea with Damp-Cold in the pelvis. Beyond simply choosing any *analgesic*, *spasmolytic* oil at random for temporary pain relief, oils that address the whole congestive Damp-Cold pelvic terrain – such as the primarily *decongestant*, *warming* and *stimulant* Geranium and Rosemary – would be chosen as well for a much more effective and holistic treatment.

*Pharmacology*

We can apply *a posteriori* logic making whole-oil pharmacology, as proposed by C. Duraffourd and J.-C. Lapraz, or making the energetic functions of oil fragrance (see Appendix A) a context for chemistry-based pharmacology. For example, oils dominant in a sweet fragrance usually have a high content in either esters, monoterpenols or sesquiterpenes. Or conversely, oils high in any of these constituents usually possess a sweet fragrance (lemony-sweet, rosy-sweet, green-sweet, etc.).

If the connection between the therapeutic character of an essential oil and its particular chemical composition is not made, the possibility may arise of poor or even wrong oil selection in practice. Marjoram oil is one such acute example. A time-tested remedy in tincture and essential oil form for treating painful spasmodic conditions of all smooth and striped muscles, Marjoram is essentially a *systemic relaxant*. The fundamental character of Marjoram is expressed in the key sweet, green and somewhat pungent qualities of its fragrance energy. Relying on the *a priori* structure–function approach of basing its character on its chemical composition alone would belie its strongly relaxant character. Despite the oil's 90% dominance in monoterpenols and monoterpenes, for reasons unknown it still acts as though esters were dominant – as in Roman camomile, which tellingly also expresses a sweet, green fragrance profile. By relating Marjoram's chemical composition to both its clinically proven character and its signature fragrance qualities of sweet and green, a more accurate profile of its essential character and therapeutic functions is obtained.

In each of these areas, the advantages of engaging the synergy of both systems' modalities are clear: to obtain a larger, more dynamic and detailed picture of the patient's complaint, to arrive at a more accurate diagnostic conclusion, to formulate a comprehensive treatment plan tailored to the individual, and to select essential oils with a judicious juxtaposition of known vitalistic functions with scientifically proven specific actions. Any treatment that ventures to take this integrated approach is bound to obtain superior results.

## The Concept of Essential Remedy Actions

Despite their intrinsic differences, the close relationship between the functional and specific actions of essential oil remedies needs to be explored in more detail. Examining the characteristic fragrance qualities and chemical constituents of essential oils will clarify their juxtaposition in the profiles of the materia aromatica. Cardamom oil, for instance, has two functional actions, primarily *relaxant* and primarily *restorative* and *stimulant*; it is dominant in sweet esters and pungent 1,8 cineole and monoterpenes, respectively. The specific actions associated with each of its functional actions are then listed. An oil's functional actions are the essential, broad actions from which its specific actions are derived.

Practitioners of Western, Chinese and Ayurvedic herbal medicine have all searched for ways of simplifying the broad range of therapeutic effects demonstrated by natural remedies. Going beyond remedy tropism, they have always sought to classify them according to their simplest, broadest therapeutic effects. The motivation behind their search was as pragmatic as it is theoretical: in any period when herbal medicine has flourished, practitioners have needed to organize the large number of single and compound remedies at their disposal in a way that is manageable in clinical practice – i.e. well organized in their pharmacy draws and medicine jars. In written manuals too, such as herbal materia medicas and formula pharmacopeias, they strove to organize the clinical information based on broad, systemic classifications.

Moreover, when all is said and done about the nature and functions of the remedies themselves, Western practitioners on the whole have followed the approach of classifying remedies based on their essential functional qualities and effects in actual treatment. The classic example is the text *Peri Kraseos Kai Dynameos Ton Haplon Pharmakon* (*On the Mixture and Effective Qualities of Simple Remedies*) written in about 165 by the eminent Greek physician Claudios Galenos (Galen). This work lists remedies according to their basic natural qualitative functions of warming, cooling, drying, moistening, astringing, softening, restoring and relaxing (Holmes 2007). Later, practitioners such as Lémery, Ettmueller and De Tournefort took this one step further: they realized that remedies ultimately remain just expressions of a few basic treatment principles and extended the older categories to include the more therapy-oriented remedy actions of causing sweating, causing urination, causing expectoration, causing menstruation and a few others – all of which had also been developed by Chinese doctors at least 1,000 years previously – an interesting case of independent causation.

In Chinese herbal medicine, a clear example of the therapeutic orientation to remedy classification is that of Cheng Zhong-ling, still in use today for both single herbs and formulas. This early-18th-century physician divided remedies into eight fundamental types according to the therapeutic strategies of causing sweating, causing vomiting, purging, harmonizing, warming, clearing, tonifying and reducing. An interesting earlier classification, found in the 12th-century text *Shen Ji Jing* (*Classic of Sagacious Remedies*), is similar, although based more on the nature of the remedies themselves. Here the herbs and prescriptions are organized according to their ability to disperse, unblock, tonify, purge, make slippery, astringe, dry, moisten, lighten or make heavy.

However, just a few practitioners in both West and East went beyond even these basic remedy classifications, distilling them further into two or three template types. The prolific historian Cornelius Celsus in first-century Rome, in his landmark *De Re Medicina*, significantly mentions the classification of herbal (including aromatic) remedies in a Greek medical lineage that categorized remedies according to whether they tightened or relaxed tissues, i.e. heightened or decreased tissue tone (these are the basic actions for treating Weak and Tense conditions). Likewise, the Chinese doctor

Zhang Zi-he reduced Cheng Zhong-ling's eight treatment methods down to just three: causing sweating, causing vomiting, and purging – all to be understood in their broadest sense. John Floyer in early 1700s England viewed remedies as either mainly *warming* or *cooling*, in line with the basic dyad of warmth quality in Chinese herbal and dietary medicine. In the early 1800s in North America, Thomsonian practitioners and Eclectic and Physiomedical physicians generally classified remedies as *stimulants* or *relaxants*, which again connoted warming and cooling effects. Historically the common denominator among Western practitioners certainly came to be the twin polar categories of *stimulating/warming* remedies and *relaxing/cooling* remedies, which crystalized during the late Eclectic era of herbal medicine in North America.

In both West and East, there clearly exist many variations on the theme of essential remedy actions and treatment strategies. What they all have in common is one, two or more complementary/opposite dyads or pairs: *warming* versus *cooling*, *tightening* versus *relaxing*, *stimulating* versus *sedating*, *moistening* versus *drying*, *raising* versus *sinking*, and so on. Some remedy actions are based purely on tissue states, such as the *astringing/relaxing* dyad of the early Physiomedicalists (Cook, Thurston) and the closely related *consolidating/dispersing* dyad found in some traditions of Chinese herbal medicine. The latter pair of actions, although it is also based on the effects of remedies on tissue states, is ultimately broader in practice because it includes functions based on energy movement as well as tissue states. Other remedy actions are based on autonomic nervous activity, such as the *stimulating/sedating* dyad of Physiomedical practitioners (Thurston, Priest). Some are squarely based on circulatory dynamics, such as Floyer's *warming/cooling* axis, also expressed in Chinese medicine as *dispelling cold/clearing heat*. Yet others are based on the physiological cycle of assimilation and rejection, such as the *tonifying/eliminating* (*restoring/purging*) pair used by both Chinese and Galenic-Greek practitioners.

Because essential oils have been an integral part of herbal prescribing in the West, we now have a clear opportunity to classify their basic actions according to the same principles. The rich and ever-growing indications of symptoms and disorders for those oils now in common use require nothing less than the systemic, functional approach that herbal medicine practitioners have always maintained. We can now classify the core essential oil materia aromatica, like the herbal materia medica, according to fundamental remedy functions. This will allow us to benefit from an integrated treatment approach that includes both vitalistic and analytic modes of treatment, and benefit (without prejudice) from both empirical experience and modern scientific research. Organizing now the materia aromatica of essential oils along these lines will make the fundamental therapeutic nature of each oil clearer by any standard. Bringing it in line with vitalistic herbal medicine will also foster a true and much-needed integration with the herbal materia medica. On a practical note, it will certainly make selecting essential oils and creating formulas for treating physical conditions easier and more accurate.

The two core dyads of *restoring/relaxing* and *stimulating/sedating* established by Thurston (1900) and Priest and Priest (1981) serve as an excellent rubric of basic actions, with the additional specification that *stimulating* implies a *warming* effect and *sedating* a cooling effect. These actions clearly take on a new light when seen as functional remedy actions in the context of a broad vitalistic approach. Rather than representing particular physiological actions related to tissue state, circulation and innervation, each with their specific and limited applications, the four actions become generic and therefore more widely applicable. For instance, each action may be systemic or local, and describe function or tissue state. At the same time, its multivalency can then represent both remedy actions and treatment strategy. In short, what I propose here is not yet another physiological definition of a basic set of remedy actions, as we find in Western herbal medicine since the rise of the modern era. What is needed is a new interpretation of these actions, a new approach to their use – in other words, a whole-systems model of remedy actions that, through its multivalency, can serve a variety of different diagnostic and therapeutic goals.

The **restoring/relaxing** dyad is regulating, and remedies with either action gently bring function and structure back to normal balance by working in conjunction with the person's own vital energy. *Restoratives* and *relaxants* essentially regulate the nervous system and its dependent functions by either increasing its tension in the case of hypotonic or Weak conditions, or by relaxing its tension in the case of hypertonic or Tense conditions.

The **stimulating/sedating** dyad is directional: remedies with either action functionally and structurally, causing an alteration by directing the person's vital energy in a particular way. *Stimulants* and *sedatives* essentially operate through both nervous and arterial functions; they either greatly increase their functions, resulting in a warming effect in the case of hyposthenic or Cold conditions, or they reduce their functions in the case of hypersthenic or Hot conditions.

Moreover, keeping in mind the fact that the functions of these two basic dyads is to serve the six basic functional conditions of pathology (see Appendix B), it becomes clear that a third dyad is required to address the aspect of fluid circulation (as opposed to nervous or circulatory dynamics). The functions of *moist demulcents* and *emollients*, and *dry decongestants* and *astringents*, current in all herbal medicine traditions, are fundamental here.

The **moistening/drying** dyad is also directional and causes an alteration in function and structure. *Demulcents* and *decongestants* operate mainly by increasing or decreasing tissue hydration, with the result of either a *moistening* effect in the case of Dry conditions, or a *drying* and *decongesting* effect in the case of Damp, Congestive conditions.

**To summarize:** Each basic functional remedy action treats a primary pathological condition, which in practice can assume varying presentations. The herbal and essential oil remedies that convey each action all provide both a fundamental treatment function *and* different specific pharmacological actions. Their functional actions embody both a broad, central therapeutic theme while also including specific actions on body tissues and systems. Both these are described in relation to their pharmacology in Table 4.1 below. Many of the specific actions of essential oils are also detailed in Tables 4.2–4.6.

## The Six Functional Actions of Essential Oils

*Restorative essential oil remedies*

Restoratives are used to treat hypotonic or Weak conditions, marked by characteristics such as weakness, atonicity and hypofunctioning of function and structure. Typical symptoms include fatigue, lethargy, low endurance, dull aches and pains, distraction, brain fog, poor concentration and memory loss, low resistance, a droopy complexion, various tissue and structural weaknesses, a weak or thin pulse and a pale, swollen or trembling tongue.

Restorative essential oils are either general (systemic), i.e. *nervous restoratives*, or specific, e.g. *cerebral restoratives*, *respiratory restoratives* and *liver restoratives*. Restoratives to the circulation include a variety of different remedy types, including *venous restoratives* and *coronary restoratives*; remedies with a *mucostatic* effect are also essentially *restorative*, as are *haemostatics*. *Restoratives* include *astringents* and *demulcents* in addition to organ or tissue-specific *restoratives*.

The pharmacology of *restoratives* is dominant in monoterpenols, sesquiterpenes, monoterpenes and the oxide 1,8 cineole. These oils on the whole are either sweet or pungent in fragrance and neutral to warm in warmth quality.

- **Monoterpenol dominant restoratives with rosy-sweet or floral fragrance and moderately warming quality.** These include Palmarosa, Coriander seed, Nerolina, Geranium and Thyme ct. linalool. These *restoratives* are *nervous restoratives* in particular and *broad-spectrum anti-infectives* (*antimicrobials*); they are *immune-regulating* as well as *immunostimulant*. They are excellent for treating chronic Weak terrain with nervous weakness or neurasthenia, and immune impairment or immune dysregulation.

- **Sesquiterpene dominant restoratives with sweet-woody fragrance.** These include Atlas cedarwood, Patchouli, Sandalwood, Myrrh, Frankincense and Ylang ylang no. 1. Most are also noted for their *venous* and *lymphatic decongestant* actions, as well as for *anti-inflammatory* and *relaxant, nervous sedative* actions – often good choices for combined Weak-Tense or Damp conditions in general.

Table 4.1 The Six Functional Physiological Actions of Essential Oils

| Functional action | Main specific actions | Functional indication | Main constituents | Fragrance qualities | Essential oil examples |
|---|---|---|---|---|---|
| Restoratives | Nervous restoratives | Hypotonic, Weak conditions or terrain | Monoterpenes 1,8 cineole Monoterpenols | Pungent Sweet | **Pungent:** Cajeput, Niaouli, Rosemary, Ravintsara, Cardamom, Pine, Yarrow, Tea tree<br>**Sweet:** Geranium, Palmarosa, Rose, Thyme ct. linalool, Rosewood, Jasmine abs. |
| Relaxants | Nervous relaxants Neuromuscular relaxants | Hypertonic, Tense conditions or terrain | Esters Phenolic ethers Sesquiterpenes | Green Sweet Woody | **Green:** Lavender, Clary sage, Blue tansy, Roman/German camomile, Sambac jasmine<br>**Lemony-sweet:** Mandarin, Sweet orange, Neroli, Petitgrain, Nerolina, Ylang ylang no. 1<br>**Woody:** Cedarwood, Patchouli, Vetiver |
| Stimulants | Nervous stimulants Arterial stimulants | Hypersthenic, Hot conditions or terrain | Monoterpenes Phenols Ketones | Pungent | **Pungent:** Fennel, Tropical basil, Clove, Ginger, Nutmeg, Black pepper, Spearmint<br>**Acrid-pungent:** Pimenta berry, Oregano, Thyme ct. thymol, Ajowan |
| Sedatives | Nervous sedatives Arterial sedatives | Hyposthenic, Cold conditions or terrain | Esters Aldehydes | Green Rooty | **Sweet-green:** Lavender, Clary sage, Marjoram, Roman/German camomile<br>**Lemony-green:** Lime, Lemongrass, May chang, Kaffir lime, Coriander leaf<br>**Rooty:** Vetiver, Lovage root, Dong quai |
| Decongestants | Blood decongestants Mucus decongestants Lymphatic decongestants Kidney decongestants Liver decongestants | Congestive, Damp conditions or terrain | Monoterpenes Sesquiterpenols | Pungent Sweet Woody | **Pungent:** Niaouli, Cypress, Rosemary, Green myrtle, Juniper berry, Myrrh<br>**Sweet:** Geranium, Clary sage<br>**Woody:** Cedarwood, Patchouli, Sandalwood |
| Demulcents | Respiratory and gastric demulcents | Dry conditions or terrain | Sesquiterpenes | Sweet | Copaiba, Sandalwood |

- **Warming, monoterpene dominant restoratives with fresh-pungent fragrance.** These include Cajeput, Niaouli, Rosemary, Frankincense, and conifer oils such as Siberian fir and Grand fir. This group is both *restorative* and *stimulant*, and therefore somewhat warming, unlike the other two groups. With their particularly strong tropism for respiratory functions, they are especially effective *pulmonary/respiratory restoratives*. They address both acute and chronic Weak conditions tending to Cold.

- **1,8 cineole dominant restoratives with fresh-pungent fragrance.** These include Cajeput, Niaouli, Eucalyptus, Ravintsara, Laurel and Grand fir. These oils also are both *restorative* and *stimulant*, and on the whole somewhat warming. By stimulating numerous vascular, respiratory and digestive functions, they are also important *cerebral restoratives*, *stimulant expectorants* and *digestive stimulants* in general. They have also shown good *immunostimulant* and *antiviral* effects. In general, they are excellent for treating acute or chronic Weak conditions with some type of fluid stagnation, such as cerebral circulatory insufficiency, stagnation of bronchial phlegm and stagnant digestive functions.

*Restorative* oils include the following particular actions:

- Coriander seed, Nerolina and Sweet basil, *restoratives* to the brain and nervous system with an *antidepressant* action

- Palmarosa and Patchouli, *restoratives* to the intestinal microflora with a *prebiotic* effect

- Palmarosa, Patchouli and Helichrysum, *restoratives* to the intestines with *tissue-regenerative* and *anti-inflammatory* actions

- Geranium, Lemon and Carrot seed, *restoratives* to the liver, i.e. *hepatobiliary restoratives*

- Lavender, Palmarosa and Tea tree, *restoratives* to the heart and nervous system with *cardiotonic* and *antidepressant* actions

- Patchouli, Atlas cedarwood and Cypress, *restoratives* to the veins with a *venous decongestant* action

- Scots pine, Grand fir and Black spruce, *restoratives* to the respiratory and neuroendocrine systems

- Niaouli, Thyme ct. linalool and Thyme ct. thymol, *restoratives* to the respiratory, nervous, adrenal and immune systems

- Myrrh, Green myrtle and Atlas cedarwood, *restoratives* to the mucous membrane with *astringent*, *mucostatic* and *antiseptic* actions

Equivalent *restorative* herbal remedies include Nettle herb (*restorative* to the blood), Hawthorn berry (*restorative* to the heart and circulation), Goldenrod (*restorative* to the kidneys), American ginseng root (*restorative* to the nervous and digestive systems), Dong quai root (Dang Gui) (*restorative* to the blood), Schisandra berry (Wu Wei Zi) (*restorative* to the liver and nervous system) and Prepared rehmannia root (Shu Di Huang) (*restorative* to the blood and adrenal cortex) (Holmes 1999, 2007).

## Relaxant essential oil remedies

Relaxants treat hypertonic or Tense conditions, characterized by tension, hypertonicity and hyperfunctioning of function and structure. Typical symptoms include nervous tension, high energy, restlessness, a racing mind, overfocus, spasmodic (sharp) or erratic pain, a drawn complexion, muscle tension, a tight or wiry pulse and a thin tongue body with lateral lines.

Relaxant essential oils are also broadly either more systemic or more local and affect only particular organs. *Nervous relaxants* and *neuromuscular relaxants* are the two main systemic types that systemically relax the nervous system and both smooth and striped muscles. A more specific, local *relaxant* action is shown by *spasmolytics* and *anticonvulsants*.

The pharmacology of *systemic relaxants* is dominant in esters, sesquiterpenes and phenolic ethers. These oils are generally sweet, green or woody in fragrance, and neutral to cool in warmth quality.

- **Ester dominant relaxants with sweet-green fragrance and moderately cooling quality.** These include Lavender, Clary sage, Petitgrain, Roman camomile, Siberian fir, Helichrysum and Ylang ylang. They are excellent *nervous sedatives* with a strong *spasmolytic* action, and good *analgesic* and *anti-inflammatory* actions. These will relax both acute Tense conditions and chronic Tense terrain that tends to Heat.

- **Sesquiterpene dominant relaxants with sweet-woody fragrance.** These include Atlas cedarwood, Patchouli, Sandalwood, Myrrh, Frankincense and Ylang ylang no. 1. They are *restorative* as well as *relaxant* to the nervous system, and therefore perfect for treating chronic combined Weak-Tense terrain. They specifically possess *nervous sedative, anti-inflammatory*, and *venous* and *lymphatic decongestant* actions. Other sesquiterpene dominant *relaxants* are sweet-green in fragrance; they include German camomile, Blue tansy and Yarrow. These are also notable *anti-inflammatory* and *antiallergic* (*antihistamine*) remedies.

- **Phenolic ether dominant relaxants with sweet-pungent fragrance and a neutral to warm quality.** These include Fennel, Aniseed, Basil ct. methylchavicol, Tarragon and Laurel. They are *nervous* and *neuromuscular* *relaxants* with excellent *spasmolytic* and *analgesic* actions, and good *anti-inflammatory* actions. They are best given for acute Tense conditions of the smooth and striped muscle organs, regardless of the underlying terrain.

Other relaxant oils have a smaller net of tropism and act as effective relaxants to one or two organ functions in particular – notably:

- Cypress, Hyssop and Siberian fir, *respiratory relaxants* with a *bronchodilatant* action

- Mandarin, Spearmint and Peppermint, *digestive relaxants* with an *intestinal spasmolytic* action

- Lemon eucalyptus and Wintergreen, *cardiovascular relaxants* with *vasodilatory*, *hypotensive, anti-inflammatory, analgesic* and *spasmolytic* actions

- Fennel, Lavender and Petitgrain, *neurocardiac relaxants* with *analgesic* and *anti-arrhythmia* actions

- Fennel, Spearmint and Marjoram, *bladder/urinary relaxants* with an *analgesic* action

- Laurel, Lemongrass and Basil ct. methylchavicol, *neuromuscular relaxants* with *analgesic* and *anti inflammatory* actions

Most of the above *systemic relaxants* are also *uterine relaxants* with *spasmolytic* and *analgesic* actions on the uterus. Equivalent *relaxant* herbal remedies, in addition to some of the above, include Camomile flower, Skullcap herb, Cramp bark, Black cohosh root, Sichuan lovage root (Chuan Xiong), Chrysanthemum flower (Ju Hua), Magnolia bark (Hou Po) and Gambir vine twig (Gou Teng).

## Warm stimulant essential oil remedies

Warming stimulants treat hyposthenic or Cold conditions, characterized by insufficient warmth and presenting symptoms such as chills, dislike of cold, withdrawal, apathy, a flat affect, a pale complexion, cold skin, hands and feet, a slow pulse and a purplish tongue body.

The majority of *warm stimulants* exert a systemic stimulant effect through arterial circulatory and nervous system stimulation. Nervous stimulation divides into autonomic/smooth muscle and neuromuscular/striped muscle stimulation and is the basis for *expectorant, digestive stimulant, diuretic, emmenagogue* and *antirheumatic* remedy actions.

Circulatory stimulation divides into arterial, capillary and venous stimulation, resulting in arterial stimulants, capillary stimulants and venous decongestants; pelvic and liver decongestants are more specific decongestant actions.

Stimulation of the arterial circulation is the basis for other actions such as:

- Causing sweating with *diaphoretics*
- Promoting digestive functions with *digestive/gastrointestinal stimulants*
- Promoting bronchial elimination with *mucolytic stimulant expectorants*
- Promoting menstrual flow with *emmenagogues*
- Promoting increased urine elimination with *diuretics*
- Treating rheumatic–arthritic conditions with *antirheumatics* and *antiarthritics* (which also include *analgesic* and/or *anti-inflammatory* actions)

Clearly, stimulation can result in a large number of therapeutic effects, each of which is useful for a particular systemic, organ or local condition.

The pharmacology of *systemic warm stimulant* essential oils is dominated by monoterpenes, phenols and ketones. These oils are generally warm to hot in warmth quality, and pungent or acrid in fragrance.

- **Warming, monoterpene dominant stimulants with fresh-pungent fragrance.** These include Rosemary, Cajeput, Niaouli, Fennel, Nutmeg, Black pepper and Spike lavender. These *arterial stimulants* also possess *decongestant* (and *stimulant expectorant*) actions on bronchial phlegm and the venous and lymphatic circulation. In some of these oils, these actions are aided by the presence of 1,8 cineole. Some of these oils stimulate adrenocortical secretions, notably cortisol. They will treat both acute or chronic Weak-Cold conditions or terrain.

- **Strongly warming, phenol dominant stimulants with acrid-pungent fragrance.** These include Clove, Oregano (most types), Pimenta berry, Thyme ct. thymol, Winter savoury and Cinnamon bark (also rich in cinnamaldehyde). These *stimulants* are also noted for their outstanding *anti-infective* (*antimicrobial*) and *immunostimulant* effects, and especially for their potent *antibacterial* action. The majority do not seem to interfere with the beneficial intestinal microflora when ingested. They are reserved strictly for short-term use in acute Cold and/or infectious conditions.

- **Warming, ketone dominant stimulants with pungent-green fragrance.** These include Fennel, Hyssop, Spearmint, Peppermint and Rosemary ct. verbenone. These *stimulants* are also generally *expectorants* (*mucolytic* and *lipolytic*), *cholagogues*, *antilipaemics* and *antiparasitics*. They excel at treating Cold conditions with fluid stagnation.

A few oils are noted for their specific local *stimulant* action, usually as a result of combined nervous and circulatory stimulation:

- Cardamom, Green myrtle and Thyme ct. linalool, *gastric stimulants* with *stomachic*, *aperitive* and *carminative* actions

- Clove, Nutmeg and Black pepper, strong *intestinal stimulants* with *aperitive*, *carminative* and *antidiarrhoeal* actions

- Fennel, Spearmint, Hyssop and Green myrtle, *respiratory stimulants* with a *mucolytic expectorant* action

- Fennel, Peppermint and Basil ct. methylchavicol, *hepatobiliary stimulants* with a *cholagogue* action

- Rosemary, Juniper berry and Angelica root, *uterine stimulants* with *emmenagogue* and sometimes *parturient* actions

- Niaouli, Rosemary and Thyme ct. thymol, *nervous*, *cerebral* and *adrenal stimulants*

Equivalent *warm stimulant* herbal remedies include Cayenne pepper, Horseradish and most of the essential oil remedies mentioned; Chinese stimulant herbs include Cassia cinnamon twig (Gui Zhi), Wind-protector root (Fang Feng), Asian masterwort root (Qian Hu) and Wood aromatic root (Yun Mu Xiang) (Holmes 2007).


## *Cool sedative essential oil remedies*

Cooling sedative remedies address hypersthenic or Hot conditions, characterized by feelings of heat, throbbing pain, excitability, agitation, elation, emotivity, easy perspiration, warm skin, a flushed or red complexion, a rapid pulse and a red tongue body.

The majority of *cool sedative* essential oils exert a systemic sedative, i.e. calming, effect through arterial circulatory and nervous sedation or relaxation. Nervous sedation, like stimulation, is the basis for *nervous sedative*, *hypnotic*, *analgesic*, *refrigerant* and *antipyretic* remedy actions. In the neuromuscular organs, sedation is usually (and confusingly) termed relaxation in herbal medicine, as in *cardiovascular* or *gastrointestinal relaxants* – an example of inconsistent (but unavoidable) herbal medical terminology. Most *sedatives* are also *anti-inflammatory*, but this specific action is also found throughout the materia aromatica (see Tables 4.2–4.6 below).

The pharmacology of *systemic cool sedative* essential oils is dominated by esters and monoterpenoid aldehydes (e.g. citral). These oils are generally lemony, green or rooty in fragrance and cool to cold in warmth quality.

- **Cooling, ester dominant sedatives with sweet-green fragrance.** These include Lavender, Clary sage, Petitgrain, Roman camomile, Helichrysum and Ylang ylang. They are excellent *nervous sedatives* with a strong *spasmolytic* action, and *analgesic* and *anti-inflammatory* actions. They treat acute and chronic Tense conditions equally well.

- **Strongly cooling, aldehyde dominant sedatives with sweet-green fragrance.** These include Lemongrass, May chang, Lemon eucalyptus, Kaffir lime petitgrain and Melissa. These specifically possess excellent *anti-inflammatory* and *nervous sedative* (*hypnotic*) actions, and *analgesic* and *hypotensive* actions. They tend to also exert *gastrointestinal* and *hepatic stimulant* actions; i.e. they are paradoxically also good *digestive stimulants*. They are excellent for the short-term treatment of acute Hot-Tense conditions.

Some oils act as strong *sedatives* to one or two organ functions in particular – notably:

- Marjoram, Mandarin, Sweet orange and Roman camomile, *cerebral sedatives* with a marked *hypnotic* action

- Lemongrass, May chang, Lemon eucalyptus and Wintergreen, *neuromuscular sedatives* with strong *analgesic* and *anti-inflammatory* actions

- Vetiver, Marjoram and Wintergreen, *sexual sedatives* with an *anaphrodisiac* action

Equivalent *cool sedative* herbal remedies include Hops flower, Goldenseal root, Echinacea root, Baikal skullcap root (Huang Qin), Black figwort root (Xuan Shen) and Gypsum (Shi Gao) (Holmes 2007).

## *Moist demulcent essential oil remedies*

Moist demulcent remedies treat dehydrated or Dry conditions, characterized by dry mucosa and skin, presenting thirst, dry cough, dry skin, constipation with small hard stool, mental distraction, a rough pulse and a dry, furless tongue.

The majority of *demulcents* are herbal, not essential oil remedies. The very fine, dry and concentrated nature of essential oils prevents them in general from exerting a moistening effect, whether internally or topically. The main exceptional *demulcent* oils are those with a thick consistency, such as:

- Benzoin and Sandalwood, *respiratory demulcents* with *antitussive* and *anti-inflammatory* actions

- Vetiver, Palmarosa and Sandalwood, *intestinal demulcents* with *anti-inflammatory* and *antiallergic* actions

All demulcent oils are also *emollient* and somewhat *antipruritic* when applied topically. Equivalent *moist demulcent* herbal remedies that Chinese medicine describes as Yin tonics include Comfrey leaf, Marshmallow root, Chickweed herb, Plantain leaf, Lilyturf root (Mai Men Dong), Asian asparagus root (Tien Men Dong) and Stonebushel stem (Shi Hu) (Holmes 2007).

## Dry decongestant essential oil remedies

Dry decongestant remedies address congestive or Damp conditions, characterized by fluid congestion of some kind. This includes pelvic blood congestion with dysmenorrhoea and haemorrhoids, liver congestion with sluggish energy in the morning, venous congestion with varicose veins and ankle oedema, water retention with oedema, lymphatic congestion with swollen glands, and mucus over-production with discharges.

*Decongestant* remedies, both herbal and essential oil, generally divide according to their *decongestant* effect on blood, water, lymphatic or mucus circulation.

The pharmacology of *decongestant* essential oils is dominant in sesquiterpenes and monoterpenes. These oils are generally either sweet or pungent in fragrance. Quite a few act systemically on most body fluids, including Cypress, Niaouli, Geranium, Atlas cedarwood, Patchouli, Green myrtle and Yarrow.

- **Sesquiterpene dominant decongestants with sweet-woody fragrance.** These include Myrrh, Atlas cedarwood, Patchouli and Sandalwood. They possess excellent *venous* and *lymphatic decongestant* actions, as well as good *anti-inflammatory* and *nervous sedative* actions. They are good choices for combined congestive Damp and Tense terrain conditions in general.

- **Monoterpene dominant decongestants with fresh-pungent fragrance.** These include Cypress, Yarrow, Juniper berry, Rosemary, Green myrtle, Myrrh, Frankincense and Grand fir. This group is both *restorative* and *stimulant*, and therefore somewhat warming. In general, they are able to decongest respiratory, liver, venous circulatory and lymphatic functions, usually with a net *diuretic* and *detoxicant* (*alterative*) effect. They are perfect for treating chronic Damp conditions with sluggish elimination and toxin overload.

The following are examples of *decongestant* oils that notably act on one or two organ functions in particular:

- Juniper berry, Carrot seed and Sandalwood, *kidney/urinary decongestants* with a *diuretic* action

- Green myrtle, Myrrh and Atlas cedarwood, *mucus decongestants* with a *mucostatic* action

- Cypress, Cistus and Patchouli, *venous decongestants* for the venous return circulation of the legs

- Lemon, Grapefruit, Niaouli and Geranium, *liver decongestants*

- Yarrow, Geranium and Niaouli, *uterine* and *pelvic decongestants*

- Grapefruit, Niaouli and Lemongrass, *lymphatic decongestants* with a *detoxicant* effect

Equivalent *dry decongestant* herbal remedies include Yarrow herb, Artichoke leaf, Black haw bark, Horsechestnut seed, Butcher's broom herb, Japanese pagoda tree flower (Huai Hua) and Oriental arborvitae tip (Ce Bai Ye) (Holmes 2007).

## The Specific Actions of Essential Oils

Like their functional actions, the specific actions of essential oils too may be usefully broken down by dominance of certain constituents – always keeping in mind that we are necessarily only seeing a part of the whole synergy in an oil. The following pharmacology tables (Tables 4.2–4.6) include oils whose constituents and actions have been largely determined by the evidence of some kind of research. *Anti-inflammatory* essential oils, for example, have been shown to rely for their activity on a very wide range of molecules – variously on sesquiterpenes, sesquiterpenols, aldehydes, monoterpenols, monoterpenes and esters. Moreover, to obtain greater clinical relevance, the specific *anti-inflammatory* actions of these oils can be placed in the larger context of their *relaxant*, *restorative* or *stimulant* functions. Although their *anti-inflammatory* action would seem most congruous with a *relaxant* function – as when mediated by sesquiterpenes and sesquiterpenols, for instance – it can clearly also co-exist with a *stimulant* function – as in *warming*, *stimulant* oils that contain the key *anti-inflammatory* constituent sabinene, for example. This insight again underscores the fundamental difference between the oils' specific actions and vitalistic functions: the specific action of reducing inflammation does not correlate directly with relaxant, stimulant, cooling or warming functions; it can associate with any of these. However, the practitioner who is able to combine the logic of pharmacology with that of vitalistic functions will be in a better position to make a more precise choice of oils for treating a particular condition.

In addition to providing a pharmacological rationalization of oil actions, the actions linked to particular constituents are presented with a view to clarifying their clinical applications. The aim is also to present the spectrum of possible therapeutic indications for a single type of constituent. An overview of these tables will reveal that monoterpenols, for example, display an amazing versatility of clinical functions. Oils high in various monoterpenols are able to serve as:

- *Restorative* and *relaxant anti-inflammatories* for treating chronic inflammation: l-linalool, terpinen-4-ol, α-terpineol

- *Relaxant nervous restoratives* for chronic tension and exhaustion: l-linalool, terpinen-4-ol, α-terpineol

- *Spasmolytics* with a topical analgesic action for pain relief: menthol

- *Hypnotic cerebral sedatives* for cerebral overstimulation: l-linalool

- *Antibacterials* for bacterial infections with chronic weakness: geraniol, linalool, borneol, citronellol, terpinen-4-ol

**Table 4.2 Essential Oils for Reducing Inflammation: Anti-Inflammatories**

| Essential oils | Active constituent | Oil fragrance | Therapeutic indications |
|---|---|---|---|
| **Relaxant anti-inflammatories** | | | |
| | **Sesquiterpenes** | | |
| German camomile, Blue tansy, Yarrow | Chamazulene | Sweet, green | • A wide range of acute and chronic inflammatory conditions |
| Ylang ylang no. 1, Melissa, Black pepper | Caryophyllene | Sweet, green | • Acute inflammation from allergy, esp. with tense terrain |
| Atlas/Himalayan cedarwood, Patchouli | Cedrene, himalchene | Woody | • Excellent for topical use in skin inflammation |
| Helichrysum, Turmeric, Ginger | Curcumene | Sweet, woody | |
| Myrrh | Elemenes, copaene | Woody | |
| Patchouli, Spikenard | Patchoulenes | Woody, rooty | |
| Spikenard | Gurjunenes | Woody, rooty | |
| | **Sesquiterpenols** | | |
| German camomile, Blue tansy, Helichrysum, Neroli, Lemongrass, Vetiver, Patchouli, Atlas cedarwood, Kunzea | α-bisabolol, misc. others | Sweet, green, woody | • Acute or chronic inflammatory conditions with agitation, in tense and/or hot terrain<br>• Excellent for topical use |
| | **Aldehydes** | | |
| Lemongrass, May chang, Melissa, Lemon, Grapefruit, Lemon eucalyptus, Citronella, Kaffir lime petitgrain | Citral, citronellal | Lemony, green | • Acute inflammatory conditions with pain, with tense and/or hot terrain<br>• Damp-hot, toxicosis or infectious conditions<br>• Use low dilution topically |

*cont.*

**Restorative and relaxant anti-inflammatories**

| Monoterpenols | Odour | Indications | Source plants |
|---|---|---|---|
| l-linalool | Sweet (floral) | • Chronic inflammatory conditions with tense-weak terrain, esp. with insomnia, exhaustion | Geranium, Palmarosa, Clary sage, Lavender, Neroli, Marjoram, Petitgrain bigarade, Thyme ct. linalool, Sweet basil, Nerolina, Ho wood |
| Terpinen-4-ol, α-terpineol | | • Inflammation from immediate allergies | Tea tree, Niaouli, Marjoram, Nutmeg, Blue tansy, Plai |

**Stimulant anti-inflammatories**

| Monoterpenes | Odour | Indications | Source plants |
|---|---|---|---|
| Sabinene | Pungent | • Chronic inflammatory conditions with fatigue, esp. with weak and cold terrain<br>• Use in small to moderate doses | Nutmeg, Black pepper, Juniper berry, Laurel, Ravintsara, Plai, Yarrow |
| β-myrcene | | | Frankincense, Juniper berry, Black pepper |

| Aldehyde | Odour | Indications | Source plants |
|---|---|---|---|
| Cinnamaldehyde | Sweet, pungent | • Chronic inflammatory conditions with fatigue, esp. with weak and cold terrain<br>• Use in small doses | Cinnamon bark, Cassia bark |

| Ester | Odour | Indications | Source plants |
|---|---|---|---|
| Bornyl acetate | Fresh, pungent | • Chronic inflammatory conditions with fatigue, esp. with weak and damp terrain<br>• Use in small to moderate doses | Black spruce, Hemlock spruce, Siberian fir, Silver fir, Grand fir, Balsam fir, Douglas fir, Cistus, Rosemary ct. verbenone, Inula, Black cardamom |

**Table 4.3 Essential Oils for Reducing Spasms: Spasmolytics**

| Essential oils | Active constituent | Oil fragrance | Therapeutic indications |
|---|---|---|---|
| **Nervous sedative spasmolytics** | | | |
| | **Esters** | | |
| Lavender, Clary sage, Marjoram, Neroli, Petitgrain bigarade, Bergamot mint | Linalyl acetate | Herbaceous, sweet | • A wide range of acute and chronic spasmodic conditions |
| Roman camomile | Amyl angelate/tiglate | Herbaceous, sweet | • Spasmodic conditions with pain, agitation; esp. with tense terrain |
| Geranium, Palmarosa, Neroli, Marjoram, Ylang ylang no. 1, Thyme ct. garaniol | Geranyl acetate | Rosy-sweet | • Excellent for topical use |
| Neroli, Helichrysum | Neryl acetate | Sweet (floral) | |
| Ylang ylang no. 1, Ylang ylang extra | Methyl benzoate | Floral-sweet | |
| Spikenard, Siberian and Balsam fir, Larch | Bornyl acetate | Pungent-fresh | |
| **Stimulant spasmolytics** | | | |
| Clove, Cinnamon leaf | Eugenyl acetate | Pungent | • Spasmodic conditions with pain, fatigue; in cold and/or weak terrain |
| | **Phenolic ethers** | | |
| Fennel, Aniseed, Star anise | Anethole | Pungent, sweet | • Spasmodic conditions with pain, esp. in cold and/or damp terrain |
| Basil ct. methylchavicol, Tarragon | Methylchavicol | Pungent, sweet | |
| Nutmeg | Myristicin | Pungent | |
| **Spasmolytics with topical analgesic action** | | | |
| | **Monoterpenol** | | |
| Peppermint, Cornmint, Catmint | Menthol | Pungent, green | • Spasmodic conditions with pain<br>• For topical pain relief |

*cont.*

| Essential oils | Active constituent | Oil fragrance | Therapeutic indications |
|---|---|---|---|
| | **Phenylpropanoid** | | |
| Wintergreen | Methylsalicylate | Fresh-pungent | • Spasmodic conditions with pain<br>• Avoid in cold and weak terrain<br>• For topical pain relief |
| | **Phenol** | | |
| Laurel, Pimenta berry, Clove, Nutmeg, Black pepper | Eugenol | Spicy-pungent | • Spasmodic conditions with pain<br>• Avoid in hot and tense terrain<br>• For topical pain relief |

Table 4.4 Essential Oils for Calming the Nervous System: Nervous Sedatives

| Essential oils | Active constituent | Oil fragrance | Therapeutic indications |
|---|---|---|---|
| **Hypnotic cerebral sedatives** | | | |
| | **Esters** | | |
| Lavender, Clary sage, Marjoram, Neroli, Petitgrain bigarade, Cistus | Linalyl acetate | Sweet-green | • Acute or chronic cerebral overstimulation with agitation, pain, anxiety; in tense or tense-hot terrain |
| Roman camomile | Amyl angelate/tiglate | Sweet-green | |
| Geranium, Neroli, Marjoram, Linaloeswood, Ylang ylang no. 1 | Geranyl acetate | Rosy-sweet | |
| Neroli, Helichrysum | Neryl acetate | Rosy-sweet | |
| Ylang ylang no. 1 and extra | Methyl benzoate | Floral-sweet | |
| | **Monoterpenol** | | |
| Lavender, Clary sage, Neroli, Geranium, Marjoram, Mandarin, Bergamot, Petitgrain bigarade, Lime | l-linalool | Floral-sweet | • Cerebral overstimulation with chronic tense-weak terrain |

**Spasmolytic, relaxant nervous sedatives**

| | | | |
|---|---|---|---|
| **Esters** | | | |
| Lavender, Clary sage, Marjoram, Lime, Petitgrain bigarade, Bergamot, Neroli | Linalyl acetate | Sweet-green | • Acute or chronic spasmodic conditions with pain, esp. in tense or tense-hot terrain |
| Roman camomile | Amyl angelate/tiglate | Sweet-green | |
| Geranium, Neroli, Marjoram, Rose | Geranyl acetate | Rosy-sweet | |
| Neroli, Helichrysum, Rose | Neryl acetate | Rosy-sweet | |
| Ylang ylang no. 1 and extra | Methyl benzoate | Floral-sweet | |

**Analgesic, restorative nervous sedatives**

| | | | |
|---|---|---|---|
| **Monoterpenols** | | | |
| Lavender, Clary sage, Petitgrain bigarade, Thyme ct. linalool, Neroli, Marjoram, Mandarin | $l$-linalool | Floral-sweet | • Chronic tense-weak conditions with chronic exhaustion, insomnia, pain |
| Tea tree, Marjoram, Kunzea, Plai | Terpinen-4-ol, α-terpineol | | |

**Anti-inflammatory nervous sedatives**

| | | | |
|---|---|---|---|
| **Aldehydes** | | | |
| Lemongrass, May chang, Citronella, Melissa, Lemon eucalyptus, Lemon verbena, Lemon myrtle, Lemon tea tree, Kaffir lime petitgrain | Citral, citronellal | Green-lemony | • Acute hot or tense conditions with local or systemic inflammation, toxicosis or infection<br>• Caution with topical use |

Table 4.5 Essential Oils for Restoring the Nervous System: Nervous Restoratives

| Essential oils | Active constituent | Oil fragrance | Therapeutic indications |
|---|---|---|---|
| **Stimulant cerebral restoratives** | | | |
| | **Monoterpene oxide** | | |
| Cajeput, Niaouli, Ravintsara, Saro, Tea tree, Rosemary spp., Green myrtle, Eucalyptus spp., Spike lavender, Sage, Grand fir, Cardamom, Nutmeg, Laurel, Thyme ct. thymol | 1,8 cineole | Fresh-pungent | • Cerebral deficiency with mental fatigue in weak terrain, especially chronic<br>• Caution with long-term and excessive use |
| **Warming, arterial stimulant nervous restoratives** | | | |
| | **Monoterpenes** | | |
| Rosemary ct. cineole/camphor, Saro, Niaouli, Cajeput, Ravintsara, Ginger, Nutmeg, Cardamom, Juniper berry, Fennel, Fir spp., Cistus, Frankincense, Spike lavender, Cypress, Sage, Peppermint, Laurel, Green myrtle, Black pepper, Cinnamon leaf, Hyssop, Galbanum | α- and β-pinene, *l*-limonene, terpinenes | Fresh-pungent, balsamic | • Weak conditions with cold or congestive damp terrain, simple or infectious<br>• Caution with long-term and excessive use<br>• Caution with topical use and dilution percentage |
| Lemon, Grapefruit, Lime | *d*-limonene | Fresh-lemony | • Chronic weak conditions |
| | **Phenols** | | |
| Pimenta berry, Holy basil, Clove bud, Laurel, Thyme ct. thymol/carvacrol, Oregano spp., Cretan thyme, Winter savoury | Eugenol, carvacrol, thymol | Acrid-pungent | • Cold-weak conditions, simple or infectious; with fatigue<br>• Caution with topical and internal use |
| **Relaxant nervous restoratives** | | | |
| | **Monoterpenols** | | |
| Lavender, Clary sage, Geranium, Marjoram, Neroli, Sweet basil, Rose, Petitgrain bigarade, Sweet orange, Nerolina, Thyme ct. thujanol | *l*-linalool | Floral-sweet | • Chronic tense-weak conditions, including with developing heat, with exhaustion, insomnia |
| Tea tree, Marjoram, Thyme ct. borneol | Terpinen-4-ol, α-terpineol | Mild | |

**Neuroendocrine restoratives**

| | Monoterpenes | | |
|---|---|---|---|
| Siberian fir, Silver fir, Balsam fir, Scotch pine, Black spruce, Cypress, Rosemary ct. verbenone, Niaouli, Black pepper | Delta-3-carene, α-pinene | Woody-pungent | • Neuroendocrine weakness with debility in weak or congestive damp terrain<br>• Caution with excessive use |

**Table 4.6 Essential Oils for Treating Infections: Anti-Infectives**

| Essential oils | Active constituent | Oil fragrance | Therapeutic indications |
|---|---|---|---|
| **Antibacterials** | | | |
| | **Monoterpenols** | | |
| Tea tree, Palmarosa, Geranium, Sage, Thyme ct. *l*-linalool, Thyme ct. thujanol, Lavender, Neroli, Rose, Inula | Geraniol, linalool, terpinen-4-ol, borneol, citronellol | Sweet, herbaceous | • Bacterial infections, esp. chronic, with weak terrain and chronic immune deficiency<br>• Esp. for children, elderly and sensitive people<br>• Excellent for topical use |
| | **Sesquiterpenols** | | |
| Sandalwood (all *Santalum* species) | Santalols | | • Bacterial infections, esp. chronic, with damp/ weak terrain |
| | **Phenols** | | |
| Thyme ct. thymol, Wild thyme, Ajowan | Thymol | Pungent, acrid | • Acute bacterial infections, esp. with weak or cold terrain and immune deficiency<br>• Avoid in tense and hot terrain |
| Clove, Pimenta berry | Eugenol | Pungent, acrid | |
| Oregano spp., Thyme ct. carvacrol, Wild thyme, Capitate thyme, Winter savoury | Carvacrol | Pungent, acrid | • Combine with monoterpenol-rich oils to increase safety<br>• Use short term only<br>• Avoid topical use |

*cont.*

| Oils | Group / Constituents | Scent | Uses |
|---|---|---|---|
| | **Esters** | Rosy-sweet | • Acute or chronic infections, esp. with pain, tense terrain |
| Palmarosa, Citronella, Lemongrass, Rose, Melissa, Cardamom, Laurel | Geranyl acetate, terpenyl acetate | | |
| | **Monoterpenes** | Fresh, pungent | • Most bacterial infections<br>• Use also to increase penetration of other oils<br>• Excellent for surface infections |
| Eucalyptus spp., Cajeput, Niaouli, Ravintsara, Saro, Juniper berry, Ginger | Limonene, α-pinene | | |
| **Antivirals** | | | |
| | **Oxide** | Fresh, pungent | • Acute and chronic viral infections<br>• Use short or long term |
| Ravintsara, Saro, Cajeput, Niaouli, Eucalyptus spp., Sage, Spike lavender, Mastic thyme | 1,8 cineole | | |
| | **Miscellaneous** | Fresh-pungent | • All types of viral infections |
| Cajeput, Niaouli, Ravintsara, Saro, Eucalyptus spp., Peppermint, Lemon, Bergamot, Cistus, Black spruce, Tarragon, Basil ct. methylchavicol | Monoterpenes, phenolic ether | | |
| **Antifungals** | | | |
| | **Monoterpenols** | Sweet, herbaceous | • Chronic fungal infections, esp. with weak terrain and chronic immune deficiency<br>• Esp. for children, elderly and sensitive people<br>• Use short or long term<br>• Excellent for topical use |
| Tea tree, Palmarosa, Geranium, Lavender, Petitgrain bigarade, Thyme ct. linalool, Thyme ct. geraniol, Thyme ct. thujanol, Neroli, Nerolina, Rosalina, Plai | Geraniol, l-linalool, terpinen-4-ol, α-terpineol | | |

| | Components | Odour | Indications / Cautions |
|---|---|---|---|
| **Sesquiterpenols** | | | |
| Carrot seed, Sandalwood, Patchouli, Spikenard, Vetiver, German camomile | Carotol, santalols, patchouli alcohols, vetiverol, α-bisabolol | | • All fungal infections<br>• Excellent for topical use |
| **Aldehydes** | | | |
| Lemongrass, May chang, Lemon eucalyptus, Lemon myrtle, Lemon tea tree, Kaffir lime petitgrain | Citral, citronellal | | • All fungal infections, esp. with hot or tense-hot terrain<br>• Use low dilutions topically |
| Cinnamon bark, Cassia bark | Cinnamaldehyde | Sweet, pungent | • Fungal infections with cold, weak terrain<br>• Not for topical use |
| **Ketones** | | | |
| Peppermint, Spearmint, Hyssop, Coriander seed, Myrrh, Sage, Rosemary ct. verbenone | Menthone, carvone, piperitone, camphor, verbenone | | • Fungal infections with weak, damp terrain |
| **Phenols** | | | |
| Thyme ct. thymol, Thyme ct. carvacrol, Wild thyme, Clove, Pimenta berry, Winter savoury, Cinnamon bark, Oregano, Tree basil | Thymol, eugenol, carvacrol, methyl-chavicol | Acrid-pungent | • For all types of infections, esp. with weak or cold terrain and immune deficiency<br>• Avoid in tense and hot terrain<br>• Combine with oils rich in monoterpenols to increase safety<br>• Use short term only<br>• Avoid topical use |

# Angelica Root

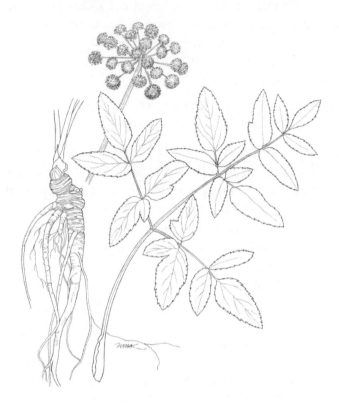

**Botanical source:** The root of *Angelica archangelica* L. (Apiaceae/Umbelliferae, carrot family), a water-loving herb of the temperate and subarctic Northern hemisphere

**Other names:** European angelica, Garden angelica, Root of the Holy Ghost; Angélique (Fr), Angelika (Ge), Angelica (It, Sp)

**Appearance:** A pale to dark yellow or amber liquid, depending on the age of the roots and the oil; the odour is warm, fresh and somewhat peppery, herbaceous, balsamic and somewhat musty, woody; the peppery notes increase with ageing

**Perfumery status:** A base note of very high intensity and excellent persistence. The root oil is considered much finer than the seed oil and herb oil.

**Extraction:** Steam distillation of the fresh or dried two-year-old roots (ideally), usually in November and December; the roots take 12–24 hours to distil

**1 kg oil yield from:** 250–350 kg, a moderate to low yield

**Production areas:** Hungary, France, Holland, Belgium, Germany

**Typical constituents:** Monoterpenes 70–91% (incl. α-pinene 24–27%, α-phellandrene 12–15%, d-limonene 13%, β-myrcene 4–12%, γ-terpenene <4%, camphene <1%, sabinene) • oxide 1,8 cineole 14% • aromatic p-cymene 4–10% • coumarins and furanocoumarins 2% (incl. umbelliferone, angelicin, archangelicin, bergapten, osthol, osthenol, imperatorin, xanthotoxol) • esters 1.5–2% (incl. bornyl acetate, trans-verbenyl acetate) • lactones <2% (incl. pentadecanolide <1%, ambrettolide <1%) • sesquiterpenes 3% (incl. β-caryophyllene <0.2%) • monoterpenols 1% (incl. linalool, borneol) • sesquiterpenols 1%

**Chance of adulteration:** Moderate, because of the high cost of production. Mainly with synthetic monoterpenes or Angelica seed oil, which is easier to produce.

**Related oils:** Angelica seed oil (see below). Of the over 60 different species of Angelica seen, the main oil commonly available is that of the Nepal angelica (*Angelica glaucens* Edgw.) produced in Nepal. This oil cannot be used interchangeably with Angelica root oil as its profile of constituents is very different. Monoterpenes are minor percentages here and the main compounds are butylidenephthalide and ligustilide (also found in Chinese and Japanese angelica root oils, Dang gui and Toki respectively). The fragrance too is less pungent and more herbaceous.

Botanically related plants in the carrot family whose root oils are often produced include Japan angelica (*A. japonica* A. Gray), Dong quai root (*A. sinensis* [Oliv.] Diehls), Lovage root (*Ligusticum levisticum* L., syn. *Levisticum off.* Koch), Sichuan lovage root (*Ligusticum wallichii* Franchet) and Parsnip root (*Pastinaca sativa* L.). Galbanum (*Ferula gummosa* Boissier, syn. *F. galbaniflua* Boiss. et Buhse) and Asafoetida (*Ferula asa-foetida* L.) are unique in this genus in being distilled from the oleoresin.

The seeds of carrot family plants are also high in essential oil; many of these are distilled for various industrial and therapeutic purposes, including Angelica seed, Fennel seed (sweet and bitter types), Aniseed, Coriander seed and leaf, Carrot seed and the seeds of Cumin, Celery, Parsley, Caraway, Dill and Khella (see below and Fennel for profiles).

## Therapeutic Functions and Indications

### SPECIFIC SYMPTOMATOLOGY – *All applications*

Disconnection, mental scatteredness, delusions, spells of anxiety and fearfulness, loss of willpower and motivation, discouragement, poor perseverance, inability to finish projects, poor decision making, nervous tension, insomnia, appetite loss, chronic indigestion with bloating, flatulence, abdominal pain, alternating constipation and diarrhoea, chronic respiratory infections, cough with productive phlegm, wheezing, painful scanty periods, absent periods, chronic muscle aches and pains, all symptoms worsen with stress

## PSYCHOLOGICAL – *Aromatic diffusion, external applications*

**Essential PNEI function and indication:** Stimulant in weakness and regulating in dysregulation conditions

**Possible brain dynamics:** Increases basal ganglia functioning

**Fragrance category:** Middle tone with woody, rooty and pungent notes

**Indicated psychological disorders:** ADD, dissociative disorders, minor depression, psychotic and schizoid conditions

### STABILIZES THE MIND AND PROMOTES INTEGRATION

- Mental instability, anxiety, fearfulness
- Disconnection, scatteredness, spaciness, oversensitivity, dissociation
- Euphoria, delusion, paranoia, agitation
- Thinking-instinct disconnection

### PROMOTES WILLPOWER AND PERSEVERANCE

- Low willpower or strength, indecisiveness
- Discouragement, low perseverance
- Mental and emotional burnout

## PHYSIOLOGICAL – *Nebulizer inhalation, gel cap, suppository, pessary, external applications*

**Therapeutic status:** Mild remedy with no cumulative toxicity

**Topical safety status:** Non-irritant, non-sensitizing; extremely photosensitizing

**Tropism:** Nervous, endocrine, reproductive, respiratory, digestive, urinary musculoskeletal systems

**Essential diagnostic function:** Restores weak/hypotonic and relaxes hypertonic/tense terrain conditions

### PRIMARILY REGULATING AND RESTORATIVE:

*autonomic nervous (PNS/SNS) regulator:* ANS dysregulation with digestive and mood disorders; alternating constipation and diarrhoea, migraine, palpitations, menopausal syndrome, hyperthyroid syndrome

*adrenal regulator:* adrenocortical dysregulation with energy swings

*nervous and cerebral restorative:* nervous exhaustion, burnout or breakdown; neurasthenia, convalescence, incl. postpartum

PRIMARILY RELAXANT:

*nervous and cerebral sedative, mild hypnotic:* chronic hypertonic/tense and cold/atonic conditions; chronic stress-related conditions in general, incl. anxiety states, insomnia, vertigo, ADD, ADHD

*uterine relaxant, spasmolytic:* spamodic dysmenorrhoea

*strong digestive/gastrointestinal relaxant, spasmolytic, analgesic, carminative:* spasmodic digestive conditions, esp. with indigestion, bloating, flatulence; colic, spasmodic IBS

*respiratory relaxant, antitussive:* spasmodic cough and dyspnoea, asthma

*analgesic:* musculoskeletal pain, sciatica, precordial pain, menstrual pain, urinary pain; headache, incl. migraine; toothache

*anticoagulant:* thrombosis, other clotting disorders

*antitoxic:* poisoning from food, toxic herbs, alcohol

PRIMARILY STIMULANT:

*uterine stimulant, emmenagogue:* amenorrhoea, oligomenorrhoea, failure to progress during labour, placental retention

*strong digestive/gastrointestinal stimulant:* atonic digestive conditions, incl. chronic gastroenteritis, chronic colitis, atonic-type peptic ulcer, anorexia

*respiratory stimulant, mucolytic expectorant:* chronic congestive bronchitis, dyspnoea

*neuromuscular stimulant, antirheumatic, analgesic:* rheumatic and arthritic disorders

*detoxicant diuretic:* anuria, metabolic toxicosis, rheumatic conditions, gout

ANTIMICROBIAL ACTIONS:

*anti-infective, leukocyte immune stimulant:* respiratory infections (incl. colds and flus), urinary infections

*antibacterial:* typhus, diphtheria, cholera, flu, bronchitis, malaria, psoriasis

*antifungal:* skin fungal infections, fungal intestinal dysbiosis, candidiasis

SYNERGISTIC COMBINATIONS

- Angelica root + Rosemary + Cajeput: strong digestive and respiratory stimulant-spasmolytic and antimicrobial in atonic digestive and respiratory conditions of many kinds, esp. with chronic indigestion, bloating, colic, IBS; in chronic bronchitis and asthma

- Angelica root + Siberian fir: stimulant expectorant and antitussive for chonic bronchitis, bronchial asthma, chronic cough

COMPLEMENTARY COMBINATIONS

- Angelica root + Bergamot + Lavender: autonomic nervous regulator for autonomic dysregulation with chronic digestive and mood disorders; alternating constipation and diarrhoea, menopausal syndrome

- Angelica root + Clary sage/Lavender: strong nervous and cerebral sedative in chronic stress-related conditions, esp. chronic anxiety, insomnia, neurasthenia

- Angelica root + Green myrtle/Petitgrain bigarade/Lavender: cerebral sedative and restorative for chronic mental fatigue, neurasthenia, nervous burnout or breakdown, ADD, convalescence

- Angelica root + Roman camomile/Laurel: strong spasmolytic and analgesic digestive relaxant in chronic spasmodic, painful digestive conditions, esp. with colitis, IBS, bloating, diarrhoea

- Angelica root + Cardamom/Fennel: digestive stimulant, carminative and aperitive for digestive atony with appetite loss, indigestion, flatulence, anorexia

- Angelica root + Juniper berry: emmenagogue for amenorrhoea, oligo-menorrhoea, long cycles

- Angelica root + Juniper berry: neuromuscular stimulant, detoxicant diuretic, antirheumatic in rheumatic and arthritic conditions, metabolic toxicosis, gout

## TOPICAL – *Liniment, ointment, cream, compress and other cosmetic*

**Skin care:** Pale, cold skin types

*tissue stimulant, rubefacient:* lifeless/cold/atonic/puffy skin

*antipsoratic:* psoriasis

**Therapeutic precautions:** Angelica root oil is a systemic warming, drying stimulant that is contraindicated in hypersthenic/hot and dry conditions, including fever, acute inflammation and dry respiratory conditions in general. Being a uterine stimulant, the oil is also contraindicated throughout pregnancy. Note also the dose-dependent action on the nervous system when absorbed internally (see below).

**Pharmacological precautions:** Angelica root oil creates skin photosensitivity and the potential for sunburn because of its content in furanocoumarins; therefore, topical use should be avoided before exposing the skin to the sun or UV light, including sunbathing. The oil is best avoided in babies and infants because of its content in monoterpenes and 1,8 cineole. It is also reported contraindicated in diabetes.

**Preparations:**

- Diffusor: 1–3 drops in water

- Massage oil: 2–3% dilution in vegetable oil

- Liniment: 2–4% dilution in vegetable oil after doing a patch test

- Gel cap: 1–2 drops with some olive oil. The small and less frequent dose is regulating and restorative on the nervous system; while the larger or more frequent dose is more sedative.

## Chinese Medicine Functions and Indications

**Aroma energy:** Pungent, woody, rooty

**Movement:** Circulating

**Warmth:** Neutral to warm

**Meridian tropism:** Liver, Stomach, Spleen, Lung

**Five-Element affinity:** Earth, Metal

**Essential function:** To activate the Qi, harmonize the Middle Warmer and calm the Shen

1. **Activates the Qi, relaxes constraint, calms the Shen and relieves pain**

   - **Qi constraint with Shen agitation**, with chronic nervous tension, insomnia, anxiety, digestive symptoms worse with stress:

     Bergamot/Lavender/Mandarin/Marjoram

   - **Liver-Spleen disharmony with Shen dysregulation**, with abdominal bloating and pain, flatulence, diarrhoea, feeling stressed, anxiousness:

     Bergamot/Yarrow/Cardamom/German camomile

   - **Qi constraint with pain**, incl. muscle, joint or nerve pain; headache, toothache, abdominal pain, chest pain

     Lavender/Roman camomile/Marjoram

2. **Warms and harmonizes the Middle Warmer, breaks up stagnation, regulates digestion and relieves pain**

- **Stomach-Spleen empty-cold** with flatulence, colic, abdominal bloating and pain, diarrhoea:

  Rosemary/Nutmeg/Ginger/Cajeput

- **Stomach-Spleen Qi stagnation** with indigestion, bloating, appetite loss, nausea, alternating constipation and diarrhoea:

  Spearmint/Peppermint/Cardamom/Fennel

3. **Warms and activates the Lower Warmer, reduces stagnation and promotes menstruation**

- **Lower Warmer Qi and Blood stagnation with internal cold**, with delayed, scanty or absent periods, painful periods, vaginal discharges, urinary irritation:

  Rosemary/Fennel/Juniper berry/Ginger

4. **Warms the Lung, diffuses Lung Qi, expels phlegm and relieves coughing**

- **Lung phlegm cold/damp** with chronic cough, sputum expectoration, chest distension, difficult breathing:

  Cajeput/Grand fir/Green myrtle/Cardamom

REMARKS

The genus *Angelica* is one of the few aromatic plants that originate in temperate and subarctic regions ranging from Lapland, Greenland and Iceland to Scandinavia, Siberia and the Russian Far East. From the 10th century onwards the European angelica was especially a favourite cooking spice (the seed) and spring vegetable (the tender leaves) in Scandinavian countries. In the 1300s, the root became extremely popular in monastic medicine in Central Europe and predictably found its way into medicinal liqueurs such as Chartreuse, Bénédictine and Eau de Carmes, and later even some gins. Angelica root and stem candied in brown sugar also became much-loved sweets. The 14th century saw the aromatic water appear, followed by the essential oil in the second half of the 16th century – as recorded in the notable herbal dispensatory of 1589, the *Dispensatorium Noricum*.

It is hard for us today to justify, let alone imagine, the stellar reputation that Angelica root enjoyed in those days. It became the supreme panacea, the magical remedy of the Holy Ghost, one might say the European ginseng. It was prepared in numerous ways and relied on for treating a large variety of conditions, much like the herb Yarrow. In modern times, and especially with the clinical exploration of the tincture and the essential oil, Angelica root's systemic physiological functions have become much clearer. They do go some way to justifying its traditional repute. Equally, they also make us wonder about the relatively minor clinical use to which the oil is put today.

Moreover, it is important to consider the clear differences between the use of Angelica root in alcoholic tincture and in essential oil form; the two preparations should always be considered separately. The tincture is more *stimulating*, *bitter* and *dispersing*, with a greater effect on the lungs, the exterior and the upper body; its bitter constituents also create a better focus for atonic digestion in general. The essential oil is more *sedating* and *regulating*, with a stronger tropism for nervous and reproductive functions, for the interior and the lower trunk; its digestive activity is on the whole more *relaxant* and *analgesic*.

Combining different constituents and actions into a complex remedy, Angelica oil is essentially both a relaxant and a stimulant with an underlying neuroendocrine regulating action. From the functional medicine perspective, it addesses **tense, weak and cold terrain**. It is almost unique in treating this particular combination of conditions. The theme that Angelica root clearly lays out is the balancing of opposites. Its tropism too expresses a polarity dance, namely between the brain and nervous functions above, and metabolic and reproductive functions below. On the brain and nervous system specifically, the oil acts both as a restorative and sedative, like the paradoxical action of Rhodiola. It excels at relieving chronic forms of anxiety and insomnia, as well as nervous exhaustion or breakdown from any cause. In balancing opposite functions, Angelica root also serves as one of the rare ANS and adrenocortical regulators for treating autonomic nervous dysregulation. It is best used for long-term dysregulation of the terrain resulting from chronic tension, weakness and cold combined, with their wide arc of symptoms.

Curious, observant practitioners in the past were not slow in realizing that the plant itself exhibits a strong structural and functional polarity. Angelica is all umbels and seeds above and deep roots below. It soaks up sunlight from above (by developing coumarins right down to its roots) and rich, humid mineral earth from below. Likewise, in its fragrance, Angelica exudes fresh, peppery top notes from its phellandrene content and musty, earthy base notes from its lactones. Light and dark, dry and damp, fresh and musty, Air and Earth, Angelica is the very emblem of the polarity and interplay between cerebral and metabolic functions.

Angelica root does have a strong tropism for the reproductive organs in both relaxant and stimulant mode, and is excellent for both spasmodic dysmenorrhoea and amenorrhoea; it is also a classic European midwife's remedy for stalled labour and placental retention. Spasmodic and chronic atonic, stagnant conditions of the lower digestive tract will also benefit with the right delivery methods for this oil, again especially with systemic tension and weakness present. Abdominal colic and pain are key indications here because of the oil's additional analgesic effect. Angelica root is a good remedy for pain and is strong enough to relieve many types of pain, including neuromuscular pain, headaches, toothache and precordial pain. In the respiratory tract, Angelica root operates in similar twin relaxant–stimulant mode and is a good choice for chronic spasmodic and/or congestive bronchitis with breathing difficulty and productive cough.

In terms of infections, Angelica root is particularly antifungal because of its umbelliferone content; coumarins are generally beneficial in skin conditions such as psoriasis and vitiligo.

When used by gentle olfaction, Angelica root again expresses the theme of balancing cerebral and metabolic functions in their psychic aspect. While its fresh, pungent notes target conscious mental functions, its rooty, woody notes have a tropism for subconscious instinctive functions. By stabilizing mental functions and boosting instinctive ones, the complex fragrance has the rare ability to integrate opposite poles of the psyche. The effect is both one of rekindling the powers of will and courage, and bringing the flights of the mind down to earth, down to a grounded centre.

Like just one or two other oils with woody, rooty notes, Angelica root is for the person who has been discouraged by setbacks and finds it difficult to justify mustering any further effort of will or perseverance to continue his or her aims; for the person who has finally become resigned to accepting failure or putting up with an unsatisfactory situation. This condition could also result from burnout from overwork, and from chronic illness, trauma or drug abuse.

**Related oils:** Several other oils in the carrot family have similar but distinct uses.

**Angelica seed** oil has a fresh, pungent, herbaceous fragrance and is used in a similar but very limited way in comparison to the root oil. Its profile of constituents is also very similar, headed by β-phellandrene at 35–72%. Small doses are used for its *restorative* properties (see above), while larger doses are more *nervous sedative* and *spasmolytic*, and are mainly given for stress-related digestive conditions and anxiety states. Angelica seed is a mild, non-toxic remedy, and non-irritant and non-photosensitizing when applied topically.

**Lovage root** (*Ligusticum levisticum*) is the steam-distilled oil from the garden plant and displays a deep sweet-root fragance with smooth oily notes. It has enjoyed use as a culinary and important medicinal plant since ancient times and was first distilled as an aromatic remedy in central Europe during the 1550s. Its chemical profile is dominated by a mix of phthalides (50–55%, incl. ligustilide) with lesser amounts of monoterpenes (<25%), sesquiterpenes (<10%), monoterpenols (<8%) and coumarins (<4%). Lovage root has mild therapeutic status and is non-irritant and non-sensitizing to the skin.

As a physiological remedy, Lovage root oil is used in a similar way to the tincture, as essentially a restorative and stimulant in hypotonic/weak and congestive/damp conditions. It is a good nervous restorative in chronic neurasthenia with fatigue or debility, and a smooth muscle restorative for smooth-muscle atony, especially in the digestive and urinary tract, and the uterus. The oil is a toner for bladder-muscle weakness presenting as frequent scanty urination, gastrointestinal weakness with indigestion, flatulence, bloating and dull epigastric pain, as in chronic gastritis; and uterine weakness with chronic scanty, absent or difficult periods.

French practitioners in particular value Lovage root highly in liver and biliary congestion with chronic toxin accumulation because of its liver-gallbladder decongestant, liver protective and detoxicant action. The oil would help phase-II detoxification of nutrients while protecting the liver from chemical insult. In tandem, Lovage root is also a good diuretic for water retention and chronic nephrosis and therefore a good all-round remedy for metabolic toxicosis in general – also considered a damp type of condition. As a systemic detoxicant, the oil is also excellent for skin eruptions, and psoriasis in particular. It has also proven very effective for acute poisoning from chemicals and drugs, as an antitoxic. It is moderately antibacterial, antifungal and antiparasitic.

Lovage root also comes with a long history of use by past European midwives and wise women practitioners of all kinds, including Trotula of Salerno and Hildegard von Bingen, as both a menstrual and obstetrical remedy (Holmes 2007). Like Angelica root oil, Lovage root is an emmenagogue, useful for amenorrhoea and scanty periods but also failure to progress during labour due to hypotonic contractions, and postpartum placental retention. This makes Lovage contraindicated during the main part of pregnancy but useful for priming the uterus for labour starting one or two weeks before the due date. The oil, like the tincture, may also be used to promote or restart labour until contractions resume. Standard dilutions and doses apply. Because of its content in coumarins, sun exposure should be avoided for 12 hours after application.

**Sichuan lovage root** (*Ligusticum wallichii*) from China is also available; the oil is extracted from a root that is much used in Chinese herbal medicine worldwide. Its fragrance is moderately spicy and herbaceous, with warm, fresh and oily notes also found in Celery seed, and some minor rooty notes. Like the closely related Lovage root, its chemical profile is dominated by a mix of phthalides, including ligustilide (20–58%) and butylidene phthalide (<1%); monoterpenes (<29%), including β-phellandrene and trans-ocimene (both c. 11%); a cluster of sesquiterpenes (<20%), including muurolene (c. 5%), caryophyllene, elemene, patchoulene and selinene (each c. 2%); a few monoterpenols, including lavandulol (4%); and the phenolic ether isomyristicin (2%). Sichuan lovage root is a mild remedy with no cumulative toxicity and is non-irritant or sensitizing to the skin.

Because this oil has only been produced very recently, no documented experience on its clinical use is available. However, the decoction of the whole root in Chinese herbal medicine has long-established therapeutic functions and indications, and the tincture extract has shown further applications (Holmes 1999). Nevertheless, in addition to the essential oil, the root does contain alkaloids, notably the alkaloid tetramethylpyrazine (aka ligustrazine, also found in the cacao fruit and therefore chocolate), which has shown a slew of actions that include anti-inflammatory, hypotensive and neuroprotective ones that clearly contribute to the remedy's overall action. With that reservation in mind, it is probable that Sichuan lovage root oil still does embody at least some of the actions of the tincture, while most likely also giving them a particular twist that differentiates it from the tincture (as is usual with essential oils).

Sichaun lovage root in tincture form is essentially a relaxant remedy to the nervous, cardiovascular and reproductive systems, with a secondary stimulant effect on the uterus. Its nervous sedative and analgesic action is used mainly for pain conditions of many kinds, especially headaches (tension and vascular) and abdominal, arthritic and rheumatic pain. The tincture is a good coronary, cerebral and systemic vasodilator with a variety of clinical applications. In addition to use for dysmenorrhoea, it is also an important uterine stimulant for treating amenorrhoea and uterine dystocia (tense-type) and placental retention. Sichuan lovage root oil is essentially a mild remedy with extremely little cumulative toxicity, despite the minor presence of isomyristicin. Still, caution is advisable with internal use in those taking the drugs MAOIs, SSRIs and pethidine. Moderate standard dilutions and doses apply.

**Dong quai** (*Angelica sinensis*) from China is steam distilled from the root of the important Chinese medicinal plant. Its odour is sweet, woody with smoky, rooty undertones. Its profile of constituents is similar to that of the two lovages above, with phthalides, including ligustilide (c. 45%), cnidilide and butylidene phthalide; monoterpenes (including p-cymene), smaller levels of sesquiterpenes, sesquiterpenols and coumarins (incl. bergapten, scopoletin and umbelliferone), and very small amounts of the phenol carvacrol and the ether safrole. Dong quai oil has mild therapeutic status and is non-irritant and non-sensitizing to the skin.

Because Dong quai oil has only been produced very recently, no documented experience on its clinical use is available. However, the decoction of the whole root in Chinese herbal medicine has long-established therapeutic functions and indications, and the tincture extract has shown further applications (Holmes 1997). However, in addition to the essential oil, the root does contain other key constituents such as ferulic acid and various phytosterols, whose activity has been well documented by Chao and Lin (2011). Nevertheless, in view of the oil's content in key active constituents, it is likely to act on its own as a *smooth-muscle relaxant* in the circulatory, respiratory, gastrointestinal and reproductive systems, addressing mainly **tense (hypertonic) conditions**, as well as possessing good *nervous sedative*, *neuroprotective*, *anti-inflammatory* and *anti-carcinogenic actions*. Like Sichuan lovage, Dong quai oil will also act as a good *coronary*, *cerebral* and *systemic vasodilator* with a variety of clinical applications. Dong quai oil is essentially a mild remedy with extremely little cumulative toxicity, despite the minor presence of carvacrol. However, because of its content in bergapten, topical application of Dong quai oil should be followed by avoiding exposure to the sun or tanning beds for at least 12 hours. Moderate standard dilutions and doses apply.

As a psychological remedy, Dong quai root oil has a pronounced grounding, centring effect that will be useful for treating mental and emotional instability and scatteredness, and for helping reconnect dissociated thoughts and ideas with an individual's physical body, especially with their senses. The oil is also psychologically supportive and nurturing without being smothering and would help with emotional loss and grief.

**Galbanum** (*Ferula gummosa*) from Iran, Afghanistan and Northwest India is steam distilled from the aromatic oleoresin that is obtained by incision from the herb's trunk. With an intense green, somewhat balsamic-fresh-pungent odour, its constituents include monoterpenes <85% (incl. α-pinene 45–50%, δ-3-carene 10–20%, l-limonene), phthalides, sulphuric aliphatic derivates, pyrazines, furanic compounds, esters, sesquiterpenes and coumarins (incl. umbelliferone, galbanic acid, gummosine). The commercial oil is sometimes adulterated with cheap oils high in monoterpenes such as Scotch pine and Rosemary. Galbanum is a mild remedy with no cumulative toxicity and is non-irritant or sensitizing to the skin.

Galbanum is an aromatic remedy whose medicinal, religious and perfumery applications go back to all known cultures of the Central and West Asia. It had the highest status among the resins, being known as the sacred mother resin in relation to frankincense, myrrh and other resins. In Hebraic culture, Galbanum was an important ingredient in sacred incense, along with myrrh and frankincense. In ancient Egypt it was a valuable resin and key component of 'green incense'.

Physiologically, Galbanum is essentially a warming stimulant remedy by nature that addresses hyposthenic/weak, atonic/cold and congestive/damp conditions. As a remedy, its main tropisms are respiratory, urinary, reproductive and musculoskeletal functions. As a stimulant mucolytic expectorant with a good anti-infective and antiseptic action, Galbanum treats chronic bronchial infections with copious phlegm, dyspnoea, wheezing and coughing. As a detoxicant diuretic, the oil treats scanty, irritated or mucousy urination, arthritic disorders and water retention. Galbanum is an emmenagogue and a strong spasmolytic analgesic for amenorrhoea or scanty, painful periods with long cycles. Its action in the upper digestive tract is again stimulant, spasmolytic and analgesic, being indicated for gastric atony with cramping pain and bloating.

Paradoxically, Galbanum is also said to balance and calm neuroendocrine functions and has been used as such in the French tradition to calm anxiety, reduce pituitary hyperfunctioning and treat menopausal hot flushes (Dupont 2002). It was much used in earlier days for 'female hysteria'.

The oil also exerts an astringent mucostatic effect on the mucosa similar to Myrrh that will benefit damp, congestive conditions (including infectious ones) such as vaginitis with leucorrhoea, blennorrhoea, mucousy stool and other discharges. Its valuable topical applications include tissue regeneration and antisepsis for wounds, sores and ulcers, and maturation for boils, abscesses and furuncles. Caution with sun exposure is in order for 12 hours after application because of its coumarin content. Galbanum is contraindicated during pregnancy and in babies and children. Moderate standard dilutions and doses apply.

**Asafoetida** (*Ferula asa-foetida*), Hing in Hindi, is also from Iran and Afghanistan. Like Galbanum, the oil is steam distilled from the dark red, aromatic oleoresin that is obtained by incision from the whole plant, herb and root. The light orange to brown oil has an intense sulphuric-pungent odour caused by aliphatic sulphur compounds, notably butylpropenyl disulfide and other propenyl di- and tri-sulfides (18–88%); small amounts of monoterpenes and ferulic and valeric acid are also found. Asafoetida is an ancient and important aromatic remedy and spice much used in Ayurveda and traditional Greek medicine, and is well described by medieval practitioners such as Ibn Baitar (Al Andalus) and Platearius (Italy). Asafoetida oil is a mild remedy with no cumulative toxicity but may be irritant and sensitizing to the skin in some because of its high content of sulphur compounds.

Asafoetida is essentially a *warming stimulant* and *relaxant* that addresses a mix of hypotonic/weak, hyposthenic/cold and hypertonic/tense conditions. Working as a digestive stimulant–relaxant, its strong spasmolytic and carminative action treats flatulence, colic, IBS and colitis. It is also used as an effective anthelmintic for roundworms and is reputed to be a liver stimulant and decongestant, as well as diuretic, emmenagogue and aphrodisiac. For respiratory functions, Asafoetida is a good pungent mucolytic expectorant, antitussive and bronchospasmolytic for bronchitis, asthma and spasmodic cough and dyspnoea conditions such as whooping cough and croup. Asafoetida also exerts a relaxant action on cardiovascular and neuromuscular functions, where it can treat palpitations, tachycardia, muscle cramps and spasms, convulsions, including in children, and hemiplegia and facial palsy. Exercise caution with topical use (see above). Moderate standard dilutions and doses apply.

# Basil ct. Methylchavicol

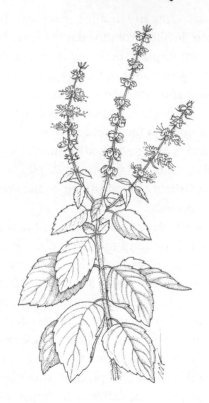

**Botanical source:** The herb of *Ocimum basilicum* L. ct. methylchavicol (Lamiaceae/ Labiatae – lipflower family), an extensively cultivated herb of subtropical and Mediterranean regions

**Other names:** Tropical basil, Exotic basil, Comoran basil, Thai basil; Basilic exotique (Fr), Basilikum (Ge), Basilico (It), Albahaca (Sp), Basilikon (Gr)

**Appearance:** A mobile pale viridian liquid with a warm, sweet, herbaceous odour with a somewhat fresh-camphoraceous, anisic top note

**Perfumery status:** A heart note of high intensity and poor persistence

**Extraction:** Steam distillation of the fresh herb in flower, usually January to June

**1 kg oil yield from:** 600–1,000 kg of the fresh herb (a very poor yield)

**Production areas:** India (native), Vietnam, Egypt, Comores, Madagascar, Réunion

**Typical constituents:** Phenolic ethers 72–90% (incl. methylchavicol [estragole] 68–87%, methyleugenol 1–3%) • oxides 2–6% (incl. 1,8 cineole, trans-ocimene oxide) • monoterpenols (incl. linalool <9%, fenchol, terpinene, terpineol, citronellol)

• sesquiterpenes (incl. β-caryophyllene <4%) • monoterpenes (limonene <3%, terpenen-4-ol <2%, β-ocimene <2%) • esters (incl. linalyl/fenchyl/bornyl acetate) • ketones 1% (3-octanone, camphor) • aldehydes 1% • monoterpenols 1% • phenols (incl. eugenol trace – 1%)

**Chance of adulteration:** Moderate, often with synthetic highlights. The more expensive Sweet basil oil is more likely to be reconstituted from this cheaper Tropical basil with synthetic linalool added.

**Related oils:** Like the Thymus, Salvia and Artemisia genera, the basil or *Ocimum* genus is highly polymorphic and expresses about 160 different species, cultivars (varieties), formas and chemotypes. Their pharmacognosical profiles represent countless variations on the proportions of five key constituents: methylchavicol, methyleugenol, eugenol, linalool and camphor. The main kinds of Basil oil currently available may be conveniently organized by their chemical dominance as follows. However, note that Basil oils rarely express a singular chemical dominance, and instead usually a plural dominance of primary and secondary constituents; these express a kaleidoscope of creative combinations among these five key constituents.

1.  **Fresh-herbaceous basil oil with methylchavicol dominant**

    • Basil ct. methylchavicol (*Ocimum basilicum* L. ct. methylchavicol), commonly known as Tropical, Exotic or Comoran basil (this profile)

2.  **Sweet-herbaceous basil oils with linalool dominant**

    • Sweet or French basil (*Ocimum basilicum* L. ct. linalool), with its characteristic intensely sweet-herbaceous fragrance, with a linalool content of 40–69% and relatively low levels of eugenol (9–15%) and methylchavicol

    • Hoary basil (*Ocimum canum* Sims ct. linalool), moderately sweet-herbaceous, containing 60–90% linalool

3.  **Spicy-herbaceous basil oils with eugenol dominant**

    • Large-leaf or Lettuce-leaf basil (*Ocimum basilicum* L. ct. eugenol), Grand basilic or Grand vert in French, high in methyleugenol (55–60%) and up to 25% methylchavicol

    • Bush basil (*Ocimum basilicum* L. var. minimum ct. eugenol), Petit basilic in French, high in methyleugenol (<60%) and up to 23% methylchavicol

    • Holy basil or Tulsi (*Ocimum sanctum* L. ct. eugenol, syn. *O. tenuifolium* L. ct. eugenol) from India and Malaysia, deeply herbaceous and somewhat sweet and spicy, with a 35–67% eugenol content. This species also yields methyleugenol and methylchavicol chemotypes.

- Tree basil, Clove basil or African basil (*Ocimum gratissimum* L. ct. eugenol) from India and Madagascar, also known as Wild basil in Hawaii, with a eugenol content of up to 85%. A further five chemotypes of Tree basil are reported: ct. thymol, ct. citral, ct. geraniol, ct. linalool and ct. methyl cinnamate. Most of these are rarely available, however.

4. **Fresh-camphoraceous basil oils with camphor dominant**

- Hoary basil (*Ocimum canum/americanum* Sims ct. camphor), containing up to 60% camphor. This is another chemotype of this species, which also expresses further chemotypes: ct. citral, also called Lemon basil, and ct. methylcinnamate.

- African blue basil (*O. kilimandscharicum x basilicum* Guerke)

In terms of clinical use, all these basil oils share many common functions and uses; however, the dominant chemotype will emphasize particular therapeutic usage for physiological or psychological conditions (see below).

## Therapeutic Functions and Indications

SPECIFIC SYMPTOMATOLOGY – *All applications*

Anxiety, worry, anxious depression, feeling chronically tired and stressed-out, sleeping difficulties, mood swings, emotional outbursts, chronic indigestion with pain and bloating, irregular stool, right subcostal pain, asthmatic breathing, spasmodic cough, urinary irritation, varicose veins, heavy legs, heavy periods with premenstrual bearing-down pains

PSYCHOLOGICAL – *Aromatic diffusion, whole-body massage*

**Essential PNEI function and indication:** Regulating in dysregulated conditions; stimulant in weakness conditions

**Possible brain dynamics:** Reduces deep limbic system hyperfunctioning

**Fragrance category:** Middle tone with sweet, green, pungent notes

**Indicated psychological disorders:** Bipolar disorder, ADD

PROMOTES EMOTIONAL RENEWAL AND CLARITY

- All pathogenic (stuck) emotions and distressed feelings in general, esp. anger

- Emotional confusion and illusion with conflict; emotional dependency

- Lethargy, drowsiness

- Mental illusions, confusion, disorientation

- Negative thinking, pessimism, depression

## PHYSIOLOGICAL – *Nebulizer inhalation, gel cap, suppository, external applications*

**Therapeutic status:** Mild remedy with no cumulative toxicity

**Topical safety status:** Mild skin irritant, non-sensitizing, non-photosensitizing

**Tropism:** Nervous, respiratory, digestive, reproductive, musculoskeletal, venous circulatory systems

**Essential diagnostic function:** Relaxes hypertonic/tense and decongests damp/congestive terrain conditions

PRIMARILY RELAXANT:

*systemic nervous relaxant, SNS inhibitor, vagotonic:* hypertonic/tense conditions with nervous tension; acute stress-related conditions in general

*strong spasmolytic and analgesic, moderate anti-inflammatory:* a large range of acute spasmodic and inflammatory conditions with pain, esp. of smooth muscles; acute and chronic pain conditions, tension headaches

- *cerebral sedative, hypnotic:* anxiety, insomnia, travel sickness, vertigo

- *strong gastrointestinal relaxant and regulator, also carminative, antiemetic:* spasmodic neurogenic digestive conditions with pain, incl. nervous indigestion, gastritis, enteritis, colic, spasmodic IBS, aerophagia; gastric pain from ulcers, hyperacidity; severe flatulence, nausea, vomiting

- *respiratory relaxant (broncho-spasmolytic/-dilatant), antitussive:* spasmodic or nervous dyspnoea, cough and dysphonia; spasmodic asthma and bronchitis, whooping cough

- *neuromuscular relaxant, also anticonvulsant:* muscle spasms and pain, neuralgia, incl. neuritis, sciatica, tendinitis; fibromyalgia, rheumatoid arthritis, gout, arteriosclerosis; seizures, dizziness, vertigo

*moderate antiallergic:* type-I allergies, incl. allergic asthma, dermatitis, colitis, duodenitis, gastritis, cholecystitis, prostatitis

PRIMARILY DECONGESTANT:

*moderate pelvic/uterine/prostate decongestant:* pelvic congestion with congestive dysmenorrhoea, haemorrhoids, prostate congestion, prostatitis, BPH

*moderate venous decongestant:* venous deficiency/congestion with varicose veins; phlebitis

*liver decongestant, cholagogue:* liver-gallbladder congestion with upper digestive indigestion, painful indigestion; liver disease

*gastrointestinal and pancreatic stimulant, carminative:* gastrointestinal and pancreatic enzyme deficiencies with severe indigestion, flatulence, bloating, pain

PRIMARILY RESTORATIVE:

*nervous and cerebral restorative, antidepressant:* chronic neurasthenia with physical and mental fatigue, depression, nervous breakdown; incl. from chronic disease or fever, in convalescence; MS and other neurodegenerative disorders

ANTIMICROBIAL ACTIONS:

*strong antiviral:* a wide range of viral infections, incl. hepatitis, croup, pleurisy, influenza, dengue fever, malaria; shingles, herpes, neuritis, encephalitis, MS, poliomyelitis

*antibacterial:* gastroenteritis, yellow fever, acute and chronic urinary infections

*antifungal:* fungal conditions, esp. with Aspergillus spp., Fusarium, Candida insecticidal: mosquitoes, flies and other insects

SYNERGISTIC COMBINATIONS

- Basil ct. methylchavicol + Fennel/Tarragon: strong gastrointestinal stimulant, relaxant and spasmolytic for upper and lower nervous digestive conditions with indigestion, colic, pain, incl. IBS

- Basil ct. methylchavicol + Tarragon: strong antiviral, analgesic and spasmolytic for viral infections in general, especially involving acute pain and spasm (e.g. croup, influenza, dengue fever, neuritis, etc.)

COMPLEMENTARY COMBINATIONS

- Basil ct. methylchavicol + Lavender/Petitgrain bigarade: nervous relaxant and cerebral restorative for chronic anxiety, insomnia and stress-related conditions in general

- Basil ct. methylchavicol + Palmarosa/Clary sage: nervous restorative for chronic neurasthenia with debility, nervous breakdown, burnout, depression

- Basil ct. methylchavicol + Peppermint: cerebral regulator for dizziness, vertigo, travel sickness, headaches; also strong antiviral in general

- Basil ct. methylchavicol + Peppermint/Fennel: strong gastrointestinal spasmolytic, stimulant and carminative for upper and lower indigestion with pain, flatulence, colic

- Basil ct. methylchavicol + Marjoram/Lemongrass: strong spasmolytic, anti-inflammtory muscle-relaxant in a wide range of spasmodic, inflammatory neuromuscular conditions with pain

- Basil ct. methylchavicol + Vetiver + Lemon eucalyptus: anti-inflammatory, analgesic for rheumatoid arthritis

- Basil ct. methylchavicol + Siberian fir/Hyssop: bronchodilator and antitussive for asthma, spasmodic dyspnoea and cough

- Basil ct. methylchavicol + Cypress: venous decongestant and anti-inflammatory for venous fatigue with varicose veins, phlebitis, ankle oedema

- Basil ct. methylchavicol + Geranium: pelvic decongestant for congestive dysmenorrhoea, haemorrhoids

- Basil ct. methylchavicol + Niaouli + Black spruce: prostate decongestant in BPH, prostatitis

- Basil ct. methylchavicol + Tea tree + Sage: antiviral for viral infections, esp. from chronic debility

TOPICAL – *Liminent, ointment, cream, compress and other cosmetic preparations*

**Skin care:** Not used

*antiseptic, anti-inflammatory, analgesic:* insect bites, boils, furuncles, abscesses, acne, eczema; muscle, sinew and joint pain of all kinds

*antiviral:* herpes (most types), warts, incl. Molluscum contagiosum (water warts) insect-repellent

**Therapeutic precautions:** Basil ct. methylchavicol oil is contraindicated in weak conditions or terrain without additional tension present causing symptoms of stagnation, such as spasm, inflammation and pain. However, it is equally effective in acute tense and chronic tense-weak terrain.

**Pharmacological precautions:** Basil ct. methylchavicol is a mild skin irritant from its high methylchavicol content; the dilutions below should not be exceeded. The oil should be avoided internally during the first trimester and used with caution during the remainder of pregnancy and lactation. Internal use of Basil ct. methylchavicol should be cautious. Although there is a theoretical risk of its minor constituent methyleugenol acting as a carcinogen, no record of a carcinogenic risk is noted in French medicine and no related prohibition exists in French pharmacy regulations.

**Preparations:**

- Diffusor: 2–3 drops in water

- Massage oil: 0.5–1% dilution in vegetable oil

- Liniment: 1–4% dilution in vegetable oil for short-term use after doing a patch test

- Gel cap: 2–3 drops with some olive oil

## Chinese Medicine Functions and Indications

**Aroma energy:** Sweet, green, pungent

**Movement:** Circulating

**Warmth:** Neutral

**Meridian tropism:** Liver, Heart, Spleen, Stomach, Lung

**Five-Element affinity:** Wood, Earth, Metal

**Essential function:** To activate Qi and Blood, calm the Liver and calm the Shen

1. **Activates the Qi, relaxes constraint, calms the Shen and relieves pain**

   - **Qi constraint with Shen agitation**, with nervous tension, irritability, agitation, mood swings, insomnia:

     Bergamot/Lavender/Marjoram/Roman camomile

   - **Heart and Liver Qi constraint with Shen agitation**, with restlessness, insomnia, palpitations, irritability, mood swings, anxiety:

     Mandarin/German camomile/Ylang ylang no. 1

2. **Regulates the Qi, breaks up stagnation, harmonizes the Middle Warmer and relieves pain**

- **Liver-Spleen disharmony with Shen agitation**, with severe nervous indigestion, abdominal pain, bloating and flatulence, irregular stool, diarrhoea, acute stress, mood swings:

  Peppermint/German camomile/Blue tansy/Roman camomile

- **Stomach Qi stagnation (Liver-Stomach disharmony)** with indigestion on eating, appetite loss, epigastric bloating, nausea, belching, irregular stool:

  Bergamot/Fennel/Spearmint/Ginger

3. **Circulates and descends Lung Qi, relaxes the chest and relieves wheezing and coughing**

- **Lung Qi accumulation** with anxiety, wheezing, coughing, chest distension and pain:

  Lavender/Marjoram/Hyssop/Tarragon

4. **Calms the Liver, descends the Yang, extinguishes wind and relieves spasms**

- **Liver Yang rising** with headache, tinnitus, dizziness, vertigo, muscle tension:

  Clary sage/Lavender/Marjoram

- **Internal Liver wind** with tremors, muscle spasms, seizures:

  Vetiver/Roman camomile/Laurel

- **Wind-phlegm obstruction** with seizures with spasms, paralysis:

  Vetiver/Ylang ylang no. 1/Tarragon

5. **Invigorates the Blood in the Lower Warmer and lower limbs, reduces stagnation and relieves varicosis**

- **Lower Warmer Blood stagnation** with heavy, painful clotted periods, headaches:

  Yarrow/Clary sage/Geranium

- **Blood stagnation in the lower limbs** with varicose veins, ankle oedema, fatigue:

  Cypress/Rosemary/Atlas cedarwood

REMARKS

Varieties of basil seen worldwide are used as both culinary herb and herbal medicine, starting with ancient Egypt and India, through to the Graeco-Roman era. Alexander the Great is said to have brought basil back to Greece from his Asian campaigns and thereby introduced the herb to the West. Basil has always enjoyed many historical associations with power and wealth – an interesting theme. Dedicated in India to the Hindu god Krishna, basil is called *Basilikon* in Greek, 'the royal herb', based on the root word *basileos*, 'king'. In different cultures basil was variously an emblem of prosperity and good luck, a source of strength during periods of fasting and a spiritual ally to assist the dying in their onward journey. Orthodox Christian churches throughout Slavic countries place pots of basil by the altar and use the sprigs to sprinkle holy water. Whatever its many uses, basil is clearly esteemed as a potent plant and a powerful medicine for body and soul – always to be respected and, if possible, harnessed for its potential healing power.

Brunschwygk's *Liber de Arte Distillandi Simplicibus* of 1500 mentions the steam-distilled Sweet basil oil that appeared in 15th-century Europe. In contrast, the tropical variety has been cultivated for its essential oil in Southeast Asia, India and the Indian Ocean islands only since the early 20th century. French colonial trading made Tropical basil very familiar to French culture and resulted in the oil being routinely used in both perfumery and medicine. In a clinical context, Tropical or Comoran basil oil is now officially known by its chemotype of methylchavicol. For treatment it is crucial to differentiate this particular oil from the other chemotypes of basil available. This is especially important as in commerce there is considerable confusion among the different types of Basil oil available.

Sweet herbaceous, and yet fresh, Basil methylchavicol, or Tropical basil for short, acts as a typical relaxant remedy for treating tense terrain. French practitioners consider it the number one oil for treating acute spasms and pain, wherever found. A good SNS inhibitor for acute stress-related conditions in general, Tropical basil is a systemic nervous and neuromuscular relaxant acting on both smooth and striped muscles. Its spasmolytic, analgesic and anti-inflammatory actions are equally appropriate for a large variety of painful spasmodic musculoskeletal, digestive and respiratory conditions. Methylchavicol, the oil's dominant constituent, is a lab-research-proven spasmolytic. For these conditions, the oil is as useful in topical preparations as for internal ones. It is especially widely applicable in the digestive tract, as it also exerts a stimulant effect on gastric and pancreatic enzymes – treating essentially weak, stagnant upper gut symptoms such as bloating and fullness on eating. Small wonder that the herb is a culinary favourite, especially in East Asian countries.

With its nervous and cerebral restorative effect, Tropical basil may equally be used in chronic tense conditions with additional symptoms of weakness present. The oil is a classic for depression and neurasthenia arising from long-term tense-weak terrain.

Tropical basil is also useful as a blood and fluid decongestant remedy for treating damp in the pelvis and legs. Venous congestion in the liver, pelvic basin, uterus and lower limbs will benefit, including the extremely common pelvic congestion in women, congestive dysmenorrhoea and male prostate congestion. Clinical experience has also shown this oil to be an excellent antiviral and is often given for a wide range of viral infections.

Tropical basil's uplifting fresh, pungent fragrance comes to psychological expression when used by gentle olfaction. With a sharp vitality, the oil cuts through mental confusion and illusion, allowing one to discern and see things clearly for what they really are. Its sweet, green fragrance energy extends that to the emotional realm, helping one cut through emotional ambiguity and release distressed emotions that remain unresolved. Tropical basil shines especially when the individual experiences difficulty with digesting and coming to terms with feelings of resentment and anger. This is especially true when these feelings arise in reaction to challenging external situations, such as negative social moods, personal reproaches and judgements, and even humiliation and degradation. In so doing, the oil can help one summon the courage and confidence to self-assert, to fully express, and will especially support the expression of righteous indignation and appropriate anger.

Tropical basil can foster emotional freedom filled with light and joy, free of emotional dependency and free of other addictions in general. The Royal Herb's traditional associations of power and wealth never ring truer than when we undersand them to support personal empowerment.

**Related basil oils:** Making clear differentiations among the many types of Basil oils is important for clinical use. They should ideally be based on their chemical constituents rather than their species or variety. As a guideline, the following dominant chemotypes will emphasize respective actions, regardless of the particular species or variety. In terms of their therapeutic status, all Basil chemotypes are essentially mild remedies with no cumulative toxicity except for the camphor chemotype.

- **Methylchavicol dominance:** Systemic relaxant, spasmolytic and anti-inflammatory actions for hypertonic/tense conditions with spasm, inflammation and pain. Basil ct. methylchavicol (Tropical basil) is the main oil of this chemotype available (this profile).

- **Linalool dominance:** Systemic restorative, nervous restorative, carminative digestive and liver stimulant, for hypotonic/weak and congestive/damp conditions with neurasthenia, fatigue, digestive and mild adrenocortical deficiency with flatulence and somnolence after meals. This type also shows uterine and prostate decongestant actions in the treatment of pelvic congestion with dysmenorrhoea and prostate swelling/hyperplasia. Linalool chemotypes are also effective antipyretics for reducing fevers and are also applied in low dilutions for dry eczema because of their anti-inflammatory and mild antipruritic action. The main linalool basil types available are Sweet basil and Hoary basil.

    For psychological use by olfaction, these sweet-green basils are excellent regulators for helping resolve distressed emotions and promote emotional balance in general.

- **Eugenol dominance:** Anti-infectious (antibacterial, antifungal, antiparasitic), spasmolytic, anti-inflammatory and analgesic, especially for bacterial digestive and respiratory infections, bacterial intestinal dysbiosis, and intestinal parasites such as giardia and hookworm. Eugenol-dominant basil oils are generally warming stimulants, like Pimenta berry, and are also about the same strength as Pimenta berry. They are also used as digestive stimulants for various forms of indigestion with abdominal pain and bloating. Because eugenol has also shown *antioxidant* and *anticancer* (*antiproliferative*) actions, these eugenol-rich basil oils may also be useful for various types of cancer.

  Large-leaf basil, Bush basil, Holy basil and Tree basil are the main representatives in this group. This last species has also shown an *antiallergic* action and is also *analgesic*, *vulnerary* and *tissue regenerative* when used topically. Low dilutions up to 2% should be used in topical preparations because of their skin-irritant quality. Holy basil has a reputation for being an adaptogen. In Southeast Asia the herb is a widely used remedy for treating infections, fevers, rheumatic pain, vomiting, motion sickness and (topically) wounds. Because production of Holy basil oil is only of recent occurrence, it has seen relatively little clinical application and research, and almost no documentation.

- **Camphor dominance:** Spasmolytic, anti-inflammatory, hypotensive and mucolytic expectorant in acute spasmodic and inflammatory cardiovascular, digestive and respiratory conditions, including neurogenic angina pectoris; also for bronchial congestion with dyspnoea and moderate hypertension.

  Camphor basil is the main oil available in this group. However, it should be used with utmost caution, as it has strong status with some acute toxicity. Camphor basil is neurotoxic, teratogenic and abortive, and is contraindicated during pregnancy and breastfeeding, and with babies and children. Oral or other internal use is not advisable; administration is best restricted to topical forms such as liniments in moderate dilution.

# Black Pepper

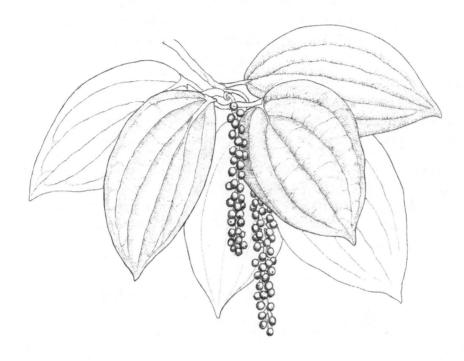

**Botanical source:** The fruit of *Piper nigrum* L. (Piperaceae – pepper family), a shrub or climbing vine of the wet Asian tropics

**Other names:** Black peppercorn; Poivre noir (Fr), Schwarzer pfeffer (Ge), Gulmirch (Hindi), Merica (Indonesian), Pepe nero (It), Pimiento negro (Sp), Filfil (Ar), Hu Jiao (Ch)

**Appearance:** A mobile clear or greenish-grey fluid with a warm-spicy, dry sweet-woody and somewhat fresh odour

**Perfumery status:** A heart note of very high intensity and good persistence

**Extraction:** Steam distillation of the dried and crushed or ground unripe peppercorns, November to February

**1 kg oil yield from:** 50–100 kg of the dried corns (an excellent yield)

**Production areas:** India (native), Sri Lanka, Indonesia, Madagascar, Tanzania, China

**Typical constituents:** Monoterpenes 55–78% (incl. d-limonene <40%, β-pinene 5–35%, α-phellandrene 1–27%, δ-3-carene 1–19%, β-phellandrene <19%, α-pinene

<19%, sabinene <20%, myrcene <10%, δ-elemene 2%, terpinene, p-cymene, terpinolene) • sesquiterpenes 20–30% (incl. β-caryophyllene 10–33%, bisabolene <5%, elemene, humulene, cubebenene, α- and β-selinene, farnesene, bergamotene, curcumene) • monoterpenols (incl. terpinen-4-ol <1%, linalool <1%, trans-carveol, elemol, trace bisabolol) • ketones dihydrocarvone, piperitone <1% • aldehyde piperonal • caryophyllene oxide • phenolic ethers • p-cymene methyl ester, traces safrole/myristicin/carvacol methyl ether • sulphur N-formyl piperidine • piperonylic acid

**Chance of adulteration:** Good, especially with the oils of Eucalyptus dives, Elemi, Schinus molle, Cubeb and Cedrella, as well as with isolated constituents such as phellandrene, limonene, pinene and Clove oil sesquiterpenes. The use of pepper dust, a by-product of pepper production, rather than whole peppercorns, will also result in an inferior oil more suitable for commercial than therapeutic use.

**Related oils:** Occasionally a White pepper oil is produced from the same but mature fruit, simply with the pericarp removed. Other related oils called pepper both in and outside of the *Piper* genus include Cubeb pepper, Long pepper, Sichuan pepper, Pink pepper and Brazilian pepper (see below). These are less often available and therefore see less clinical use.

## Therapeutic Functions and Indications

### SPECIFIC SYMPTOMATOLOGY – *All applications*

Apathy, loss of motivation, insecurity, loss of self-confidence, spaciness, oversensitivity, fearfulness, apprehension, vulnerability, mental confusion and fogginess, poor concentration, lethargy, chronic physical fatigue, low endurance, aches and pains, poor vision, scanty urination, water retention, cold hands and feet, appetite loss, indigestion, bloating, flatulence, abdominal pain, loss of sex drive, cough with hard sputum, muscle and joint pains, stiff cold joints

### PSYCHOLOGICAL – *Aromatic diffusion, whole-body massage*

**Essential PNEI function and indication:** Stimulant in weak conditions
**Possible brain dynamics:** Increases prefrontal cortex and basal ganglia functioning
**Fragrance category:** Top tone with pungent and somewhat rooty notes
**Indicated psychological disorders:** ADD, depression, dissociative disorder

PROMOTES COURAGE AND SELF-CONFIDENCE

- Discouragement with apathy, loss of motivation, self-neglect
- Low self-confidence and self-esteem, depression

PROMOTES GROUNDING AND STRENGTH

- Insecurity, fearfulness
- Mental and emotional burnout

## PHYSIOLOGICAL – *Nebulizer inhalation, gel cap, suppository, external applications*

**Therapeutic status:** Mild remedy with no cumulative toxicity

**Topical safety status:** Non-irritant, non-sensitizing

**Tropism:** Circulatory, nervous, digestive, respiratory, urogenital, musculoskeletal, reproductive systems

**Essential diagnostic function:** Warms asthenic/cold and stimulates hypotonic/weak terrain conditions

*strong central and diffusive arterial circulatory stimulant, SNS stimulant:* a wide range of asthenic (cold) and hypotonic (weak) conditions with circulatory deficiency, chronic physical fatigue; incl. convalescence, CFS

*adrenal stimulant:* adrenal fatigue syndrome with chronic afternoon or evening fatigue

*cerebral and nervous stimulant, vision enhancer:* physical and mental fatigue, dizziness, poor concentration, vision impairment

*strong musculoskeletal stimulant and sedative, antirheumatic, anti-inflammatory, analgesic:* rheumatic-arthritic conditions with aches, pains, stiffness, incl. fibromyalgia; neurological pain, incl. neuralgia, sciatica, toothache; colic pain, lumbar pain, temporary limb paralysis

*digestive stimulant, gastrointestinal pancreatic and liver stimulant, aperitive, carminative, antiemetic:* atonic digestive conditions with indigestion, appetite loss, flatulence, bloating, pain, constipation or diarrhoea, anorexia; chronic gastroenteritis, pancreatitis; acute nausea, vomiting

*respiratory stimulant, fluidifying expectorant, antitussive, antiseptic:* congestive dyspnoea and bronchitis, esp. chronic, with hardened sputum, emphysema, cough, fatigue

*reproductive/sexual stimulant, aphrodisiac:* loss of libido (frigidity, impotence)

*detoxicant diuretic:* oedema, cardiac oedema, oliguria, metabolic toxicosis antioxidant, potentially anticancer

Antimicrobial actions:

> *moderate antibacterial:* intestinal and respiratory infections, incl. with Staph. aureus, E. coli, incl. gastroenteritis, food poisoning, dysentery, cholera; bronchitis, colds, laryngitis, tonsillitis

> *antitoxic, antidotal:* fish and mushroom poisoning

Synergistic combinations

- Black pepper + Ginger: digestive stimulant, carminative, analgesic, antibacterial, antiemetic for a wide range of digestive disorders, incl. flatulence, nausea, vomiting, anorexia, gastroenteritis

- Black pepper + Cypress/Basil ct. chavicol: gastric and pancreatic stimulant for upper digestive deficiency with indigestion, bloating, epigastric pain

- Black pepper + Ginger/Thyme ct. thymol: sexual restorative for loss of libido (frigidity, impotence)

Complementary combinations

- Black pepper + Cajeput/Rosemary: strong arterial stimulant and analgesic for circulatory deficiency with cold skin and extremities, chronic rheumatic-arthritic pain

- Black pepper + Niaouli: intestinal antibacterial for gastritis, enteritis, microbial toxicosis, food poisoning

- Black pepper + Juniper berry: strong analgesic and detoxicant for acute and chronic rheumatic, arthritic and neuralgic pain

- Black pepper + German camomile/Lavender: strong anti-inflammatory and analgesic in neuralgic, rheumatic and arthritic disorders

- Black pepper + Juniper berry: detoxicant diuretic for oedema, oliguria, metabolic toxicosis

- Black pepper + Frankincense: stimulant fluidifying expectorant for bronchitis with hardened sputum

Topical – *Liniment, ointment, cream, compress and other cosmetic preparations*

**Skin care:** Pale, devitalized skin

*rubefacient, analgesic:* poor muscle tone, muscle aches and pains, sprains, strains, bruises, chilblains; to warm and tone muscles before and after sports; sore throat

**Therapeutic precautions:** Black pepper oil is a strong systemic warming, drying stimulant and therefore contraindicated in hypersthenic/hot, hypertonic/tense and dry conditions. This includes acute fever and inflammation (not chronic inflammation), agitation, insomnia and hyperadrenia. For the same reason, avoid use for babies and infants.

**Pharmacological precautions:** Although Black pepper is not a skin irritant, skin irritation may occur with topical use if the oil is oxidized. All use of the oil should be avoided in babies and infants because of its monoterpene-based fresh-pungent quality.

**Preparations:**

- Diffusor: 2–4 drops in water

- Massage oil: 2–4% dilution in vegetable oil

- Liniment: 4–7% dilution in vegetable oil

- Gel cap: 1–3 drops with olive oil

## Chinese Medicine Functions and Indications

**Aroma energy:** Pungent

**Movement:** Rising

**Warmth:** Warm to hot

**Meridian tropism:** Kidney, Spleen, Stomach, Lung, Bladder

**Five-Element affinity:** Water, Earth, Metal

**Essential function:** To tonify and raise the Yang, warm the interior and strengthen the Shen

1. **Tonifies the Yang and warms the Kidney; raises the clear Yang and strengthens the Shen and libido**

   - **Kidney Yang deficiency with Shen weakness**, with loss of sex drive, weak loins and knees, physical and mental fatigue, cold extremities, loss of self-confidence:

     Black spruce/Pimenta berry/Thyme ct. thymol

   - **Clear Yang Qi deficiency with Shen weakness**, with mental fog, confusion, loss of focus, apathy, slow response:

     Rosemary/Ravintsara/Cajeput/Peppermint

2. **Warms and harmonizes the Middle Warmer, resolves damp and relieves pain and distension**

- **Stomach-Spleen empty cold (Spleen Yang deficiency)**, with epigastric or abdominal pain, nausea, appetite loss, odourless loose stool, morning diarrhoea:

  Ginger/Clove/Pimenta berry

- **Stomach-Spleen damp-cold or toxic-damp**, with indigestion, flatulence, nausea, abdominal bloating, chronic diarrhoea:

  Nutmeg/Pimenta berry/Juniper berry

3. **Warms and harmonizes the middle warmer, descends rebellious Qi and relieves vomiting and pain**

- **Stomach-Spleen Qi stagnation**, with chronic indigestion, epigastric bloating and pain, nausea, belching:

  Fennel/Peppermint/Cardamom

- **Stomach cold with Qi rebellion**, with nausea, appetite loss, hiccups, vomiting, epigastric or abdominal pain:

  Fennel/Ginger/Clove

4. **Warms the Lung, resolves phlegm and relieves coughing**

- **Lung phlegm-cold/damp**, with cough, copious expectoration of sputum, chest pain, cold hands and feet, chronic fatigue:

  Scotch pine/Grand fir/Green myrtle

- **Lung wind-cold** with chills, coughing, chest pain, sore throat, aches and pains:

  Silver fir/Ravintsara/Rosemary

5. **Warms and opens the meridians, dispels wind-damp-cold and relieves pain**

- **Wind-damp-cold obstruction**, with muscle aches and pains, joint stiffness:

  Rosemary/Niaouli/Juniper berry/Frankincense

6. **Drains water-damp, promotes urination and relieves swelling**

- **Water-damp accumulation**, with leg and ankle oedema, fatigue:

  Juniper berry/Fennel/Geranium

REMARKS

The most sought-after spice in human history, Black pepper is native to Southwest India and Sri Lanka and by cultivation spread to Indonesia and the Philippines to the East, and Madagascar to the south. The world traveller Marco Polo around 1290 documented pepper production all along the Malay and Indonesian archipelago, noting that the crop was all destined for Chinese ports. From the 10th century on, the tentacles of Arabic maritime trade effectively distributed this valuable aromatic from the Malabar coast not only to Chinese but also to Middle Eastern and European trade centres.

In the West, Greek and Roman writers such as Theophrastus, Dioscorides and Plinius eulogized its benefits; Rome itself had to erect dedicated pepper warehouses to cope with its large-scale consumption. The spice achieved its pinnacle of desirability in the European Middle Ages in the 13th century when it assumed the status of monetary currency and was traded against gold itself. Called 'black money', pepper became the twin condiment to the equally vauable seasalt, 'white money'. Spice traders were even called 'pepperers' after the Latin *piperarii*, as it was their chief trade. Following Vasco da Gama forging the first European sea path to India in 1498, the Portuguese then opened further pepper plantations in Indonesia to create a trade monopoly they were to maintain up to the 18th century. Already in 1504, Portuguese cutters first sailed down the Thames loaded with a black pepper cargo valued at an astronomical price. In a déjà-vu scene, in 1797 the New England schooner *Rajah* sailed into New York's East River carrying a pepper consignment from Sumatra worth over $100,000.

Black pepper essential oil is first mentioned in the key early text of the Italian apothecary Saladin, the *Compendium aromatorium* of 1488; this was followed by entries in the writings of Valerius Cordus and Della Porta. Winther von Andernach in 1571 then fully documented the specific techniques for steam distilling spice oils such as Clove, Cardamom, Cinnamon and Black pepper. In the early 18th century, the renowned biochemist Caspar Neuman developed the oil's initial pharmacognosy.

Like Cinnamon, Black pepper has always been an essential remedy in Ayurvedic and traditional Greek (Tibb Unani) medicine and is considered hot and dry in the second degree. However prepared, Black pepper is a classic systemic warming stimulant for treating conditions underpinned by a cold, weak and damp/congestive terrain. Working as an arterial circulatory stimulant and a twin sympathetic nervous and adrenocortical stimulant, Black pepper excels at treating fatigue and cold, especially when chronic and when involving adrenal fatigue. As with the similar oil Nutmeg, Black pepper also achieves an excellent detoxicant effect in resolving damp conditions, especially at the level of the GI tract, the bronchi, the kidneys (a nice diuretic here) and the sinews. This, coupled with a strong analgesic and anti-inflammatory action on joints, muscles and peripheral nerves, makes the oil a prominent remedy for chronic, cold, damp-type rheumatic and arthritic disorders with key symptoms of pain and stiffness. Topical preparations for treating these conditions will here include a useful rubefacient and capillary stimulant action.

Perhaps it is Black pepper's main image as a spice that has turned it into an important remedy for digestive problems. As with so many oils, it is hard to tell whether its use as a condiment has led to this status or whether research has impartially confirmed its multiple benefits to digestive functions more than to others. Either way, Black pepper certainly displays a strong tropism for both the large and small intestine, stimulating, detoxifying, disinfecting and increasing nutrient uptake as it is absorbed. The remedy should often be combined with others for treating intestinal conditions, including gut dysbiosis, food poisoning, enteritis and colic. Further up the digestive chain, Black pepper acts as a comprehensive gastric-pancreatic stimulant for treating all atonic, cold states of the upper gut. It has also shown moderate liver-protective and liver-detoxicant actions. Certain French practitioners even go so far as to claim that, when absorbed in the gut, the oil will increase the bioavailability of other oils' constituents, thereby enhancing their functions.

Black pepper is no less useful as a psychological aromatic when used by olfaction. Like some other spices, this oil has an intimate relationship to issues of the lower gut related to self-preservation. Warm and spicy, Black pepper is able to connect us to our instinctive, gut-felt feelings of safety and security in the face of the unknown. In so doing, the fragrance can help us build self-confidence and self-esteem built on courage and full belief in ourselves and our personal decisions rather than on external actions. Black pepper is for those who, lacking strong boundaries from weakened internal resources, tend to be easily swayed by others and by life circumstances in general. In the process of ignoring their healthy fears, they become prone to confusion, mistrust or anxiety. Over time, it can support turning that vulnerability into a true inner strength.

**Related oils:** Of the approximately 1200 pepper species, the following types are also available as essential oil and may be useful for clinical practice.

**Cubeb pepper** (*Piper cubeba* L.), Tailpepper or Java pepper, with its warm, spicy-woody fragrance, is high in sesquiterpenes (cubebene) and sesquiterpenols (cubebol). Originating in Sumatra, Malaysia and Sri Lanka, Cubeb was an important aromatic spice and remedy during the Middle Ages following importation from India in the 12th century. Cubeb essential oil was first distilled in the 16th century in Central Europe. It is a mild remedy with no cumulative toxicity and is not skin-irritant or sensitizing. Its pharmacognosy is typically sesquiterpenes c. 50% (incl. δ-cadinene 10%, α- and β-cubebene 10%, α-copaine 7%, germacrene 3%, β-caryophyllene 2%); sesquiterpenols c. 20% (incl. cubebol 7%, epicubebol 6%, globulol, nerolidol 3%); monoterpenes c. 14%; monoterpenols (incl. α-terpineol 4%, linalool 1%); ketone cis-asarone 4%; and 1,8 cineole <1%.

Like Black pepper, Cubeb oil from Indonesia is suited for treating cold and weak terrain. It is a systemic stimulant, especially to cerebral, nervous, arterial circulatory, neuromuscular and digestive functions. The oil's main use by internal delivery is as a strong digestive stimulant and a urogenital anti-infective. Cubeb pepper exerts excellent aperitive and carminative actions for upper digestive stagnation with indigestion, flatulence, distension and appetite loss. It is considered anti-inflammatory for enterocolitis and also rheumatic conditions. Its good antibacterial and diuretic actions have a good tropism for the urogenital organs and are effective for both acute and chronic infections and inflammations, including cystitis, prostatitis, gleet, urethritis, bacterial vaginitis with leucorrhoea, and gonorrhoea. For these, the remedy works quickly from the third day of use onward.

Cubeb pepper is traditionally much used in both essential oil and tincture form together with or instead of Copaiba. Like Black pepper, Cubeb pepper may also be used as a stimulant expectorant for congestive, infectious bronchial conditions. Cubeb pepper is contraindicated for long-term use as it may cause overexcitement, agitation or diarrhoea by overstimulating the nervous, circulatory and digestive systems. When used as a single remedy, an 8–10-day course is usual. Moderate standard doses apply.

Spicy, pungent, warming, stimulating and uplifting in aroma, Cubeb pepper can be used by olfaction as a psychological remedy for loss of self-confidence, loss of motivation and depression, especially in those prone to brain fog and spaciness.

**Long pepper** (*Piper longum* L.), from the Indian Ocean islands, South India and Indonesia, is a spicy, pungent, warm-to-hot systemic stimulant and very similar in status, nature, functions and indications as Black pepper. The oil is high in β-caryophyllene (18%) and piperine. Long pepper was the first known pepper in the Mediterranean and was even more highly valued by Romans than Black pepper. It became a much-used spice and aromatic remedy during the Middle Ages and Renaissance, but eventually fell into disuse in favour of Black pepper. Long pepper is considered especially analgesic, anti-inflammatory, bronchospasmolytic and antitussive, and is also known as an antiproliferative anticancer remedy. The oil is contraindicated in pregnancy because of its antifertility action. The same precautions, dilutions and doses apply as for Black pepper.

**Sichuan pepper** (*Zanthoxylum bungeanum* Maximovicz), in the citrus or rue family (Rutaceae), Chuan Jiao in Chinese, originates in the mountain valleys of Sichuan. The fruit is also sourced from *Z. simulans* Hance in Eastern China and Taiwan. With a fresh, lemony, green fragrance, Sichuan pepper contains d-limonene 40–50% and β-myrcene, along with other non-volatile constituents. The Sichuan peppercorn has a long history of important spice use in China with a unique, distinctive piquancy when ingested; it is an ingredient in the classic Sichuan five-spice powder. Chinese medicine makes use of Sichuan pepper as a spicy, heating analgesic herb for treating epigastric and abdominal pain, diarrhoea and vomiting, either from infection or from intestinal parasites (especially from roundworms, Ascaris). The essential oil has these same indications plus others not yet explored or documented. Moderate standard dilutions and doses of this mild, non-toxic oil apply.

**Pink pepper** (*Schinus molle* L.) is from the Peruvian pepper tree in the sumac family (Anacardiaceae); the fruit (peppercorn) contains <20% myrcene and other analgesic constituents such as d-limonene, p-cymene and α- and β-phellandrene. The related Brazilian pink pepper (*Schinus terebinthifolius* Raddi) also contains many analgesic constituents such as d-limonene, α-phellandrene, δ-3-carene and terpenen-4-ol.

# Cardamom

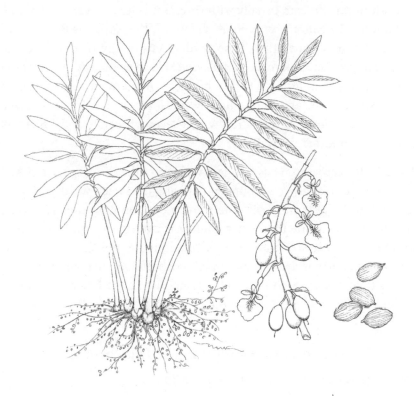

**Botanical source:** The fruit pods of *Elettaria cardamomum* (L.) Maton (Zingiberaceae – ginger family), a plant of the wet Southeast Asian tropics

**Other names:** Mysore cardamom, Green/Small cardamom; Cardamomo (It, Sp), Chhoti elachi (Hindi), Elekkai (Tamil, Malay), Bai dou kou (Ch)

**Appearance:** A colourless to pale yellow liquid with a warm, sweet-spicy odour with some fresh-spicy overtones and mild musty-rooty undertones

**Perfumery status:** A head note of medium intensity and persistence

**Extraction:** Essential oil by steam distillation or $CO_2$ extraction from the seed. An oleoresin is also produced in small quantities.

**1 kg yield from:** 100–150 kg of the dried fruits (a moderate yield)

**Production areas:** South India (native), Sri Lanka, Guatemala

**Typical constituents:** Esters 30–52% (incl. α-terpinyl acetate <51%, linalyl acetate <8%) • 1,8 cineole 23–48% • monoterpenes 5–17% (incl. d-limonene 2–10%, sabinene <5%, β-myrcene <2%, α-pinene <1.6%) • monoterpenols 2–16% (incl. linalool 1–7%, α-terpineol 1–4%, terpinen-4-ol 1–3%, geraniol <1.6%) • sesquiterpenols <4%

(incl. trans-nerolidol, cis-nerolidol) • aldehydes <5% (incl. neral <2%, geranial) • p-cersol • methyl ethers • ketones, methyl heptenone • acids (incl. acetic, butanoic, decanoic, nerylic and perillic acid)

**Chance of adulteration:** Fair, usually with several species and varieties of the related black cardamom (*Amomum costatum*, *A. villosum*), the Nepal or Bengal cardamom (*A. subulatum*) and various other 'false' cardamoms, many from Sri Lanka. These include round or Java cardamom (*A. compactum* Soland ex Maton) from Western Java, bastard cardamom (*A. xanthioides*) and Chinese cardamom (*A. globosum*). These are often used to stretch Cardamom oil, thereby considerably altering its pharmacology and therapeutic functions. Adulteration with α-terpinyl acetate and 1,8 cineole from cheaper sources is another possibility.

**Related oils:** 'False' cardamom oils distilled from any of the above species of Amomum. These oils are more strongly fresh-pungent, missing the sweet, warm, spicy fragrance profile of Elettaria Cardamom oil. Their levels of monoterpenes are consistently much higher (<70%), while their ester content is extremely low. In practice, 'False' cardamom oils are more stimulant than Cardamom and possess no relaxant action. Round cardamom and bastard cardamom oils are both high in camphor and borneol; the former is used as a spice in Java and Sumatra, while the latter is an Indian spice. Both also have different characteristics than Cardamom oil.

## Therapeutic Functions and Indications

SPECIFIC SYMPTOMATOLOGY – *All applications*

Insecurity, loss of self-confidence, emotional inhibition, discouragement, pessimism, moodiness, fatigue, loss of mental focus, chronic anxiety and depression, insomnia, nervous breakdown, hot spells, chills, appetite loss, chronic indigestion, abdominal bloating and pain, flatulence, nausea, vomiting, alternating constipation and diarrhoea, heartburn, chronic productive cough

PSYCHOLOGICAL – *Aromatic diffusion, whole-body massage*

**Essential PNEI function and indication:** Regulating in dysregulated conditions
**Possible brain dynamics:** Reduces deep limbic system hyperfunctioning
**Fragrance category:** Top tone with pungent and sweet notes
**Indicated psychological disorders:** Bipolar disorder, minor depression

PROMOTES SELF-CONFIDENCE AND COURAGE

- Loss of self-confidence with insecurity, inhibited emotional expression

- Discouragement with apathy, pessimism

PROMOTES EMOTIONAL STABILITY AND INTEGRATION

- Moodiness, emotional instability, repetitive emoting
- Feeling-thinking disconnection and conflict

## PHYSIOLOGICAL – *Nebulizer inhalation, gel cap, suppository, pessary*

**Therapeutic status:** Mild remedy with no cumulative toxicity

**Topical safety status:** Mild skin irritant, non-sensitizing

**Tropism:** Nervous, digestive, urinary, respiratory systems

**Essential diagnostic function:** Relaxes hypertonic/tense and warms hyposthenic/cold terrain conditions

PRIMARILY RELAXANT:

*nervous and cerebral sedative, PNS stimulant:* anxiety states, esp. chronic; insomnia

*strong gastrointestinal relaxant, spasmolytic, carminative:* spasmodic digestive conditions, esp. nervous indigestion with gas, colic

*antiallergic:* type-I and III allergies, including food allergies and sensitivities; intestinal hyperpermeability

*antiemetic:* nausea, vomiting, motion sickness

*respiratory relaxant:* spasmodic dyspnoea, asthma

*neuromuscular analgesic, anti-inflammatory:* muscle spasms, cramps

*antibacterial, antifungal, anthelmintic*

PRIMARILY RESTORATIVE AND STIMULANT:

*nervous and cerebral restorative:* fatigue, low vitality, loss of focus, disorientation, depression, esp. with anxiety; chronic neurasthenia, nervous breakdown; ANS dysregulation with mood, digestive and temperature disorders; alternating constipation and diarrhoea

*strong gastric stimulant, stomachic, aperitive:* upper digestive atony with indigestion, epigastric distension, pain, nausea; anorexia, halitosis, aerophagia with heartburn

*stimulant expectorant, antitussive:* chronic bronchitis with productive cough

*mild aphrodisiac*

*mild emmenagogue*

*antioxidant*

*mild antibacterial, antifungal, antiparasitic*

SYNERGISTIC COMBINATIONS

- Cardamom + Petitgrain bigarade/Coriander seed: nervous and cerebral sedative, restorative and regulator for chronic neurasthenia with physical and mental exhaustion, insomnia, anxiety, depression, nervous breakdown; ANS dysregulation

COMPLEMENTARY COMBINATIONS

- Cardamom + Ginger/Pimenta berry: strong digestive stimulant, aperitive and stomachic for upper digestive atony with indigestion, appetite loss, flatulence, bloating

- Cardamom + Ginger: antiemetic for nausea and vomiting, travel and altitude sickness

- Cardamom + Basil ct. chavicol/Fennel/Nutmeg: strong digestive relaxant, spasmolytic and carminative for spasmodic digestive conditions, esp. nervous indigestion with gas, colic

- Cardamom + Patchouli: digestive antiallergic for food sensitivities and allergies

- Cardamom + Ravintsara/Cajeput: stimulant expectorant, antitussive, antiseptic and nervous restorative for chronic congestive bronchial conditions with productive cough, chronic fatigue

## TOPICAL – *Liniment, ointment, cream, compress and other cosmetic preparations*

**Skin care:** Not used

**Therapeutic precautions:** Cardamom oil is both a relaxant and stimulant and should be avoided in hypersthenic/hot and dry conditions in general.

**Pharmacological precautions:** Avoid using this pungent oil on babies and infants because of its 1,8 cineole content.

**Preparations:**

- Diffusor: 2–3 drops

- Massage oil: 1–3% dilution in vegetable oil

- Liniment: 2–8% dilution in vegetable oil
- Gel cap: 2–3 drops with olive oil

## Chinese Medicine Functions and Indications

**Aroma energy:** Sweet, pungent

**Movement:** Circulating, rising

**Warmth:** Neutral to warm

**Meridian tropism:** Heart, Liver, Stomach, Spleen, Lung

**Five-Element affinity:** Fire, Earth, Metal

**Essential function:** To nourish Heart Blood, regulate the Qi and harmonize the Shen

1. **Nourishes Heart Blood, settles the Heart and harmonizes the Shen**

   - **Heart Blood deficiency** with Shen disharmony, with chronic physical and mental fatigue, depression, anxiety, insomnia:

     Petitgrain/Palmarosa/Lavender/Clary sage

2. **Regulates the Qi, reduces stagnation, harmonizes the Middle Warmer and relieves distension**

   - **Liver-Stomach/Spleen disharmony** with indigestion, epigastric fullness, abdominal distension and pain:

     Mandarin/Basil ct. methylchavicol/Peppermint

   - **Stomach-Spleen Qi stagnation** with indigestion, bloating, appetite loss, nausea, vomiting:

     Spearmint/Peppermint/May chang/Basil ct. chavicol

3. **Descends Stomach Qi, harmonizes the Stomach and relieves vomiting**

   - **Stomach cold with Qi rebellion**, with hiccups, nausea, vomiting:

     Ginger/Fennel/Black pepper/Clove

4. **Warms the Lung, expels phlegm and relieves coughing**

   - **Lung phlegm-cold/damp** with cough, copious expectoration of sputum, chest distension:

     Cajeput/Grand fir/Black pepper

REMARKS

Unlike nutmeg to the East and coriander to the West, cardamom is a tropical Indian spice through and through. It is one of just a few herbal remedies that found its way not only into Ayurvedic medicine, still flourishing in its native Kerala and Sri Lanka, but also into traditional Chinese medicine to the East and traditional Greek medicine to the West. The Chinese pharmacopeia actually includes three kinds of cardamom: the white (Bai dou kou), the black (Cao guo) and the wild cardamom (Sha ren). Botanists and herbalists of those countries were well acquainted with the various types of cardamom since earliest days, carefully distinguishing their appearance and medical uses.

Cardamom was known in all cultures of antiquity, including Egyptian: hieroglyphs of 700 BC depict its use as a spice, perfume and an aromatic ingredient for ritual fumigations. Considered 'the queen of spices' because of its refined, noble scent, cardamom has long been a perennial staple for Indian spice blends and spiced teas. Arabic and Jewish traders in early Medieval times moved the spice from the Malabar Coast to Mediterranean ports such as Alexandria, Constantinople and later Genoa; it also became a staple in the cuisines of most Arabic countries. Although it enjoyed some reputation as an aphrodisiac in Medieval European love potions, this aspect is now considered only mild.

Like the oils of Ginger and Fennel, Cardamom oil is dominated by the theme of balanced opposites. Fresh, sweet-spicy and uplifting, its fragrance is underpinned by a unique musty, almost earthy depth not found in other spice oils. Its complex pharmacological profile too bears the imprint of complementary opposites, its vitalizing 1,8 cineole balanced with calming esters – as with Laurel and Green myrtle. In therapeutic terms, this opposition translates as stimulation balanced with relaxation.

As a warming, stimulating oil, Cardamom is a classic aromatic for treating cold conditions of the digestive and respiratory tract, and weakness of the nervous system with mental fatigue and depression. Tellingly, each black seed does resemble a miniature brain – somewhat. As a relaxant, spasmolytic nervous sedative remedy, however, Cardamom also addresses tense conditions, typically involving anxiety and insomnia. In terms of energetic medicine, Cardamom settles and comforts the Heart under long-term unproductive stress, while also gently boosting mental and physical vitality. Acting bivalently on the nervous system, the oil is tailor-made for the individual suffering from chronic depression with anxiety, and chronic neurasthenia with exhaustion, anxiety and poor-quality sleep, in turn followed by low energy the next morning. For the same reason, Cardamom should be considered for balancing systemic autonomic nervous dysregulation, alongside Petitgrain.

With digestive functions, Cardamom again shows true brilliance: this is one of the best carminative spasmolytics and aperitives rolled into one. It is one of the few aromatic remedies able to treat cold and tension focused on the gut; and a classic for stress-induced indigestion with bloating, flatulence and poor appetite. Research also shows promise for Cardamom as an antiallergic agent and again should find application for gut-related allergies of many kinds.

Clearly, Cardamom is ultimately a harmonizing remedy: creating a balance between the head and the heart, and the head and the gut. In psychological terms, Cardamom by olfaction is particularly useful for promoting emotional self-confidence and expression. With its clear pungent fragrance underpinned with sweet and somewhat rooty notes, the oil may help those with emotional inhibition arising from insecurity and a deeper inability for taking care of their own emotional needs and self-nurturance. Here Cardamom will support the instinct for developing healthy needs rather than neediness arising from emotional lack – needs compensating for lack of emotional satisfaction. Ultimately, Cardamom is able to kindle a true desire, a true passion for life based on the pleasure principle, supporting the universal human issue of healthy self-gratification.

# Carrot Seed

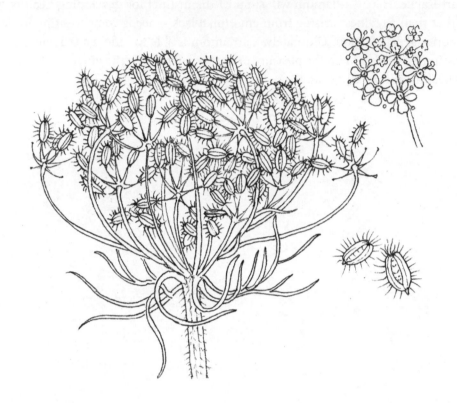

**Botanical source:** The fruit of *Daucus carota* L. subsp. *carota* (Apiaceae/Umbelliferae – carrot family), a widespread temperate herb

**Other names:** Cultivated carrot seed; Seme di carota (It), Semilla de zanahoria (Sp)

**Appearance:** A mobile yellow to amber liquid with a mild sweet-herbaceous and dry woody odour

**Perfumery status:** A heart note of medium intensity and medium persistence

**Extraction:** Steam distillation of the crushed dried seeds

**1 kg oil yield from:** 70–100 kg of the seeds (a good yield)

**Production areas:** France, Hungary, Morocco, India

**Typical constituents:** Sesquiterpenol carotol 36–73% • sesquiterpenes <19% (incl. β-bisabolene <2–10%, β-caryophyllene 1–6%, daucene 2%, α-bergamotene) • monoterpenes <32% (incl. α-pinene 2–14%, β-pinene <6%, sabinene 2–7%, l-limonene 3%, β-myrcene 2%, β-carotene) • esters (incl. geranyl acetate 3%) • monoterpenols (incl. linalool <3%, geraniol <2%) • caryophyllene oxide <3%, oxide daucol 1–4% • phenolic methylether asarone

**Chance of adulteration:** Moderate, although additives may include d-limonene and synthetic components such as α-pinene and other monoterpenes. Possible adulteration or even substitution with Wild carrot seed oil (*Daucus carota* var. *maximum*) also exists. The latter oil contains only traces to none of the key constituent carotol, instead being high in geranyl acetate and sabinene, and with therapeutic actions quite different from the cultivated carrot seed oil.

**Related oils:** Other seed oils in the carrot family, including Coriander seed, Celery seed, Cumin seed and Caraway seed (see also below)

## Therapeutic Functions and Indications

### SPECIFIC SYMPTOMATOLOGY – *All applications*

Spaciness, oversensitivity, delusions, feelings of insecurity, fearfulness, worry, compulsivity, repetitive thinking, poor motivation, pessimism, lethargy, malaise, water retention, urinary irritation, aches and pains, chronic physical and mental fatigue, distraction, energy improves late morning, nervous exhaustion, depression (often for no reason), right flank pain, recurrent urinary infections, chronic indigestion, abdominal bloating, mucus in stool

### PSYCHOLOGICAL – *Aromatic diffusion, whole-body massage*

**Essential PNEI function and indication:** Regulating in dysregulation conditions; relaxant in overstimulation conditions

**Possible brain dynamics:** Reduces basal ganglia and cingulate system hyperfunctioning

**Fragrance category:** Middle tone with woody and sweet notes

**Indicated psychological disorders:** ADHD, dissociative disorder, obsessive-compulsive disorder

#### STABILIZES THE MIND AND PROMOTES INTEGRATION

- Disconnection, scatteredness, spaciness, oversensitivity, dissociation
- Euphoria, delusion, paranoia, agitation

#### PROMOTES STABILITY AND STRENGTH

- Emotional instability with anxiety, fearfulness
- Loss of emotional security and strength

PROMOTES COGNITIVE FLEXIBILITY

- Worry, obsession, compulsivity
- Repetitive thinking, inability to let go

## PHYSIOLOGICAL – *Nebulizer inhalation, gel cap, suppository, external applications*

**Therapeutic status:** Mild remedy with no cumulative toxicity
**Topical safety status:** Non-irritant, non-sensitizing

**Tropism:** Nervous, hepatobiliary, digestive, urinary, musculoskeletal systems

**Essential diagnostic function:** Restores hypotonic/weak terrain conditions

*thyroid/thyroxine restorative and regulator:* hypothyroid syndrome

*nervous restorative and regulator:* chronic fatigue (physical and mental), depression, nervous exhaustion, neurasthenia

*hypertensive:* mild hypotension (esp. from liver congestion)

*strong liver trophorestorative, decongestant, detoxicant and protective:* liver and biliary congestion, jaundice, all liver disease, incl. hepatitis, cirrhosis; metabolic toxicosis, drug and all chemical toxicosis

*kidney restorative and decongestant:* nephrosis, all chronic kidney disorders

*detoxicant diuretic, alterative, mild anti-inflammatory:* metabolic toxicosis with fatigue, malaise; eczema, psoriasis, gout, cystitis, prostatitis; oedema

*antilipaemic, mild anticoagulant:* hyperlipidaemia, incl. high blood cholesterol; atherosclerosis

*antianaemic:* anaemia

*contraceptive*

ANTIMICROBIAL ACTIONS:

*strong antifungal:* fungal infections, incl. dermatophytes, Candida albicans

*antibacterial*

SYNERGISTIC COMBINATIONS

- Carrot seed + Atlas cedarwood: nervous restorative for chronic physical or mental fatigue, neurasthenia

- Carrot seed + Patchouli: antifungal detoxicant and anti-infective for fungal intestinal dysbiosis and hyperpermeability with Candida
- Carrot seed + German camomile: mucosal regenerator for gastric and duodenal ulcers

COMPLEMENTARY COMBINATIONS

- Carrot seed + Pimenta berry: thyroid/thyroxine regulator for hypothyroid syndrome
- Carrot seed + Lemon/Grapefruit + Lavender: nervous restorative for chronic mental fatigue, depression
- Carrot seed + Petitgrain/Lavender: nervous restorative and regulator for chronic neurasthenia, insomnia
- Carrot seed + Lemon/Rosemary ct. verbenone: strong liver restorative and detoxicant in all chronic liver conditions, incl. liver toxicosis; in all drug abuse
- Carrot seed + Lovage root/Celery seed: strong liver detoxicant and protective, diuretic for toxicosis from drugs, chemicals and metabolism
- Carrot seed + Fennel/Juniper berry: diuretic kidney detoxicant for kidney deficiency, metabolic toxicosis with malaise, eczema, urinary infections
- Carrot seed + Helichrysum: antilipaemic for hypercholesterolaemia, hyperlipidaemia
- Carrot seed + Lemongrass + Geranium: antifungal for fungal infections

TOPICAL – *Liminent, ointment, cream, compress*
*and other cosmetic preparations*

**Skin care:** Sensitive and mature skin types

*skin toner and elasticizer:* tired or irritated skin, wrinkles

*skin regenerator, vulnerary:* chronic wounds, chronic rodent/non-healing/ gangrenous ulcers; burns, boils, furuncles, abscesses, dermatitis, eczema, psoriasis; ageing spots, scars, stretch marks, UV damage

*strong antifungal:* fungal skin infections, incl. mycoses, tinea, athlete's foot, jock itch

*antitumoural(?):* skin and mucosal cancer

*antibacterial:* acne, impetigo, rosacea

**Therapeutic precautions:** None

**Pharmacological precautions:** Carrot seed oil has shown a female contraceptive action by reputation and research, and an antigestational effect during pregnancy that may be based on uterine stimulation. Like the tincture, Carrot seed oil is therefore best avoided during pregnancy.

**Preparations:**

- Diffusor: Not used
- Massage oil: 2–5% dilution in vegetable oil
- Liniment: 5–20% dilution in vegetable oil
- Gel cap: 2–3 drops with olive oil

# Chinese Medicine Functions and Indications

**Aroma energy:** Sweet, woody

**Movement:** Stabilizing

**Warmth:** Neutral

**Meridian tropism:** Heart, Liver, Spleen

**Five-Element affinity:** Wood, Earth

**Essential function:** To nourish the Blood, resolve damp and strengthen the Shen

1. **Nourishes the Blood, animates the Heart, strengthens the Shen and relieves depression**

    - **Heart and Liver Blood deficiency** with mental and physical fatigue, depression, low motivation, pessimism:

      Geranium/Clary sage/Coriander seed

2. **Resolves damp, harmonizes the Middle Warmer and relieves distension and swelling**

    - **Spleen toxic-damp** with chronic indigestion, abdominal bloating, mucus in stool:

      Thyme ct. linalool/Patchouli/Palmarosa

    - **General damp** with lethargy, heaviness of body, water retention:

      Lemongrass/Grapefruit/Fennel

Remarks

In contrast to its use in herbal medicine as a tincture, Carrot seed in essential oil form is a major remedy for the liver and kidneys, and in that sense it is the equivalent aromatic remedy to Dandelion root. Carrot seed has shown its worth as a premier oil for chronic liver problems, regardless of the particular condition, combining detoxicant, protective and trophorestorative actions. Working in tandem with the kidneys as a detoxicant diuretic, this oil is an important alterative remedy for a chronic terrain of toxicosis, the accumulation of metabolic or chemical toxins. Like any good alterative, Carrot seed works on the level of blood and interstitial fluids, systemically altering the body's internal fluid environment for the better and promoting toxin removal. Skin conditions in particular will benefit from this effect, as with cerain herbal alteratives. The oil's reputation for helping hypothyroid syndrome is an interesting bonus and makes one wonder about its mechanism of action. It certainly deserves to see more clinical experience.

The skin will benefit from the topical use of Carrot seed as much as from internal use. European doctors have relied on this remedy for around a century for its superb, deep regenerating action on skin cells in conditions as varied as chronic ulcers and abscesses through to cancer of the skin and mucous membrane. Today cosmetologists also swear by its ability to tone and elastisize tired, irritated or mature skin. Fungal skin infections will also yield under its strong antifungal action.

Carrot seed oil may also be used as a psychological remedy by olfaction. Its woody, dry notes signal a centring, stabilizing effect similar to that of Atlas cedarwood. Carrot seed is for the individual who feels insecure, vulnerable and anxious, and mentally scattered, easily distracted and distraught or fearful. The oil's sweet, mildly herbaceous notes extend its use to conditions of loss of cognitive flexibility, manifesting as chronic worry, repetitive thinking, and even obsessions and compulsivity. At the extreme end, Carrot seed could help with dissociative conditions, including excessive euphoria and delusions.

**Related oils:** The following oils all from the carrot (Apiaceae) family have over the centuries also found specific therapeutic applications. Their uses are similar to the tincture preparation but often more focused. Almost all of them have their therapeutic roots in traditional Greek medicine (Tibb Unani) practised in the Eastern Mediterranean through to modern Iran and North India.

**Celery seed** (*Apium graveolens* var. *dulce* L.) is the steam-distilled oil from the seed of the culinary vegetable. With a warm, intense spicy sweet, oily fragrance, its major constituents are monoterpenes 55% (incl. d-limonene 35–78%) and sesquiterpenes 40% (incl. selinene 10–33%), with smaller amounts of phthalides (5–15%) and coumarinic ethers. Celery seed oil is clinically used in a similar but also different way to the tincture, essentially addressing hypotonic/weak and congestive/damp terrain with toxin accumulation. It is considered a nervous and adrenocortical restorative for chronic weak conditions with chronic fatigue, loss of stamina, debility and burnout. Along with that, Celery seed is a metabolic and smooth-muscle stimulant for metabolic stagnation and insufficient gastrointestinal secretions; it is also an emmenagogue and parturient, sometimes used in liniments to prime the uterus in preparation for labour.

Like so many other oils in the carrot family, Celery seed is a major alterative that exerts an important detoxicant and decongestant action on the liver and kidneys; it is specifically liver protective and diuretic, and indicated in liver and kidney congestion with poor phase-II detoxification, metabolic and exogenous toxicosis (incl. chemicals, drugs) and all chronic kidney conditions in general. In tandem with this, Celery seed exerts a good detoxicant effect on the skin, with good results in psoriasis and the removal of lipofuscin pigments (a type of metabolic toxin) specifically; this has implications not only for flat age spots on the skin but also for macular degeneration and various neurodegenerative conditions such as Alzheimer's and Parkinson's disease.

Other uses for Celery seed include cystitis and other urinary infections resulting from a combined diuretic and antiseptic action; a pelvic decongestant action for pelvic congestion, including haemorrhoids; and possibly a dissolvent and analgesic effect on arthritic, urinary and arterial mineral deposits, including acute joint pain, urinary stones, bone spurs, gout and arteriosclerosis. Although completely non-toxic, non-irritant and non-sensitizing, Celery seed is slightly photosensitizing. As a uterine stimulant, it is best avoided during pregnancy until pre-labour. The oxidized oil should be avoided. Standard dilutions and doses apply.

**Cumin seed** (*Cuminum cyminum* L.) is the steam-distilled oil from the seed of the West Asian plant. Its fragrance is warm, sweet-spicy, like the crushed seed. Its chemistry is dominated by cumin aldehyde (20–40%) and various monoterpenes (notably terpinene 11–32%). Cumin oil is systemically both relaxing and stimulating, like Cardamom, and in herbal medicine was considered one of several warming seeds. The oil is a good nervous and cerebral sedative, SNS inhibitor, hypnotic and analgesic for hypertonic/tense conditions with insomnia, anxiety and acute and chronic pain. Its smooth-muscle relaxant, spasmolytic, anti-inflammatory action on the gut will treat stress-related indigestion, colic, IBS, colitis and IBD. At the same time, its gastrointestinal stimulant, carminative and aperitive actions address flatulence, distension and appetite loss. Both types of action together make Cumin a valuable all-round aromatic digestive remedy. As with Carrot seed, some success has also been noted with use as a thyroid/thyroxine regulator for hypothyroid syndrome. Cumin has also shown a good *antifungal* action, especially against Candida, and a *radiation-protectant* effect by increasing glutathione-S-transferase activity and CP450 liver enzymes.

**Caution:** Cumin is moderately photosensitizing, so exposure to sunlight should be avoided for 12 hours after application. Otherwise, normal dilutions and doses of this mild, non-toxic remedy apply. Avoid use during pregnancy and with babies and infants.

**Caraway seed** (*Carum carvi* L.) is the steam-distilled oil of the culinary plant with a warm, sweet, spicy odour similar to the dried seed; the oil is sometimes rectified to improve its odour. Its chemical profile is dominant in ketones 50–60% (incl. d-carvone <58%), monoterpenes 36–45%, d-limonene 26–46% and monoterpenols (incl. cis-carveol <6%). Caraway is a mild remedy with no cumulative toxicity and no skin irritation or sensitization. Essentially a warming stimulant for weak conditions, the oil is an excellent digestive stimulant and carminative for upper indigestion, distension, flatulence and aerophagia, and counteracts intestinal fermentation (like Laurel and others). Equally hepatobiliary stimulant, decongestant, choleretic and cholagogue, it addresses acute or chronic liver-gallbladder congestion with indigestion and right flank pains. Caraway is also valued for atonic/weak-type constipation, as it aids colonic contractions. It is also antiparasitic and specifically antiamoebic. In the respiratory system, Cumin acts as a mucolytic and expectorant, drying up congestion of excess mucus and sputum. The oil has also shown oestrogenic and galactagogue actions. Avoid use of the oxidized oil and all use during pregnancy. Moderate standard dilutions and doses of this mild, non-toxic remedy apply.

**Dill seed** (*Anethum graveolens* L.) is the steam-distilled oil of the culinary plant with a fresh, spicy fragrance similar to the crushed seed. Its name is said to derive from the Old Norse *dilla*, 'to lull', as in calming infant colic – but note that traditionally the seed was used by infusion, not the essential oil, which is contraindicated for infants. Dill seed oil highlights monoterpenes 25–50% (incl. d-limonene, phellandrene), ketones 40–60% (incl. carvone <50%) and coumarins <4%. Like traditional Greek medicine, modern practice values both seed and oil for its stimulant action on upper digestive functions. The oil's profile of constituents and therapeutic uses closely mirror that of Caraway as an upper digestive stimulant and carminative, and a liver-gallbladder stimulant decongestant. Dill seed is clearly another comprehensive remedy for most acute forms of upper indigestion. It can also be used for its mucolytic expectorant action in acute bronchitis with copious sputum, and its mild draining diuretic action for kidney weakness with mild toxicosis. Avoid use of the oxidized oil and all use during pregnancy, as well as with babies and infants. Moderate standard dilutions and doses of this mild, non-toxic remedy apply.

Two **Parsley seed** oils are worth noting. It is clinically crucial to distinguish Parsley oil distilled from the curly parsley, which contains little apiol, from the apiol-dominant Italian parsley. However, in case of unavailable analytical identification, both oils should be avoided.

Parsley seed or herb ct. pinene (*Petroselinum crispum* Mill. ct. pinene) is the fresh, woody-herbaceous steam-distilled oil of cultivated varieties of parsley, commonly called curly parsley. Both Parsley seed and Parsley herb oil are in limited production and used interchangeably or combined into a single oil. It is a medium-strength remedy with moderate cumulative toxicity, like Nutmeg oil: both oils contain myristicin, which may cause potential neurotoxicity. The oil shows high levels of monoterpenes (<75%), with α-pinene, β-pinene and β-phellandrene especially prominent, as well as myristicin (5–17%) and small amounts of sesquiterpenes, monoterpenols (incl. linalool <6%) and aldehydes.

Parsley seed is sometimes used in French medicine as a neuromuscular relaxant for treating epileptic seizures and similar nervous disturbances. Its good spasmolytic and anti-inflammatory actions are used in colitis, kidney colic, neurogenic bladder with dysuria and strangury, and spasmodic dysmenorrhoea. Like the tincture, Parsley seed oil also has a detoxicant diuretic action for oedema and metabolic toxicosis, and an emmenagogue action. Topical uses in 1–4% dilutions include the treatment of wounds, contusions, swollen glands and skin parasites such as head lice, tinea and scabies. Internal use should proceed with caution with a daily maximum of only 2 drops per day. The oil is contraindicated during pregnancy and breastfeeding, as well as generally in babies, infants and sensitive individuals.

Parsley seed ct. apiol (*Petroselinum sativum* L. ct. apiol) is the steam-distilled seed oil of Italian or flat-leaf parsley. It is a strong remedy with acute toxicity from its combined content in the constituents parsley apiol (11–68%), a phenol, and the phenolic ether myristicin (1–48%); it also contains <35% monoterpenes. Apiol is toxic to the liver and kidneys, and abortifacient, while myristicin is a neurotoxin. The oil is also a moderate skin irritant. Parsley seed ct. apiol might occasionally be used by trained practitioners for its strong emmenagogue action in chronic amenorrhoea, its spasmolytic action on smooth muscles and a fluidifying expectorant effect. However, because of its high toxicity, the oil is generally avoided, like the majority of Artemisia oils, and certainly never used during pregnancy and breastfeeding.

# Cinnamon Bark

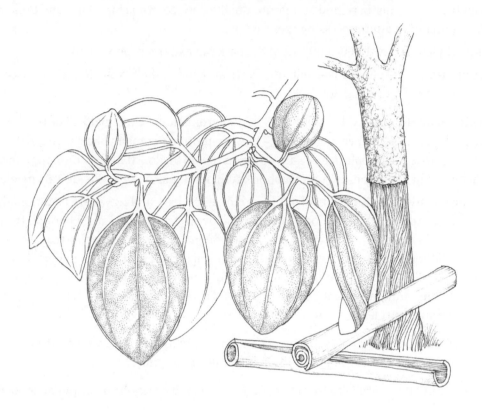

**Botanical source:** The bark of *Cinnamomum zeylanicum* Blume (syn. *Cinnamomum verum* J.S. Presl) (Lauraceae – laurel family), a tree of the humid tropics of Sri Lanka, India and Southeast Asia. Although various species of Cinnamomum are cultivated in other tropical regions, including Jamaica and various African countries, an oil from these is not usually distilled.

**Other names:** Ceylon cinnamon, Madagascar cinnamon, Seychelles cinnamon; Canelle de Ceylan (Fr), Zimt (Ge), Cinnamomo (It), Canela (Sp), Kayu manis (Indonesian, Malay), Dar sini (Ar)

**Appearance:** A mobile yellow-brown fluid that tends to darken and thicken with age and exposure to air; the odour is intensely sweet, spicy and tenacious

**Perfumery status:** A heart note of very high intensity and good persistence

**Extraction:** Steam or hydrodistillation of the bark, usually May and June or October and November; cohobation is often used to maximize oil yield and quality (as with Rose oil). The pieces of bark are usually dried in the sun for ten days, causing them to roll up into the familiar quills; after that they are also often soaked in cold water overnight to slightly ferment them before distillation the following morning.

Two qualities of Cinnamon oil are generally recognized: a superior type extracted from the tree's inner bark; and an inferior quality derived from chips, bark and broken quills remaining after processing these as spice.

**1 kg oil yield from:** 1,500–3,000 kg of the bark (an extremely poor yield)

**Production areas:** Sri Lanka (native), Southwest India, the Seychelles, Madagascar, the Comores, Burma and South Africa

**Typical constituents:** Aldehydes 62–78% (incl. aromatic cis-cinnamaldehyde 60–76%, benzaldehyde 2%) • phenol eugenol 2–13% • ester trans-cinnamyl acetate 0.3–10% • sesquiterpene β-caryophyllene 1–4% • monoterpenol linalool 0.2–5% • monoterpenes pinene, β-phellandrene 1–2% • camphor <1.4% • coumarins <1% • oxide 1,8 cineole

**Chance of adulteration:** Considerable, as cinnamon bark and leaves are traditionally often co-distilled. Cinnamon bark oil may also be stretched with Cassia bark oil from China or Vietnam (Cinnamomum spp.), itself often adulterated or reconstructed (see below). Other common adulterants of Cinnamon oil include synthetic cinnamaldehyde and eugenol, as well as the oils of Canella bark (*Canella winterana*), Clove (*Syzygium aromaticum*) and Laurel leaf (*Laurus nobilis*). Further diluents may include fuel oil, kerosene and petroleum.

**Related oils:** Of the 300-plus species of Cinnamomum found worldwide, the following are also produced as essential oils in their country of origin:

- Cinnamon leaf (also from *C. zeylanicum*) with its phenolic fresh-pungent notes

- Cassia bark (*C. cassia* J.S. Presl) from South China; this is by far the most common type of Cassia oil available

- Saigon or Vietnamese cassia bark (*C. loureirii* C. Nees) from Vietnam, Laos and Cambodia

- Indonesian or Korintje cassia bark (*C. burmannii* [C. Nees & T. Nees] Blume) from Indonesia, Malaysia and Borneo

All of these cheaper Cassia bark oils contain 75–85% cinnamaldehyde and are much more commonly used in the food and beverage industries, as well as in the spice trade, than the Ceylon cinnamon that is preferred for clinical practice. Virtually all of commercial cinnamon spice worldwide is derived from one or other type of Cassia cinnamon, not Ceylon cinnamon (see also 'Related oils' at the end of this 'Cinnamon Bark' section).

# Therapeutic Functions and Indications

## Specific symptomatology – *All applications*

Emotional coldness, withdrawal, apathy, discouragement, loss of motivation, listlessness, depression, loss of sex drive, low self-confidence, chronic physical and mental fatigue, debility, somnolence, cold hands and feet, cold skin, dizziness, palpitations, cold abdomen, weak low back, scanty or stopped periods, painful periods, chronic vaginal discharges, indigestion with bloating and constipation, digestive colic, diarrhoea with undigested food, chronic or recurring infections

## Psychological – *Aromatic diffusion*

**Essential PNEI function and indication:** Stimulant in weakness conditions, sensory integrating in sensory disintegration conditions

**Possible brain dynamics:** Increases basal ganglia functioning

**Fragrance category:** Middle tone with sweet and pungent notes

**Indicated psychological disorders:** Depression, catatonia, schizoid states, sensory integration disorder

### Promotes courage and self-confidence

- Discouragement with apathy, poor motivation, emotional burnout
- Low self-confidence and self-esteem, self-neglect, depression

### Promotes disinhibition and integration

- Emotional, sensual and sexual repression and inhibition; loss of libido
- Sensing/feeling disconnection and conflict
- Sensory deprivation, disconnection or disintegration

## Physiological – *Gel cap, suppository, external applications*

Use with caution.

**Therapeutic status**: Mild remedy with no cumulative toxicity

**Topical safety status**: Strong skin irritant, sensitizing, possibly slightly photosensitizing

**Tropism:** Circulatory, nervous, digestive, urinary, reproductive systems

**Essential diagnostic function:** Stimulates and warms asthenic/cold and restores hypotonic/weak terrain conditions

PRIMARILY STIMULANT AND WARMING:

***strong systemic nervous and central arterial circulatory stimulant, SNS stimulant, peripheral vasodilator, capillary stimulant:*** a wide range of chronic hypotonic (weak) and asthenic (cold) conditions with circulatory deficiency, cold extremities (esp. the feet), chronic physical and mental debility and fatigue; incl. convalescence, hypothermia, Raynaud's disease, CFS

- ***cerebral stimulant:*** mental debility, neurasthenia, depression, somnolence

- ***gastrointestinal stimulant, carminative, antifermentative, antiseptic:*** digestive atony with indigestion, flatulence, constipation; intestinal dysbiosis

- ***gastrointestinal relaxant, spasmolytic, analgesic:*** diarrhoea, IBS, colic, colitis

- ***reproductive stimulant, aphrodisiac:*** sexual debility, frigidity, impotence

- ***strong uterine stimulant, emmenagogue:*** amenorrhoea, oligomenorrhoea

- ***respiratory stimulant, expectorant:*** chronic bronchitis

- ***strong antioxidant***

MISCELLANEOUS ACTIONS:

***antipyretic:*** malaria, dengue, typhoid and other tropical fevers

***astringent mucostatic:*** vaginitis with leucorrhoea

***astringent haemostatic:*** passive haemorrhage, esp. from lungs or intestines, incl. haemoptysis, haematuria, haemafecia, metrorrhagia

***progesteronic:*** progesterone deficiency syndrome with low libido, dysmenorrhoea, fatigue

***anticoagulant***

***antitoxic:*** toxic animal bites and stings

ANTIMICROBIAL ACTIONS:

***broad-spectrum anti-infective, antimicrobial, detoxicant:*** a wide range of infections, esp. chronic, gastrointestinal, urinary

- ***strong broad-spectrum antibacterial:*** bacterial infections both gram-positive and gram-negative, incl. H. pylori, Staph. aureus, Strep. faecalis, Pseudomonas aeruginosa, incl. gastroenteritis, colitis, dysentery, microbial enterotoxicosis, food poisoning, intestinal toxicosis; cystitis, nephritis, vaginitis; malaria, typhoid; bronchitis, pharyngitis/strep throat, pyorrhoea

- *strong antiparasitic, anthelmintic (larvicidal):* amoebiasis, amoebic dysentery, roundworms (Ascaris), tapeworms (Taenia), pinworms/enterobiasis, scabies, pediculosis

- *broad-spectrum antifungal:* fungal infections, incl. Candida spp., Aspergillus spp., fungal cystitis, lung and kidney TB

- *antiviral:* misc. viral infections, esp. respiratory, gastrointestinal, urogenital; incl. influenza, colds, SARS

SYNERGISTIC COMBINATIONS

All for short-term use only: see 'Therapeutic precautions' below.

- Cinnamon bark + Thyme ct. thymol: strong nervous, cerebral and arterial stimulant for severe chronic asthenic/cold conditions, esp. with depression, debility

- Cinnamon bark + Thyme ct. thymol: strong broad-spectrum antibacterial, antifungal and antiparasitic for a wide range of severe acute or chronic bacterial, fungal and parasitic infections, esp. respiratory, intestinal, with colitis, gastroenteritis, dysentery, parasites

- Cinnamon bark + Clove bud: strong broad-spectrum antibacterial, antifungal and antiparasitic for a wide range of severe acute bacterial, fungal and parasitic infections, especially gastrointestinal, in cold, weak terrain

COMPLEMENTARY COMBINATIONS

All for short-term use only: see 'Therapeutic precautions' below.

- Cinnamon bark + Juniper berry/Laurel: gastrointestinal stimulant, detoxicant and antifermentative for chronic digestive atony with intestinal bacterial dysbiosis and microbial toxicosis, intestinal sepsis or putrefaction; with flatulence, colic, diarrhoea

- Cinnamon bark + Nutmeg: intestinal relaxant, broad-spectrum antimicrobial, spasmolytic, analgesic and antidiarrhoeal for acute intestinal infections with painful colic, diarrhoea; food poisoning, enteritis, colitis, dysentery

- Cinnamon bark + Tea tree: strong antipyretic and antimicrobial for acute and chronic tropical infections with fever, incl. dengue, malaria, typhoid

- Cinnamon bark + Cistus: astringent haemostatic for passive haemorrhage, incl. haemoptysis, haematuria, haemafecia, metrorrhagia

- Cinnamon bark + Ginger/Juniper berry: strong uterine stimulant, emmenagogue for chronic amenorrhoea, oligomenorrhoea in asthenic/cold conditions with poor circulation

- Cinnamon bark + Scotch pine/Nutmeg: reproductive stimulant, aphrodisiac for chronic loss of libido

## TOPICAL – *Liniment, lotion*

See 'Pharmacological precautions' below.

**Skin care:** Not used

*rubefacient, analgesic:* local pain conditions

*antiparasitic, antiviral:* skin parasites, incl. lice; warts

*ant repellent, mosquito repellent (A. aegypti)*

**Therapeutic precautions:** Cinnamon bark oil is a strong warming stimulant to nervous, circulatory and most organ functions, and is therefore contraindicated in hypersthenic/hot, hypertonic/tense and dry conditions; this includes high fever, acute inflammation, hypertension, agitation and insomnia. Cinnamon is best kept for treating chronic, not acute, asthenic/cold and hypotonic/weak conditions. Because of this, and because it is a uterine stimulant, Cinnamon bark is also contraindicated during pregnancy and breastfeeding, as well as in babies, infants, children under age five, and sensitive individuals.

Internal use is best limited to a single eight-day course, and then always within a formula rather than on its own. Long-term, full-dose internal use is discouraged as it may also cause liver damage; the adjunctive use of liver restorative oils, herbs or nutrients in a formula is recommended. Inhalation with an essential oil nebulizer is not recommended to avoid serious irritation to the mucous membrane.

**Pharmacological precautions:** Cinnamon bark oil is highly irritant and sensitizing to the skin and mucosa because of its content in cinnamaldehyde and eugenol; topical, dermal and aroma-atomizer use should therefore be entirely avoided. Again, all use of Cinnamon is contraindicated in babies, infants and young children, and only with caution in patients on anticoagulant (blood-thinning) or diabetic medication, or with peptic ulcer and bleeding disorders.

**Preparations:**

- Diffusor: 1 drop in water

- Massage oil: None

- Liniment: 0.25–1% dilution in vegetable oil as part of a blend for short-term use

- Gel cap: 1–2 drops with some olive oil for short-term use, e.g. an eight-day course; and usually as part of a formula; the maximum daily dose is 5 drops. Like all strongly stimulant oils, Cinnamon bark should always be combined with other oils to soften its intensity and enhance treatment results; especially with sweet, monoterpenol-rich oils such as Palmarosa, Tea tree, Lavender or Thyme ct. linalool.

## Chinese Medicine Functions and Indications

**Aroma energy:** Pungent, sweet, woody

**Movement:** Circulating

**Warmth:** Warm to hot

**Meridian tropism:** Kidney, Spleen, Lung

**Five-Element affinity:** Earth, Water

**Essential function:** To tonify the Yang, warm the interior and strengthen the Shen

1.  <u>Tonifies the Yang, warms the Kidney and strengthens the Shen and libido</u>

    - **Yang deficiency with Shen weakness**, with physical and mental fatigue, cold hands and feet, dizziness, palpitations, recurrent infections, apathy:

      Rosemary/Black spruce/Ginger/Thyme ct. thymol

    - **Kidney Yang deficiency** with low sex drive, frigidity, impotence, weak loins and knees, fatigue, cold skin and extremities, vaginal discharges:

      Ginger/Black spruce/Clove bud

2.  <u>Warms and harmonizes the Middle Warmer, resolves damp and relieves pain and distension</u>

    - **Stomach-Spleen empty cold (Spleen Yang deficiency with cold)** with nausea, vomiting, epigastric or abdominal pain, chronic loose stool, morning diarrhoea:

      Juniper berry/Ginger/Nutmeg/Clove

    - **Stomach-Spleen damp-cold** with chronic diarrhoea, undigested food in stool, cold limbs:

      Patchouli/Nutmeg/Black pepper

    - **Stomach-Spleen toxic-damp** with indigestion, abdominal bloating, diarrhoea:

      Patchouli/Niaouli/Thyme ct. linalool

3. **Warms and activates the Lower Warmer, breaks up stagnation and promotes menstruation**

- **Lower Warmer Blood and Qi stagnation with cold**, with scanty or absent periods, loss of sex drive, cold extremities:

  Rosemary/Niaouli/Juniper berry

REMARKS

Cinnamon is one of the very few aromatics that are an integral part of all the world's major traditional cultures and medical systems. As always, Cinnamon today is an essential – perhaps the most essential – remedy in Chinese, Ayurvedic and traditional Greek medicine. This is partly because, practically speaking, the presence of two major sources of Cinnamon, the Ceylon (Sri Lanka) type and the Chinese cassia type, made and still make possible almost worldwide availability. Ceylon cinnamon is native to Western Sri Lanka and the Malabar Coast of Southwest India, while Cassia cinnamon is native to the South China provinces of Guangdong, Guangxi and Yunnan. Moreover, what make Cinnamon equally essential is the very fundmental nature of the spice remedy itself: supporting human warmth in all its aspects – physical, emotional and spiritual. Cinnamon is nothing less than the iconic aromatic that has fostered and sustained human warm-bloodedness since prehistory and is thus totally embedded in our collective warmth psyche both conscious and unconscious.

The presence of these two major sources of Cinnamon makes it historically difficult to identify which type is actually being referred to in most of past literature; and in most cases this is not an issue because of their similarity. However, it is known that medieval Arabic and Jewish traders of cinnamon in their best interest kept their Eastern sources under wraps, and vague at best; some of them might not even have known their distant sources. Many of the fantastic stories they invented for this purpose are retold in the nightly tales of *One Thousand and One Nights*. Although there are Arabic texts that specify Ceylon cinnamon as coming from that island in the 13th century, it seems that the two cinnamon types were clearly differentiated only in late 16th-century Europe. Nervertheless, certain practitioners throughout history had always been very clear about the two main types. The celebrated Greek physician Claudios Galenos (Galen for short), for example, declared using five types of Cinnamon in his practice. The Roman historian Pliny describes both main types in his first-century *Historia Naturalis*. Regardless, the barks of both Ceylon and Cassia cinnamon have been extensively valued and traded since known history.

Because of its iconic status, cinnamon (either type) has always been associated with monarchy, often as political gifts, and with worship of the human and cosmic divine in the form of ceremonial perfumes and sacred aromatic offerings to the gods and goddesses. The important ancient port town of Alexandria in Egypt imported cinnamon around 2000 BC by way of the Arabian Peninsula and the Red Sea; cinnamon was a key ingredient in Kyphi, the sacred incense offered daily in huge quantities to the Egyptian gods. The Hebrew Bible contains numerous mentions of both cinnamon types, the 'sweet cinnamon' qinnamon and the cassia cinnamon ketsiah. The latter was part of the holy anointing oil and the Ketoret, the consecrated incense burnt on the incense altar at the original Temple service in Jerusalem. The Greek temple of Apollo at Miletos on the West coast of Anatolia (Turkey today) still shows an inscription recording the gift of Kinamonon (cinnamon) and Malabathron (a herbal formula) from its Athenian rulers. It was the Greek poetess Sappho, however, who (perhaps not surprisingly) penned the first Greek reference to Kasia (cassia) in the seventh century BC.

Since the days of those ancient cultures, however, both cinnamons have more often been associated with culinary needs rather than divine aspirations. The long history of its sourcing in South China and the Malabar Coast, and their trading along the desert and maritime Silk Roads, involves Arabic and Jewish traders (up to the end of the overland Silk Roads in Izmir or Alexandria), Venetian traders (from Alexandria to Venice), Ottoman traders (along the desert Silk Roads), Dutch traders (maritime from their colonial plantations in Ceylon since 1556) and the British East India Company since 1796 (Nabhan 2014). Certainly, cinnamon, and especially the far more common Cassia cinnamon, has found its way into most of the world's great spice mixes, including Chinese five-spice powder, Middle Eastern baharat and Mexican moles and recaudos.

However, when using Cinnamon as an aromatic remedy in essential oil form, it becomes crucial to use Ceylon cinnamon oil, not Cassia oil. Although both types are routinely adulterated (see above), Ceylon cinnamon is less so. As was usual, the aromatic water of Ceylon cinnamon was being produced long before the essential oil itself, certainly during the 14th century. As the aromatic water came over during distillation, attentive distillers noticed the heavy oil sinking to the bottom of their Florentine flask instead of floating to the top, as do most oils. Eventually they decided to separate that heavy, deep-orange liquid. By 1540, Valerius Cordus was recording Cinnamon oil production and use in herbal medicine. By 1582, the oil was a taxable remedy in established Berlin apothecaries; it has remained a pharmaceutical staple ever since. Numerous compound formulas in tincture form include a small amount of cinnamon bark or oil to make them more warming, stimulating and moving.

As a physiological remedy, Cinnamon oil is accompanied by several important considerations if it is to be used successfully. Firstly, any topical or oral use needs to take into account its extremely skin-irritant (dermocaustic) and sensitizing nature. Consequently, the oil is infrequently used topically, and only in gel caps, combined with other oils, and at the right minimal dosage internally. Secondly, internal use needs to consider its extremely warming, stimulating nature and adhere to its attached therapeutic and pharmacological cautions.

With those caveats stated, Cinnamon remains an excellent systemic stimulant working strongly through both central nervous and arterial stimulation. The combination of high-level cinnamaldehyde and eugenol is considered key here.

Its essential indication in functional medicine is cold and weak terrain conditions, regardless of symptoms. Chronic physical and mental debility and fatigue are its major indications here. The Chinese medicine idiom here is a warming tonification of the Kidney Yang, the fire of ming men, with all its implications for sustained health. Cinnamon is a particularly strong uterine stimulant or emmenagogue for chronic amenorrhoea, especially in a woman with cold-weak terrain, and will also act as an aphrodisiac for chronic loss of sexual drive. Cold, atonic conditions of the gut, especially the intestines, will also hugely benefit, all the more so if a bacterial or parasitic infection is present, or if the microfloral terrain is dysbiotic in any way.

Cinnamon is one of the very best broad-spectrum antibacterial remedies, whether given on its own or combined with other oils or herbs. As such, it can act as either a terrain remedy when the infection is chronic, or a symptom remedy when it is acute. The oil is now known to selectively act against gut pathogens only, leaving healthy blooms undisturbed. However, Cinnamon is certainly not the only oil with this characteristic, despite the common assumption that phenol-rich oils will to some degree inhibit all commensal intestinal strains.

Lesser but no less effective indications for Cinnamon are tropical intermittent fevers, such as dengue and malaria; French doctors used to combine it with Cinchona bark (containing quinquina) for treating and preventing malaria. Likewise, its astringent and haemostatic actions for passive haemorrhage and vaginal discharges. For haemorrhage, Cinnamon water (hydrosol) was much used in herbal pharmacy, as well as for correcting the unpleasant taste of other remedies in a tincture. There are certainly better oils for treating vaginal discharges. Concerning a purported hypoglycaemiant action, it turns out that Cassia cinnamon, not Ceylon cinnamon, was probably used for the study in question (Henriette's Herbal 2006); strictly speaking therefore, the result remains inconclusive.

Cinnamon by olfaction is also an important psychological remedy for cold and weakness on the emotional and soul level. Its intensely sweet, pungent aromatic qualities rarely fail to impart a deep warmth to heart and spirit – promoting courage and self-confidence in those discouraged, demoralized and often isolated by a setback in life, especially in matters of love. In these withdrawn and often depressed individuals, Cinnamon is able to stoke the missing emotional fire – the nurture, motivation and courage needed to make positive changes for a more fulfilled existence. Here the fragrance fosters the healthy pleasure principle for individual fulfilment, including the promise of a fully embodied sensuality as well as a heart-centred love. Like Jasmine absolute and other oils that integrate the senses, Cinnamon is also for sensory as well as emotional disconnection and disintegration.

In a larger context, Cinnamon supports a genuine desire for life itself. Where discouragement and disorientation result from severe emotional loss or betrayal, the fragrance can be nothing less than deeply life- and self-affirming for those unable to meet these challenges.

**Related oils:** The following two kinds of Cinnamon oil should be clearly differentiated from the bark oil.

**Cinnamon leaf**, sweet, spicy, pungent, and somewhat clove-like in fragrance, has the phenol eugenol (68–87%) as its main constituent, not cinnamic aldehyde, present only <2% in the leaf; the other notable constituent is a cluster of esters <9%. Like Pimenta berry and Pimenta leaf oils, Cinnamon leaf oil is a wide-acting antimicrobial and a deeply warming stimulant remedy. Like Pimenta berry/leaf, it stimulates nervous, circulatory and neuromuscular functions, and should be considered for internal conditions with chronic cold and weak terrain. A strong anti-infective and immune stimulant, it is much used locally for mouth, throat and bronchial infections, as well as internally for urogenital and intestinal infections. In addition to being antibacterial, it has a good antifungal action and is moderately antiviral and antiparasitic. Cinnamon leaf excels with chronic infections of all kinds seen in devitalized, weak-cold terrain. Because generally far less skin irritant (dermocaustic) than Cinnamon, Clove or Oregano, the same precautions, dilutions and doses as for Pimenta berry apply.

**Cassia bark** (*C. cassia* J.S. Presl) from South China, Vietnam, Laos and Burma, also simply known as Cassia, Chinese cinnamon, or Rou gui in Mandarin, appears as a dark-brown liquid with an intense spicy-sweet, warm, somewhat woody odour. Its cinnamaldehyde levels are always 75–90%, possessing a virtually identical character and use as Cinnamon bark oil. Unfortunately, commercial Cassia bark is very common and often adulterated with Himalayan cedarwood oil, Gurjun balsam oil, rosin (colophonium) and/or petroleum; and occasionally completely reconstructed with synthetic cinnamaldehyde as the main constituent. Selection and therapeutic use of Cassia oil should clearly be approached with great circumspection.

# Cistus

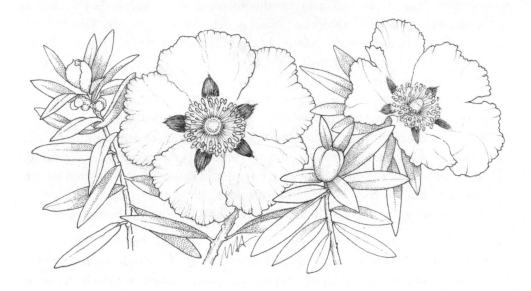

**Botanical source:** The leafy twigs of *Cistus ladaniferus* Curtis, *C. creticus* L. (Cistaceae – rockrose family), a shrub of dry Mediterranean and Middle East regions

**Other names:** Gum rockrose; Ciste ladanifère (Fr)

**Appearance:** A viscous dark yellow or amber liquid with a warm, sweet, spicy, balsamic, ambery, woody odour

**Perfumery status:** A base note of high intensity and good tenacity

**Extraction:** The leafy twigs of the rockrose bush in flower are collected in late summer. Extraction of the essential oil usually occurs in two stages. First is the steam distillation of the flowering twigs into essential oil. Next, the distillation water is redistilled with hexane and the resultant oil added to the steam-distilled oil. This is a variation on the classic cohobation method used in Rose oil production.

**1 kg yield from:** 18–25 kg (an excellent yield)

**Production areas:** Spain, Portugal, Morocco and Italy, although the plant is native to the mountain islands of the Eastern Mediterranean

**Typical constituents:** Monoterpenes 15–67% (incl. α-pinene 3–50%, camphene <10%, p-menthatriene 3%, d-limonene 2%, γ-terpinene 1.6%, p-cymene <4%, α-dimethyl styrene 1.6%) • ketones 3–10% (incl. trimethylcyclohexanone 2–6%, isopinocamphone <3%, verbenone 2%, fenchone 1%, acetophenone 1.5%) • monoterpenols 6–10% (incl. pinocarveol 3%, borneol 2%, linalool <3%) • sesquiterpenes 5% (incl. aromadendrene

1%, α-amorphene 1%, sabinene) • sesquiterpenols 6% • esters 3–5% (incl. bornyl acetate <4%, linalyl acetate, methyl benzoate) • oxide 1,8 cineole • phenols eugenol 1%, thymol

**Note:** The levels of one of Cistus's key constituents, α-pinene, can vary widely. This is a natural variation, not a chemotype phenomenon.

**Chance of adulteration:** Fair; possibly with other oil sources of α-pinene if levels are low; possibly with Gurjun balsam (*Dipterocarpus turbinatus* C.F. Gaertn.)

**Related oils:** Labdanum resin or crude labdanum is a separate product of the rockrose and the base for production of both an absolute and an essential oil. Labdanum absolute is produced by solvent extraction of the resin by way of the concrete for perfumery purposes; it is a thick, semi-solid mass with a soft, sweet, balsamic odour. Labdanum oil is distilled either from the absolute or (more rarely) directly from the resin. It has a complex sweet, soft, ambra, woody note. Its chemistry is complex and variable, but similar to that of Cistus oil. Its therapeutic uses too have been suggested to resemble those of Cistus (Rhind 2012). Labdanum resin is also obtained from other Cistus species, most notably *C. incanus* and other subspecies.

## Therapeutic Functions and Indications

### SPECIFIC SYMPTOMATOLOGY – *All applications*

Discouragement, apathy, insecurity, anxiety, unknown fears, negative thoughts, insomnia, feels easily stressed or overwhelmed, poor perseverance, poor willpower and motivation, loss of self-confidence, poor emotional boundaries, self-neglect, diarrhoea with bloody stool, menstrual flooding, varicose veins, chronic cough with expectoration, autoimmune disorders, all symptoms worse from stress

### PSYCHOLOGICAL – *Aromatic diffusion, whole-body massage*

**Essential PNEI function and indication:** Stimulant in weakness conditions

**Possible brain dynamics:** Increases prefrontal cortex and basal ganglia functioning

**Fragrance category:** Base tone with woody and pungent notes

**Indicated psychological disorders:** ADD, depression, psychotic and schizoid conditions

### PROMOTES WILLPOWER AND PERSEVERANCE

- Low willpower or strength, indecisiveness
- Discouragement, low perseverance
- Mental and emotional burnout, shock

PROMOTES SELF-CONFIDENCE AND MOTIVATION

- Low self-confidence and self-esteem, self-neglect, negativity
- Loss of motivation with apathy, procrastination

## PHYSIOLOGICAL – *Gel cap, suppository, external applications*

**Therapeutic status:** Mild remedy with no cumulative toxicity

**Topical safety status:** Non-toxic, non-irritant, non-sensitizing

**Tropism:** Nervous, respiratory, digestive, musculoskeletal systems

**Essential diagnostic function:** Restores hypotonic/weak and decongests congestive/damp terrain conditions

PRIMARILY RESTORATIVE AND DECONGESTANT:

*strong astingent, tissue regenerator and haemostatic:* diarrhoea with bloody stool; dysentery, ulcerative colitis, rectocolitis, inflammatory bowel disease, incl. Crohn's disease; bleeding haemorrhoids; menorrhagia, metrorrhagia; nosebleed

*strong astringent venous restorative and pelvic decongestant:* varicose veins, phlebitis; pelvic congestion with haemorrhoids, menorrhagia, prostate congestion (BPH)

*anti-inflammatory, analgesic, immune regulator:* dermatitis; autoimmune conditions, incl. rheumatoid arthritis, Crohn's disease, arteritis, MS

*stimulant and mucolytic expectorant, antitussive:* chronic bronchitis, coughs with copious sputum

*diuretic*

PRIMARILY RELAXANT:

*mild nervous and cerebral sedative, PNS stimulant:* chonic mild to moderate anxiety, insomnia, chronic stress-related conditions

ANTIMICROBIAL ACTIONS:

*antiviral, immunostimulant:* common cold, flu, childhood viral infections, incl. measles, chickenpox, whooping cough, scarlet fever; dysentery; HIV

*antibacterial:* bacterial infections incl. Escherichia coli, staphylococcus aureus; urinary tract and gastrointestinal infections

*anti-fungal:* fungal infections, incl. Candida albicans

SYNERGISTIC COMBINATIONS

- Cistus + Myrrh: strong astringent, haemostatic, anti-inflammatory, anti-infective and tissue regenerator for diarrhoea with bloody or mucopurulent stool; incl. enteritis, dysentery, ulcerative colitis

- Cistus + Cypress: strong haemostatic for bleeding haemorrhoids, haemafecia, metrorrhagia, epistaxis

- Cistus + Mastic: strong astringent pelvic and venous decongestant for pelvic blood congestion, varicose veins, haemorrhoids

- Cistus + Scotch pine/Mastic: mucolytic expectorant and respiratory restorative for chronic bronchitis with copious sputum

- Cistus + Frankincense: anti-inflammatory autoimmune regulator in autoimmune conditions, incl. rheumatoid arthritis, lupus, Crohn's disease, arteritis, MS

COMPLEMENTARY COMBINATIONS

- Cistus + Atlas cedarwood: nervous sedative for chronic insomnia, anxiety, unknown fears, chronic stress-related conditions

- Cistus + Tea tree: antiviral and antipyretic in childhood viral fevers, incl. chickenpox, measles, German measles

- Cistus + Geranium: strong uterine haemostatic for menorrhagia and metrorrhagia

- Cistus + Vetiver: immune regulator and anti-inflammatory in autoimmune conditions, incl. rheumatoid arthritis, Crohn's disease, rectocolitis, IBD, MS

- Cistus + Lavender: nervous and cerebral sedative for chonic anxiety, insomnia

- Cistus + Geranium: strong astringent and haemostatic tissue regenerator for wounds, sores, ulcers, etc., incl. with bleeding (topical use)

- Cistus + Spike lavender + Laurel: tissue regenerator for scars (topical use)

## TOPICAL – *Liminent, ointment, cream, compress and other cosmetic preparations*

**Skin care:** Mature skin type

*vulnerary, tissue regenerator, astringent, antiseptic:* wounds, fissures, sores, ulcers, esp. chronic, non-healing, painful, purulence; wrinkles, scars *styptic:* bleeding (incl. from wounds), haemorrhage

*analgesic, anti-inflammatory:* muscle aches and pain

*tick repellent:* ticks (Borrelia burgdorferi)

**Therapeutic precautions:** Cistus oil is very drying and is generally contraindicated in dry conditions, especially dry respiratory conditions with dry cough, dry mouth and constipation.

**Pharmacological precautions:** Nebulizer inhalation is contraindicated for Cistus because of its neurotoxic ketone constituents. Using caution during pregnancy is traditional. Avoid use in babies and infants because of its pungent, high-monoterpene nature. Rare reports of dermatitis and photosensitivity also exist with topical use, possibly from the use of an oxidized oil.

**Preparations:**

- Diffusor: 1 drop in water

- Massage oil: 1–3% in vegetable oil

- Liniment: 5–10% dilution in vegetable oil

- Gel cap: 2–3 drops with olive oil

- 1–3% dilution in Cistus tincture for best haemostatic action

## Chinese Medicine Functions and Indications

**Aroma energy:** Woody, pungent

**Movement:** Stabilizing

**Warmth:** Neutral

**Meridian tropism:** Lung, Large Intestine, Heart, Triple Heater

**Five-Element affinity:** Metal, Fire

**Essential function:** To astringe fluids, resolve damp and stop bleeding

1. **Astringes the Lung, expels phlegm, dries damp and relieves coughing**

   - **Lung phlegm-damp** with expectoration of thick viscous sputum, full cough with chest pain, blood in sputum:

     Cypress/Myrrh/Green myrtle

2. **Astringes the Lower Warmer, astringes fluids and stops bleeding and discharge**

   - **Large Intestine damp-heat/damp-cold** with bloody diarrhoea, purulent bloody stool:

Myrrh/Black spruce/Sandalwood/Tea tree/Cinnamon

- **Menorrhagia and metrorrhagia:**

Geranium/Rose

REMARKS

Cistus oil is distilled from the gum rockrose bush native to Cyprus, Rhodes, Crete and other islands of the Eastern Mediterranean Sea. In its native Cyprus, the rockrose was sacred to the goddess Aphrodite in Paphos. In the intense Mediterranean sun the shrub spreads a warm, earthy fragrance around itself as it develops a sticky, brown protective resin in its glandular hairs to maintain hydration. While today Cistus oil is distilled directly from the resinous leaves and twigs, it was the resin itself, called crude Labdanum, that was traditionally used in medicine and perfumery. The Greek historian Herodotus described how shepherds collected the valuable resin either by manually sweeping rockrose shrubs with leather-thonged rakes or simply by allowing their sheep and goats to graze freely among them and then later by combing their beards to separate the resin.

Labdanum resin is one of the earliest aromatic substances of ancient Asia Minor, along with Myrrh, Mastic and Spikenard. It finds mention in the Bible most likely as Shecheleth and was a key ingredient of Egyptian perfumes and sacred incense mixes, including the famous Kyphi. The resin was also highly esteemed in ancient Arabic and Andalusian culture. Whether used to scent homes or to stage a fragrant sacred space by censing, the crude resin was traditionally almost always mixed with Benzoin – and still is today. The resin was used medically since earliest days for its strong astringent, haemostatic and vulnerary properties, both topically and internally. Cistus oil shares all of Labdanum's functions and actions so prized by generations of Western herbalists and pharmacists. Like many essential oils, its origins go back to the Renaissance period, when Cistus oil was distilled from the crude resin with wine or wine spirits (then called Aqua Vitae).

Like the traditional remedy Labdanum, Cistus oil is recognized today as the most effective astringent, haemostatic and vulnerary aromatic remedy of the materia aromatica. It enjoys all the indications common to any effective herbal remedy of the same kind and finds extensive internal and topical use. Cistus's key indications are discharge and haemorrhage, as in dysentery or other diarrhoea with bloody stool; inflammatory bowel disease, vaginal bleeding of all kinds and bleeding haemorrhoids. In rectocolitis, Cistus's valuable immune regulating action also comes into play. Autoimmune conditions with chronic inflammation of many kinds will respond to it, including multiple sclerosis (MS). The remedy is also a prime astringent decongestant to pelvic and venous congestion; it should often be included in formulas for varicosities of any kind as it has shown to increase the elasticity of the large veins (Faucon 2015).

Although Cistus clearly excels for symptom relief both acute and chronic, it is nevertheless possible to pin down a systemic effect through its action on the nervous system. Cistus essentially treats terrain that is weak, damp and tense. Acting as a sedative for anxiety and insomnia, the oil is especially useful when discharge and congestion involve chronic negative stress. In the chest area, Cistus with its abundant pungent monoterpenes is an excellent drying, mucolytic expectorant for wet, productive coughs. French practitioners also make extensive use of its excellent antiviral action for viral childhood infections in particular. Topically, the oil finds applications in both a medical and cosmetic context, its key action being tissue regeneration – an important action in any skin lesion.

It comes as no surprise that Cistus also makes for a valuable psychological remedy. Sweet, woody and spicy, the oil by olfaction exerts a strong centring and strengthening effect that is soon followed by a feeling of calm upliftment and protection. For instance, Cistus can provide strength and comfort in cases of shock or acute burnout with feelings of cold and emptiness. In terms of terrain treatment, Cistus is for the individual who is oversensitive to others and to the environment. Lacking both emotional and sensory boundaries, this person becomes overly influenced by others and therefore vulnerable to emotional and sensory overwhelm. Cistus is an invaluable ally for the process of reclaiming the truth of one's true and essential convictions, and for helping one fully embrace and embody those inner convictions. In so doing, the oil can help foster a self-identity founded on inner source rather than on external role models, allowing one's true personality to shine and one's innate warmth to radiate – a function that is traditionally linked to the thymus gland.

Like Frankincense, Cistus manages the complex task of helping us be fully embodied while reaching for spirit. In ancient Hebrew and Egyptian cultures, its fragrance in a sacred or ritual context allowed for connection to the divine – not just divine beings, but also divinity within.

**Mastic** (*Pistacia lentiscus* L.) has very similar uses to Cistus. The viscous, greenish-brown oil is steam-distilled from the twigs and branches, and sometimes from the oleoresin, of a shrubby tree in the cashew (Anacardaceae) family. These are collected in countries around the Mediterranean, especially Morocco, Spain and the Greek island of Chios. The resin has a long history of use in ancient Middle Eastern cultures that resembles Myrrh: for censing, anointing and other purification rituals, for embalming and as an aromatic remedy and spice. Venetian and Genovese aromatarii imported the resin during the Middle Ages; the distilled oil was first produced in the 1450s. It soon became established within herbal medicine and pharmacy, alongside the tincture, as an important aromatic astringent and haemostatic remedy. In the East Mediterranean, the resin is traditionally used as a masticatory to freshen the breath and strengthen the gums, as a flavouring agent for liqueurs such as ouzo (Greece), raki (Turkey, Crete) and mastika (Chios, Macedonia, Bulgaria), as well as for sweet things such as sweets, pastries, puddings and ice creams. Like Turpentine resin, Mastic resin also furnishes a traditional perfume, varnish and paint thinner. The resin is also used in traditional dentistry as a tooth filling, often with alum and Clove oil, for tooth decay.

Mastic has a fresh, pungent, balsamic odour and shows high levels of monoterpenes <55% (incl. α-pinene 8–18%, myrcene 5–15%, sabinene 3–10%, d-limonene and δ-3-carene), with smaller amounts of sesquiterpenes and their alcohols <8%, and the monoterpenol terpinene-4-ol <5% and bornyl acetate <2%. It has mild therapeutic status with no cumulative toxicity and is non-irritant and non-sensitizing to the skin.

Mastic's main use is for its strong astringent venous, lymphatic and venous restorative actions in severe congestive conditions such as pelvic blood congestion and its typical symptoms, including haemorrhoids; venous and lymphatic congestion with varicose veins, phlebitis and varicose ulcers. This coupled with its diuretic action makes it also useful for leg oedema and cellulite. Mastic is specifically also a strong prostatic decongestant for prostate congestion with swelling (BPH). Here the remedy is also anti-inflammatory and useful for thrombophlebitis. As an antiseptic stimulant and mucolytic expectorant, the oil treats congestive bronchitis with copious sputum, and as an antiseptic mucostatic diuretic, urinary infections with mucous discharges. Atonic gut conditions also respond well to Mastic's stimulant, carminative action, especially flatulence, colic and gastric ulcers. Topically, the oil acts as a vulnerary and antihaematoma agent for bruises and haematoma. By inhalation, Mastic exerts a good nasal decongestant effect, like other fresh pungent, monoterpene-rich oils. The same dilutions, doses and precautions as for Cistus oil apply.

# Clove Bud

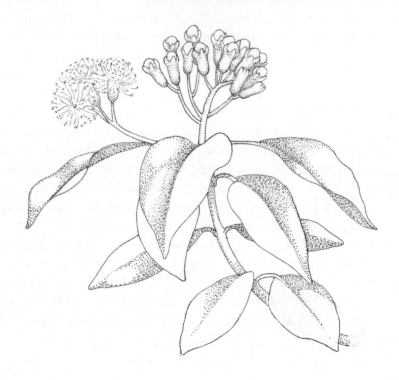

**Botanical source:** The flowerbud of *Syzygium aromaticum* (L.) Merr. & Perry (syn. *Eugenia aromatica* Kuntze, *E. caryophyllata* Thunb.) (Myrtaceae – myrtle family), a forest tree of the lowland maritime tropics of Indonesia and the Indian Ocean islands

**Other names:** Clou de girofle (Fr), Gewürznelke (Ge), Chiodo di garofano (It), Clavo (Sp), Cengkeh (Indonesian, Malay), Ding xiang (Mandarin), Qaranful (Ar)

**Appearance:** A mobile clear yellow liquid with a deep, spicy warm, sweet odour with delicate vanilla-like overtones

**Perfumery status:** A heart note of high intensity and good persistence

**Extraction:** Steam or water distillation of the sun-dried whole or comminuted flowerbuds, usually June through August; October through January in Madagascar, Réunion and Ndzwani

**1 kg oil yield from:** 8–12 kg of the dried flower cloves (an extremely high yield)

**Production areas:** Indonesia (native to the Moluccas), Madagascar, Pemba (Tanzania), Comores, La Réunion, Mauritius, Seychelles, Sri Lanka. During the 19th century, the small island of Pemba supplied the largest amount of cloves worldwide.

**Typical constituents:** Phenols 60–96% (incl. eugenol 50–95%, isoeugenol, methylchavicol, methyleugenol) • esters 16–25% (incl. eugenyl acetate 11–27%, terpenyl acetate, methyl benzoate, methyl salicilate) • sesquiterpenes (incl. α- and β-caryophyllene 4–14%, cubebene, copaene, calamenene, α-ylangene, α-humulene) • caryophyllene and humulene oxide • ketones 1% (incl. methyl allyl ketone, 2-undecanone) • monoterpenols <1% • sesquiterpenols <1% • aldehydes

**Chance of adulteration:** Common, mainly with Clove leaf or Clove stem oil, various oils of the Pimenta species, and sometimes with isolated or synthetic eugenol and eugenyl acetate. Clove leaf oil itself is sometimes adulterated with Aromatic ravensara (Clove-nutmeg) oil (*Ravensara aromatica* Gmel.). Even in the case of a pure Clove oil, the use of poor plant material, e.g. clove dust (a by-product of clove production) rather than whole cloves, will also result in an inferior oil more suitable for commercial than therapeutic use.

**Related oils:** Clove leaf, a brown liquid with a woody, earthy and somewhat cinnamon-like odour, also high in eugenol (up to 88%) but with little eugenyl acetate to balance it. Also Brazil clove (*Dicypellium caryophyllatum*), also known as Clove-cassia or Clove-bark oil, distilled from the wood and bark.

## Therapeutic Functions and Indications

### Specific symptomatology – *All applications*

Discouragement, apathy, hopelessness, low self-esteem, poor self-confidence, emotional coldness, loss of motivation, low willpower, feelings of insecurity and vulnerability, helplessness, spaciness, oversensitivity, physical and mental fatigue, debility, cold extremities, low resistance with chronic infections, digestive problems with bloating, constipation, appetite loss, loss of sexual drive, absent periods

### Psychological – *Aromatic diffusion, whole-body massage*

Use with caution.

**Essential PNEI function and indication:** Stimulant in weak conditions

**Possible brain dynamics:** Increases basal ganglia functioning

**Fragrance category:** Middle tone with pungent, sweet, woody notes

**Indicated psychological disorders:** ADD, depression, dissociative disorder, psychotic and schizoid conditions

### Promotes motivation and self-confidence

- Loss of motivation, discouragement
- Low self-confidence and self-esteem, depression, self-neglect

Promotes strength, stability and integration

- Insecurity, vulnerability

- Mental and emotional instability, anxiety, fearfulness

- Mental and emotional burnout

## Physiological – *Gel cap, suppository, external applications*

Use with caution.

**Therapeutic status:** Mild remedy with no cumulative toxicity

**Topical safety status:** Skin irritant, sensitizing

**Tropism:** Circulatory, nervous, digestive, urinary, reproductive systems

**Essential diagnostic function:** Stimulates and warms asthenic/cold and hypotonic/weak terrain conditions

Primarily stimulant and warming:

*strong systemic nervous and central arterial circulatory stimulant, SNS stimulant:* a wide range of asthenic (cold) and chronic hypotonic (weak) conditions with circulatory deficiency, chronic physical and mental debility and fatigue; incl. convalescence, CFS

- *cerebral stimulant:* mental debility, neurasthenia, depression, postpartum depression

- *thyroid/thyroxine restorative:* hypothyroid syndrome, thyroxine resistance, low metabolic rate, esp. with cold, fatigue, depression

- *adrenal stimulant, hypertensive:* adrenal fatigue syndrome (esp. with afternoon or evening fatigue), low stamina, hypotension

- *reproductive stimulant, aphrodisiac:* sexual debility, loss of libido, impotence

- *uterine stimulant, emmenagogue, parturient:* amenorrhoea, oligomenorrhoea; prelabour treatment, stalled labour (uterine dystocia)

- *gastrointestinal stimulant, carminative, antifermentative:* atonic lower gastrointestinal indigestion with bloating, appetite loss, constipation; intestinal dysbiosis, intestinal fermentation

- *strong antioxidant, antitumoural, anticancer:* cancerous conditions

PRIMARILY RELAXANT:

*strong spasmolytic, anti-inflammatory, analgesic:* acute spasmodic and inflammatory

conditions, incl. intestinal colic, spasmodic IBS, asthma, spasmodic dysphonia, pleurisy, neuralgia, arthritis

*moderate antihistamine:* type-I allergic disorders

*anti-oestrogenic:* oestrogen accumulation syndrome

ANTIMICROBIAL ACTIONS:

*broad-spectrum anti-infective, immunostimulant, anti-inflammatory, deep lymphatic stimulant:* a wide range of infections, esp. neurological, gastrointestinal, urinary, female reproductive, dental

- *strong antiviral:* shingles, viral neuritis, HSV-1, MS, polio, enteritis, enterocolitis, dengue fever, viral hepatitis, pleurisy, AIDS, SARS

- *strong broad-spectrum antibacterial:* both gram-positive and gram-negative bacterial infections, incl. with Staph. aureus, Strep. pneumoniae/pyogenes/faccalis, Salmonella, Esch. coli, Pseudomonas, H. pylori, incl. gastroenteritis, food poisoning, microbial toxicosis, severe dysbiosis, mucous colitis, cholera, amoebic dysentery; pneumonia; malaria; urinary infections, salpingitis; tonsillitis, dental infections, abscesses

- *strong broad-spectrum antifungal:* fungal infections with Candida spp., Trichophyton spp., Microsporum spp., Aspergillus spp., Sporotrychium spp., Fusarium spp., incl. candidiasis, athlete's foot, nail-bed fungus, tinea/ringworm, jock itch

- *anthelmintic:* intestinal parasites

- *pediculicidal:* head lice (Pediculus capitis)

SYNERGISTIC COMBINATIONS
All for short-term use only: see 'Therapeutic precautions' below.

- Clove bud + Thyme ct. thymol: strong broad-spectrum anti-infective, immunostimulant, anti-inflammatory and detoxicant in a large range of acute infections, bacterial, viral, fungal and parasitic; esp. with debility, cold-weak terrain

- Clove bud + Winter savoury/Thyme ct. carvacrol: strong broad-spectrum anti-infective in severe acute urinary and reproductive organ infections, esp. cystitis, nephritis, gonorrhoea, prostatitis

COMPLEMENTARY COMBINATIONS

All for short-term use only: see 'Therapeutic precautions' below.

- Clove bud + Ravintsara: strong nervous stimulant and antiviral for chronic neurasthenia in weak, cold terrain, with poor circulation, fatigue, debility, cold, depression; shingles, viral neuritis, CFS, etc.

- Clove bud + Hyssop + Rosemary (all chemotypes): neurotonic and hypertensive for chronic neurasthenia with poor arterial circulation or hypotension

- Clove bud + Scotch pine/Black spruce: thyroxine restorative in chronic hypothyroid syndrome or thyroxine resistance, with deep cold, fatigue

- Clove bud + Nutmeg: strong adrenal stimulant, hypertensive for chronic adrenal fatigue with loss of endurance, afternoon fatigue, cold extremities, low blood pressure

- Clove bud + Niaouli/Tea tree: strong broad-spectrum anti-infective, anti-inflammatory and lymphatic stimulant/detoxicant in a large range of viral and bacterial infections of all body systems

- Clove bud + Laurel + Black pepper: strong antifermentative, antibacterial, lymphatic stimulant, detoxicant and spasmolytic for severe intestinal fermentation, dysbiosis, microbial toxicosis, food poisoning

- Clove bud + Cajeput: strong gastrointestinal stimulant-relaxant, spasmolytic and anti-infective in a wide range of infectious upper and lower digestive disorders, esp. with colic, diarrhoea, bloating, vomiting

- Clove bud + Cinnamon/Nutmeg: strong antibacterial and spasmolytic for severe gastrointestinal infections, incl. colitis, enteritis, dysentery; esp. with colic, tenesmus

- Clove bud + Black spruce: broad-spectrum anthelmintic for a wide range of intestinal parasites

- Clove bud + Peppermint: analgesic for neuralgias, abdominal and intestinal pain

- Clove bud + Lavender: partus preparator to prime the uterus for labour and delivery, starting two weeks before the due date

TOPICAL – *Liniment, lotion*

---

See 'Pharmacological precautions' below.

**Skin care:** Not used

> *vulnerary, antibacterial:* chronic infected wounds, ulcers, boils, furunculosis, infected acne

> *antifungal:* fungal skin conditions, incl. athlete's foot

> *pediculicidal:* lice, autumn mites

> *anesthetic/analgesic:* toothache, insect bites, arthritic and rheumatic pain

> *rubefacient, counterirritant:* arthritic and rheumatic pain

> *insect repellent, moderate tick repellent, larvicidal:* mosquitoes, moths, flies, mites, ticks

> *deodorant*

**Therapeutic precautions:** Clove bud is a strong warming stimulant to nervous, adrenal, thyroid and circulatory functions, and is therefore contraindicated in hypersthenic/hot and hypertonic/tense terrain; this includes high fevers, acute inflammation, hypertension, hyperthyroid, agitation and insomnia. The oil should also be avoided in dry terrain (e.g. with thirst, dry cough or constipation) and in babies, infants, sensitive individuals and during breastfeeding in general. Clove bud is best kept for treating chronic, not acute, asthenic/cold and hypotonic/weak conditions. Because it is a uterine stimulant, it is also contraindicated during pregnancy.

Internal use is best limited to 8–10-day courses, and then always within a formula rather than on their own, as with all high-phenol oils. Long-term internal use may cause liver damage and inhibit the healthy microflora; this should be prevented with the adjunctive use of liver restoratives and prebiotic foods, supplements or oils. Inhalation of Clove oil alone with an essential oil aroma-nebulizer is not recommended to avoid irritation to the mucous membrane.

**Pharmacological precautions:** Although Clove oil is somewhat irritant to the skin and mucosa, it is essentially non-irritant to the skin when used in proper dilution. Still, care should be taken to avoid any potential long-term sensitization in some individuals. Use with caution in those taking anticoagulant medication or presenting peptic ulcer or bleeding disorders.

**Preparations:**

- Diffusor: 1–2 drops in water

- Massage oil: 0.5% dilution in vegetable oil, preferably in combination with other oils

---

- Counterirritant liniment: 1–2% dilution in vegetable oil after first doing a patch test

- Gel cap: 1–2 drops with olive oil for short-term use, e.g. an eight-day course; and usually as part of a formula; the maximum daily dose is 5 drops. Like all phenolic oils, Clove should always be combined with other oils to reduce its intensity and enhance treatment results, especially with sweet, monoterpenol-rich oils such as Palmarosa, Thyme ct. linalool, Tea tree or Lavender.

## Chinese Medicine Functions and Indications

**Aroma energy:** Pungent, sweet, woody

**Movement:** Stabilizing

**Warmth:** Warm to hot

**Meridian tropism:** Kidney, Spleen, Stomach

**Five-Element affinity:** Water, Earth

**Essential function:** To tonify the Yang, warm the interior and strengthen the Shen

1. <u>**Tonifies the Yang, warms the Kidney and strengthens the Shen and libido**</u>

   - **Yang deficiency with Shen weakness**, with physical and mental fatigue, cold extremities, apathy, loss of self-confidence:
   Rosemary/Ginger/Black spruce/Thyme ct. thymol

   - **Kidney Yang deficiency** with loss of sex drive, frigidity, impotence, weak loins and knees, fatigue, cold skin and extremities:
   Ginger/Black spruce/Cinnamon bark

2. <u>**Warms and harmonizes the Stomach, descends rebellious Qi and relieves vomiting and pain**</u>

   - **Stomach cold with Qi rebellion**, with nausea, appetite loss, hiccups, vomiting, epigastric or abdominal pain:
   Cardamom/Ginger/Black pepper

   - **Stomach cold with shan qi**, with sharp abdominal pain:
   Fennel/Peppermint/Nutmeg

3. <u>**Warms and harmonizes the Middle Warmer, resolves damp and accumulation, and relieves pain and distension**</u>

   - **Stomach cold with food stagnation/accumulation** with acute indigestion, epigastric and/or abdominal bloating, belching, appetite loss:
   Cypress/Juniper berry/Fennel

- **Stomach-Spleen toxic-damp** with chonic indigestion, abdominal bloating, diarrhoea:

Patchouli/Juniper berry/Black pepper

- **Stomach-Spleen empty cold (Spleen Yang deficiency with cold)** with epigastric or abdominal pain, chronic constipation or loose stool, morning diarrhoea:

Ginger/Nutmeg/Black pepper

4. **Warms and activates the Lower Warmer, breaks up stagnation, promotes menstruation and relieves pain**

- **Lower Warmer Blood and Qi stagnation with cold**, with late, scanty or absent periods, painful periods, loss of sex drive:

Ginger/Fennel/Juniper berry

REMARKS

Like nutmeg and mace, clove – the 'nail aromatic' – is a gift of the spice islands to the world, the Molucca (Maluku) Islands in the Malay Archipelago. The trade of dried clove buds with Han China goes back to the 3rd century BC. Surfing the Indian Ocean with Arabic maritime trade during long medieval centuries, the costly spice by human transport eventually reached the westerly islands of Mauritius in 1753, and soon the Seychelles, Sri Lanka, La Réunion and the Comores, eventually beaching off the East African coast on Pemba and Zanzibar. To this day, clove essential oil is still produced in almost all of these Indian Ocean islands. The exotic spice gained Mediterranean ports, including stellar Alexandria, in the first century through Phoenician traders. The guild of multilingual Radhanite Jews then became instrumental in moving the valuable spice from Middle Eastern ports to major European cities through their highly developed trade networks (Nabhan 2014). The Venetian world traveller Marco Polo in his journals, published c. 1300, gives full details of a bustling clove trade with Moluccan spice traders in Chinese ports on the East China Sea. The later colonial Portuguese and then Dutch monopoly of the Moluccas is well documented: in 1605 it strategically slashed the thriving multi-island clove plantations down to only the island of Ambon and three minor nearby islands; on Ternate an enormous 350-year-old tree stemming from the Portuguese era still survives. In 1768, cuttings of the clove tree were sequestered to Ile-de-France (Mauritius) and in 1793 westward on to La Réunion, and finally to the Caribbean territories of French Guyana, Trinidad, Dominica, St. Vincent and Martinique – bringing the spice's global journey almost full circle.

Clove is a well-established remedy in both Ayurvedic and Chinese medicine since over two millennia. The essential oil itself only emerged in 15th-century Europe and, like other aromatic spices, soon became an important remedy in pharmacy. Today, the oil distilled from high-quality cloves is an essential remedy in the materia aromatica for both physiological and psychological purposes.

Deeply stimulating and warming to both central arterial and nervous systems, Clove oil is an important remedy for treating chronic cold terrain, especially with debility and infection present. In the Chinese medicine idiom, this is a deficiency of the Kidney Yang, the fire of ming men. Physiologically, this often involves hypothyroid functioning, whether from thyroxine resistance or insufficiency. Clove has a notable beneficial effect in these syndromes, especially with cold, fatigue and depression present.

Rarely used on its own and usually within a formula, Clove focuses on stimulating the organs of the lower trunk and pelvis, particularly digestive and reproductive. Chronic amenorrhoea and loss of libido, chronic adrenal fatigue with debility, and chronic intestinal atonicity are key indications here. The plant itself was named after Saint Eugenia, patron saint of midwives: one of its time-honoured uses is for preparing a woman for labour by priming the uterus; traditional Indonesian use is to insert one clove a day vaginally starting about two weeks before the due date. The oil is an excellent partus preparator in the first phase of labour. Moreover, the oil yields particularly high mileage in the gut: to the GI stimulant action is added a good relaxant spasmolytic, anti-inflammatory one. Its constituent eugenyl acetate has shown a spasmolytic effect comparable to the alkaloid papaverine. The result is a superb remedy for the lower gut not only in atonic, cold conditions, but also in tense inflammatory conditions – both presenting painful spasms.

Attentive clove growers on plantations a long time ago observed Clove trees' ability, when transported, to keep down tropical diseases; after the trees were felled, they noted a greater spread of these diseases. Layered over Clove's two basic actions is a superb wide-spectrum anti-infective effect, which includes stimulation of deep lymphatic functions and antifermentative and detoxicant actions. The oil is indicated not only in all frank intestinal and other infections, whether viral, bacterial or fungal, but also in all dysbiotic, fermentative conditions of the microbiome. Clove's excellent antiviral action has been applied successfully in a large range of viral disorders, including the herpes simplex virus. Most of its actions have been linked to its combined content in the phenol eugenol and the caryophyllenes. Among eugenol's many tested actions is a notable anticancer action and an oestrogen-inhibiting effect that may be put to use in oestrogen-accumulation syndrome.

Clove works no less deeply as a psychological remedy when used by gentle olfaction. The deeply warming, sweet, woody, spicy fragrance is centring and strengthening, reaching deep into the body's physical core. Clove encourages full embodiment of our being and full connection with our inner resources. In supporting the self to fully tap into his or her source of true power and inner strength, Clove is for disempowerment causing insecurity, constant vulnerability and the need to dissociate. In bolstering deep resources and an embodied sense of self, the fragrance can support those who are too easily influenced by outside forces and prone to feeling insecure, helpless and victim to the whims of circumstances. It is interesting that Clove in traditional cultures was specific for providing protection against evil influences. Clove essentially connects the unconscious with the conscious, and gut feelings with conscious feelings and willpower. In so doing, Clove can be a valuable ally in the basic human task of developing self-acceptance and taking full responsibility for oneself – for nothing less than building the inner foundation of true self-esteem.

# Coriander Seed

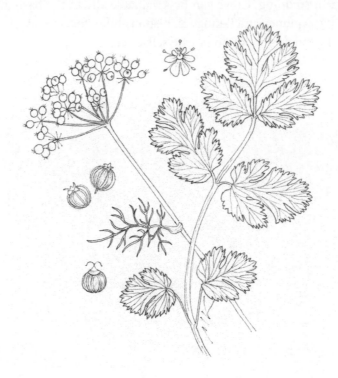

**Botanical source:** The fruit of *Coriandrum sativum* L. (Apiaceae – carrot family), a herb from temperate Eastern Europe and West Asia

**Other names:** Coriandre doux (Fr), Koriander (Ge)

**Appearance:** The steam distilled oil: a mobile pale yellow liquid with a light sweet-spicy and somewhat woody, musky odour; the essential oil extracted by CO2: a viscous pale amber liquid with deep, warm, spicy notes with some lemony high and earthy low notes

**Perfumery status:** A heart note of high intensity and medium persistence

**Extraction:** Steam distillation of the air-dried seeds. The longer the drying process (ideally up to about 12 weeks), the less their unpleasant animalic aroma is released when the seeds are crushed and distilled.

**1 kg oil yield from:** 100–120 kg (a good yield)

**Production areas:** Ukraine, Crimea, Poland, Romania, Hungary, India

**Typical constituents:** Monoterpenols 60–80% (incl. linalool 55–75%, geraniol, borneol) • ketones <9% (incl. camphor <3%, carvone, anethone) • monoterpenes 10–20% (incl. γ-terpinene 8%, p-cymene 3%, d-limonene 2%) • coumarins and furano-coumarins (incl. umbelliferone, bergaptene) • decylaldehyde

**Chance of adulteration:** Moderate, possibly with additional synthetic or other-oil derived linalool; possibly with the oils of Sweet orange and Cedarwood

## Therapeutic Functions and Indications

SPECIFIC SYMPTOMATOLOGY – *All applications*

Fatigue, nervous exhaustion, grief, apathy, loss of motivation, depression, loss of appetite, indigestion with bloating and flatulence after eating small amounts, malaise, chronic headaches, dry skin, urinary irritation

PSYCHOLOGICAL – *Aromatic diffusion, whole-body massage*

**Essential PNEI function and indication:** Regulating in dysregulated conditions

**Possible brain dynamics:** Reduces deep limbic system hyperfunctioning, stimulates basal ganglia hypofunctioning

**Fragrance category:** Middle tone with sweet and spicy-pungent notes

**Indicated psychological disorders:** Bipolar disorder, minor depression

PROMOTES EMOTIONAL STABILITY AND INTEGRATION

- Moodiness, emotional instability, repetitive emoting

- Feeling-thinking disconnection and conflict

PROMOTES SELF-CONFIDENCE AND COURAGE

- Loss of self-confidence with insecurity, inhibited emotional expression

- Discouragement with apathy, pessimism

PHYSIOLOGICAL – *Nebulizer inhalation, gel cap, suppository, pessary, external applications*

**Therapeutic status:** Mild remedy with no cumulative toxicity

**Topical safety status:** Non-irritant, non-sensitizing, photosensitizing

**Tropism:** Nervous, digestive, urinary, musculoskeletal systems

**Essential diagnostic function:** Restores hypotonic/weak conditions, stimulates hyposthenic/cold conditions

PRIMARILY RESTORATIVE:

*nervous and cerebral restorative, antidepressant:* chronic hypotonic (weak) conditions with fatigue, exhaustion, depression, anxiety; neurasthenia, nervous exhaustion and breakdown, incl. postpartum

*gonadal/ovarian restorative, progesteronic:* low progesterone syndrome with PMS with depression, anxiety, frigidity (low libido)

*adrenocortical restorative and regulator:* hypoadrenia, dysadrenia

PRIMARILY STIMULANT:

*gastrointestinal stimulant, carminative:* chronic hypotonic digestive conditions with distension, flatulence, colic; intestinal fermentation, dysbiosis, chronic gastroenteritis

*stomachic, aperitive:* appetite loss (anorexia), esp. with distension on eating

*kidney stimulant, detoxicant diuretic, alterative:* metabolic toxicosis with rheumatic or arthritic pain, dysuria, gout; nephritis

*liver detoxicant and protective:* metabolic, drug and chemical toxicosis, chemotherapy

*analgesic, spasmolytic, anti-inflammatory, antirheumatic, antiarthritic:* neuromuscular pain and swelling, incl. muscle cramps, neuralgia, intestinal colic, cystalgia; rheumatoid arthritis with joint swelling; migraine headaches; dysuria

ANTIMICROBIAL ACTIONS:

*broad-spectrum antibacterial:* misc. bacterial infections, incl. with Staph. aureus, S. haemolyticus, Pseudomonas aeruginosa, Helicobacter pylori, Eschericia coli, Listeria monocytogenes, Campylobacter jejuni, Acinetobacter baumannii

*antifungal:* fungal infections

*antiviral:* influenza, measles

*anthelmintic, larvicidal:* intestinal parasites

SYNERGISTIC COMBINATIONS

- Coriander seed + Palmarosa/Petitgrain: nervous restorative and antidepressant for chronic neurasthenia with mental fatigue, depression, burnout

- Coriander seed + Lavender: nervous restorative, euphoric for acute trauma, shock, nervous breakdown

- Coriander seed + Geranium: progesteronic ovarian restorative in low progesterone syndrome with PMS with depression, anxiety, loss of libido

- Coriander seed + Palmarosa: antifungal for all fungal infections (incl. topical use)

COMPLEMENTARY COMBINATIONS

- Coriander seed + Cardamom/Fennel: gastric stimulant, carminative, stomachic and aperitive for upper digestive atony with indigestion, distension, pain; anorexia, aerophagia

- Coriander seed + Fennel/Black pepper: analgesic, spasmolytic for abdominal colic, spasmodic dysuria

- Coriander seed + Tea tree: antibacterial, analgesic for cystitis with dysuria from E. coli

- Coriander seed + Juniper berry/Lemon: detoxicant, alterative and antirheumatic for metabolic toxicosis with rheumatic or arthritic pains, gout, dysuria

## TOPICAL – *Liminent, ointment, cream, compress and other cosmetic preparations*

**Skin care:** Combination skin type

*skin regenerator, vulnerary*: scars, stretch marks, sores, ulcers, chronic wounds

*antibacterial, antifungal, mild anti-inflammatory:* a wide range of bacterial and fungal infections (see above)

*UV-protectant: ultraviolet radiation* (as sunscreen)

**Therapeutic precautions:** Only low doses are required for Coriander oil's nervous restorative action to engage; in higher doses the oil may act as a nervous sedative.

**Pharmacological precautions:** The coumarins in Coriander seed oil make it photosensitizing: exposure to sunlight or sunbeds should be avoided for 12 hours after topical application.

**Preparations:**

- Diffusor: 2–3 drops in water

- Massage oil: 2–5% dilution in vegetable oil

- Liniment: 5–10% dilution in vegetable oil

- Gel cap: 1–3 drops with olive oil

# Chinese Medicine Functions and Indications

**Aroma energy:** Sweet, pungent

**Movement:** Circulating, rising

**Warmth:** Neutral to warm

**Meridian tropism:** Heart, Stomach, Spleen, Liver

**Five-Element affinity:** Fire, Earth, Metal

**Essential function:** To nourish the Blood, harmonize the Middle Warmer and strengthen the Shen

1. **Nourishes the Blood, animates the Heart, strengthens the Shen and relieves depression**

   - **Heart Blood deficiency with Shen weakness**, with chronic physical and mental fatigue, depression, somnolence:

     Petitgrain/Palmarosa/Clary sage

   - **Uterus Blood deficiency** with chronic fatigue, low stamina, thirst, vaginal dryness, withdrawal, PMS with low self-worth, depression, anxiety, loss of sex drive:

     Vetiver/Rose/Jasmine

2. **Harmonizes the Middle Warmer, reduces stagnation and relieves distension**

   - **Stomach Qi and food stagnation** with indigestion on eating, flatulence, appetite loss, epigastric bloating with possible pain, nausea:

     Spearmint/Cardamom/Fennel

3. **Warms the meridians, dispels wind-damp-cold and relieves pain**

   - **Wind-damp-cold obstruction** with chronic muscle or joint pain and swelling:

     Siberian fir/Juniper berry/Rosemary/Spike lavender

REMARKS

With its historical roots in ancient Mesopotamia, the Fertile Crescent, coriander is almost unique in having its origins in West Asia. The library of Assyrian king Ashurbanipal already contained texts that describe coriander cultivation. Ancient Anatolians were the first to lay out coriander plantations for their spice crop on a large scale, in time causing the plant to disperse widely, especially to Armenia, Georgia, Crimea, Ukraine, Southeast Europe, the Levant and Egypt. Coriander is mentioned in an Egyptian papyrus dating from c. 2000 BC. During the long Al Andalus period, this aromatic eventually took well-worn North African trade routes to the Iberian peninsula, along with most other Arabic spices. Here again it enjoyed extensive cultivation.

With its playful light, sweet-spicy, lemony aroma, coriander soon became a favourite spice in refined Andalusian culture (Nabhan 2014). Today the seed is still an essential ingredient in various Arabic spice mixtures, such as baharat and the Moroccan ras el hanout. Although it never caught on as a major cooking spice in Europe, coriander was eventually adopted in major herb-based medicinal liqueurs such as Bénédictine and Chartreuse; it was finally distilled into an essential oil in the early 1400s.

The musty scent of fresh coriander belies the delicate sweet, spicy fragrance of the essential oil locked in its small seeds – the plant was called Koriandron in old Greece, from *koris andron*, 'bug's husband'. With its rich, sweet monoterpenol content, Coriander seed is a classic terrain oil for individuals presenting chronic weakness with stagnation. Key symptoms for its use are depression, chronic fatigue, somnolence and loss of stamina and sex drive, often associated with either states of grief, hypoadrenia or hypoprogesterone syndrome in women. The individual with Coriander terrain will benefit here from the oil's combined nervous, adrenocortical and ovarian restorative actions (as also in Niaouli). Paul Dupont (2002) considers it even a pineal restorative that may boost psychic energy. The oil's hormonal effects together make this a good woman's remedy and may be summarized in Chinese medicine as a deficiency of Blood and fluids. Coriander is one of the very few oils that will address this particular syndrome.

Coriander seed also exerts an excellent, well-known tropism for the gut, acting as a stimulant to both stomach and intestines. Like Cardamom, Juniper berry and other spice oils, its strong carminative and aperitive actions will relieve most forms of digestive stagnation that originate in digestive weakness with insufficient gastric secretions. Its all-round antimicrobial action also contributes nicely here. A wide range of bacteria respond to its broad antibacterial action. In topical applications, Coriander seed has been found to have the advantage of combining good antimicrobial actions with extremely low sensitizing potential. Equally a kidney stimulant, the aromatic remedy acts as a useful detoxicant diuretic for removing metabolic toxins from the joints and muscles, where its analgesic, anti-inflammatory actions also engage; ketones and monoterpenes are noted in respect of these actions.

When used purely by olfaction as a psychological remedy, Coriander seed clearly expresses sweet, pungent properties that target our instinctive emotions related to the gut. Able to create a sense of deep security and emotional self-nurturing, the fragrance is supportive for those who have felt discouraged for a long time. Not motivated to connect with their true gut-felt feelings, these individuals instead remain prone to mood swings and emotional outbursts. Gently stimulating and uplifting, Coriander seed is also indicated for individuals stuck in habit-bound routine and predictability, fearful of change and spontaneity, and therefore unable to move forward in their lives. It will encourage them to express feelings with confidence and less inhibition. It comes as no surprise that, from a wider perspective, Coriander has traditionally been linked to creativity and imagination, as well as a true, embodied zest for living life to the fullest.

Coriander leaf oil should be clearly distinguished from the seed oil. With the characteristic green, lemony, somewhat oily fragrance of the freshly crushed leaves, its dominant constituents are aldehydes (75–95%) such as 7-dodecanal 25%, dodecanal 16%, decanal 10%, octanal, undecadienal and tetradecanal. Others include monoterpenols (5–25%, mostly linalool), geranyl acetate 1% and camphor 1–3%. Like other oils high in aldehydes, Coriander leaf essentially addresses hypertonic/tense and hypersthenic/hot conditions. It exerts a good sedative action on the nervous system that will benefit states of anxiety, insomnia and feelings of stress. Along with that, it shows a relaxant action on smooth muscles, as well as being a carminative digestive stimulant, indicating use for digestive pain and colic, as well as stress-related forms of indigestion. Its anti-inflammatory action is especially useful for gastric and intestinal inflammation, and stomach and duodenal ulcers. In terms of endocrine functions, Coriander leaf (like the seed) is sometimes used as a moderate progesteronic remedy for low progesterone syndrome and as a moderate stimulant to thyroid and adrenal functions. The oil is also a good antiviral with good results in shingles and chickenpox. Avoid Coriander leaf on sensitive or damaged skin, and watch out for possible sensitization with repeated use. Standard dilutions and doses apply.

In terms of its psychological applications by olfaction, Coriander leaf embodies the green-lemony fragrance qualities of promoting mental alertness, optimism and good judgement. It may also help with getting over negative past experiences by supporting the resolution of distressed emotions and feelings.

# Cypress

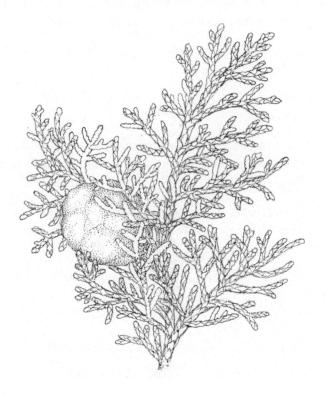

**Botanical source:** The twig and needle of *Cupressus sempervirens* L. (Cupressaceae – cypress family), a tree of dry montane Mediterranean regions

**Other names:** Italian/Mediterranean cypress; Cyprès (vert) (Fr), Zypresse (Ge), Cipresso (It), Ciprés (Sp), Kuparissi (Gr)

**Appearance:** A mobile pale yellow or pale viridian liquid with a fresh-camphoraceous and balsamic-woody odour with some fruity-green notes

**Perfumery status:** A heart note of medium intensity and fair persistence

**Extraction:** Steam distillation of the twigs and needles, usually October to March

**1 kg oil yield from:** 60–100 kg of the twigs (a good yield)

**Production areas:** France, Spain, Morocco, Greece

**Typical constituents:** Monoterpenes (incl. α-pinene 35–59%, β-pinene 1–1.5%, δ-3-camphene 10%, δ-3-carene 10–24%, l-limonene 1–3%, terpinolene 3%, p-cymene, sabinene 1–28%) • monoterpenols <11% (incl. borneol 1–9%, terpinen-4-ol 1–2%, sabinol) • sesquiterpenes 1–5% (incl. δ-cadinene, α- and β-cedrene, ocimenes)

• sesquiterpenol cedrol 1–21% • esters (incl. α-terpinyl acetate 4–6%, terpinen-4-l acetate) • traces of 1,8 cineole, manoyl oxide

**Chance of adulteration:** Moderate, usually with other raw materials for distillation, such as cypress cones, other conifer twigs from pine, juniper and such like, as well as the addition of synthetic pinenes, camphene, etc. to the final oil

**Related oils**: Other species in the worldwide cypress family are occasionally distilled for their essential oil:

- Kenya/Madagascar/Portuguese cypress (*Cupressus lusitanica* Miller), with its fresh, green aroma

- Hinoki or Japanese cypress (*Chamecyparis obtusa* Siebold et Succ.) from Japan, with its characteristic sweet-woody aroma; however, the status of this tree is highly endangered

- Sugi or Japanese cedarwood (*Cryptomeria japonica* D. Don) from Japan, Korea and Northeast China; this is the Japanese national tree; the status of this tree is highly endangered, however

- Asunaro or Hiba arborvitae (*Thujopsis dolabrata* Siebold et Succ.) from Japan, related to Arborvitae (Thuja spp.)

## Therapeutic Functions and Indications

SPECIFIC SYMPTOMATOLOGY – *All applications*

Lethargy, apathy, discouragement, indecisiveness, poor willpower, low self-confidence, low perseverance, fatigue, malaise, heavy difficult periods, dribbling or painful irritated urination, chronic joint and muscle aches, bedwetting, swollen lymph glands, varicose veins, haemorrhoids, water retention in legs and ankles, abnormal day or night sweating

PSYCHOLOGICAL – *Aromatic diffusion, whole-body massage*

**Essential PNEI function and indication:** Stimulant in weakness conditions

**Possible brain dynamics:** Increases basal ganglia and prefrontal cortex functioning

**Fragrance category:** Base tone with woody and pungent-fresh notes

**Indicated psychological disorders:** ADD, minor depression, dissociative disorder, psychotic and schizoid conditions

PROMOTES SELF-CONFIDENCE AND MOTIVATION

- Low self-confidence and self-esteem, self-neglect

- Loss of motivation with apathy, procrastination

PROMOTES WILLPOWER AND PERSEVERANCE

- Low willpower or strength, indecisiveness
- Discouragement, low perseverance
- Mental and emotional burnout

## PHYSIOLOGICAL – *Nebulizer inhalation, gel cap, suppository, external applications*

**Therapeutic status:** Mild remedy with no cumulative toxicity

**Topical safety status:** Non-irritant, non-sensitizing

**Tropism:** Neuroendocrine, respiratory, urogenital, digestive systems

**Essential diagnostic function:** To restore hypotonic/weak, decongest congestive/damp and relaxes hypertonic/tense terrain conditions

PRIMARILY RESTORATIVE:

*neuroendocrine restorative and regulator:* atonic (weak) conditions with fatigue, debility; neurasthenia, CFS, menopausal syndrome

*adrenocortical restorative:* hypoadrenia syndrome, menopausal syndrome

*ovarian restorative, oestrogenic:* hypo-oestrogen conditions, incl. menopausal syndrome, oestrogen-deficient PMS, dysmenorrhoea

*digestive and pancreatic enzyme stimulant, carminative:* atonic indigestion with abdominal bloating and swelling; pancreatic enzyme deficiency

PRIMARILY DECONGESTANT:

Strong astringent blood and fluid decongestant, esp. in the pelvis, lower limbs:

*venous restorative and decongestant:* venous deficiency with congestion, with varicose veins; varicose ulcers

*pelvic decongestant, uterine restorative, haemostatic:* pelvic congestion with congestive dysmenorrhoea, menorrhagia, mild metrorrhagia, ovarian cysts; haemorrhoids with bleeding

*prostatic decongestant:* prostate congestion with hyperplasia (BPH), prostate adenoma

*lymphatic decongestant:* lymphatic congestion with swollen glands *fluid decongestant, astringent diuretic:* oedema, incl. ankle and leg oedema; urinary incontinence, enuresis

*detoxicant diuretic:* kidney metabolic toxicosis with rheumatic and arthritic conditions, dysuria

*peripheral vasoconstrictor, anhydrotic:* excessive day or night-time sweating, sweaty feet

PRIMARILY RELAXANT:

**Smooth and striped muscle relaxant and spasmolytic:** a large range of spasmodic conditions

- **strong respiratory relaxant, antitussive:** spasmodic cough and dyspnoea, spasmodic dysphonia; whooping cough, croup, tracheitis

- **urinary relaxant:** strangury, neurogenic bladder, spasmodic dysuria, incontinence, enuresis

- **gastrointestinal relaxant:** digestive colic, IBS

- **uterine relaxant:** spasmodic dysmenorrhoea

- **neuromuscular relaxant:** muscle spasms

ANTIMICROBIAL ACTIONS:

**antibacterial, antimycobacterial:** bronchitis, whooping cough, lung TB; E. coli

SYNERGISTIC COMBINATIONS

- Cypress + Niaouli/Black spruce: strong prostate decongestant for prostate congestion or benign prostate hyperplasia

- Cypress + Juniper berry: gastric and pancreatic enzyme stimulant for upper digestive deficiency

- Cypress + Juniper berry/Carrot seed: diuretic detoxicant for kidney metabolic toxicosis, incl. arthritis, gout

- Cypress + Grapefruit: lymphatic decongestant for chronic swollen lymph glands

- Cypress + Cistus: strong astringent haemostatic for moderate to severe haemorrhage, incl. haemafecia, haematuria, metrorrhagia, bleeding haemorrhoids

- Cypress + Sage: strong neuroendocrine restorative for chronic neurasthenia with fatigue, exhaustion, burnout, menopausal syndrome

- Cypress + Hyssop: bronchodilator and antitussive for asthma and spasmodic coughs, including croup, whooping cough

- Cypress + Geranium: astringent uterine restorative and haemostatic for menorrhagia, metrorrhagia

- Cypress + Geranium/Mastic: strong venous restorative and decongestant for varicose veins, haemorroids

- Cypress + Rosemary: strong pelvic decongestant for congestive dysmenorrhoea, haemorrhoids

- Cypress + Wintergreen: strong anti-inflammatory prostatic decongestant for prostate congestion with hyperplasia, prostatitis, haemorrhoids

- Cypress + Tarragon/Marjoram: urinary spasmolytic and analgesic for strangury, spasmodic dysuria, incontinence, enuresis

## TOPICAL – *Liminent, ointment, cream, compress and other cosmetic preparations*

**Skin care:** Oily skin type (facial steam)

*capillary stimulant, detoxicant, skin toner:* tired devitalized skin, overhydrated skin, skin impurities, cellulite, frostbite

*astringent, mild antiseptic, vulnerary:* broken veins and capillaries, couperose, acne, wet eczema, seborrhoea, varicose veins, acne, boils, rosacea, wounds

*body deodorant, antiperspirant*

**Hair and scalp care:** Slow hair and scalp activity, hair loss, dandruff

**Therapeutic precautions:** Cypress oil is a dry astringent and is contraindicated in all types of dry conditions, especially dry respiratory conditions with dry, unproductive cough and dry form of constipation. Because the oil is considered oestrogenic by some practitioners (Duraffourd, D'Hervicourt and Lapraz 1988), it is contraindicated in oestrogen-dependent cancers and other high-oestrogen conditions. However, it is equally possible, but not proven, that Cypress acts more as a hormonal balancer, like Geranium, with only a potential oestrogenic action in oestrogen-deficiency conditions.

**Pharmacological precautions:** Cypress should only be used with caution in babies and infants because of its fresh-pungent, high-monoterpene nature. Cypress is traditionally contraindicated internally during pregnancy because of its uterine relaxant action; and also with mastitis.

**Preparations:**

- Diffusor: 2–4 drops in water
- Massage oil: 2–5% dilution in vegetable oil
- Liniment: 5–10% dilution in vegetable oil after doing a patch test
- Gel cap: 2–3 drops with olive oil
- Foot bath: 3–6 drops in warm water with 2 tsp. sea salt for sweaty feet, tired legs and feet

## Chinese Medicine Functions and Indications

**Aroma energy:** Pungent, woody

**Movement:** Stabilizing, circulating and rising

**Warmth:** Neutral

**Meridian tropism:** Lung, Spleen, Liver

**Five-Element affinity:** Metal, Earth

**Essential function:** To tonify the Qi, activate Qi and Blood, and strengthen the Shen

1. **Tonifies the Qi, strengthens the Lung and relieves coughing; strengthens the Shen and relieves fatigue; consolidates the exterior and stops sweating**

   - **Qi deficiency with Shen weakness**, with fatigue, weariness, distraction, poor focus, daytime sweats, weak cough:

     Ravintsara/Rosemary/Tea tree/Sage

   - **Lung Qi deficiency** with chronic weak cough, shallow breathing, fatigue, voice loss:

     Green myrtle/Hyssop/Niaouli

   - **Day or night-sweats** from Qi or Yin deficiency:

     Cypress/Tea tree

2. **Diffuses and circulates Lung Qi, and relieves coughing**

   - **Lung Qi accumulation** with spasmodic coughing, chest tightness, difficult breathing:

     Siberian fir/Fennel/Basil ct. methylchavicol

3. **Activates the Qi, harmonizes the Middle Warmer and relieves distension**

   - **Stomach-Spleen Qi stagnation** with indigestion, epigastric bloating, appetite loss:

     Spearmint/Cardamom/May chang

   - **Liver-Spleen disharmony** with epigastric or abdominal pain, cramps, colic, flatulence:

     Spearmint/Mandarin/Peppermint

4. **Activates the Lower Warmer, breaks up stagnation, harmonizes urination, relieves pain and moderates menstruation**

   - **Lower Warmer Qi stagnation** with bladder Qi constraint, with difficult, irritated, painful, dripping urination; incontinence, menstrual cramps:

     Fennel/Carrot seed/Marjoram

   - **Lower Warmer Qi and Blood stagnation** with premenstrual pain and bloating, clotted periods, improvement with onset of flow:

     Rosemary/Niaouli/Clary sage

5. **Invigorates the Blood in the Lower Warmer and lower limbs, and reduces varicosis**

   - **Blood stagnation in the lower limbs** with varicose veins, ankle oedema, fatigue:

     Clary sage/Geranium/Rosemary

6. **Drains water-damp, promotes and harmonizes urination, and relieves pain**

   - **Water-damp accumulation** with water retention (esp. in legs/ankles), painful, dripping or difficult urination:

     Juniper berry/Fennel/Carrot seed

REMARKS

A tall, spire-like evergreen tree originally from the islands of the Eastern Mediterranean, Cypress comes steeped in a patina of Greek mythology. Not only in the tale of Kyparissos, the boy who from terminal grief turned into a cypress tree, but also in the many stories of Artemis, goddess of everything wild; of Hades, master of hell; and of Cyprian Aphrodite, goddess of love. Already then, the cypress was an established emblem of the passing of life into death and the promise of a next life. The tree has an exceptional longevity of up to 2,000 years and has always stood for longevity and immortality. In consistency and because of its notable durability and incorruptability, ancient Egyptians used cypress wood to build mummy sarcophagi.

Like the sandalwood tree in Asia, the cypress has always been considered a sacred tree associated with the divine, an emblem of the transcendent. Cypress is seen as helping not only departed souls in their onward journey, but also the living in their aspirations and prayers to a greater spirit. One might think of sandalwood, the Asian tree, as inducing meditation on the divine and cypress, the Western tree, contemplation. Likewise, whereas sandalwood embodies the divine within, cypress expresses the longing for union with the divine without.

Like most other Western aromatics, Cypress the wood and then the essential oil has always been a mainstay of herbal medicine and pharmacy. Cypress Wine is a classic diuretic preparation from days past. Cypress oil is especially valued by French practitioners for its broad decongestant and astringent effects in those presenting congestive terrain. Working on the venous blood, lymphatic and fluid circulation, Cypress has a strong affinity for the pelvis and lower limbs, like the herbal remedy Red root (Ceanothus). Its central indication is any type of fluid congestion, including pelvic blood congestion, venous blood stagnation and lymphatic and water congestion in the lower parts. Like Bilberry and Horsechestnut, Cypress is also known to increase the elasticity of the veins: it is a venous restorative as well as decongestant. Topically, Cypress is used in both a medical and cosmetic context as a good toning astringent and vulnerary – it is reputedly more effective than Witchhazel.

As a pelvic decongestant, Cypress has been a major remedy for haemorrhoids (including with bleeding) since ancient times. Also in the pelvis, it is a classic prostate and uterus decongestant for hyperplasia of those organs. The oil has a special action on the uterus as both an astringent uterine restorative (think Black haw bark, Viburnum prunifolium) and an oestrogenic ovarian restorative. Toning and astringing, Cypress is invaluable for congestive dysmenorrhoea, heavy periods, ovarian cysts and bleeding haemorrhoids. Being hormonally active, this aromatic remedy is also effective for menopausal syndrome, when oestrogen levels dip. Its adrenocortical restorative action, in view of its good levels of δ-3-carene, here also comes nicely into play. In those with chronic nervous weakness or neurasthenia, Cypress can also provide long-term support. This remedy's underlying neuroendocrine restorative action makes it especially indicated in those presenting chronic underlying weakness.

Cypress also displays an excellent relaxant aspect for more acute conditions, with a particularly effective spasmolytic action on the smooth muscles of the respiratory and urinary tract. All types of spasmodic coughs and spasmodic, irritated bladder symptoms will find relief. Cypress is also a classic oil for urinary incontinence and enuresis.

When used purely by olfaction, Cypress embodies pungent and woody fragrance qualities. As a time-honoured sacred aromatic, Cypress tends to evoke contemplation on the existential issues of life, punctuated by times of radical transition in our lives, such as death, birth, bereavement and other radical changes. At this type of juncture,

Cypress will create a safe, intimate sanctuary that gently supports inner fortitude and stability. Guiding us to stay centred on essential issues, not superficial ones, the fragrance will bring focus and clarity to confusion and loss of direction. At first centring and stabilizing, the fragrance soon becomes energizing and uplifting. Cypress is for those beset with doubt, discouragement, low self-confidence and fearfulness. It can assist when life's challenges require inner strength and the courage to express one's convictions. On that basis, Cypress allows new decisions to arise authentically from within and conscious intentions to be made with complete self-assurance. Like the tree emblem itself, Cypress supports the process of radical transformation and renewal. In helping us cope with challenges in times of major life transitions, Cypress may well connect us more deeply with our destiny.

**Related oils:** In the Cypress family they include the following.

**Blue cypress** (*Callitris intratropica* Baker and Smith) from northern Australia is a sweet, woody, somewhat earthy and balsamic-scented oil steam distilled from the wood, bark and leaves of the tree in the cypress family. Its colour is a clear, deep cobalt blue from its content in the sesquiterpenes guaiazulene and chamazulene; other sesquiterpenes include guaienes, selinenes and β-elemene (all <18%); the sesquiterpenols guaiol (13–28%) and various eudesmols are also present (<35%). Blue cypress is essentially a relaxing, cooling remedy, being valued mostly for its anti-inflammatory, antihistamine, analgesic and antipruritic actions in treating immediate allergies such as dermatitis with itching, insect bite allergies and insect stings, burns and scalds in general, as well as joint inflammation and pain. The oil's antiviral action is excellent against cold sores, shingles – i.e. both forms of herpes – and common warts; it often works when nothing else will. Its use is contraindicated during pregnancy and breastfeeding because of its eudesmol levels. Standard dilutions and doses apply.

As an aromatic remedy for the psyche, Blue cypress embodies classic sweet-woody energy that centres and stabilizes. Individuals with mental-emotional instability, agitation, disconnection or spaciness will benefit from its olfaction. Like other similar oils, Blue cypress may also promote cognitive flexibility with obsessions, compulsions and states of repetitive thinking. It may be helpful in cases of ADHD and dissociative disorder.

**Siam wood** (*Fokienia hodginsii* Henry et Thomas) or Peimou oil is steam distilled from a cypress indigenous to Vietnam and South China. Its fragrance is sweet, woody, with a mild fruity note. Its constituent profile is dominated by an array of sesquiterpenes (<76%) and sesquiterpenols (<52%), chief among them being δ-cadinene (33%), γ-cadinene (16%), nerolidol (35%) and fokienol (26%). Siam wood is a nervous restorative and sedative for chronic hypotonic/weak and hypertonic/tense conditions with debility, burnout, adrenal deficiency, mental hyperactivity and other symptoms arising from chronic stress. The oil is specifically for sexual debility as it also stimulates the HPT (hypothalamus-pituitary-testicular) and the HPA (hypothalamus-pituitary-adrenal) axis. Its chemical profile further suggests anti-inflammatory, antiallergic, mucosal restorative and venous and lymphatic decongestant actions.

Siam wood is a mild remedy with no cumulative toxicity or topical irritation or sensitization; standard dilutions and doses apply.

# Fennel

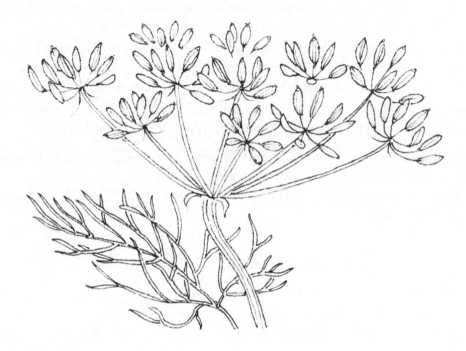

**Botanical source:** The fruit of *Foeniculum vulgare* Miller subsp. *vulgare* var. *dulce* and *F. vulgare* Miller subsp. *vulgare* var. *vulgare* (Apiaceae/Umbelliferae – carrot family); a hardy Mediterranean plant of dry ocean and littoral river areas; widely naturalized

**Other names:** *F. vulgare* subsp. *vulgare* var. *dulce*: Sweet fennel, Garden fennel, Holmboe; Fenouil doux (Fr), Fenchel (Ge), Finocchio (It), Inojo (Sp), Xiao hui xiang (Mandarin)

*F. vulgare* subsp. *vulgare* var. *vulgare*: Bitter or wild fennel; Fenouil amer/long/sauvage

**Appearance:** *F. vulgare* subsp. *vulgare* var. *dulce* (Sweet fennel): A very pale yellow or viridian liquid with a warm pungent, sweet anise-like odour

*F. vulgare* subsp. *vulgare* var. *vulgare* (Bitter fennel): A pale orange-brown liquid with a warm, rich herbaceous, camphoraceous and somewhat sweet odour

**Perfumery status:** A heart note of medium intensity and medium persistence

**Extraction:** Steam distillation of the fresh crushed seeds, usually in April to May

**1 kg oil yield from:** 30–50 kg of the seeds (an excellent yield)

**Production areas:** Croatia, Hungary, Egypt, France

**Typical constituents (Sweet fennel):** Phenolic ethers (incl. trans-anethole 46–89%, methylchavicol 1–5%, trace cis-anethole) • monoterpenes 30–46% (incl. d-limonene 2–21%, α-pinene 2–4%, cis-ocimene 12%, terpinene 10%, phellandrene <2%, myrcene, sabinene, p-cymene, thujene, camphene) • monoterpenol fenchol 3–4% • ketone fenchone 1–8% • oxide 1,8 cineole traces–6% • (furano)-coumarins bergaptene, psoralene, seseline; umbelliferone, esculetine • trace anisaldehyde

**Note:** Bitter fennel oil has slightly lower levels of trans-anethole (40–70%) and limonene (<5%), and usually somewhat higher levels of fenchone (4–24%) and α-pinene (<15%), making its fragrance less sweet (anethole) and more herbaceous and pungent.

**Chance of adulteration:** Moderate, typically with synthetic additions such as trans- and cis-anethole, fenchone, limonene and methylchavicol (Lis-Balchin 2006)

**Related oils:** Limited amounts of other varieties of fennel oil are sometimes also produced, e.g. German/Russian/Indian/Japanese fennel.

Fennel water or hydrosol enjoys traditional use in herbal medicine for treating conjunctivitis topically.

## Therapeutic Functions and Indications

SPECIFIC SYMPTOMATOLOGY – *All applications*

Moodiness, emotional brooding, emotional inhibition, discouragement, pessimism, malaise, chronic headaches, poor vision, aches and pains, scanty dribbling urination, urinary irritation and incontinence, water retention, painful scanty periods, muscle spasms, neuralgic pains, low-back pain, indigestion with bloating and flatulence, abdominal colic, bronchial congestion with cough, wheezing, palpitations, chest pain, out of breath on exertion

PSYCHOLOGICAL – *Aromatic diffusion, whole-body massage*

**Essential PNEI function and indication:** Regulating in dysregulated conditions

**Possible brain dynamics:** Reduces deep limbic system hyperfunctioning

**Fragrance category:** Middle tone with sweet, pungent notes

**Indicated psychological disorders:** Bipolar disorder, minor depression

PROMOTES EMOTIONAL STABILITY AND INTEGRATION

- Moodiness, emotional instability, repetitive emoting
- Feeling-thinking disconnection and conflict

PROMOTES SELF-CONFIDENCE AND COURAGE

- Loss of self-confidence with insecurity, inhibited emotional expression
- Discouragement with apathy, pessimism

## PHYSIOLOGICAL – *Nebulizer inhalation, gel cap, suppository, external applications*

**Therapeutic status:** Mild remedy with no cumulative toxicity

**Topical safety status:** Non-irritant, non-sensitizing

**Tropism:** Reproductive, digestive, respiratory, urinary systems

**Essential diagnostic function:** Warms asthenic/cold, stimulates hypotonic/weak and relaxes hypertonic/tense terrain conditions

PRIMARILY STIMULANT AND RESTORATIVE:

> *systemic moderate arterial circulatory and smooth-muscle stimulant:* a wide range of chronic asthenic and hypotonic conditions, esp. of reproductive, digestive, respiratory and urinary organs

> – *strong uterine stimulant and restorative, oestrogenic ovarian stimulant, emmenagogue:* low-oestrogen conditions, incl. amenorrhoea, oligomenorrhoea, dysmenorrhoea, PMS, menopausal syndrome

> – *parturient:* stalled labour, atonic and spasmodic uterine dystocia

> – *galactagogue:* insufficient postpartum breastmilk

> – *kidney-bladder stimulant, draining diuretic, anti-inflammatory:* general oedema, lower limb oedema; oliguria, dysuria; urinary infections, incl. cystitis, urethritis

> – *diuretic metabolic detoxiant:* metabolic toxicosis, incl. arthritis, gout, urinary stones, obesity, vision impairment

> – *urinary restorative:* incontinence (leakage), enuresis

> – *digestive stimulant, choleretic, cholagogue, carminative, aperitive, antiemetic:* upper digestive atony with indigestion, flatulence, appetite loss; aerophagia, constipation, anorexia, vomiting

> – *liver-protective*

> – *respiratory stimulant, expectorant:* congestive bronchial conditions, incl. congestive dyspnoea, bronchitis

- *cardiac restorative:* heart weakness (incl. from stress, disease, old age)

- *antilipaemic:* hyperlipidaemia

- *antioxidant*

PRIMARILY RELAXANT:

**systemic nervous relaxant, SNS inhibitor, spasmolytic, analgesic, moderate hypnotic:** a wide range of hypertonic (tense) conditions with spasms and pain, including:

- **neuromuscular relaxant, anti-inflammatory, analgesic:** menstrual pain, labour pain, precordial pain, lumbar pain, dysuria, muscle spasms, myalgia, neuralgia, incl. sciatica

- **neurocardiac relaxant, analgesic:** palpitations with precordial pain, tachycardia, mild anxiety and other neurogenic heart conditions; neurogenic/ Prinzmetal's angina; PMS from electrolyte imbalance

- **digestive relaxant, spasmolytic, analgesic, carminative:** spasmodic intestinal conditions, incl. colic, IBS, colitis, diarrhoea, gastrocardiac syndrome, aerophagia

- **respiratory relaxant, bronchodilator:** spasmodic bronchial conditions with spasmodic dyspnoea and cough; asthma, whooping cough, croup

- **bladder relaxant:** spasmodic dysuria

ANTIMICROBIAL ACTIONS:

**broad-spectrum antifungal:** fungal infections with Candida albicans, Trichophyton spp., Aspergillus, etc.

**anthelmintic:** intestinal parasites, esp. hookworm (Ankylostoma)

SYNERGISTIC COMBINATIONS

- Fennel + Basil ct. methylchavicol: strong smooth-muscle relaxant, spasmolytic and analgesic in all hypertonic (tense) and spasmodic conditions of the respiratory and digestive tract

- Fennel + Hyssop: mucolytic expectorant, bronchodilator and antitussive for all types of dyspnoea and cough; bronchitis, asthma

COMPLEMENTARY COMBINATIONS

- Fennel + Marjoram/Roman camomile: systemic relaxant, spasmolytic, analgesic and anti-inflammatory in all hypertonic (tense) and spasmodic conditions in general

- Fennel + Mandarin/Petitgrain: neurocardiac relaxant for heart conditions of nervous or stress-related origin, incl. tachycardia, neurogenic angina pectoris, anxiety; in PMS from electrolyte imbalance

- Fennel + Palmarosa: cardiac restorative for chronic heart weakness; for heart support in all chronic disease

- Fennel + Grand fir/Silver fir: stimulant mucolytic expectorant for bronchitis and other respiratory infections with congestion, dyspnoea, sputum production

- Fennel + Siberian fir/Cypress: bronchodilator, antitussive in asthmatic conditions with apnea, cough, dispnoea

- Fennel + Spearmint/Cardamom: choleretic, cholagogue, aperitive and carminative for acute upper digestive indigestion with bloating, flatulence, nausea, vomiting

- Fennel + Peppermint + Lavender: intestinal relaxant, spasmolytic and analgesic for colic, IBS, irregular stool, diarrhoea

- Fennel + Juniper berry: stimulant warming emmenagogue for amenorrhoea, scanty periods, esp. with cold

- Fennel + Geranium: uterine restorative, oestrogenic in oestrogen deficiency conditions, incl. PMS, amenorrhoea, menopausal syndrome

- Fennel + Juniper berry: draining diuretic for water retention with oedema, esp. of legs; scanty, irritated urination

- Fennel + Juniper berry: metabolic detoxicant and diuretic in metabolic toxicosis with arthritis, gout, urinary stones, poor vision

- Fennel + Spike lavender: rubefacient and analgesic circulatory stimulant for cold or tired muscles, hair loss (topical use in liniment)

## TOPICAL – *Liniment, ointment, cream, compress and other cosmetic preparations*

**Skin care:** Dry and mature skin types

*rubefacient:* devitalized, tired, cold or water-retentive skin; wrinkles, bruises, cellulite, hair loss; cold tired muscles: to prepare or finish activity and sports

*decongestant:* mild mastitis, breast engorgement

*antifungal:* fungal skin infections

**Therapeutic precautions:** Fennel oil is best avoided in systemic hypotonic/weak and hypersthenic/hot conditions. As it promotes oestrogen with its content in oestrogen-like molecules, Fennel by internal use is contraindicated in all high-oestrogen conditions, including oestrogen accumulation syndrome, uterine fibroids, endometriosis and oestrogen-dependent cancers. For the same reason, the oil is also contraindicated during the first seven months of pregnancy and because of its uterine stimulant action, as well as during breastfeeding.

**Pharmacological precautions:** Both Sweet and Bitter fennel oils are generally contraindicated in babies, infants and young children under five, and in those prone to migraine headaches and epilepsy. Because of their anethole content, internal use should also be avoided in liver disease, peptic ulcer, haemophilia, and those taking anti-diabetic or anticoagulant medication. Although there is a theoretical risk of its minor constituent methyleugenol acting as a carcinogen, limonene is anticarcinogenic. No carcinogenic risk is noted in French medicine and no related prohibition exists in French pharmacy regulations.

**Preparations:**

- Diffusor: 1–3 drops in water

- Massage oil: 1–3% dilution in vegetable oil

- Liniment: 3–6% dilution in vegetable oil for short-term use

- Gel cap: 1–2 drops with olive oil

## Chinese Medicine Functions and Indications

**Aroma energy:** Sweet, pungent

**Movement:** Circulating

**Warmth:** Neutral to warm

**Meridian tropism:** Liver, Spleen, Stomach, Lung, Heart

**Five-Element affinity:** Earth, Metal, Wood

**Essential function:** To activate Qi and Blood, resolve damp, harmonize the Shen and relieve pain

1. **Activates the Lower Warmer, breaks up stagnation, promotes menstruation and relieves pain**

   - **Lower Warmer Blood and Qi stagnation** with delayed, scanty or stopped periods, painful periods, PMS:

     Rosemary/Yarrow/Juniper berry/Angelica root

2. **Activates the Qi, harmonizes the Middle Warmer, regulates digestion and relieves pain**

   - **Liver-Stomach/Spleen disharmony** with epigastric and/or abdominal pain, indigestion, flatulence, diarrhoea and/or constipation, mood swings, feeling stressed:

     Bergamot/Peppermint/German camomile/Roman camomile

   - **Stomach Qi and food stagnation** with indigestion on eating, appetite loss, epigastric bloating, nausea, belching, constipation:

     Spearmint/Mandarin/May chang/Lemongrass

3. **Resolves and drains damp, harmonizes urination, and relieves leakage and swelling**

   - **Lower Warmer turbid-damp (damp, stone lin)** with frequent, scanty, dribbling urination, incontinence, irritation, bedwetting:

     Lemon/Yarrow/Juniper berry

   - **Water-damp accumulation** with general oedema, leg oedema, fatigue:

     Geranium/Juniper berry/Grapefruit

4. **Warms the Stomach, descends Stomach Qi and relieves pain**

   - **Stomach cold with Qi rebellion**, with nausea, appetite loss, belching, vomiting:

     Peppermint/Cardamom/Ginger/Clove

   - **Stomach cold with shan qi**, with sharp abdominal pain:

     Roman camomile/Peppermint/Marjoram

5. **Warms the Lung, diffuses and descends Lung Qi, relaxes the chest and relieves wheezing**

   - **Lung phlegm-cold with Qi accumulation**, with stuffy chest, difficult breathing, sternum pain, wheezing, cough:

     Siberian fir/Hyssop/Thyme ct. linalool

6. **Regulates Heart Qi, harmonizes the Shen and relieves precordial pain**

- **Heart Qi constraint with Shen dysregulation**, with chest pains, palpitations, anxiety, feeling stressed:

  Mandarin/Lavender/Petitgrain/Neroli

REMARKS

The seed of this perennial aromatic plant from the Mediterranean basin is appreciated for its culinary uses, as in fish and seafood dishes, and is still an ingredient in common liqueurs such as pastis. The word 'fennel' itself derives from the Latin *foeniculum*, literally meaning 'little hay', most likely because of its grassy aroma when chewed – fennel has always been a gratifying postprandial carminative. The seed found wide use in ancient Egypt and, once channelled eastwards throughout Asia through the network of land and ocean Silk Roads, quickly became a familiar spice and herbal remedy in two other culinary and medical environments, Indian and Chinese. In Europe, Fennel made the typical transition from an Italian medicinal herb to an aromatic water to a distilled essential oil in the course of the 14th- and 15th-century Renaissance. Both types of Fennel oil, the sweet and the bitter, may be used interchangeably – and have been all along. However, Sweet fennel oil is preferred in England, while Bitter fennel oil is standard in the French and most other European pharmacopeias.

It is interesting to note that Chinese medicine values Fennel for its stimulant, warming functions, while Western herbal medicine makes more use of its relaxant effects. With Fennel's entry as an essential oil remedy, its therapeutic applications have become even more divergent and eventually appear somewhat enigmatic. The best approach today would be to weigh the evidence of traditional experience with the facts of pharmacology. From both perspectives, Fennel comes out as a twin stimulant and relaxant for most of its indicated conditions. It displays this more dramatically than most other bivalent remedies of the same type. A glance at its chemistry profile reinforces this view, with its stimulating constituents roughly balanced by relaxing ones: the balance of monoterpenes and phenolic ethers. This thumbnail description holds true for both Sweet and Bitter fennel, as the different levels of a few constituents are relatively minor.

From the functional medicine perspective, Fennel essentially treats chronic weak-tense terrain with all its resultant stagnation. Looking at its most common traditional uses, it is clear that Fennel mainly addresses reproductive, urinary, digestive, respiratory and neuromuscular functions. In each of these areas, the oil is able to act bivalently in stimulation or relaxation mode, all depending on the need of the individual terrain.

As an important female reproductive remedy, Fennel excels as both an oestrogenic uterine stimulant for amenorrhoea, and a spasmolytic uterine relaxant for spasmodic dysmenorrhoea. The same in the gut and bronchi. Like Cardamom, the remedy is valued as a virtual panacea for digestive disorders, especially as an analgesic carminative with indigestion, pain, bloating and nausea. Again, Fennel is both a good stimulant expectorant for congestive bronchial conditions, and a spasmolytic bronchodilator in spasmodic bronchial conditions of all types – a use especially espoused by some French practitioners, who consider it second only to Basil ct. methylchavicol in this regard. They note that trans-anethole is actively spasmolytic and analgesic, as well as oestrogenic (Faucon 2015). In terms of neuromuscular functions, Fennel again acts as both a stimulant and relaxant, and is often chosen for its spasmolytic neuromuscular analgesic functions that address both neuralgic and myalgic pain.

However, this oil truly shines when tension appears together with weakness; when the two conditions need to be reconciled. This makes Fennel an excellent choice for the above-mentioned conditions once they become chronic and present secondary forms of stagnation with pain as their chief symptom expression – e.g. chronic forms of dysmenorrhoea or scanty periods with uterine weakness underpinned by low levels of oestrogen. Likewise, chronic urinary, digestive, respiratory and neuromuscular disorders that combine symptoms of tension and weakness.

Topically, Fennel is a good choice for both fungal skin infections and as a versatile, non-irritant and non-sensitizing warming rubefacient for a cluster of dermal and muscular uses.

Used by olfaction for its psychological functions, Fennel strongly targets the realm of instinctive feeling. Sweet and pungent, the fragrance helps bring to emotional awareness unconscious instinctive feelings, especially those associated with nurture, safety and belonging. Fennel is for the individual burdened with the discomfort of unresolved stuffed feelings in general. The result is a key oil for encouraging emotional expression in those unable to access what they feel on a deeper level. Fennel can encourage letting go of unresolved emotions and repetitive emoting rather than expressing genuine emotions with confidence and clarity. Moreover, by helping release unconscious feelings related to nurture and safety, the oil will help integrate repressed issues of emotional hunger and therefore heal deep vulnerability within the whole personality.

**Related oils:** The following oils are similar to Fennel and share many of its uses.

**Aniseed** (*Pimpinella anisum* L.) from Egypt and India has the typical warm, sweet-spicy fragrance of the crushed seed. It has always been used as a spice and herbal remedy in Middle Eastern cultures, and figures in numerous liqueurs throughout Mediterranean countries. The oil is produced mainly in Egypt, Turkey, Hungary and Spain. It contains the phenolic ether trans-anethole (90–96%) as major constituent, supported by d-limonene and methyl chavicol (both <5%), and some coumarins. Aniseed's therapeutic status, functions and actions are very similar to those of Fennel, except that its systemic neuromuscular and other relaxant actions for treating hypertonic/tense conditions are much stronger than its restorative actions. With a dominant tropism for the digestive tract, the oil is an excellent carminative and aperitive stomachic as well as a gastrointestinal spasmolytic. Major indications include indigestion with flatulence, appetite loss, nausea, hiccups, aerophagia, colic and colitis. It also promotes gastric secretions, reduces intestinal fermentation and is a cholagogue and choleretic. As a bronchial relaxant, Aniseed treats bronchial asthma and spasmodic coughs of all types. In gynaecology, the oil is valued for its emmenagogue and oestrogenic actions in amenorrhoea, hypo-oestrogen syndrome and menopausal syndrome. It is parturient during labour and a galactagogue during breastfeeding. The precautions are the same as for Fennel, but the physiological dose is lower, e.g. maximum 1 drop twice daily by gel cap, if ever taken as a single remedy.

**Star anise** (*Illicium verum* Hook. f.) oil from Vietnam, South China and the Philippines has the typical warm, sweet-liquorice, spicy fragrance of the crushed fruit. The fruit's use as a digestive spice and herbal remedy in Chinese medicine goes back to ancient times. Star anise oil also contains the phenolic ether trans-anethole (70–93%) as a major constituent with small amounts of d-limonene, terpenes, anisaldehyde and methylchavicol (<3.5%). The same functions, actions and precautions as for Aniseed apply.

**Khella** (*Amni visnaga* Lam.) from Morocco is the oil distilled from the fruits ('seeds') of a carrot-family plant. Its fragrance is herbaceous-green with rooty, oily notes; its chemical profile is dominant in monoterpenols (linalool 29%, borneol) and a slew of esters c. 32% (incl. isoamyl methylbutyrate and amyl isobutyrate), rounded off with small amonts of coumarins (including khellin, visnadin and visnagin), pulegone <2% and possibly chromones. Khella is valued mainly for its strong spasmolytic and analgesic action on smooth muscles that has been compared to that of the alkaloid papaverine. Its main physiological indications are acute, painful intestinal, gallbladder, kidney and uterine colic/spasms. Khella is also strongly bronchodilatant in acute asthma and vasodilatant in acute spastic and congestive angina, and somewhat anticoagulant. The only precaution is reports in the French literature of possible photosensitization and allergic reactions with topical use arising from its coumarin content. Moderate dilutions and doses apply.

**Butterbur** (*Petasites officinalis* Moench, syn. *P. hybridus* Gaertner, Meyer et Scherbius) is the oil distilled from the root of this temperate biome plant in the sunflower (Asteraceae) family. Its fragrance displays complex warm, hay-herbaceous and musty-rooty notes with lingering mild sweet-honey notes. Chemically the oil consists largely of sesquiterpenol esters (incl. petasin, petasyle and isopetasyle angelate), a sesquiterpenol (petasol) and sesquiterpene lactones (incl. eremophilanolides and philanolides). Butterbur is a traditional European herbal remedy that relies on its content in both essential oil and the pyrolizidine alkaloid platyphyllin for its renowned efficacy. Prepared in tincture form, it is a medium-strength remedy with some cumulative toxicity arising from its alkaloid.

The oil itself has seen little to no research except for clinical use as a strong analgesic and anti-inflammatory spasmolytic that is considered stronger than the alkaloid papaverine. French practitioners have achieved good results with its bronchodilatant and fluidifying expectorant actions in asthma and spasmodic/asthmatic bronchitis with spasmodic dyspnoea, cough and hard sputum. When absorbed internally, Butterbur also acts equally relaxant to the smooth muscles in spasmodic intestinal colic and gallbladder colic. It has also shown notably good results in the treatment of migraines, considered by many to be mini-seizures. The oil is also hypotensive for hypertension conditions and topically analgesic and antihistamine for relief of allergic dermatitis with pruritus, and other painful skin conditions. For both asthma prevention and treatment, a 5–10% dilution liniment is often applied, in between episodes, on the chest, nape, the upper back between the shoulderblades, and along the spine.

In tincture form, Butterbur root enjoys many other traditional uses, including the treatment of acute neuralgic and rheumatic pain (especially of the lumbars and loins), spasmodic dysmenorrhoea, amenorrhoea, dysuria and anuria, and also cardiac insufficiency and skin cancer pain (Holmes 2007). While it is very possible that Butterbur oil may address these other indications, there is currently insufficient evidence for certainty. What is certain is that the plant's alkaloid also contributes to its therapeutic synergy, despite being somewhat hepatotoxic and teratogenic. Nevertheless, for lack of clearer knowledge and because of the oil's strong tropism for the uterus, it should still be avoided during pregnancy and breastfeeding, as well as in babies and infants. Moderate dilutions and doses apply.

# Frankincense

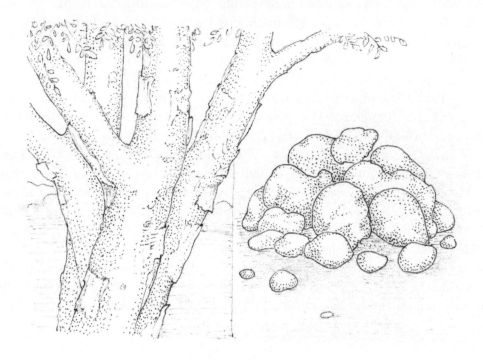

**Botanical source:** The oleo-gum-resin of *Boswellia sacra* Flückiger (syn. *Boswellia carterii* Birdw.) (Burseraceae – torchwood or incense-tree family), a hardy tree from desert regions of East Africa and Saudi Arabia. The frankincense tree of Somalia, hitherto identified as *Boswellia carterii*, is now considered to be *B. sacra*.

**Other names:** Olibanum; Luban (Arabic), Encens (Fr), Weihrauch (Ge), Incenso (It), Olibano (Sp), Ru xiang (Mandarin)

**Appearance:** A mobile pale yellow or yellow-green fluid with a sweet, woody-balsamic odour with camphoraceous and slightly lemony top notes, and rich sweet-woody basenotes

**Perfumery status:** A base note of medium intensity and good persistence

**Extraction:** Steam distillation of the oleo-gum-resin, usually in September to November. A resinoid absolute of Frankincense is also produced for the perfumery industry by solvent extraction.

   1 kg of the resinoid absolute is obtained from only about 2 kg of the resin.

**1 kg oil yield from:** 15–20 kg of the resin tears (an excellent yield)

**Production areas:** Somalia, Ethiopia, Oman, Yemen (Hadramawt). The resin is actually distilled or solvent extracted mostly in Europe and the US.

The resin itself is produced by making shallow scrapes into the tree trunk, from which a milky gum-resin soon exudes and slowly solidifies. About two or three weeks later, when the resin has sufficiently hardened, the white resin tears are collected first, as they are considered the best quality; the portion that ran down the trunk or fell to the ground is considered inferior. In the Dhofar Confederate of South Oman the green resin is considered superior and is taken internally. The dry tears are usually brittle, and pear or club shaped, and transparent whitish-yellow in colour; through friction they also acquire a thin white patina. This resin generally consists of 56–65% acid resin, 20–36% gum and 4–8% essential oil. The Roman writer Plinius the Elder (*Historiae Naturalis*) noted that mammose (breast-shaped) pieces are 'most esteemed of all', a widespread belief that also contributed the resin's Chinese name from the Tang era, Ju xiang, 'teat aromatic'.

**Typical constituents (Somalian sample):** Monoterpenes 40% (incl. α-pinene 36%, d-limonene 8%, α-thujene 24%, p-cymene 6%, sabinene 6%, camphene, β-myrcene 4%, α-terpinene, β-pinene 3%, δ-3-carene <3%, β-caryophyllene 2%, γ-terpinene, terpinolene) • sesquiterpenes (incl. α-gurjunene, α-guaiene, α- and β-phellandrene, copaene) • monoterpenols (incl. borneol, transpino-carveol, terpinenol) • sesquiterpenol (farnesol) • ketone (verbenone) • esters (incl. octyl acetate 18%, incensole acetate, octyl formate) • triterpenes (incl. boswellic acid)

Oman and Yemen frankincense has the same profile, but without the triterpenes.

**Chance of adulteration:** Moderate, usually by the addition of synthetic components such as α-pinene. With its much higher yield, Frankincense resinoid dissolved in alcohol is also sometimes passed off as the distilled oil in commerce.

**Related oils:** Of the 20 or so species of Boswellia found in rough, inhospitable areas of West Africa, Arabia and India, those yielding other types of Frankincense oil include:

- *Boswellia papyrifera* (Delile ex Caill.) Hochst. from Ethiopia and Sudan; it has a similar profile of constituents to *B. sacra*, but is much lower in monoterpenes (<9%) and high in octyl acetate (50–60%)

- *Boswellia rivae* Engler from Ethiopia; its profile is also similar to *B. sacra*, but its d-limonene levels are <28% and its δ-3-carene <17%

- *Boswellia frereana* Birdw. from Somalia (the Horn of Africa), with monoterpenes <77%

- *Boswellia serrata* Roxb. ex Colebr. from Rajasthan in India, known as Indian frankincense, Guggul or Salai guggul, with monoterpene levels <90% (65% α-thujene); it is mainly given for its anti-inflammatory and analgesic actions.

# Therapeutic Functions and Indications

## SPECIFIC SYMPTOMATOLOGY – *All applications*

Despondency, grief, listlessness, depression, discouragement, low perseverance and willpower, mental and physical fatigue, mental fog and confusion, scattered thinking, insecurity, anxiety, frequent infections, weak lungs, chronic coughing and wheezing with expectoration, genital discharges, scanty or absent periods, muscle and joint aches and pains with swelling and stiffness

## PSYCHOLOGICAL – *Aromatic diffusion, whole-body massage*

**Essential PNEI function and indication:** Stimulant in weakness conditions; regulating in dysregulation conditions

**Possible brain dynamics:** Increases prefrontal cortex functioning and regulates basal ganglia hyper- or hypo-functioning

**Fragrance category:** Middle tone with pungent, woody notes

**Indicated psychological disorders:** ADD, depression, dissociative disorder, psychotic and schizoid conditions

### PROMOTES WILLPOWER AND PERSEVERANCE

- Low willpower or strength, loss of personal boundaries

- Discouragement, low perseverance, despair, depression

- Mental and emotional burnout, shock

### STABILIZES THE MIND AND PROMOTES SECURITY

- Mental instability and scatteredness, anxiety

- Insecurity, fearfulness

## PHYSIOLOGICAL – *Nebulizer inhalation, gel cap, suppository, external applications*

**Therapeutic status:** Mild remedy with no cumulative toxicity

**Topical safety status:** Non-irritant, non-sensitizing

**Tropism:** Nervous, respiratory, digestive, muscular systems

**Essential diagnostic function:** Restores and stimulates hypotonic/weak terrain conditions

PRIMARILY RESTORATIVE:

**nervous and cerebral restorative, antidepressant:** chronic hypotonic (weak) conditions with mental and physical fatigue, incl. neurasthenia, depression, cognitive impairment, CFS

**respiratory restorative:** chronic lower respiratory weakness and congestion, incl. weak lungs, any chronic respiratory disorder

**mucosal restorative, subastringent mucostatic:** mucoid diarrhoea, leucorrhoea, gonorrhoea, gleet, mucous cystitis

PRIMARILY STIMULANT:

**respiratory stimulant and decongestant, mucolytic and fluidifying expectorant, anti-inflammatory:** chronic congestive respiratory conditions, incl. bronchitis, asthma emphysema; esp. with copious sputum, dyspnoea, apnoea

**uterine stimulant, emmenagogue:** amenorrhoea, dysmenorrhoea

**diuretic**

**pineal stimulant**(?)

PRIMARILY RELAXANT:

**strong anti-inflammatory, analgesic:** acute tissue trauma, rheumatic/arthritic pain and swelling; menstrual pain; throat, chest, epigastric and abdominal pain; sore nipples

**anti-inflammatory, immune regulator:** inflammation in type-III and type-IV immune sensitivity, incl. most autoimmune disorders, incl. rheumatoid arthritis, lupus, acute glomerulonephritis, inflammatory bowel disease

**respiratory relaxant, bronchospasmolytic:** spasmodic respiratory conditions, dyspnoea, asthma

**sinew relaxant:** joint stiffness or cramping

MISCELLANEOUS ACTIONS:

**antioxidant, antitumoural:** cancer

**immunostimulant, antiviral:** immune deficiency conditions with frequent infections, esp. viral

**moderate antibacterial:** bacterial infections, esp. respiratory, urogenital

SYNERGISTIC COMBINATIONS

- Frankincense + Black pepper/Nutmeg: strong anti-inflammatory and analgesic for musculoskeletal inflammation and pain of any kind; arthritic and tendino-rheumatic disorders with pain and cramping, esp. in weak-cold terrain

- Frankincense + Ravintsara/Thyme ct. thymol: nervous-cerebral restorative and antidepressant for chronic neurasthenia, depression, debility and cognitive impairment

- Frankincense + Black spruce: nervous and immune restorative/stimulant in all chronic immune deficiency conditions with frequent or recurring infections

- Frankincense + Ravintsara/Saro: antiviral, immunostimulant and nervous restorative in chronic, recurring or dormant viral infections in weak terrain, incl. herpes viruses, CFS, CNV, EBV

- Frankincense + Scotch pine/Black spruce: respiratory restorative, expectorant for weak lungs, any chronic respiratory disorder, incl. with dyspnoea, sputum production

COMPLEMENTARY COMBINATIONS

- Frankincense + Green myrtle/Spearmint: mucolytic expectorant for chronic bronchitis with copious sputum

- Frankincense + Hyssop/Cypress: stimulant expectorant, antitussive for chronic bronchial conditions with coughing (esp. spasmodic), dyspnoea, chronic apnoea, asthma

- Frankincense + Juniper berry: emmenagogue for amenorrhoea, esp. from cold

- Frankincense + Geranium + Myrrh: mucostatic mucosal restorative for chronic vaginitis with leucorrhoea and other reproductive and urinary discharges

- Frankincense + Cistus: anti-inflammatory immune regulator for autoimmune disorders, incl. rheumatoid arthritis, lupus, IBD, Crohn's disease, acute glomerulonephritis

TOPICAL – *Liniment, ointment, cream, compress and other cosmetic preparations*

**Skin care:** Dry and mature skin types

*skin regenerator:* wrinkles, scar tissue

*vulnerary, anti-inflammatory, detergent, antiseptic, astringent, subhaemostatic:* wounds (incl. deep injuries), chronic ulcers, varicose ulcers, non-suppurating sores, swollen gums; psoriasis; minor bleeding

*analgesic, anti-inflammatory:* acute tissue trauma, pain of dermatitis, rheumatism, arthritis, menstruation; throat, chest, epigastric and abdominal pain; sore nipples

*rubefacient:* poor hair growth

*detumescent, resolvent:* swollen boils, traumatic oedema and swelling, acne, carbuncles, abscesses, lymphadenitis

**Therapeutic precautions:** Frankincense oil is contraindicated during pregnancy because of its emmenagogue action. It is somewhat drying and should generally be avoided in all dry conditions, and especially with dry cough.

**Pharmacological precautions:** Being high in monoterpenes, oxidized Frankincense oil may cause skin sensitization. Avoid use in babies and infants.

**Preparations:**

- Diffusor: 2–4 drops in water

- Massage oil: 2–5% dilution in vegetable oil

- Liniment: 3–10% dilution in vegetable oil

- Gel cap: 2–3 drops with olive oil

# Chinese Medicine Functions and Indications

**Aroma energy:** Pungent, woody

**Movement:** Rising, circulating

**Warmth:** Neutral to warm

**Meridian tropism:** Lung, Heart, Triple Heater, Bladder

**Five-Element affinity:** Metal, Fire

**Essential function:** To tonify the Qi, activate Blood and Qi, and strengthen the Shen

1. **Tonifies the Qi, animates the Heart, strengthens the Shen and relieves depression**

    - **Qi deficiency with Shen weakness**, with mental and physical fatigue, depression, debility:

    Sage/Black spruce/Ravintsara

- **Heart and Lung Qi deficiency with Shen weakness**, with mental and physical fatigue, mental confusion, depression, pessimism, grief:
  Rosemary/Palmarosa/Hemlock spruce

2. **Resolves and eliminates phlegm, diffuses Lung Qi and relieves coughing**

- **Lung phlegm-damp/cold with Qi accumulation**, with sputum expectoration, coughing, difficult breathing, fatigue:
  Grand fir/Hyssop/Laurel

3. **Circulates and descends Lung Qi, and relieves pain and wheezing**

- **Lung Qi accumulation** with wheezing, tight chest, sternum pain, cough, fatigue:
  Fennel/Basil ct. methylchavicol/Cypress

4. **Activates Blood and Qi, breaks up stagnation and relieves pain and swelling**

- **Blood stagnation from acute trauma** with pain, swelling, discoloration:
  Geranium/Helichrysum/Myrrh/Wintergreen

- **Qi and Blood stagnation** with pain, incl. muscle and joint pain, menstrual pain, chest and abdominal pain:
  Roman camomile/Peppermint/Marjoram/Frankincense

5. **Opens the meridians, dispels wind-damp, relaxes the tendons and relieves pain**

- **Wind-damp obstruction** with stiff, painful joints of the extremities:
  Ravintsara/Niaouli/Rosemary ct. cineole or camphor/Wintergreen

REMARKS

The sticky resin secreted by the small, hardy frankincense tree of the harsh deserts of Somalia and Saudi Arabia has been harvested by Somalian, Arabic and Bedouin collectors for many a millennium. Once sorted and graded, the hardened tears of resin were sold to a relay of Arab traders who ferried them north along the overland spice trail. Frankincense thereby eventually reached the major cultural centres of Mesopotamia to the northeast and Egypt to the northwest where, like myrrh resin, it became an extremely precious commodity – at times worth more by weight than silver or gold.

Like myrrh and benzoin, frankincense was a precious aromatic in the ancient cultures of Sumeria, Babylon, Egypt, Assyria, Phoenicia, Egypt, Greece and Rome. It typified both their cultural scentscape and their archetypal soul scent – a legacy that modern Judaic and Christian societies inherited. Along with myrrh, frankincense is the most consistently used aromatic in Western religious practice, both ceremonial and meditational; it is specifically the timeless incense of the Western solar deities. The resin was censed on one hand to create an aromatic human connection to the divine in a desire for transcendental union. With a twin uplifting and calming effect, Frankincense can induce the state of focused contemplation necessary for aspiration to spirit. Conversely, the resin was traditionally also burnt to bless and inspire humans with the very fragrance of divinity. Its spiritual power would effectively disperse the forces of evil or negative energy that were responsible for disease and bad karma among humans. It was the iconic scent of divine purification.

Sumerians are known to have incorporated frankincense in their extensive range of aromatics, most of which were cultivated in what is thought to be the original biblical Garden of Eden. According to Greek historian Herodotus, Babylonians used to burn huge quantities of various resins in their sacred rites to their pantheon of gods, especially to the sun god Bael. They also developed the science of aromatic astrology to unprecedented heights, as interpretive astronomy was one of their core sciences. We may assume that frankincense was an important aromatic in ceremonies in which the king consummated his sacred marriage with the goddess at the summit of the ziggurat, the pyramidal temple palace that represented the sacred point of contact between heaven and earth.

The Egyptians continued the time-worn tradition of bringing down the divine favours of the sun gods by censing specific aromatic blends at dawn, midday and dusk throughout the kingdom. Frankincense was an important component of Kyphi, the temple incense burnt in Heliopolis every sunset to honour the setting of the sun god Rê. Queen Hatshepsut was not only a big-scale importer of resins such as myrrh, frankincense and opopanax from the land of Punt (Somaliland), but also began her own cultivation of Boswellia trees in the Nile river delta, where they apparently still grow today. Her tomb of 1480 BC contains large murals of frankincense plants. Although for most of Egyptian civilization the sacred resins and plant oils were in the domain of the priests, in the reign of Ramses III the latter started making them available to the upper classes. Eventually, like the Sumerians before them, the Egyptians incorporated most aromatics into their everyday life. The extravagant use of fragrance by late-dynasty queen Cleopatra is well documented – for example, her encounter with Mark Anthony, from the aromatic billows of her reception ship to the seductive scents of her bed chamber.

Frankincense resin in most ancient cultures was also an important aromatic in perfumery, hygiene, skin care and medicine. Resins such as myrrh, galbanum and frankincense saw widespread secular as well as sacred applications, which included extensive individual and social fragrancing. Beauty care and perfumery uses for frankincense, some of which survive to this day, also date back to the highly developed Sumerian civilization in the third or fourth millennium BC. Cosmetic applications of frankincense dating to ancient times include the use of kohl, which consisted of several resins ground and charred, for a black eyeliner that originally served to ward off the evil eye; the use of a multi-ingredient paste to perfume the hands; and, according to historian Herodotus, the use of molten frankincense for a depilatory paste.

Just as in Arabic society to this day, frankincense in Hebraic culture was originally considered the most effective scent for attracting divine blessings and dispersing evil spirits. It was (and sometimes still is) censed to purify living and work quarters as well as synagogues and mosques – with the optional addition of some benzoin and aloeswood. Ever since the edict of the prophet Moses to the Hebrews around 1500 BC to make sacred aromatic offerings, Levonah or frankincense was burnt in braziers on the incense altar morning and evening – and eventually in the main Temple sanctuary in Jerusalem, and in outlying synagogues. Together with other ingredients composing the sacred incense, the precious resin was kept in a great chamber within the Temple. Its use according to the prescribed proportions was forbidden for secular purposes. Later sacred incense recipes from the Talmud always include frankincense, along with about 16 other ingredients. However, unlike myrrh, frankincense was not used in any anointing oil recipes, such as the one found in the Book of Wisdom: anointing oils have associations with the sensuous biblical Song of Songs and the visit to Solomon by the beguiling queen of Sheba. Frankincense was also traditionally offered on its own as a supplement to sacrifice for first fruits, for the meal offering and the sabbath showbread.

The oldest Temple incense recipe, according to the Book of Exodus, was Stacte (possibly myrrh), Onycha (musk), galbanum and frankincense. Christian church incense has always made frankincense the main component, with optional secondary amounts of myrrh and/or benzoin. The Russian orthodox church, in contrast, uses mainly benzoin with optional myrrh, frankincense and others.

Frankincense saw only restrained use in Greece, being appropriately offered mainly to the sun-god Apollo in his various temples. The same was true in early Rome, when the physicians Celsus and Galenus (Galen) discussed the resin Olibanum or Mascula thura (as it was then known) in their many textbooks on remedies and aromatics. In later imperial Rome, however, this was no longer true. Benefiting from both the Silk Roads from China and Central Asia, and the Spice Road from Saudi Arabia, Rome imported ever-increasing amounts of aromatics from all corners of the globe, spending them on endless prodigal social banquets and ceremonies, both secular and sacred. To emperor Nero belongs the dubious distinction of once spending four million sestertii (over £90,000 or $120,000 in today's currency) to fragrance a single party. Rome's lavish expenditure on frankincense alone rivalled that of any previous culture: during the first century, Rome managed to burn up almost 3,000 tons of the costly resin. And surpassing even himself, on the death of his beloved wife Poppaea, the emperor Nero at her funeral decided to burn more than the entire annual output of Arabian frankincense. We can understand why, to the Romans, Saudi Arabia was *Arabia felix*, Arabia the Blessed.

All three extant classical systems of medicine, traditional Greek, Indian (Ayurveda) and Chinese, include Frankincense as an important remedy in their materia medicas (allowing for variations in the species used). However, it is very likely that its medicinal use goes back to the early Levant cultures. The medieval Persian physician Ibn Sina (Avicenna) documents using Frankincense for ulcers, tumours, fevers, dysentery and vomiting, for example, and in India and the West the remedy has been extensively used both in internal medicine and for trauma care and dermatology.

Chinese medicine employs Frankincense mainly for topical applications in conditions involving pain or tissue trauma. Here it is usually compounded with other remedies in an ointment, plaster or liniment to reduce pain, inflammation and bleeding from injury, as well as for ulcerative, arthritic, rheumatic or menstrual pain. Frankincense oil possesses all of these uses and counts as one of the top oils for tissue trauma and skin lesions in general. Today its boswellic acid is said to be a potent inhibitor of inflammation via the complement pathway, making a wide range of inflammatory disorders, including autoimmune ones, indications for its use. This same acid has also shown antioxidant and anticancer properties; it is said to suppress cancer tumour cells without fragmenting DNA and activate the genes that inhibit the growth of cancer cells (Khan *et al.* 2016).

The oil also shares Frankincense's traditional Greek and Ayurvedic medical uses, where it is described as a drying, astringing, solidifying remedy for damp or kapha conditions of the digestive, respiratory and urogenital organs. These usually involve discharges, such as excessive phlegm production in bronchitis, and leucorrhoea in vaginitis. Frankincense's stimulant and relaxant effects, based on its pungent, warm qualities, also engage in these conditions, and specifically also address amenorrhoea as well as congestive and spasmodic forms of dyspnoea with bronchitis or asthma. Because the remedy exerts a strong tropism for respiratory functions, its additional restorative effect on the lung makes it a strong candidate for treating chronic respiratory conditions, whatever their name.

Modern practice has extended the range of Frankincense's indications to include the treatment of chronic neurasthenic disorders, such as depression and chronic fatigue, and immunodeficiency conditions marked by frequent or chronic infections. The individual terrain is clearly one of chronic weakness with tendency to either hypofunctioning or dysregulated functioning – as in the case of autoimmune disorders, where it functions more as an immune regulator than as an immune enhancer and stimulant.

Clearly, Fankincense is one of the world's major remedies for gentle olfactory use by ambient diffusion. Its original French name is *Franc encens*, literally 'pure incense', denoting the 'pure censing aromatic'. With a twin uplifting and stabilizing effect, inhaling the pungent, sweet, balsamic fragrance of Frankincense can induce a state of focused contemplation or meditation that is ideal for inviting spiritual inspiration. Inspiring or literally breathing in its fragrance lifts and connects us to spirit, the divine, while yet not letting go of our body. Fankincense is all inspiration and in-breathing to connect to something greater and purer than ourselves.

In so doing, the 'pure incense' can help us transcend worldly concerns and resolve anxiety and worry in particular. In supporting us to become temporarily removed from adverse worldly circumstances, it can act as an effective palliative for soul conditions that are painful, debilitating and life-diminishing. This may include conditions of chronic psychic or physical pain, including the pain of chronic or severe illness, chronic grief from loss, depression with loss of hope and despair, burnout or nervous breakdown, and suicidal tendencies. In these conditions, Frankincense can support the suffering individual in maintaining mental and soul balance, and in regaining a positive feeling of connection to others, despite past hurts, wrongs and trauma, and despite a continued sense of innate human vulnerability.

Ultimately, Frankincense is a key essential oil for helping us cross the Rainbow Bridge along our path of developing consciousness towards wholeness. With its seven colours, the Rainbow Bridge connects heaven and earth, like the seven stoles of the Egyptian goddess Isis, or the winged, perfumed Greek goddess Iris who conveyed the gods' messages to humans. Frankincense can thus promote the integration of the two basic embodied life movements: the upward movement of liberation through transcendence with the downward movement of manifestation through immanence. Resolving these polarities into wholeness, this sacred oil can help us connect the mundane with the sacred, the ego self with the spirit self, and the human with the cosmic.

**Related oils:** The following oils, predominantly from the torchwood family, have similar uses to Frankincense.

**Palo santo** (*Bursera graveolens* Triana & Planch.) from a small and unfortunately endangered tree in the torchwood (Burseraceae) family in Central and South America has a warm, woody, somewhat pungent fragrance. The wood enjoys wide traditional use in smudging ceremonies by shamans or medicine men for clearing negative energy. Significant constituents of its essential oil are l-limonene 58%, α-terpineol 11%, menthofuran 7% and carvone. Rhind (2014) suggests anti-inflammatory, analgesic, vulnerary and antifungal actions for these constituents which could be engaged in the treatment of conditions such as rheumatic and arthritic disorders, wounds and fungal infections.

**Guaiac** or **Guayacol** is the oil extracted from Argentine or Paraguay lignum vitae (*Bulnesia sarmienti* Lorenz) in the caltrop (Zygophyllaceae) family, a tree of the Gran Chaco area in South America; its name refers to the true lignum vitae of the genus *Guaiacum* from which the celebrated traditional European remedy for syphillis was prepared. Unfortunately, the Argentine lignum vitae is also ambiguously called palo santo. With its soft, rosy, woody notes, Guaiac oil is mainly produced for flavouring soaps and perfumes. It is high in a slew of sesquiterpenes and their alcohols and may be used therapeutically for its venous and lymphatic decongestant action. It has found good use in pelvic and general venous congestion with heavy periods, haemorrhoids and varicose veins. Topical uses are expected to resemble those of Patchouli and Copaiba oil. No cautions are noted.

**Linaloeswood** (*Bursera delpechiana* Poisson) in the torchwood (Burseraceae) family is native to Mexico; the oil is distilled there for the flavouring industry, mainly from the wood and to a lesser extent the berries. Its soft rosy, lemony fragrance signals a 30–37% linalool content, along with α-terpineol <9%; other constituents include linalyl acetate <47% and geranyl acetate <31%. Linaloeswood is used by French practitioners mainly for its spasmolytic, analgesic and autonomic nervous regulating actions for painful spasms in general, as well as for more long-term ANS dysregulation in chronic digestive and mood disorders. Its significant content in linalyl acetate, as in Petitgrain and Lavender, would also suggest use in chronic conditions where nerve support is needed, and especially for neurasthenia. The oil is also generally anti-infective. No cautions are known. Linaloe leaf oil is reported to contain <70% linalyl acetate.

# Grand Fir

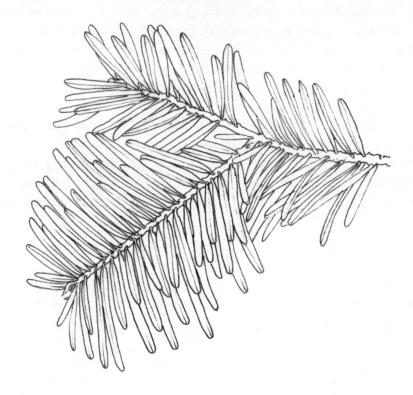

**Botanical source:** The twigs and needles of *Abies grandis* (Douglas ex D. Don) Lindley (Pinaceae – pine family), an evergreen coniferous tree from temperate boreal forests

**Other names:** Giant fir, Vancouver fir, Lowland white fir; Sapin géant (Fr), Grosstanne (Ge), Abete gigantesco (It), Abeto gigante (Sp)

**Appearance:** A mobile clear fluid with a fresh conifer, lemony-green odour

**Perfumery status:** A head note of medium intensity and poor persistence

**Extraction:** Steam distillation of the fresh end-twigs and needles, usually October to April

**1 kg oil yield from:** 130–160 kg of the fresh needles (a moderate yield)

**Production areas:** France, Austria, Bosnia-Herzegovina; possibly Western Canada where this tree is native

**Typical constituents:** Monoterpenes <66% (incl. β-pinene 25%, α-pinene 6%, β-phellandrene 12%, camphene 8–14%, l-limonene 3–6%, β-myrcene 1%) • esters (incl. bornyl acetate 16%) • 1,8 cineol 12% • monoterpenols (incl. citronellol <3%)

**Chance of adulteration:** Moderate, possibly with other cheaper types of fir oil such as Balsam fir (*Abies balsamea*) and Siberian fir (*Abies sibirica*). Large-scale commercial productions of fir oils destined for the flavouring industries may also suffer cutting with gross diluents such as turpentine.

**Related oils:** See the Siberian fir profile in Volume 1 for other essential oils often distilled from the *Abies* genus.

# Therapeutic Functions and Indications

### SPECIFIC SYMPTOMATOLOGY – *All applications*

Apathy, low self-confidence, pessimism, discouragement, loss of motivation, depression, mental confusion, poor insight, poor concentration, mental and physical fatigue, lethargy, poor stamina, cold hands and feet, muscle and joint aches and pains, chronic cough with expectoration, chronic reproductive organ discharges

### PSYCHOLOGICAL – *Aromatic diffusion, whole-body massage*

**Essential PNEI function and indication:** Stimulant in weakness conditions
**Possible brain dynamics:** Increases basal ganglia and prefrontal cortex functioning
**Fragrance category:** High tone with lemony, sweet, pungent notes
**Indicated psychological disorders:** ADD, minor depression

PROMOTES MOTIVATION, SELF-CONFIDENCE AND OPTIMISM

- Loss of motivation with apathy, negativity, self-neglect
- Loss of self-confidence and self-esteem, depression
- Discouragement, low perseverance

PROMOTES GOOD JUDGEMENT AND FORESIGHT

- Poor judgement with loss of insight and critical thinking
- Loss of foresight, inability to envision or plan

### PHYSIOLOGICAL – *Nebulizer inhalation, gel cap, external applications*

**Therapeutic status:** Mild remedy with no cumulative toxicity
**Topical safety status:** Somewhat skin irritant, non-sensitizing
**Tropism:** Nervous, circulatory, respiratory, neuromuscular, urinary systems
**Essential diagnostic function:** Restores hypotonic/weak terrain conditions

PRIMARILY RESTORATIVE AND STIMULANT:

**nervous and cerebral restorative and mild regulator:** chronic hypotonic (weak) conditions with chronic mental and physical fatigue, debility, poor memory; neurasthenia, chronic depression, CFS

**arterial circulatory stimulant:** asthenic (cold) conditions with poor circulation

**adrenal restorative, mild hypertensive:** adrenal dysregulation, hypotension

**respiratory stimulant, mucolytic expectorant, antitussive, antiseptic:** chronic congestive lower and upper respiratory conditions with cough and dyspnoea; incl. chronic bronchitis, sinusitis, rhinitis, common cold

**urogenital restorative, mucostatic:** chronic mucous discharges, incl. leucorrhoea, gonorrhoea, blennorrhoea, gleet, mucous diarrhoea

PRIMARILY RELAXANT:

**neuromuscular analgesic, anti-inflammatory:** chronic painful arthritic and rheumatic conditions, incl. fibromyalgia

**diuretic, antiseptic:** urinary infections, esp. chronic, incl. cystitis, urethritis, nephritis, prostatitis, dysuria

**mild antilithic:** urinary stones

ANTIMICROBIAL ACTIONS:

**antibacterial, immunostimulant(?):** bacterial respiratory infections, incl. colds, sinusitis, bronchitis, whooping cough

SYNERGISTIC COMBINATIONS

- Grand fir + Silver fir + Grapefruit: nervous and cerebral restorative for chronic neurasthenia, mental weakness, depression

- Grand fir + Rosemary/Black spruce: nervous, adrenal and cerebral restorative, circulatory stimulant for chronic neurasthenia, with physical and mental weakness, poor circulation with hypotension, adrenal dysregulation or fatigue

- Grand fir + Frankincense/Black spruce: respiratory restorative, mucolytic expectorant for chronic bronchitis or emphysema with chronic cough, dyspnoea, expectoration, chest pain

- Grand fir + Eucalyptus (narrow-leaf): antiseptic nasal decongestant for congestive sinusitis, rhinitis, common cold

- Grand fir + Thyme ct. thymol: strong antiseptic mucolytic expectorant for chronic bronchitis with cough and dyspnoea

- Grand fir + Juniper berry: diuretic, urinary antiseptic in urinary infections of all types

- Grand fir + Green myrtle: mucostatic, antiseptic for chronic discharges, incl. leucorrhoea, mucous diarrhoea, gleet

- Grand fir + Cajeput: analgesic and rubefacient for chronic rheumatic-arthritic conditions, esp. of upper back and shoulders

COMPLEMENTARY COMBINATIONS

- Grand fir + Spearmint + Thyme ct. linalool: antiseptic mucolytic expectorant for bronchitis with cough, copious sputum, fatigue, esp. recent, in children

TOPICAL – *Liniment, ointment, cream, compress and other cosmetic preparations*

**Skin care:** Oily, dry or mature skin types

*vulnerary:* wounds, sores, ulcers, esp. chronic

*rubefacient, analgesic:* cold, lifeless skin; muscle aches and pains

**Therapeutic precautions:** As Grand fir oil is a warming, drying stimulant, avoid use with hypertonic/tense and hypersthenic/hot conditions, including hypertension, fever, and dry respiratory conditions with dry, unproductive cough.

**Pharmacological precautions:** Grand fir oil may be a mild skin irritant as it is rubefacient. Avoid use with sensitive skin.

**Preparations:**

- Diffusor: 2–4 drops in water

- Massage oil: 2–4% dilution in vegetable oil

- Liniment: 5–10% dilution in vegetable oil

- Gel cap: 2–3 drops with olive oil

## Chinese Medicine Functions and Indications

**Aroma energy:** Pungent, lemony

**Movement:** Rising, dispersing

**Warmth:** Neutral to warm

**Meridian tropism:** Lung, Bladder, Kidney

**Five-Element affinity:** Metal, Water

**Essential function:** To tonify the Qi, dispel wind-damp-cold and strengthen the Shen

1. **Tonifies the Qi, strengthens the Shen and relieves fatigue**

   - **Qi deficiency with Shen weakness**, with fatigue, lethargy, poor concentration, listlessness, confusion, depression:

   Grapefruit/Rosemary/Black spruce

2. **Warms the Lung, dispels wind-cold, expels phlegm, diffuses Lung Qi and relieves coughing**

   - **Lung wind-cold** with cough, sore throat, aches and pains, fatigue, sinus congestion:

   Eucalyptus (narrow-leaf)/Cajeput/Black pepper

   - **Lung phlegm-cold** with chest congestion, productive cough with expectoration, some breathing difficulty, wheezing:

   Hyssop/Siberian fir/Cardamom

3. **Warms and opens the meridians, dispels wind-damp-cold and relieves pain**

   - **Wind-damp-cold obstruction** with chronic muscle aches and pains, cold extremities:

   Niaouli/Cajeput/Black pepper/Laurel

REMARKS

While Siberian fir and Scotch pine oils were historically the most commonly found in healthcare settings such as medical spas and sanatoriums, a cluster of different and interesting fir oils are currently finding increased use among practitioners. Grand fir is just one of several fir oils that have finally established themselves in the materia aromatica, even though they share much in common with the others.

Grand fir oil nicely embodies the major themes of all fir oils in treating respiratory, urinary and musculoskeletal conditions. In functional medicine terms, Grand fir addresses the chronic weak terrain of these systems with some cold and damp present. It has become a classic stimulant expectorant with mucolytic, antitussive and antiseptic actions for all chronic congestive respiratory conditions, especially when these are chronic and cold, and involve poor arterial circulation, weak lungs and a tired nervous system. With urogenital functions too, Grand fir acts as a mucostatic restorative, checking chronic mucous discharges of all kinds.

While all fir oils are cellular oxygenators and energy boosters with high levels of monoterpenes, Grand fir is the only one with any real amount of 1,8 cineole present and can therefore be considered the most energizing. The oil acts as an excellent restorative not only to the lungs but also to the brain and central nervous system. In the musculoskeletal system Grand fir is a relieble analgesic and anti-inflammatory for chronic inflammation of all muscle tissues and arthritic pain, especially arthrosis in the shoulders and scapula. This may be linked to its content in bornyl acetate and β-myrcene.

Grand fir presents an almost unique grouping of properties when used as a psychological remedy by olfaction. Combining deep balsamic, woody notes with fresh, lemony green notes, its effect is centring and strengthening on one hand and uplifting and mentally stimulating on the other. Grand fir is for the individual who lacks inner strength and resilience, along with diminished self-esteem, but who at the same time lacks the clarity to see his/her weakness and therefore the motivation to change their situation. Inviting us to let go of the past and dispel stubborn regrets, Grand fir can help us summon the strength to open up to the future with its rich potential of fresh possibilities.

**Related oils:** There is much overlap in the fragrance, chemical contituents and clinical uses of the various fir needle oils available today. However, as a general rule the following differentiations with Grand fir can be made.

**Silver fir** (*Abies alba*), Weisstanne or Edeltanne in German, Sapin baumier in French, has identical therapeutic status, functions and uses to Grand fir. Despite its softer, sweeter odour profile, this fir species is actually higher in monoterpenes (90–95%), especially l-limonene (31–47%), α-pinene (18–28%), camphene (14–20%) and δ-3-carene (14%), and somewhat lower in esters (5–10%) than Grand fir. Like the latter, Silver fir essentially addresses hypotonic/weak conditions that tend towards cold, with a focus on stimulating arterial, bronchial and neuromuscular functions. For psychological purposes by olfaction, Silver fir as a gentle fresh-pungent oil exerts a gentler effect in stimulating the mind, motivation and self-confidence. It is ideal for children, sensitive individuals and mild cases. The same preparations, precautions and dilutions as for Grand fir apply.

Silver fir cone oil, properly known as Templin oil, is steam distilled from the one-year-old cones of the silver fir in Tyrol, Austria. In addition to the usual balsamic notes, its odour is strongly citrusy, a mix of lemon and orange, from its good levels of l-limonene (28–35%) and bornyl acetate (1–13%). No therapeutic uses are reported, although similarities with other fir oils are to be expected.

**Balsam fir** (*Abies balsamea*) from Canada and the American Pacific Northwest has a very piney-green, balsamic conifer fragrance that suggests an excellent emotional balancing effect from the psychological perspective. The fragrance is less sweet than

Silver fir, less lemony than Grand fir or Nordman's fir, and less deep-balsamic than Douglas fir. It has mild status with no cumulative toxicity or skin irritation. With very similar physiological functions and uses to Grand fir, Balsam fir has also found use as an anthelmintic for thread worms (Ascarides) and has shown antitumoural activity. Like Grand fir, the oil is high in monoterpenes (75–90%), including β-pinene (28–56%), δ-3 carene (0–27%) and α-pinene (<20%); the remainder includes esters (10–25%), including bornyl acetate (5–16%), and small amounts of the monoterpene ketones camphor and piperitone. The same preparations, precautions and dilutions as for Grand fir apply.

**Douglas fir** (*Pseudotsuga menziesii* [Beissn.] Franco) from the Pacific Northwest of North America, from British Columbia down to Northern California, is actually a variety of spruce, not a member of the fir (*Abies*) family. The oil has deep balsamic conifer and lighter citrus notes and shows monoterpenes dominant (60–80%) with minor esters (including citronellyl acetate) and monoterpenols (including terpinen-4-ol). It has mild status with no cumulative toxicity or skin irritation. Its physiological and psychological applications are approximately the same as those of Grand fir. The same preparations, precautions and dilutions as for Grand fir apply. As a psychological remedy, its uses are also somewhat similar to those of Grand fir but with less mental stimulation.

**Larch** (*Larix decidua* Miller) from Austria and France is steam distilled from the needles and end-twigs of this conifer that grows at high alpine altitudes; it is a pale yellow oil that displays typical balsamic fresh-needle and some sweet notes. Like most other conifer oils, Larch is dominated by monoterpenes (<73%, with α-pinenes 40%, camphene 6%), the ester bornyl acetate (12%) and sesquiterpenes (10%). It has mild status with no cumulative toxicity or skin irritation. Its uses are broadly similar to those of Grand fir, with good anti-infectious actions in respiratory infections, especially with Streptococcus pneumoniae. Used in small doses, it has a nervous and cerebral restorative action that will benefit mental and physical fatigue, depression, etc., but in medium doses will act as a nervous relaxant and in high doses as a euphoric or hypnotic sedative. Topical applications in c. 5% dilution have been found helpful for increasing joint mobility in bone dystrophy and chronic arthitis. The same preparations, precautions and dilutions as for Grand fir apply. As a psychological remedy, its uses are similar to those of Grand fir.

# Grapefruit

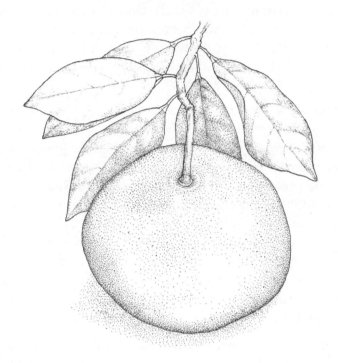

**Botanical source:** The rind of *Citrus x paradisi* Macfad. (Rutaceae – citrus family), a widely cultivated tree of warm to hot climates. Grapefruit is a hybrid of the pomelo (*Citrus grandis*) and the sweet orange (*Citrus x sinensis*); it has numerous cultivars

**Other names:** Pamplemousse (Fr), Grapefruit (Ge), Pompelmo (It), Toronja (Sp), Liu zi (Mandarin)

**Appearance:** A mobile yellow to pale-orange liquid with a warm, fresh, fruity-sweet odour

**Perfumery status:** A head note of low intensity and poor persistence

**Extraction:** Cold expression of the fresh fruit rind (but see below), usually November to March or April; a steam distilled oil is also manufactured (see below)

**1 kg oil yield from:** 250 kg of the fresh fruits (a moderate yield)

**Production areas:** USA, South Africa, Israel, Argentina, Brazil

**Typical constituents:** Monoterpenes 95% (incl. d-limonene 82–95%, α-pinene <1.6%, β-pinene, β-myrcene 1–4%, sabinene) • aldehydes (incl. octanal, nonanal, decanal, citral, citronnellal, neral, sinensal, octyl aldehyde) • coumarins and furanocoumarins (incl. aesculetine, auraptene, limettine, meranzine, bergaptole) • monoterpenols (incl. geraniol) • esters • sulphuric sesquiterpene ketone (nootkatone) trace–1%

**In the non-volatile fraction:** Flavonoids, carotenoids, steroids, coumarins, furano-coumarins. Oil composition does vary somewhat with different cultivars. The main cultivars produced are the Pink and the White grapefruit. Pink grapefruit oil is a little sweeter and generally preferred as a single oil. Pink grapefruit also contains some linalool, while White grapefruit is higher in aldehydes.

**Chance of adulteration:** Very high, because of the main use of Citrus oils in the soft-drink and perfume industry. Like most other Citrus oils, the commercial Grapefruit oil is the result of distillation of the peel and fruit once the juice is extracted: it is a by-product of juice production. Because of this, the distilled oil is generally considered inferior to the cold-pressed oil, and is sometimes blended with the cold-pressed oil (Weiss 1997). In addition, the commercial oil is usually deterpenated (i.e. has the terpenes removed), thereby further robbing it of therapeutic potency, as well as undergoing further admixtures with other citrus or terpene sources such as the far cheaper orange oil, and possibly synthetic purified or natural limonene, citral, etc. (Lis-Balchin 2006). Finally, the commercial oil will usually have UV absorbers and antioxidants such as BHA and BHT added to prevent spoilage from oxidation. Distilled Grapefruit oil should clearly be avoided for therapeutic use.

**Related oils:** With the large number of citrus oils available, it can be advantageous to obtain an overview of these in terms of their fragrance and major constituents. Because of their widespread commercial production for the soft drinks industry, especially in Italy, Argentina, South Africa and the United States, most citrus oils are available from numerous sources worldwide. The exceptions are noted. Most of these oils have separate profiles.

- **Lemony, sweet citrus oils with limonene dominant**
  This generally gives them a relaxant, calming character therapeutically, with the partial exception of Lemon oil.

  – Grapefruit (*Citrus x paradisi* Macfad.) (this profile)

  – Lemon (*Citrus limonum* [L.] Burm. fil.) (see separate profile)

  – Mandarin (*Citrus reticulata* Blanco) (see separate profile)

  – Sweet orange (*Citrus x sinensis* [L.] Osbeck) (see separate profile)

  – Bitter orange (*Citrus aurantium* subsp. amara L.) (see Sweet orange)

  – Yuzu (*Citrus junos* Sieb. et Tanaka)

- **Sweet citrus oils with limonene and esters dominant**
  Their general character is relaxant and calming to various degrees:

  - Neroli (*Citrus aurantium* subsp. amara L.) (see separate profile)

  - Bergamot (*Citrus x bergamia* L.) (see separate profile)

  - Petitgrain bigarade (*Citrus aurantium* subsp. amara L.) (see separate profile)

  - Mandarin petitgrain (*Citrus reticulata* Blanco) (see Petitgrain bigarade)

  - Italian lime (*Citrus limetta* Risso) (see Lime)

  - Persian lime (*Citrus x latifolia* Tanaka) (see Lime)

- **Lemony, green citrus oils with limonene and aldehydes dominant**
  This gives them an overall calming and cooling (refrigerant) character:

  - Lime (*Citrus x aurantifolia* L.) (see separate profile)

  - Bergamot petitgrain (*Citrus x bergamia* L.) (see Petitgrain bigarade)

  - Kaffir lime or Combava (*Citrus hystrix* DC.) (see Lime)

  - Kaffir lime petitgrain or Combava petitgrain (*Citrus hystrix* DC.) (see Petitgrain bigarade)

  - Citron (*Citrus medica* L.) (see Lime)

## Therapeutic Functions and Indications

SPECIFIC SYMPTOMATOLOGY – *All applications*

Mood swings, moodiness, morbid thoughts, pessimism, emotional and mental fatigue, poor concentration, distractibility, disorientation, listlessness, depression, low energy in the morning, poor appetite, indigestion with upper abdominal fullness, pale sluggish or oily skin, swollen glands, water retention, weight gain, abdominal obesity

PSYCHOLOGICAL – *Aromatic diffusion, whole-body massage*

**Essential PNEI function and indication:** Regulating in dysregulation conditions
**Possible brain dynamics:** Reduces deep limbic system hyperfunctioning
**Fragrance category:** Middle tone with sweet and lemony notes
**Indicated psychological disorders:** Bipolar disorder, ADHD, minor depression

PROMOTES EMOTIONAL STABILITY

- Emotional instability, mood swings
- Mental/emotional (thinking/feeling) conflict

PROMOTES OPTIMISM AND JOY

- Pessimism, negative (distressed) emotions, esp. guilt and shame
- Mild depression

MILDLY STIMULATES THE MIND AND PROMOTES ALERTNESS

- Distractibility, poor focus, poor short-term memory
- Mental fogginess, disorientation

## PHYSIOLOGICAL – *Nebulizer inhalation, gel cap, suppository, external applications*

**Therapeutic status:** Mild remedy with no cumulative toxicity

**Topical safety status:** Non-irritant, mildly sensitizing, mildly photosensitizing

**Tropism:** Nervous, digestive, lymphatic systems

**Essential diagnostic function:** Restores hypotonic/weak and decongests congestive/damp terrain conditions

PRIMARILY RESTORATIVE:

*nervous and cerebral restorative:* mental fatigue, memory loss, depression, exhaustion; neurasthenia

*liver decongestant, detoxicant, diuretic:* liver congestion, metabolic and liver toxicosis, incl. from drugs; oedema

PRIMARILY DECONGESTANT:

*lymphatic decongestant:* lymphatic congestion with swollen glands, oedema

*gastrointestinal stimulant, aperitive, carminative, cholagogue:* appetite loss, anorexia, upper indigestion

*antiplethoric:* general plethora with weight gain, abdominal obesity

*anti-inflammatory, analgesic:* rheumatic and arthritic pain

*antioxidant, antitumoural(?)*

- Grapefruit + Lemon: detoxicant diuretic in metabolic and liver toxicosis with rheumatic conditions

- Grapefruit + Juniper berry: detoxicant diuretic in metabolic toxicosis with oedema and skin, rheumatic or urinary symptoms

- Grapefruit + Rosemary: nervous restorative for mental and physical fatigue, depression

Complementary combinations

- Grapefruit + Fennel: aperitive, carminative, cholagogue for gastric indigestion, anorexia

- Grapefruit + Geranium/Lemongrass: lymphatic decongestant for lymphatic congestion with swollen glands

- Grapefruit + Lemongrass: aperitive, carminative for upper gastric indigestion, anorexia

## Topical – *Liminent, ointment, cream, compress and other cosmetic preparations*

**Skin care:** Oily skin type

*subastringent, mild antiseptic:* tired, congested skin; acne

*rubefacient, detoxicant, skin and muscle toner:* devitalized cold skin, skin impurities and blemishes, poor hair growth, hair loss; muscle and tendon fatigue (e.g. from work, sports)

*lymphatic stimulant:* swollen glands, lymph stagnation, oedema

*connective tissue and epidermal restorative, antioxidant:* slack skin, wrinkles, cellulite, stretch marks, sprains, strains, poor muscle tone

*deodorant, environmental antiseptic:* air-borne infections

**Therapeutic precautions:** Distilled Grapefruit oils should be avoided (see above).

**Pharmacological precautions:** Grapefruit oil is somewhat photosensitizing, so avoid exposure to direct sunlight after topical applications for 12 hours. Avoid continuous topical use at high dilutions because of possible skin irritation. Because Grapefruit oil, like all citrus oils, degrades easily on contact with oxygen through oxidization, it is important in skin-care especially to use fresh, non-oxidized Grapefruit oil.

The generally accepted shelf-life of genuine Grapefruit oil at room temperature is about 12 months, or 24 months if stored in a refrigerator (assuming no preservatives have been added in the first place).

**Preparations:**

- Diffusor: 5–7 drops in water

- Massage oil: 1–4% dilution in vegetable oil

- Liniment: 3–5% dilution in vegetable oil for short-term use

- Gel cap: 2–3 drops with olive oil

## Chinese Medicine Functions and Indications

**Aroma energy:** Lemony, sweet

**Movement:** Expanding, rising, circulating

**Warmth:** Neutral

**Meridian tropism:** Liver, Spleen, Stomach

**Five-Element affinity:** Wood, Earth

**Essential function:** To resolve damp, regulate the Qi and strengthen the Shen

1. **Resolves damp, harmonizes the Shen and relieves bloating and swelling**

   - **General damp with Shen dysregulation**, with lethargy, mood swings, malaise, heaviness of body, water retention, swollen glands:

     Lemongrass/Lemon/May chang

   - **Spleen toxic-damp** with appetite loss, indigestion, bloating, lethargy, weight-gain, irregular stool:

     Patchouli/Niaouli/Palmarosa

2. **Harmonizes the Middle Warmer, reduces stagnation and relieves distension**

   - **Stomach-Spleen Qi stagnation** with epigastric bloating and fullness, poor appetite, indigestion on eating:

     Lemon/Spearmint/Peppermint/Grapefruit

3. **Raises the clear Yang and strengthens the Shen**

   - **Clear Yang Qi deficiency with Shen weakness**, with mental fatigue, poor focus, distractibility, fogginess, headaches:

     Lemon/Rosemary/Cajeput

REMARKS

The grapefruit originates in the long archipelago of Malaysia, Indonesia and New Guinea and was introduced to China and India in early centuries BC. It is possible that the fruit was hybridized in its original Southeast Asian cradle, although a natural (or further?) hybridization is said to have occurred in Barbados (1750) and Jamaica (1789); certainly, the word 'grapefruit' itself first appears in Jamaica in 1814. In the 12th century, the fruit was brought as a mere curiosity to Europe and in the early 19th century to Florida by command of Napoleon's fleet physician, Philippe Odet.

Enjoyed as a dessert in China since earliest times, the grapefruit is a popular gift at the Mid-autumn festival, alongside the even more popular moon cakes. This equinox festival, which corresponds exactly to the Hebrew festival Sukkoth, is a celebration of the full moon on the 15th day of the eighth lunar month; the Chinese have always considered this moon to be the clearest and brightest full moon of the whole year.

As a physiologic remedy, Grapefruit can be seen as a variant on Lemon. It is a restorative to the brain and nervous system; and a good stimulant-decongestant to hepatic, upper GI and lymphatic functions, and may well include a venous and capillary stimulant action as well. Like Lemon also, Grapefruit as a result obtains a good alterative action that is ideal for those with symptoms of toxicosis and damp resulting from poor detoxification and elimination functions. These actions are duplicated on the skin and excel with applications to tired, devitalized, congested skin. Interestingly, Grapefruit is considered by some cosmetologists to act as a restorative to the connective tissue – something to be expected of Lemon as well but certainly not documented. Regardless, the two oils combine well, whether used by internal or topical delivery methods. It comes as no surprise to see their pharmacology profile as virtually identical, with dominant monoterpenes in terms of quantity; and aldehydes, monoterpenols, esters and coumarins providing nice support in terms of qualitative effects.

The traditional association of grapefruit with the moon is an apt one. As a psychological remedy, Grapefruit by olfaction is oriented to promoting emotional stability, mental poise and spiritual joy. In simple terms, this oil combines the psycho-olfactory qualities of Mandarin and Lemon. Like Mandarin, Grapefruit is able to touch our emotional innocence and lighten the emotional heart, dispelling long-held disappointment and resignation. Like Lemon, Grapefruit can open mental clarity and optimism, gently illuminating negative thoughts and helping to focus distracted, scattered thoughts. Because Grapefruit promotes a gentle mental clarity, not a sharp spotlight like Lemon, it allows the mind to remain linked to the emotions, to the heart. This oil essentially promotes emotional and mental clarity combined, thereby harmonizing conflict between them. It is one of the best oils for healing the head-heart connection.

# Green Myrtle

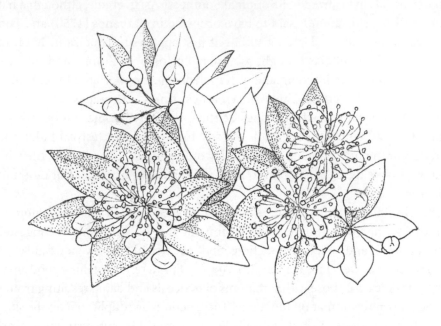

**Botanical source:** The leaf of *Myrtus communis* L. ct. cineole (Myrtaceae – myrtle family), an evergreen shrub or small tree of the Mediterranean and West Asia; widely cultivated

**Other names:** Corsican pepper; Myrte (Fr, Ge), Mirto (It, Sp)

**Appearance:** A mobile pale greenish yellow fluid with a fresh camphoraceous and fruity-sweet-herbaceous odour; later slight warm, balsamic spicy-woody notes appear

**Perfumery status:** A head note of high intensity and medium persistence

**Extraction:** Steam distillation of the fresh leaves of the flowering shrub, usually June through to August. Some producers will include end twigs along with the leaves, which impart woody notes to the oil that detract from the sweet-fresh odour profile.

**1 kg oil yield from:** 120–170 kg of the leaves (a good yield)

**Production areas:** Morocco, Algeria, Tunisia, Spain, South France, Albania

**Typical constituents:** Monoterpenes <62% (incl. α-pinene 14–58%, limonene 5–14%, β-pinene, camphene) • oxides (incl. 1,8 cineole 19–42%, caryophyllene oxide, 2-methylfurane) • esters 18–31% (incl. myrtenyle acetate <21%, linalyl/terpenyl/neryl/geranyl/bornyl/trans-carvyl acetat, methyl myrtenate) • monoterpenols (incl. linalool 1–10%, myrtenol, α-terpineol, geraniol, terpinen-4-ol, nerol) • sesquiterpenes (incl. β-caryophyllene, azulene, humulene, dihydroazulene) • aldehydes (incl. n-decanal, trans-hexanal, furfural, methylebutanal, myrtenal) • lactones myrtucommulones A and B • methyleugenol <0.8% • estragole trace–1.4%

**Chance of adulteration:** Moderate, possibly with other cheaper oils high in monoterpenes and oxides such as Cajeput, Niaouli and Eucalyptus species

**Related oils:** Red myrtle, so called from its deep orange to red colour. The constituents and clinical uses of the two types of myrtle oil are widely confused in the literature, most likely arising from poor organoleptic, i.e. sensory, identification (see below).

In a wider sense, two large botanical groups of oils belong to the myrtle family: the *Eucalyptus* and the *Melaleuca* (Cajeput, Niaouli, Tea tree, etc.) genus. Myrtle is not to be confused with Wax myrtle (*Myrica cerifera*) or Bog myrtle (*Myrica gale*), both of which yield neurotoxic oils that are not used clinically.

## Therapeutic Functions and Indications

SPECIFIC SYMPTOMATOLOGY – *All applications*

Low self-confidence, poor self-expression, confusion, indecision, mood swings, sorrow, sadness, low vitality, mental and physical fatigue, lethargy, lack of follow-through, depression with anxiety, cold extremities, shallow breathing, undeveloped or constricted chest, chronic cough with sputum, chronic runny nose or sinus congestion, chronic indigestion with bloating, chronic vaginal discharges, urinary irritation with mucus in urine, scanty or stopped periods

PSYCHOLOGICAL – *Aromatic diffusion, whole-body massage*

**Essential PNEI function and indication:** Stimulant in weakness conditions; regulating in dysregulation conditions

**Possible brain dynamics:** Increases basal ganglia functioning and reduces deep limbic system hyperfunctioning

**Fragrance category:** Middle tone with pungent, sweet, green notes

**Indicated psychological disorders:** ADD, depression, bipolar disorder, addiction

STIMULATES THE MIND AND PROMOTES ALERTNESS

- Lethargy, drowsiness, stupor
- Mental confusion, disorientation, lack of focus

PROMOTES SELF-CONFIDENCE AND PERSEVERANCE

- Low self-confidence and self-esteem, pessimism
- Poor perseverance

PROMOTES EMOTIONAL STABILITY

- Emotional confusion with conflict; distraction, mood swings, emotivity
- Negative distressed emotions, addictions in general

## PHYSIOLOGICAL – *Nebulizer inhalation, gel cap, suppository, pessary, liniment*

**Therapeutic status:** Mild remedy with no cumulative toxicity

**Topical safety status:** Non-irritant, non-sensitizing

**Tropism:** Neuroendocrine, respiratory, digestive, urinary, reproductive systems

**Essential diagnostic function:** Restores hypotonic/weak conditions and decongests congestive/damp terrain conditions

PRIMARILY RESTORATIVE:

*nervous and cerebral restorative and mild relaxant:* chronic hypotonic (weak) and hypertonic (tense) conditions with mental and physical fatigue, concentration loss, somnolence; chronic cerebral deficiency, nervous or anxious depression, neurasthenia, insomnia

*thyroid/thyroxine restorative:* hypothyroid syndrome, thyroxine resistance

*female hormonal and uterine restorative:* chronic amenorrhoea

*astringent mucosal restorative, mucostatic, antiseptic:* chronic and subacute mucous membrane weakness with mucus overproduction and discharge, simple or infectious, esp. respiratory, intestinal and urogenital, incl.:

- chronic bronchitis with copious sputum, rhinitis, post-nasal drip
- mucousy stool, diarrhoea, dysentery
- chronic mucous cystitis, blennuria
- vaginitis with leucorrhoea, urethritis with gleet
- antioxidant

PRIMARILY STIMULANT AND DECONGESTANT:

*strong respiratory stimulant and decongestant, mucolytic expectorant, antitussive, antiseptic:* acute and chronic congestive lower and upper respiratory conditions with mucous overproduction, productive cough, congestive dyspnoea; incl. bronchitis, emphysema; sinusitis, rhinitis, otitis media, common cold

*gastrointestinal stimulant, carminative, antiseptic:* chronic atonic gastroenteritis with abdominal bloating, indigestion, mucousy diarrhoea

*liver and pancreatic stimulant and decongestant, mild hypoglycaemiant:* liver congestion, pancreatic deficiency, hyperglycaemia

*pelvic, prostatic and lymphatic decongestant:* chronic pelvic congestion with haemorrhoids, urinary incontinence and irritation, discharges, chronic prostate hypertrophy (BPH)

*mild anti-inflammatory, analgesic and spasmolytic:* muscle and joint pain and cramps; intestinal colic, prostatitis, cystitis, urethritis

ANTIMICROBIAL ACTIONS:

*antibacterial:* bacterial infections (respiratory, digestive, urinary; see above)

*broad-spectrum antifungal:* fungal infections, esp. with Trichoderma viride, Candida spp., Aspergillus niger

SYNERGISTIC COMBINATIONS

- Green myrtle + Eucalyptus, blue-gum or narrow-leaf/Niaouli: strong antiseptic nasal decongestant, stimulant expectorant, immunostimulant for all upper and lower respiratory infections, esp. with copious sputum or nasal discharge; with recurring infections

- Green myrtle + Thyme ct. thymol/Laurel: strong mucolytic respiratory anti-infective and expectorant for chronic lower respiratory infections, esp. with dyspnoea, copious sputum, fatigue, depression

- Green myrtle + Cypress: gastrointestinal stimulant and spasmolytic for chronic digestive atony with mucousy stool, colic, IBS, irregular stool

- Green myrtle + Cypress: strong pelvic, urinary and prostatic decongestant for chronic pelvic congestion with haemorrhoids, urinary incontinence and discharges, prostate hyperplasia, prostatitis

- Green myrtle + Patchouli/Thyme ct. linalool: antiseptic gastrointestinal stimulant for chronic gastroenteritis with abdominal bloating, mucousy diarrhoea

COMPLEMENTARY COMBINATIONS

- Green myrtle + Nutmeg/Rosemary: nervous and cerebral restorative for mental/cerebral deficiencies, neurasthenia, somnolence, psychosis

- Green myrtle + Lavender/Petitgrain bigarade: nervous and cerebral sedative for chronic insomnia (onset and maintenance types), neurasthenia, nervous or anxious depression

- Green myrtle + Pimenta berry: thyroid restorative/stimulant in chronic hypothyroid syndromes, thyroxine resistance

- Green myrtle + Clary sage: uterine restorative for chronic amenorrhoea

- Green myrtle + Spearmint/Hyssop: strong respiratory decongestant and mucolytic expectorant for acute and chronic bronchial congestion with dyspnoea, continuous expectoration

- Green myrtle + Clary sage/Myrrh: mucostatic astringent for vaginal and intestinal mucus discharges, incl. leucorrhoea, mucousy stool

- Green myrtle + Sage: urogenital antiseptic and mucostatic astringent for chronic urinary and vaginal discharges, simple or infectious, incl. blennuria, mucous cystitis, vaginitis, mucous colitis

- Green myrtle + Atlas cedarwood: mucostatic mucosal restorative for chronic vaginitis with leucorrhoea, mucous cystitis, blennuria, gleet

- Green myrtle + Geranium: pelvic and lymphatic decongestant for chronic pelvic congestion with haemorrhoids, urinary incontinence, dysmenorrhoea

- Green myrtle + Black spruce: prostatic decongestant for chronic BPH, prostatitis with fatigue, urinary incontinence

TOPICAL – *Liniment, ointment, cream, compress and other cosmetic preparations*

**Skin care:** Oily or combination skin

*skin revitalizer and regenerative, capillary stimulant:* devitalized, underactive cold skin, wrinkles; chronic sores, ulcers and wounds

*skin detoxicant (cleanser), mild astringent:* skin impurities of all types, open pores

*antiseptic:* acne, eczema

**Hair and scalp care:** poor hair growth, hair loss, dandruff, seborrhoea, short or insufficient eyebrows

**Therapeutic precautions:** Green myrtle oil is a drying, astringent stimulant that is contraindicated in dry conditions of all kinds, especially dry respiratory conditions with dry unproductive cough.

**Pharmacological precautions:** Green myrtle should be used with caution in those taking diabetic medication. Although Green myrtle oil has shown some anticancer action, it does contain the carcinogenic constituents methyleugenol and estragole, as well as the anticarcinogenic limonene (Tisserand and Young 2013).

**Preparations:**

- Diffusor: 3–5 drops in water
- Massage oil: 2–5% dilution in vegetable oil
- Liniment: 5–10% dilution in vegetable oil
- Gel cap: 1–3 drops with olive oil. The small dose is more nervous sedative, the larger dose more restorative, stimulant and decongestant.

## Chinese Medicine Functions and Indications

**Aroma energy:** Pungent, sweet, green

**Movement:** Rising

**Warmth:** Neutral to warm

**Meridian tropism:** Lung, Bladder, Spleen

**Five-Element affinity:** Metal, Earth

**Essential function:** To tonify the Qi, resolve damp and harmonize the Shen

1. **Tonifies the Qi, harmonizes the Shen and relieves fatigue**

   - **Qi deficiency with Shen dysregulation**, with morning lethargy, fatigue, mental confusion or dullness, mood swings, shallow sleep, mild depression:
     Niaouli/Thyme ct. linalool/Nerolina

2. **Resolves and expels phlegm, dries damp and relieves coughing**

   - **Lung phlegm-damp** with expectoration of thick viscous sputum, full cough:
     Spearmint/Hyssop/Atlas cedarwood/Sage

   - **Lung phlegm-cold with underlying Lung Qi deficiency**, with fatigue, chronic weak or full cough, mucous expectoration:
     Grand fir/Scotch pine/Hyssop

3. **Resolves damp and turbidity, and relieves distension; harmonizes urination and stops discharges**

- **Spleen toxic-damp** with chronic indigestion, poor appetite, abdominal bloating, loose mucousy stools, irregular bowel movement:

  Patchouli/Thyme ct. linalool/Pimenta berry

- **Lower Warmer turbid-damp** with chronic vaginal discharges, chronic irritated, dribbling urination:

  Geranium/Atlas cedarwood/Silver fir/Myrrh

4. **Invigorates the Blood in the Lower Warmer and reduces stagnation**

- **Lower Warmer Blood stagnation** with pelvic weight or dragging sensation, irritated, urgent dribbling urination:

  Niaouli/Cypress/Geranium

REMARKS

Hardy, adaptive and long-lived, the flowering myrtle announces its presence in the warm Mediterranean air with elegant wafts of floral, herbaceous notes lined with inklings of honey and frankincense. Its lingering, complex fragrance mixes well with the fresh resinous scents of Aleppo pine and mastic – its comon companions all over the Mediterranean.

In all of recorded history, the sweet flowering myrtle has always been associated with love – but not with love as a state of passion, embodied in the rose, but love lyrically and authentically expressed. Greek goddess Aphrodite cherished her myrtle bushes: the love she gave and sought was about the expression of true feelings and joyful authentic connection. Erato, Greek muse of lyric and erotic poetry, wore a head garland of myrtle and roses. In Roman times, newly-weds wore crowns of myrtle to celebrate their shared new step in life's journey. Designed for rest and rejuvenation, most traditional Arabian gardens, from Baghdad and Isfahan in the East to Andalusian Cordoba and Granada in the West, included the beloved fresh myrtle in their floral scentscape, along with the playful orange and the sensuous jasmine. In a wider sense, myrtle has always conveyed the qualities of purity, beauty, even innocence – it certainly lifted spirits. It is no accident that its leaves and flowers were a main ingredient in a rejuvenating 16th-century skin-care lotion known as Angel Water.

Like Laurel, with which Myrtle shares much in common, Myrtle is a remedy of several facets. Its complex, refined fragrance is an expression of its wide rainbow of constituents. In the words of medical herbalist André Bitsas (2009), 'L'arome de la myrte est balsamique, frais, oxygenant…mais avec un raffinement supplémentaire qui est, comme toujours dans ce cas, l'image d'une biochimie complexe et d'un intense pouvoir de synergie interne' – 'The fragrance of myrtle is balsamic, fresh and oxygenating…but with an additional refinement that, as always, is the image of a complex biochemistry and intense potency of internal synergy.' Dominant monoterpenes, oxides and esters are here rounded off with representatives of all the other major chemical families.

The flowers, leaves and berries are all common in the folk practices of Mediterranean islands such as Cyprus, Corsica and Sardinia – practices which today are reflected in the use of the essential oil. Doctors of traditional Greek medicine valued Myrtle essentially as a drying astringent and expectorant remedy in patients presenting Phlegm as the dominant toxic fluid. Today, this would translate as a remedy for damp terrain presenting as congestion and discharges. Myrtle is more specifically a classic restorative, astringent and decongestant for chronic weak and damp terrain. The remedy is a restorative to the nervous system, thyroid and uterus in chronic weak conditions. With its combined cerebral restorative and sedative action, Green myrtle is one of the best aromatics for chronic insomnia, neurasthenia and nervous or anxious depression – a little like Petitgrain bigarade oil and herbs such as Skullcap (*Scutellaria laterifolia*) and Rhodiola (*Rhodiola rosea*). To all organs of the mucous membrane – especially the bronchi, GI tract and vagina – it is an excellent *restorative astringent* for chronic mucosal discharges. Green myrtle also combines a toning action on the uterus with an unspecified hormonal action that shines in cases of chronic amenorrhoea.

Congestive conditions with damp terrain also need stimulation as much as astringing. Many of Green myrtle's remaining functions make sense in terms of a systemic stimulant decongestant and antibacterial action. This oil works deeply into the bronchi and lungs, clearing obstructing phlegm, resolving dyspnoea and productive coughs, and superbly managing chronic respiratory conditions and infections in general. Likewise, it excels in treating chronic urinary infections with mucous discharges. In the abdominal region, Green myrtle is decongestant to the uterus, prostate, liver, pancreas and lymphatic circulation. French practitioners have been using Myrtle for centuries for haemorrhoids, including topically in St. John's wort oil.

As a psychological remedy by olfaction, Green myrtle again picks up Aphrodite's theme of authentic expression. Its pungent, sweet-green, herbaceous fragrance is stabilizing, clarifying and energizing all at the same time. Green myrtle is one of the best oils for balancing the mind and the solar plexus, thereby promoting clarity, inspiration and emotional stability. The oil encourages increased perception and intuition, supporting us in gently reflecting on what is actually and authentically true for us. Having done that, Green myrtle then may give us just enough courage, confidence and sense of good timing to express our truth in a clear, timely and well-considered way.

Green myrtle is for the confused, conflicted and easily influenced individual who lacks healthy self-assertiveness. It is gentle enough to support a sensitive person gain internal balance and emotional poise, yet powerful enough to support the breaking of bad habits and addictions, whether related to pathogenic emotions or drugs.

**Red myrtle oil** (*Myrtus communis* ct. myrtenyl acetate) is less frequently distilled as the more common Green myrtle. Mainly produced in Morocco, it also occurs in Corsica, South France and Turkey. This oil should be carefully distinguished from Green myrtle. Red myrtle is a somewhat viscous oil with a deep orange to red colour presenting dry, sweet wood and fresh pine notes; it is clearly easy to differentiate its appearance from Green myrtle. Despite being commonly described as chemically dominant in myrtenyl acetate, Red myrtle is actually equally dominant in three constituents: the ester myrtenyl acetate 13–36%, monoterpenes 28–36% (mainly α-pinene and limonene) and 1,8 cineole <35%. Smaller amounts of monoterpenols, sesquiterpenes and methyleugenol complete its profile.

However, for physiological treatment, Red myrtle can be used almost interchangeably with Green myrtle. It has mild status with no cumulative toxicity or skin irritation. Its main clinical value lies in its good venous and lymphatic decongestant action on the circulation of the legs and pelvis. Its main indications are venous deficiency with symptoms such as varicose veins, pelvic congestion with haemorrhoids, prostate hypertrophy, and urinary incontinence and irritation. Here it combines well with such oils as Cistus, Cypress and Atlas cedarwood. Red myrtle is also a good astringent mucosal restorative for acute and chronic respiratory and genitourinary discharges. The same precautions and preparations as for Green myrtle apply.

For psychological purposes by olfaction, Red myrtle exerts a centring, strengthening and uplifting effect based on its pungent-woody fragrance. It is useful for promoting grounded, centred stimulation, alertness and self-confidence.

# Hyssop

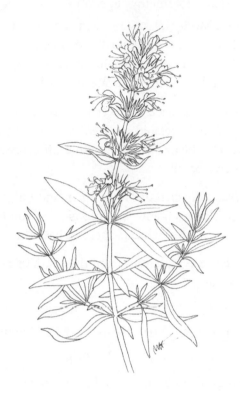

**Botanical source:** The herb of *Hyssopus officinalis* L. ssp. officinalis (Lamiaceae/ Labiatae – lipflower family), a widespread perennial temperate, Mediterranean and Central Asian herb

**Other names:** Hysope (Fr), Ysop (Ge), Hisopo (Sp), Ezob (Hebrew)

**Appearance:** A mobile pale viridian fluid with a sweet-herbaceous, somewhat fresh odour with warm-spicy and sweet-honey base notes

**Perfumery status:** A heart note of medium intensity and medium persistence

**Extraction:** Steam distillation of the partially dried herb in flower, usually in July and August

**1 kg oil yield from:** 200–300 kg of the fresh herb (a poor yield)

**Production areas:** France, Italy, Hungary, England

**Typical constituents:** Ketones, incl. monoterpenones 35–80% (incl. pinocamphone 12–56%, isopinocamphone 25–39%, trace α-thujone) • monoterpenes 25–30% (incl. β-pinene 12–23%, limonene 6–10%, β-phellandrene 6%, myrcene 5%, sabinene 4%)

• sesquiterpenes 12% (incl. germacrene D <3%, β-caryophyllene <3%, aromadendrene)
• monoterpenols 5–10% (incl. borneol, geraniol, terpinen-4-ol, α-terpineol, myrtenol)
• esters bornyl acetate, methyl myrtenate • phenolic ethers 4% (incl. myrtenyl methyl ether 1–4%, methylchavicol <1%, methyleugenol) • 1,8 cineole 0.6%

**Chance of adulteration:** Moderate, usually with a cocktail of cheaper oils such as Camphor, Cedarleaf, Lavandin, Green myrtle or Sage, or with the other subspecies below. Any strong fresh-pungent odour would indicate a high cineole content, which is never found in Hyssop oil; this often indicates Spanish hyssop (see below).

**Related oils:** The variety Hyssop decumbens (*Hyssopus officinalis* var. *decumbens* Briq. a.k.a. *H. montana*) is the main related oil used in practice (see below). The oils of various subspecies may also be available sometimes, if properly identified. They are also used to adulterate Hyssop oil.

- *Hyssopus officinalis ssp. aristatus* from Spain and Bulgaria, with a 40–50% 1,8 cineole content. This pungent-herbaceous oil is sometimes sold as Spanish hyssop or Hyssop ct. 1,8 cineole; it does not have the same uses as Hyssop

- *Hyssopus officinalis ssp. canescens* from the south of France, high in both 1,8 cineole and linalool

## Therapeutic Functions and Indications

SPECIFIC SYMPTOMATOLOGY – *All applications*

Moodiness, mood swings, ruminations, trouble letting go, chronic shame feelings, mental fog, poor focus, depression, lethargy, fatigue, cold hands and feet, appetite loss, indigestion, abdominal bloating, chronic weak cough, shallow breathing, cough with copious fetid sputum, chest pain, hard dry cough with difficult expectoration and chest distension, wheezing, scanty, late or stopped periods, water retention

PSYCHOLOGICAL – *Aromatic diffusion, whole-body massage*

**Essential PNEI function and indication:** Regulating in dysregulation conditions; mild stimulant in weakness conditions

**Possible brain dynamics:** Reduces deep limbic system hyperfunctioning

**Fragrance category:** Middle tone with sweet, green notes

**Indicated psychological disorders:** Bipolar disorder

PROMOTES EMOTIONAL RENEWAL, STABILITY AND INSIGHT

- All pathogenic (stuck) emotions and distressed emotions in general

- Irritability, moodiness, negative feelings, incl. guilt

- Emotional conflict or instability, shame

PROMOTES MENTAL STABILITY

- Mental confusion, distraction

- Negative thoughts, pessimism, cynicism, repetitive thinking


## PHYSIOLOGICAL – *Gel cap, suppository, external applications*

**Therapeutic status:** Medium-strength remedy with some cumulative toxicity

**Topical safety status:** Non-irritant, non-sensitizing

**Tropism:** Nervous, circulatory, respiratory, digestive, urinary systems

**Essential diagnostic function:** Restores hypotonic/weak and decongests damp/congestive terrain conditions

PRIMARILY RESTORATIVE:

*nervous and cerebral restorative, antidepressant:* hypotonic (weak) conditions with fatigue, poor circulation, depression, neurasthenia, CFS, cerebral deficiency, MS and other neurodegenerative disorders

PRIMARILY STIMULANT AND DECONGESTANT:

*arterial circulatory stimulant and equalizer:* poor circulation, hypotension, hypertension(?)

*strong respiratory stimulant and decongestant, fluidifying and mucolytic expectorant, antitussive, antiseptic:* all congestive respiratory conditions, acute or chronic, with copious or hardened sputum, congestive dyspnoea and cough

*gastrointestinal stimulant, aperitive:* atonic indigestion, anorexia, gastroenteritis

*uterine stimulant, emmenagogue:* amenorrhoea, oligomenorrhoea

*moderate bronchial and pulmonary relaxant, anti-inflammatory:* chronic and acute spasmodic or congestive dyspnoea and asthma; all inflammatory lung conditions

*resolvent antilithic, diuretic:* urinary stones (oxalic and phosphatic)

*lipid metabolism regulator, antilipaemic:* hyperlipidaemia, atherosclerosis

*misc.:* MS

ANTIMICROBIAL ACTIONS:

*anti-infective, antimicrobial, anti-inflammatory:* a wide range of lower and upper respiratory infections, esp.:

- *antibacterial:* bacterial infections, esp. chronic, with cough, dyspnoea, sputum; bronchitis, whooping cough, enphysema, pneumonia, lung TB; rhinitis, sinusitis, pharyngitis, intestinal dysbiosis, leprosy

- *antiviral:* viral infections, incl. common cold, sinusitis, acute bronchitis, croup, pleurisy, pneumonia, herpes

- *antifungal:* fungal infections, esp. with Aspergillus spp., incl. aspergillosis

- *anthelmintic:* intestinal parasites, esp. Lamblia

SYNERGISTIC COMBINATIONS
Usually for short-term use: see 'Therapeutic precautions' below.

- Hyssop + Rosemary ct. verbenone: strong nervous restorative, hypertensive and antidepressant for chronic neurasthenia, fatigue, depression, hypotension

- Hyssop + Cypress: antitussive for cough of any kind, congestive or spasmodic

- Hyssop + Spearmint/Green myrtle: strong mucolytic stimulant expectorant, antiseptic and antitussive for chronic bronchitis or emphysema with dyspnoea, cough and copious sputum

- Hyssop + Siberian fir + Frankincense: strong bronchodilator for acute asthmatic episodes with severe apnoea

COMPLEMENTARY COMBINATIONS
Usually for short-term use: see 'Therapeutic precautions' below.

- Hyssop + Thyme ct. thymol: strong nervous restorative, arterial stimulant, hypertensive and antidepressant for chronic neurasthenia, fatigue, depression, hypotension, poor circulation

- Hyssop + Niaouli: strong antiviral expectorant for acute viral respiratory infections, incl. bronchitis, croup, RSV, pleurisy

- Hyssop + Scotch pine/Black spruce: strong mucolytic expectorant, antitussive and respiratory restorative for chronic congestive respiratory conditions with fatigue, cough, copious or hard sputum, congestive dyspnoea

- Hyssop + Fennel/Basil ct. methylchavicol: bronchodilator and antitussive for spasmodic respiratory conditions with spasmodic cough and dyspnoea, chronic asthma

- Hyssop + Peppermint/Rosemary: hypertensive for hypotension

- Hyssop + Lemon: antilithic for urinary stones

- Hyssop + Sage: antilipaemic for hyperlipidaemia, atherosclerosis

- Hyssop + Helichrysum: vulnerary, antihaematomal for all soft tissue trauma with haematoma (topical use)

## TOPICAL – *Liniment, ointment, cream, compress and other cosmetic preparations*

**Skin care:** Combination skin type

> ***vulnerary:*** bruises, wounds, cuts, scars, contusions, sprains, strains

**Therapeutic precautions:** Only those relating to internal dosage and length of intake.

**Pharmacological precautions:** Hyssop is a medium-strength remedy with some potential cumulative neurotoxicity when absorbed internally because of its combined pinocamphones and thujone content (although the latter is only present in trace amounts). It is therefore contraindicated for use with all nebulizers and in those with a tendency to migraines or epileptic seizures, as well as in babies, infants, children under 3, the elderly and pregnant women. For all types of internal use, exercise care with respect to dosage and length of intake (see below).

**Preparations:**

- Diffusor: 2–4 drops in water

- Massage oil: 1–2% dilution in vegetable oil

- Liniment: 2–5% dilution in vegetable oil

- Gel cap: 1 drop with olive oil, and no more than 3 drops total per day, for a single 10-day course maximum, and always in combination with other oils. For more long-term use, Hyssop oil should be combined with other oils in a formula at no more than 10% of the whole formula.

## Chinese Medicine Functions and Indications

**Aroma energy:** Sweet, green, pungent
**Movement:** Circulating

**Warmth:** Neutral to warm

**Meridian tropism:** Lung, Spleen, Bladder

**Five-Element affinity:** Metal, Earth

**Essential function:** To tonify the Qi, resolve phlegm-damp and strengthen the Shen

1. **Tonifies the Qi, strengthens the Lung, uplifts the Shen and relieves depression**

   - **Qi deficiency with Shen weakness**, with physical and mental fatigue, listlessness, depression:

     Rosemary/Niaouli/Thyme ct. thymol

   - **Lung Qi deficiency** with chronic weak cough, shallow breathing, fatigue, grief:

     Rosemary/Grand fir/Saro/Black spruce

2. **Resolves and expels phlegm, dries damp, diffuses Lung Qi and relieves coughing**

   - **Lung phlegm-damp/cold** with productive cough, copious sputum, fatigue:

     Scotch pine/Atlas cedarwood/Spearmint/Thyme ct. thymol

   - **Lung phlegm-dryness** with hard dry cough, difficult expectoration:

     Copaiba

   - **Lung phlegm-heat** with copious fetid, yellow or pink sputum, chest pain:

     Blue-gum eucalyptus/Lemon eucalyptus/Tea tree

3. **Releases the exterior, dispels wind, opens the sinuses and relieves congestion; boosts the protective Qi**

   - **External wind-cold/heat with Qi deficiency**, with sneezing, sinus congestion, fatigue, possible fever:

     Cajeput/Ravintsara/Laurel

   - **Lung wind-cold/heat** with chills, sore throat, cough with slight expectoration, nasal congestion:

     Grand fir/Niaouli/Ravintsara

4. **Circulates and descends Lung Qi, relaxes the chest and relieves wheezing**

   - **Lung Qi accumulation** with chest distension, wheezing, fatigue:

     Siberian fir/Fennel/Cypress

5. **Resolves damp and turbidity, and relieves distension**

   - **Spleen toxic-damp** with appetite loss, indigestion, abdominal bloating, flatulence:

     Patchouli/Thyme ct. linalool/Green myrtle/Juniper berry

**6. Activates the Lower Warmer, reduces stagnation and promotes menstruation**

- **Lower Warmer Blood and Qi stagnation** with scanty/late/stopped periods, menstrual cramps, scanty urination:

Clary sage/Fennel/Cypress/Yarrow

REMARKS

A widespread culinary and medicinal plant, Hyssop was originally found from Central Asia to the East Mediterranean. This fragrant lipflower thrives in dry, well-drained rocky soil and warm, sunny dispositions. In the still, dry heat of a summer's day, its blue, purple, pink or white flowers attract swarms of bees who will greedily suck its pollen dust. A fine aromatic honey is the result of their utilitarian passion. Savouring the delights of hyssop honey was a major motivation for medieval European monks to cultivate the plant in their polynia-like physick gardens – even though it was not their only inducement. They sincerely did value Hyssop as a herb for relieving coughs and treating damp, congestive respiratory conditions, living as they usually did in cold, damp old monastic buildings. This is emblematic for the therapeutic use of Hyssop both in herbal and essential oil form.

But Hyssop's monastic associations go deeper than that. Ancient Hebraic culture in the Levant esteemed the herb for ritual and purification purposes; Ezob, the 'holy herb', is mentioned in the Old Testament for purifying the Temple by censing, and for rituals such as Passover. The Eastern Orthodox Church adopted the practice of sprinkling hyssop water to ritually cleanse people and objects (including churches); this is the origin of the Roman Catholic asperges, the special sprinkling of holy water to bless a congregation on important feast days. Tellingly, the standard Gregorian chant intoned at the start of asperges goes *Asperges me, Domine hyssopo et mundabor*, 'sprinkle me, Lord, with hyssop and I will be purified'.

Of all the aromatic remedies with a strong tropism for respiratory functions, Hyssop perhaps has this strongest tropism of all. Since the beginnings of traditional Greek medicine on the islands of the East Mediterranean, it has been a highly esteemed compehensive respiratory and restorative remedy. The essential oil itself is listed in Berlin city tax records of 1574 and, along with the tincture, continues to be a staple in respiratory formulas of herbal medicine practitioners in the West.

Note that Hyssop oil is normally used in formulas rather than on its own: Hyssop's potential neurotoxicity does impose restrictions to its use (see above). The interesting issue here is, simply, how to keep those powerful volatile molecules, the ketones, under control while they carry out their deep regenerating and revitalizing activities on the mucous membranes. Once again, the lesson to be learnt here is to develop a positive attitude of caution arising from respect for a powerful plant rather than succumbing to negative caution stemming from fear of potential toxication.

In simplified form, Hyssop is a one-size-fits-all aromatic for treating congestive phlegm conditions arising from damp terrain – elegantly described in Chinese medicine as various phlegm syndromes of the Lung. Its key function is resolving mucus overproduction in the chest and eliminating congestion by loosening hardened phlegm and promoting expectoration. As a bonus, Hyssop will relieve most types of cough and reduce dyspnoea, even in spasmodic asthma, where its anti-inflammatory action also engages.

Hyssop is especially indicated for individuals with a history of chronic nervous system and respiratory weakness. Its nervous and cerebral restorative action has always been valued for physical and mental fatigue, and depression. Not only acute but long-term respiratory conditions will all benefit from its respiratory restorative action – as with conifer oils such as Scotch pine and Black spruce. Although the weight of Hyssop's anti-infective use is on the treatment of respiratory infections, some practitioners will also make use of its various antimicrobial actions for intestinal and dermal infections.

Hyssop also exerts an arterial stimulant effect that is felt not only in the upper trunk as a stimulant expectorant, but also in the digestive tract as a digestive stimulant, the uterus as an emmenagogue and the kidneys as a diuretic – where it has a reputation for helping dissolve urinary stones. Eclectic practitioners in 19th-century North America also relied on Hyssop in tincture form to 'equalize the circulation' (as they nicely put it), i.e. to regulate blood pressure – but it is still unclear whether this action carries over to the essential oil itself.

Hyssop used purely as a psychological remedy by olfaction displays the typical virtues of a sweet, green oil. It has the potential for helping resolve and transform emotional stagnation, thereby resolving inner conflicts and negative emotions. Its deep, rich, herbaceous honey fragrance has the particular ability to draw us inward, allowing us to explore discord in our emotional realm with due patience and humility. Hyssop may potentially open us to nothing less than reclaiming our true integrity and resolving shame by supporting the process of accepting, understanding and forgiving ourselves. The olfactory blessing of this oil is indeed a purification, as several traditions have recognized. However, it is clearly not a cleansing involving any expulsion of external negative energies, as with other sacred herbs, but rather a purification that can only arise from a sincere inner reconciliation and a recreation of our integrity.

Hyssop thrived for centuries in a monastic milieu where it yielded a sweet, herbaceous honey; it enhanced the complex production of liqueurs, such as Chartreuse, as well as treating damp, congestive respiratory conditions. However, this was clearly not the only reason for the herb's enduring success in a monastic setting. On an energetic and spiritual level, Hyssop was a perfect companion to those men and women who sought to explore the path of reclusion and who subconsciously benefited from its enduring support of their contemplative practices.

**Hyssop decumbens** (*Hyssopus officinalis* var. *decumbens*, a.k.a. *H. montana*) has the same actions and indications as *Hyssopus officinalis*, except that it may be a stronger nervous restorative and antidepressant for neurasthenic or chronic fatigue conditions with depression, fatigue and so on. This is attributed to its high content (48–60%) of d-linalool and trans-linalool oxide, and its relatively low content in ketones (<1.5%). This oil is also higher in 1,8 cineole (12–15%). French practitioners often reserve Hyssop decumbens for treating children's upper and lower respiratory conditions, especially viral infections such as bronchitis, croup, pleurisy and pneumonia. Here the oil also acts as a good mucolytic expectorant. It is also a good liver decongestant and gastrointestinal stimulant for liver congestion, hepatitis, intestinal stagnation and parasites (including Lamblia).

Physiologically, Hyssop decumbens enjoys mild status with no cumulative toxicity or skin irritation because of the much lower level of ketones. It can therefore be dosed at the standard 2–3 drops per gel cap, for instance. None of the Hyssop oil precautions apply.

# Jasmine

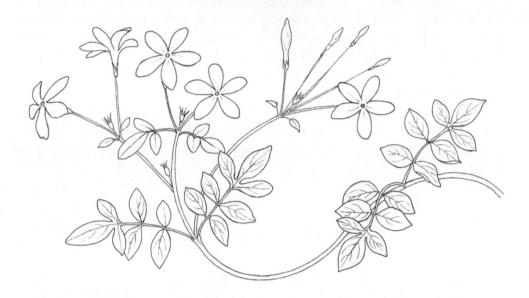

**Botanical source:** The flower of *Jasminum grandiflorum* L. (Oleaceae – olive family), an evergreen shrub or climber of the subtropics also adapted to a Mediterranean climate

**Other names:** Royal jasmine, Spanish/Catalonian/Tuscan/Italian jasmine; Jasmin (Fr, Ge, It, Sp), Chameli (Urdu), Jati (Hindi, Sanskrit), Yasmin (Persian, Arabic)

**Appearance:** A viscous ochre or dark amber fluid with an intense, warm, caramel sweet-floral odour with oily, tea-leaf green and fruity notes; the odour varies somewhat depending on the time of harvest and country of origin

**Perfumery status:** A heart note of high intensity and good persistence

**Extraction:** Solvent extraction of the fresh flowers with hexane, usually June to October; the first extract produces Jasmine concrete, which is thoroughly washed with hot ethanol to produce Jasmine absolute. Both products are almost exclusively used in perfumery and food flavouring.

**1 kg oil yield from:** 800–1,000 kg of fresh flowers (a very low yield); in contrast, 400 kg of flowers yield 1 kg of Jasmine absolute

**Production areas:** Egypt, Morocco, India. Production of Jasmine absolute first began in Egypt when Charles Garnier brought solvent extraction equipment there in 1912.

**Typical constituents:** Esters <47% (incl. benzyl acetate 15–35%, linalyl acetate, methyl anthranilate, methyl jasmonate, phytyl acetate <7%) • monoterpenols <42%

(incl. d-linalool 3–16%, geraniol <10%, α-terpineol <5%, phytol 7–12%) • aromatic alcohols (incl. benzyl benzoate 3–20%, benzyl alcohol <6%) • azoturic compounds (incl. indole <4%) • squalene oxide 6–12% • squalene <6% • ketones (incl. cis-jasmone 1–4%) • eugenol 1–3% • methyl jasmonate <0.5% • jasmolactone • phenylacetic acid • benzaldehyde traces

**Chance of adulteration:** Very high. Synthetic additives include indole, cinnamic aldehyde, benzyl acetate and benzoate, α-amyl cinnamic aldehyde, jasmone and fractions of Ylang ylang.

The quality of Jasmine absolute depends not only on lack of adulteration, but also in the first place on how well the solvent hexane has been removed from the concrete extract (see 'Extraction' above).

**Related absolutes:** Of the over 200 species of jasmine growing worldwide, only three species are regularly produced as an absolute extract: Royal jasmine (this profile), Sambac jasmine (*J. sambac* – see separate profile) and Indian jasmine (*J. auriculatum*, also known as needle-flower jasmine). *J. officinale*, known as white or poet's jasmine, is not extracted, although the grandiflorum species is often grafted onto *J. officinale* rootstocks.

The fragrant flowers of several other vines are also variously called 'jasmine', but are not made into an absolute or essential oil:

- Winter jasmine (*Jasminum nudiflorum*) originally from North China

- Pink or white jasmine (*Jasminum polyanthum*) from Southeast Asia, whose white flowers exude a sweet, musky fragrance at night

- Angelwing jasmine (*Jasminum laurifolium*) from the Southwest Pacific Islands

- Hong Kong jasmine (*Jasminum lanceolarium*) from South China

- Madagascar or bridal jasmine, or Hawaiian wedding flower (*Stepanotis floribunda*), widely cultivated in the Polynesian Islands and the Caribbean, with white, waxy, tubular flowers

- Gardenia or Cape jasmine (*Gardenia jasminoides*) from East Asia, with its strongly fragrant white flowers

- Crape jasmine, East India rosebay or double jasmine (*Ervatamia divaricata*) from the Philippines, China and India, whose waxy white flowers exhale fragrance at night

- Night-blooming jasmine (*Cestrum nocturnum*) originally from the Antilles, with its greenish-white flowers and intense, sweet nocturnal perfume, occasionally also prepared into an absolute in India

- Star, Chinese or confederate jasmine (*Trachelospermum jasminoides*) from subtropical Southeast Asia with fragrant white flowers, also widely cultivated in California and the Southeastern United States

- Yellow or Carolina jasmine/jessamine (*Gelsemium sempervirens*) from Central America and the Southeastern United States, whose flowers are occasionally used in herbal medicine

# Therapeutic Functions and Indications

## SPECIFIC SYMPTOMATOLOGY – *All applications*

Withdrawal, discouragement, pessimism; feelings of emotional insecurity, shame and guilt; low self-worth, listlessness, depression, fearfulness, low sex drive, slow-mindedness, spaciness, physical and emotional fatigue or exhaustion, cynicism, despair, self-destructive tendencies

## PSYCHOLOGICAL – *Aromatic diffusion, whole-body massage*

**Essential PNEI function and indication:** Sensory integrating in sensory disintegration conditions; euphoric in acute overstimulation conditions

**Possible brain dynamics:** Reduces deep limbic system and cingulate gyrus hyperfunctioning

**Fragrance category:** Middle tone with sweet note

**Indicated psychological disorders:** Minor depression, PMS, HSDD, shock, PTSD, dissociative disorder, sensory integration disorder, addiction disorders, codependency

### PROMOTES EMOTIONAL SECURITY AND STRENGTH

- Loss of emotional security and safety; anxiety

- Emotional withdrawal, discouragement, pessimism, disconnection

- Emotional wounding, including loss, betrayal, deprivation

### PROMOTES DISINHIBITION AND INTEGRATION

- Emotional, sensual and sexual repression and inhibition; loss of libido

- Sensing/feeling disconnection and conflict

- Sensory deprivation and disintegration

PROMOTES EUPHORIA AND RESOLVES SHOCK AND TRAUMA

For short-term use in acute conditions.

- Severe guilt, shame, recrimination, cynicism, despair, self-destructiveness

- Melancholic depression, especially with pessimism, grief, fear, despair

- Acute shock from trauma (mental/emotional/physical)

SYNERGISTIC COMBINATIONS – FOR OLFACTION AND TOPICAL APPLICATIONS

- Jasmine + Clary sage: hormonal reproductive restorative, spasmolytic, analgesic for hormonal imbalance with frigidity, PMS, dysmenorrhoea, amenorrhoea

COMPLEMENTARY COMBINATIONS – FOR OLFACTION AND TOPICAL APPLICATIONS

- Jasmine + Coriander seed/Lavender: restorative and antidepressant for mental and emotional fatigue and exhaustion; depression, incl. postpartum

- Jasmine + Sandalwood: restorative, euphoric, integating and disinhibiting for sexual debility or nervous exhaustion with worry or depression; loss of libido and self-esteem

- Jasmine + Neroli: restorative, nurturing, antidepressant and euphoric for emotional withdrawal, esp. from shock; severe discouragement, pessimism, despair

- Jasmine + Helichrysum: nurturing and euphoric for emotional withdrawal, wounding or trauma, with negative or distressed emotions

- Jasmine + Rose: nurturing, euphoric and stabilizing for emotional loss or wounding with loss of security and self-esteem, severe shame, negative or distressed emotions, suicidal tendencies

- Jasmine + Patchouli: restorative, disinhibiting, integrating and euphoric for emotional insecurity and loss of safety; sensory-emotional repression and inhibition, loss of libido

- Jasmine + Ylang ylang: strong euphoric, disinhibiting, aphrodisiac for sensual and sexual repression and inhibition, loss of sexual self-image or identity, loss of libido, repressed anger

- Jasmine + Sambac jasmine: strong euphoric for severe acute shock from trauma; for severe guilt, shame and depression

PHYSIOLOGICAL – *External applications only*

**Therapeutic status:** Mild remedy with no cumulative toxicity

**Topical safety status:** Non-irritant, non-sensitizing

**Tropism:** Reproductive, respiratory, digestive, nervous systems

**Essential diagnostic function:** Restores hypotonic/weak terrain conditions

*nervous and cerebral restorative:* mental fatigue, burnout, nervous breakdown, depression; esp. from emotional causes, trauma, acute transitions, postpartum

*uterine stimulant, spasmolytic, mild analgesic:* amenorrhoea, dysmenorrhoea, uterine dystocia, labour pain

*hormonal stimulant(?):* hormonal insufficiency, PMS, frigidity, infertility, impotence

*galactagogue:* scanty or absent lactation

*agalactic:* excessive lactation, for weaning

*mucostatic:* leucorrhoea, mucoid diarrhoea, mucous colitis, otorrhoea

*stimulant expectorant:* bronchitis with dry or moist cough, with sputum or pain

*demulcent:* hoarseness, voice loss, sore throat

*antibacterial*

*antitumoural*

*antioxidant*

TOPICAL – *Liniment, lotion*

See 'Pharmacological precautions' below.

**Skin care:** Sensitive, dry and mature skin types

*emollient, mild anti-inflammatory, antipruritic:* skin irritation and inflammation, acute eczema or dermatitis, neurogenic pruritus

*skin regenerative, vulnerary:* sores, ulcers, acne, scars, stretch marks; wrinkles

*mild analgesic:* muscle and joint aches and pains, esp. chronic; sprains

**Therapeutic precautions:** All use of Jasmine absolute is contraindicated in babies, infants and young children. Internal absorption is contraindicated during pregnancy as Jasmine is a uterine stimulant. However, it also reduces serum prolactin levels (like Chasteberry) to also support labour functions and later reduce lactation if used for weaning.

**Pharmacological precautions:** An allergic reaction is very occasionally seen with topical use of Jasmine absolute, most likely from a poor-quality product, i.e. one that is chemically adulterated or simply poorly produced with measurable remnants of hexane used in the production of the concrete. For both these reasons, internal use is discouraged and should only be considered with a high-quality absolute.

**Preparations:**

- Diffusor: 1 drop in water

- Massage oil: 0.5–3% dilution in vegetable oil

- Liniment: 3–4% dilution in vegetable oil

# Chinese Medicine Functions and Indications

**Aroma energy:** Sweet

**Movement:** Circulating

**Warmth:** Neutral to warm

**Meridian tropism:** Heart, Pericardium, Liver, Chong, Ren

**Five-Element affinity:** Fire, Wood

**Essential function:** To nourish the Blood, animate the Heart and strengthen the Shen

1. **Nourishes the Blood, regulates menstruation and strengthens the Shen**

    - **Blood deficiency with Shen weakness,** with scanty periods, amenorrhoea or long cycles, mental fatigue, menstrual cramps, PMS with depression, negative emotions:

        Geranium/Palmarosa/Petitgrain bigarade/Coriander seed

    - **Uterus Blood deficiency with Chong and Ren Mai Essence deficiency,** with amenorrhoea, vaginal dryness, frigidity, sterility:

        Vetiver/Rose/Black spruce

2. **Nourishes Heart and Liver Blood, animates the Heart, strengthens the Shen and relieves depression**

    - **Heart Blood deficiency with Shen weakness,** with chronic depression with anxiety, mood swings, negativity:

        Palmarosa/Coriander seed/Clary sage

    - **Liver Blood deficiency with Shen weakness,** with depression, pessimism, insecurity, shame feelings, loss of sex drive:

        Geranium/Neroli/Rose

### 3. Glosses the Shen and suspends emotions

- **Shock, acute trauma, acute emotions**:
  Rose/Lavender/Atlas cedarwood

- **Depression in general** (symptom relief for all types of depression):
  Neroli/Ylang ylang/Clary sage

REMARKS

The royal jasmine shrub is native to the broad region spanning Western South Asia, the Arabian Peninsula, Northeast Africa and the African Great Lakes region. Its name drives from the Persian *yasmin*, meaning fragrant. Royal jasmine has long been an integral part of life in India for personal and community uses. Like several other tropical flowers, such as champaca also in India, gardenia in Tahiti and sampaguita in the Philippines, the heady, sweet jasmine flowers are traditionally infused in coconut oil; the infused oil is widely used as a hair and body oil, and as a base for perfumes and ointments. Hindu and Buddhist temples both use the flowers lavishly. It is interesting that jasmine is also the official symbol of the city of Damascus in Syria, known as the City of Jasmine – this despite having originally lent its name to the Damask rose (up to the 16th century since unknown ancient times, Damascus was actually the most important production and distribution centre for rosewater).

Royal jasmine has long been cultivated as a fragrant ornamental in the Mediterranean, especially in Spain and Italy, where it became Spanish or Catalonian jasmine. Equally beloved in Italy during the Renaissance, the flower's sensuous, seductive fragrance contributed largely to the sensory awakening from the long, torpid sleep of the Middle Ages – possibly along with the elevating aroma of bitter orange flowers. It therefore indirectly fuelled the original development of perfumery as an aesthetic art distinct from herbal medicine. With the rise of chemical plant extraction around the turn of the 20th century, jasmine quickly became an essential aroma in modern perfumery, along with rose, narcissus and several others. As a potent aromatic with intriguing olfactory potential, Jasmine absolute then became a reliable 'oil' in the emerging British aromatherapy of the 1970s. Today, Jasmine absolute is emerging as a key aromatic remedy for psychological applications quite separate from any physiological action.

It is unfortunately difficult to pin down the exact physiological effects of Jasmine absolute. There are three reasons for this. Firstly, because taking Jasmine absolute by direct method of internal administration is not encouraged (see above); this in itself has discouraged clinical experimentation as a physiological medicine. Secondly, because the absolute extract has hardly been used medicinally, only the flower infusion in Indian Ayurvedic medicine. Thirdly, because extremely little research has been conducted on Jasmine in any preparation form; this goes especially for its clinically effective hormonal action.

Despite this drawback, Jasmine has a minor reputation as woman's remedy for regulating non-specific hormones, and for stimulating uterine functions, as in amenorrhoea and failure to progress in the first stage of labour. In Ayurvedic medicine it is also known as a nervous restorative for chronic mental fatigue, burnout and depression; it certainly works well in postpartum depression. Jasmine has a good twin effect on depression, both physiological and psychological, by olfaction. In terms of functional conditions, Jasmine addresses essentially a weak terrain that tends to damp and cold.

Topically, Jasmine is a useful emollient for soothing and moistening dry, irritated, itchy skin conditions; it is also reputedly skin-regenerative and somewhat analgesic. Jasmine has a reputation among some cosmetologists for its ability to aid dry, mature and sensitive types of facial skin.

However, as a result of its limitations as a physical medicine, practitioners have focused largely on the aromatherapeutic uses of Jasmine absolute. It is classically described as a floral-sweet, euphoric, sensory integrating aromatic. Even when prescribing for dermal, gynaecological or respiratory conditions, and regardless of the delivery method, a practitioner such as Bitsas (2009) will add a small amount of Jasmine to his blends when emotional causes are involved.

Possibly the key function of Jasmine by olfaction is its disinhibiting and integrating effect on the personality, with the net result of bolstering self-esteem. Chronic states of personal inhibition of any kind, especially involving a degraded self-image and often resulting from an overly strict, moralistic upbringing, will benefit from Jasmine. Here the fragrance seems to have a special affinity for integrating what we sense with how we feel emotionally. It can help those whose life situation no longer matches their feelings, who simply feel stuck in their suffering, experiencing distressed emotions such as shame and fear, and unable to change their situation. Depression is often the result, along with cynicism, despair and self-destructive tendencies.

Acute depression is another key indication for Jasmine by olfaction. The fragrance creates euphoria – a feeling of bliss and carefreeness – but it does not sedate. Unlike Rose and Clary sage, also mild euphorics, Jasmine engenders a wide-awake state of temporary bliss. With acute depression, shock and any traumatic experience, this is exactly the kind of emotional band-aid that is required. Creating a temporary cocoon around the wounded self, Jasmine will help the process of resolving an acute negative experience in all safety and security. In the healing process, emotions will begin to stabilize and aspects of the self will become more integrated.

# Laurel

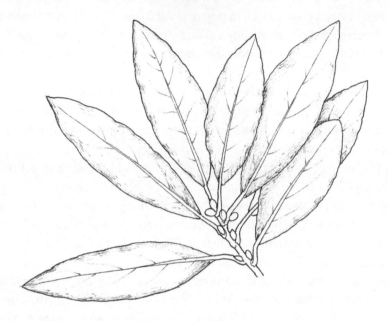

**Botanical source:** The twig and leaf of *Laurus nobilis* L. (Lauraceae – laurel family), a hardy East Mediterranean tree widely introduced elsewhere

**Other names:** Bay/Roman/noble laurel; Laurier (noble) (Fr), Lorbeer (Ge), Lauro (It, Sp)

**Appearance:** A mobile pale green-yellow to olive-green fluid with a fresh, warm-camphoraceous and rich sweet-green odour

**Perfumery status:** A heart note of strong intensity and medium persistence

**Extraction:** Steam distillation of the half-dry twigs and leaves, late August to October; sometimes also in spring

**1 kg oil yield from:** 50–100 kg of the leaves (a good yield)

**Production areas:** Slovenia, Croatia, Bosnia-Herzegovina, Hungary, Turkey, South France, Morocco

**Typical constituents:** Oxides (incl. 1,8 cineole 35–50%, dehydro-1,8 cineole) • monoterpenes 12–19% (incl. α-pinene 4–16%, β-pinene 3–5%, sabinene 4%) • mono-terpenols 13–21% (incl. linalool 8–18%, α-terpineol, terpinen-4-ol 3%, geraniol, borneol, cis-thujanol-4) • esters 17% (incl. terpenyle/linalyle/bornyle/geranyle/eugenyl acetate) • phenols (methyleugenol 2–7%, eugenol 1–5%, cis-eugenol) • sesquiterpenes 4% (incl. β-elemene, β-caryophyllene, α- and β-phellandrene) • sesquiterpenols 2% •

sesquiterpene lactones <3% (incl. costunolide, artemorine) • ketone camphor • traces lauric acid

**Chance of adulteration:** Quite commonly with Blue-gum eucalyptus, Cajeput and Green myrtle, as well as various synthetic components such as 1,8 cineole, α-terpenyl acetate and methyleugenol

**Related oils:** In the large and diverse laurel family of oils belong Ravintsara, Camphor, Cinnamon, May chang and Rosewood. Laurel oil should not be confused with the oil of Bay rum leaf (*Pimenta racemosa*) in the myrtle family (see the Pimenta berry profile). The commercial designation 'Bay oil' is therefore ambiguous and unsatisfactory, especially in a therapeutic context, even though it properly refers to Bay rum leaf oil.

## Therapeutic Functions and Indications

### SPECIFIC SYMPTOMATOLOGY – *All applications*

Emotional confusion and conflict, low self-esteem, insecurity, shyness, easily frightened, timidity, feeling stuck in a rut; long-term physical and mental fatigue, exhaustion, depression with anxiety, chronic worry, mental fogginess; mood swings, chronic headaches; chronic indigestion worse from stress with bloating, flatulence, pain, poor appetite; chest distension and congestion, chronic productive cough, wheezing; chronic or recurring infections, swollen lymph glands; muscle cramps, aches and pains; stiff painful joints

### PSYCHOLOGICAL – *Aromatic diffusion, whole-body massage*

**Essential PNEI function and indication:** Stimulant in weakness conditions
**Possible brain dynamics:** Increases basal ganglia functioning and reduces deep limbic system hyperfunctioning
**Fragrance category:** Middle tone with sweet, green, pungent notes
**Indicated psychological disorders:** ADD, depression, bipolar disorder

PROMOTES EMOTIONAL RENEWAL AND CLARITY

- All pathogenic (stuck) emotions and distressed feelings in general
- Emotional confusion with conflict; emotional illusions

PROMOTES WILLPOWER, COURAGE AND SELF-CONFIDENCE

- Loss of willpower or strength, poor personal boundaries
- Discouragement, pessimism, negativity

- Loss of self-confidence with insecurity, anxiety

- Mental and emotional burnout

## PHYSIOLOGICAL – *Nebulizer inhalation, gel cap, suppository, external applications*

**Therapeutic status:** Mild remedy with no cumulative toxicity

**Topical safety status:** Non-irritant, possibly mildly sensitizing

**Tropism:** Nervous, respiratory, digestive, urinary, reproductive systems

**Essential diagnostic function:** Restores hypotonic/weak conditions and relaxes hypertonic/tense terrain conditions

### PRIMARILY RESTORATIVE AND STIMULANT:

*strong central nervous restorative and regulator:* hypotonic (weak) conditions with fatigue, debility, incl. neurasthenia, CFS, ANS dysregulation; incl. from chronic disease, convalescence, postpartum

*cerebral restorative and mild sedative:* cerebral/mental deficiency with cognitive impairment, fatigue, depression, esp. with anxiety; MS and other neurodegenerative disorders

*strong respiratory stimulant, mucolytic expectorant, mucosal restorative (anticatarrhal):* congestive bronchial conditions with dyspnoea, expectoration, incl. chronic bronchitis, emphysema; rhinitis (see below)

*gastrointestinal stimulant and detoxicant, stomachic, carminative, antifermentative:* atonic digestive conditions with appetite loss, upper indigestion, bloating; microbial toxicosis, intestinal putrefaction or fermentation

*lymphatic stimulant/decongestant:* lymphatic congestion, swollen glands from infections

*uterine stimulant, emmenagogue:* atonic amenorrhoea; uterine dystocia

*diuretic*

*antioxidant, anticancer*

### PRIMARILY RELAXANT:

*spasmolytic, analgesic, anti-inflammatory:* spasm and pain conditions in general, of smooth and striped muscles; local pain conditions, incl. sciatica, tendinitis, CTS; paralysis, Raynaud's disease

***antiarthritic, antisclerotic, analgesic:*** arthritic and rheumatic conditions (all types) with joint stiffness, deformity, muscle contracture, incl. osteoarthritis; muscle cramps and spasms; arteriosclerosis(?)

***bronchodilator, antitussive:*** spasmodic dyspnoea and cough, incl. asthma, croup, whooping cough; spasmodic dysphonia

***coronary dilator, hypotensive:*** spasmodic angina/coronary disease; hypertension, arteriosclerosis

***gastrointestinal relaxant, analgesic:*** indigestion with flatulence, pain; colic, IBS

***antiemetic:*** nausea, vomiting, travel sickness

***uterine relaxant and analgesic:*** spasmodic dysmenorrhoea, esp. with severe cramps

***bladder relaxant and analgesic:*** spasmodic dysuria

***mild cerebral sedative:*** anxiety, obsessive-compulsive disorder, psychotic states

ANTIMICROBIAL ACTIONS:

***anti-infective, antimicrobial, immunostimulant, anti-inflammatory, detoxicant, analgesic:***

- ***antiviral:*** viral infections in general, incl. upper respiratory (acute flu, rhinitis, sinusitis, bronchitis, tonsillitis, otitis media, pneumonia); hepatitis, enteritis, neuritis, aphthous sores, stomatitis; urinary infections

- ***antibacterial:*** upper and lower respiratory infections, esp. chronic; chronic bronchitis, gastrointestinal infections, incl. intestinal sepsis/fermentation, microbial toxicosis, colitis, intestinal TB and cancer; lung abscess; urinary and skin infections

- ***antifungal:*** intestinal dysbiosis, candidiasis (Candida albicans/tropicalis/ pseudotropicalis)

- ***antimalarial, antipyretic:*** malaria, other tropical fevers

SYNERGISTIC COMBINATIONS

- Laurel + Eucalyptus, blue-gum/Green myrtle: strong antiseptic stimulant expectorant and nasal decongestant in chronic bronchitis with dyspnoea, cough and dysphonia; emphysema, rhinitis, sinusitis

- Laurel + Eucalyptus, narrow-leaf/Ravintsara: antiviral, expectorant for all viral upper and lower respiratory infections, influenza

- Laurel + Rosemary: analgesic, antirheumatic for painful rheumatic-arthritic conditions

- Laurel + Rosemary/Niaouli/Ravintsara: strong nervous and cerebral restorative in neurasthenia with chronic fatigue, depression, amnesia, mental impairment

- Laurel + Green myrtle: strong anti-infective mucolytic expectorant for all lower respiratory infections with congestive dyspnoea, cough and copious sputum

- Laurel + Green myrtle: digestive stimulant-relaxant for chronic gastroenteritis, colitis

### COMPLEMENTARY COMBINATIONS

- Laurel + Nutmeg + Clary sage: strong nervous and cerebral restorative for neurasthenia with chronic fatigue, depression, anxiety, dizziness, headaches, memory loss

- Laurel + Basil ct. methylchavicol/Petitgrain bigarade: strong nervous restorative and regulator in deficiency and dysregulated ANS conditions, incl. chronic neurasthenia, ANS dysregulation; in chronic disease, convalescence

- Laurel + Cypress/Basil ct. chavicol: bronchodilator and antitussive in all spasmodic respiratory conditions, incl. spasmodic dyspnoea, cough, asthma, spasmodic dysphonia

- Laurel + Thyme ct. linalool/Thyme ct. thymol: strong anti-infective expectorant for all upper and lower respiratory infections, viral and bacterial; esp. chronic, with fatigue

- Laurel + Atlas cedarwood: mucostatic expectorant for congestive bronchial conditions with copious sputum, dyspnoea, cough

- Laurel + Sage/Winter savoury: urinary antiseptic, analgesic and spasmolytic for urinary tract infections with dysuria

- Laurel + Juniper berry/Nutmeg: intestinal detoxicant and antiputrefactive for gut microbial toxicosis, intestinal sepsis or putrefaction

- Laurel + Atlas cedarwood: lymphatic stimulant for chronic lymphatic congestion

- Laurel + Lemon eucalyptus/May chang: analgesic, anti-inflammatory, antiarthritic in acute, painful arthritic and rheumatic conditions

- Laurel + Black pepper/Nutmeg: analgesic, anti-inflammatory, antiarthritic, stimulant in chronic painful arthritic and rheumatic conditions

- Laurel + Roman camomile: spasmolytic and analgesic for severe painful spasms and cramps of most kinds

- Laurel + Ylang ylang/Spikenard/Tarragon: coronary dilator, hypotensive for spasmodic angina pectoris, hypertension

## TOPICAL – *Liniment, ointment, cream, compress and other cosmetic preparations*

**Skin care:** Atonic, congested and oily skin types

*capillary stimulant, rubefacient:* slow hair and scalp activity, dandruff, loss of eyebrows, chilblains

*vulnerary, skin regenerator, antiputrefacient:* ulcers, bedsores, abscesses, esp. chronic, non-healing; necrosis, gangrene

*antiseptic, antifungal, antibacterial, detumescent:* acne, boils, furuncles, milia, fungal skin conditions

*analgesic, anti-inflammatory, spasmolytic:* local pain, incl. sprains, strains, muscle and joint pain, spasm and stiffness; sciatica, tendinitis, toothache, earache

*insectifuge, antiparasitic:* lice, scabies, insects in general

**Therapeutic precautions:** Laurel oil is a warming, drying stimulant that is contraindicated in hypersthenic/hot and dry conditions of all kinds, including agitation, acute fever, acute anxiety and dry respiratory conditions with dry unproductive cough. Internal and intensive use of Laurel, including in a nebulizer, is also contraindicated during pregnancy, as Laurel is a uterine stimulant.

**Pharmacological precautions:** The sesquiterpene lactones in Laurel oil are known to cause a contact allergy with inflammation in some individuals. Because Laurel oil varies widely in its levels of these lactones, doing a patch test before any topical application is strongly advised. For the same reason, Laurel is contraindicated for topical use on sensitive or broken skin as it may act as a mild sensitizer. However, various tests also showed no irritation or sensitization for Laurel at 2–10% dilution.

Laurel should be avoided in babies, infants and children because of its high levels of 1,8 cineole. The oil's content in methyleugenol may also be of concern in cancer conditions. However, only very high levels of methyleugenol have shown carcinogenic activity, while low levels of it have tested anticarcinogenic (Tisserand and Young 2013). Laurel notably also contains the anticarcinogenic constituent eugenol.

**Preparations:**

- Diffusor: 2–4 drops in water

- Massage oil: 1–3% dilution in vegetable oil

- Liniment: 2–8% dilution in vegetable oil after doing a patch test and preferably in a blend

- Gel cap: 1–2 drops with olive oil

# Chinese Medicine Functions and Indications

**Aroma energy:** Pungent, sweet, green

**Movement:** Rising and circulating

**Warmth:** Neutral to warm

**Meridian tropism:** Lung, Bladder, Spleen, Liver

**Five-Element affinity:** Metal, Earth, Wood

**Essential function:** To tonify the Qi, activate Qi and Blood, and strengthen the Shen

1. **Tonifies the Qi, raises the clear Yang, animates the Heart, strengthens the Shen and relieves fatigue and depression**

   - **Qi and protective Qi deficiency with Shen weakness**, with chronic physical and mental fatigue, chronic or recurring infections, lethargy, depression, grief:
     Niaouli/Ravintsara/Sage/Tea tree

   - **Clear Yang Qi deficiency with Shen weakness**, with mental fogginess, poor focus, depression, dizziness, confusion, slow response:
     Rosemary/Peppermint/Grand fir/Cajeput

2. **Activates Qi and Blood, breaks up stagnation, resolves damp, harmonizes the Middle Warmer and relieves distension**

   - **Stomach-Spleen Qi and Blood stagnation** with chronic dull or sharp epigastric or abdominal pain, distension, colic, diarrhoea:
     Lavender/Peppermint/Roman camomile

   - **Stomach Qi and food stagnation** with indigestion on eating, appetite loss, nausea, epigastric bloating, eructations, flatulence:
     Fennel/May chang/Lavender

   - **Spleen toxic-damp** with indigestion, abdominal bloating, flatulence, lethargy:
     Niaouli/Patchouli/Black pepper/Thyme ct. linalool

3. **Activates the Lower Warmer, breaks up stagnation, promotes menstruation and relieves pain**

   - **Lower Warmer Qi and Blood stagnation** with late, scanty, painful periods; or stopped periods:

     Juniper berry/Rosemary/Angelica root

4. **Warms the Lung, resolves and expels phlegm, and relieves coughing; diffuses and descends Lung Qi, and relieves wheezing**

   - **Lung phlegm-damp/cold with Qi accumulation**, with severe cough, chest distension, copious sputum expectoration, wheezing:

     Green myrtle/Spearmint/Hyssop/Rosemary ct. verbenone

   - **Lung Qi accumulation** with wheezing, cough, chest distension, pain:

     Fennel/Cypress/Basil ct. methylchavicol

5. **Warms and releases the exterior, dispels wind-cold and relieves pain and coughing; boosts the protective Qi**

   - **External wind-cold** with sneezing, chills, mild nasal congestion, aches and pains:

     Eucalyptus, narrow-leaf/Ravintsara/Niaouli

   - **Lung wind-cold** with fatigue, coughing, chills, nasal congestion, aches and pains:

     Eucalyptus, narrow-leaf/Siberian fir/Niaouli/Cajeput

6. **Warms and opens the meridians, dispels wind-damp-cold, relaxes the tendons and relieves pain**

   - **Wind-damp-cold obstruction** with muscle or joint pains, cramping, stiffness:

     Nutmeg/Siberian fir/Black pepper/Frankincense

REMARKS

A hardy evergreen shrub, laurel originates in the Taurus mountains of Asia Minor, from where it spread by cultivation around the Mediterranean. Its leaves have infused many a spice mix and were once used as packing material for the formerly famous liquorice bars produced in Turkey and Italy. Laurel leaves and berries have always been used as herbal remedies throughout East Mediterranean countries. The essential oil of the leaves is still distilled in Southeast Turkey to this day, being a common ingredient in soap manufacture throughout the Middle East – an extremely appropriate use, considering its multiple benefits to the skin. It is unclear at which time period the essential oil was first produced or when it became widely available. However, William Salmon, the ever-reliable prolific writer-practitioner, records fairly early use (1707) and specifies the best distillation method for both the leaves and berries. Certainly, by the early 19th century, Laurel oil was being produced in numerous Balkan countries and then later in the Moroccan Maghreb – although always in moderate quantities. To this day, Laurel oil does not find extensive use in either perfumery or food flavouring.

Laurel's name in ancient Greece was Daphne, so-named after the Greek goddess Daphoene; laurel leaves were chewed by her priestesses in the valley of Tempe for inducing ecstatic trance states and oracular prophecy. To this day the plant remains the emblem of poetic inspiration and distinction. Early European universities, for instance, would title an inspired writer Poet Laureate – a tradition that still survives. Building further on the laurel emblem, graduates were called Bachelors from the Latin *baccalaureus*, a berry of laurel: they possessed the berries, but not the coveted leaves. By extension, anyone unmarried became later known as a bachelor, as single graduates were forbidden to marry as a means of preventing distraction from their studies. In the late Hellenic period, however, the traditional symbolism of Laurel Daphne, the plant of ecstatic insight conferred by Daphoene, became taken over by cool-headed Apollo and changed to symbolize courage and valour in games and warfare.

The laurel is a plant of extreme vitality: if cut down, it will regrow from roots that remain alive. Its essential oil expresses the same strength and vitality when put to therapeutic use. Laurel is able to strongly revitalize and regulate a chronically weak and dysregulated nervous system and is indicated in most chronic conditions presenting as exhaustion, debility, depression or neurasthenia, regardless of cause. Laurel combines a strong nervous restorative action with a mild sedative one, ending up with a superb balancing, regulating effect. A glance at the oil's pharmacology will confirm its deeply restorative potential: its constituents are dominated by a rich cocktail of the vitalizing oxide 1,8 cineole, energizing monoterpenes and, in the base range, deeply tonifying, warming phenols. Both energetically and pharmacologically, Laurel belongs to the high-cineole oils, alongside the likes of Cajeput, Niaouli and Rosemary – all oils with essentially potent revitalizing ability and a typical fresh-pungent fragrance quality.

Laurel's action on living tissue also continues this energetic theme of revitalization and regeneration. Working deeply, strongly but always gently, this oil is one of the best for treating tissue putrefaction, sepsis and necrosis – all chronic or degenerative conditions. As a skin regenerator and capillary stimulant, it treats chronic wounds, ulcers and abscesses, especially when non-healing. As a nervous restorative and immune stimulant, it is especially indicated for treating chronic or recurrent infections. In this role, Laurel is absolutely on a par with the herbal remedy Echinacea, even down to stimulation of the superficial lymphatic microcirculation. Laurel is much used for upper and lower respiratory and gastrointestinal infections of all kinds, again especially when chronic and unresolved. In the gut, the oil is also detoxicant and antifermentative for microbial toxicosis and chronic microfloral dysbiosis.

However, Laurel could be thought of as the most balanced, or yin, of all the yang natured, warming, stimulating, fresh-pungent high-cineole oils. Like its sister oil Niaouli, it carries considerable yin with its yang, thereby showing a particularly gentle, non-forceful strength. This is apparent in its rich, sweet-green fragrance as much as in its relaxant and balancing constituents, such as esters and alcohols. With about a quarter proportion of these, Laurel is as much a potential neuromuscular relaxant as a stimulant, able to relax tense, spasmodic, painful conditions of the gut, bronchi, uterus, bladder and coronary circulation in particular. Perhaps because it is so reliable here as elsewhere, many European practitioners prefer to use Laurel mainly as a relaxant rather than a stimulant remedy. Regardless, the final spectrum of its indications is quite large and the combining possibilities with other oils almost endless. Still, in the end the oil will always shine in conditions of the above body systems when they present a combined terrain of chronic weakness and tension.

Promoting gentle strength is also a key theme to the use of Laurel by olfaction. Laurel is for individuals who are unable to develop their true potential because of confusion, self-doubt or low self-worth; for those unable to assert and express their true convictions, regardless of external criticism; and for those who lack the courage to resolve their burden of distressed emotions. Kindling a gentle but fearless inner warrior, Laurel can help one cultivate a persistent but calm inner strength and self-esteem – a true self-esteem arising from deep conviction and expressed with clarity and confidence. In tandem, the sweet-green oil is deeply revitalizing on the emotional level, able to transform long-held distressed emotions, thereby resolving emotional conflict. The theme of deep regeneration appears again here in the form of inner renewal and carries the potential for a fresh, authentic opening to the world.

# Lemon Eucalyptus

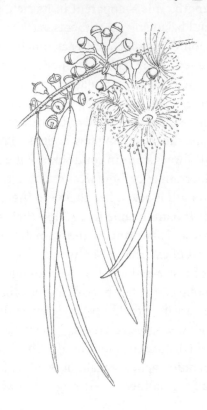

**Botanical source:** The leaf of *Corymbia citriodora* (Hook.) K.D. Hill & L.A.S. Johnson (syn. *Eucalyptus citriodora* Hook.) (Myrtaceae – myrtle family), a widespread (sub) tropical tree

**Other names:** Lemon-scented gum, Lemon spotted gum; Eucalyptus citronné (Fr)

**Appearance:** A mobile colourless to pale yellow fluid with a sweet-lemony and slightly green fragrance. The sweet, round note is dependent on high levels of citronellal relative to citronellol.

**Perfumery status:** A heart note of high intensity and poor persistence

**Extraction:** Steam distillation of the fresh leaves and twiglets, usually August and September

**1 kg oil yield from:** 30–60 kg of the leaves (an excellent yield)

**Production areas:** Australia, South Africa, Tanzania, Brazil, Vietnam, China

**Typical constituents:** Aldehydes (incl. monoterpenoid citronellal 60–85%, isovaleric aldehyde) • monoterpenols (incl. citronellol 5–42%, isopulegol 2–20%, geraniol, transpinocarveol, cis- and trans-p-menthan-3.8-diols, linalool) • monoterpenes (d-limonene <15%, β-pinene) • esters (citronellyl butyrate and citronellate) • ketone menthone <4% • 1,8 cineole 0.6%

**Chance of adulteration:** Rare, because of its abundant yield and low price

**Related oils:** The large eucalyptus family in general, and specifically the fresh-lemony group high in citral or citronellal (see the Eucalyptus profile in Volume 1), as well as various other oils with the same characteristics (see below)

## Therapeutic Functions and Indications

### SPECIFIC SYMPTOMATOLOGY – *All applications*

Pessimism, negative outlook, listlessness, depression, loss of insight and foresight, loss of good judgement and critical thinking, flat affect, irritability, hot spells, palpitations, mild anxiety and insomnia, indigestion, muscle, joint or tendon aches and pains, cough with expectoration, chest pain and distension

### PSYCHOLOGICAL – *Aromatic diffusion, whole-body massage*

**Essential PNEI function and indication:** Stimulant in deficiency conditions
**Possible brain dynamics:** Increases prefrontal cortex functioning
**Fragrance category:** Middle tone with sweet, lemony and green notes
**Indicated psychological disorders:** ADD, depression

PROMOTES EMOTIONAL RENEWAL AND OPTIMISM

- All pathogenic (unproductive, stuck) emotions and distressed feelings in general, especially from past negative experiences

- Pessimism, depression

PROMOTES GOOD JUDGEMENT, INSIGHT AND FORESIGHT

- Poor judgement with loss of insight, emotional confusion with conflict

- Loss of foresight, inability to envision or plan

### PHYSIOLOGICAL – *Nebulizer inhalation, gel cap, external applications*

**Therapeutic status:** Mild remedy with no cumulative toxicity
**Topical safety status:** Non-irritant, possibly sensitizing
**Tropism:** Nervous, cardiovascular, respiratory, digestive, urinary systems

**Essential diagnostic function:** Cools and relaxes hypersthenic/hot terrain conditions

*nervous and vascular relaxant, refrigerant, antipyretic:* hypersthenic (hot) conditions in general, esp. with inflammation, pain, palpitations, hot spells, hot flushes, fevers

*cardiovascular relaxant, vasodilator, hypotensive:* palpitations, arrhythmia, hypertension

*mild cerebral sedative:* insomnia, anxiety

*strong anti-inflammatory and analgesic, mild spasmolytic:* acute pain and inflammation conditions in general, tendino-muscular, articular and vascular:

- tendinitis, tennis elbow, epicondylitis; all rheumatic conditions, incl. fibromyalgia; tissue trauma

- arthritis (all types)

- pericarditis, coronaritis

- acute pharyngitis, laryngitis, bronchitis, pneumonia, asthma, pleurisy

- inflammatory bowel disease, Crohn's

- pelvic inflammatory disease, cystitis (incl. interstitial)

*stimulant expectorant:* lower respiratory congestion, esp. acute, incl. bronchitis, emphysema

*pancreatic restorative/regulator:* diabetes

*diuretic*

*antioxidant*

*mild antiviral*

A<small>NTIMICROBIAL ACTIONS</small>:

*antifungal:* fungal infections, incl. with Aspergillus niger, A. ochraeus, Candida albicans, Trichophyton, Microsporum; incl. athlete's foot, candidiasis, tinea/ringworm

*antiviral:* shingles, herpes, chickenpox

*mild antibacterial:* acute bacterial infections, esp. with Staph. aureus, P. acnes; respiratory and urinary infections

SYNERGISTIC COMBINATIONS

- Lemon eucalyptus + Lemongrass/May chang/Citronella: neurovascular relaxant, refrigerant, antipyretic: in hot conditions with agitation, hot spells, hot flushes, fever

- Lemon eucalyptus + Lemongrass/May chang/Citronella: cardiovascular relaxant, vasodilator, hypotensive for palpitations, arrhythmia, hypertension, anxiety

- Lemon eucalyptus + Lemongrass/May chang: strong neuromuscular sedative, anti-inflammatory and analgesic in acute arthritic, rheumatic and tendon conditions, incl. arthritis, fibromyalgia, tendinitis

- Lemon eucalyptus + Lemongrass: antifungal in a wide variety of fungal infections

- Lemon eucalyptus + May chang + German/Roman camomile: strong anti-inflammatory, spasmolytic and analgesic in all inflammatory and spasmodic gastrointestinal, urinary and reproductive disorders, incl. colitis, inflammatory bowel disease, interstitial cystitis, pelvic inflammatory disease

COMPLEMENTARY COMBINATIONS

- Lemon eucalyptus + Bergamot/Petitgrain bigarade: nervous sedative and regulator for acute stress-related conditions, esp. anxiety, insomnia

- Lemon eucalyptus + Wintergreen: neuromuscular sedative, anti-inflammatory and analgesic in acute arthritic, rheumatic and tendon conditions, incl. arthritis, tendinitis, fibromyalgia

- Lemon eucalyptus + Eucalyptus (blue-gum) + Niaouli: stimulant expectorant, anti-inflammatory, antipyretic, antimicrobial for acute bronchitis (bacterial, viral), croup or pleurisy, with cough, dyspnoea, chest pain, fever

- Lemon eucalyptus + Lavender/Helichrysum: analgesic, anti-inflammatory for tissue trauma with pain and inflammation, incl. sprains, strains, injuries (also topically)

- Lemon eucalyptus + Geranium: pancreatic restorative, blood-sugar regulator in hypoglycaemia, diabetes

- Lemon eucalyptus + Citronella: insect repellent, esp. mosquitoes (topical use)

TOPICAL – *Liniment, lotion*

See 'Pharmacological precautions' below.

**Skin care:** Oily, dry or mature skin types

> *analgesic, anti-inflammatory:* injuries, strains, sprains, insect bites; muscle, tendon and joint pain, inflammation; tissue elongation and contraction (see above)

> *antiseptic, mild vulnerary:* wounds, cuts, sores, acne, dandruff

> *insect repellent, insecticidal, deodorant (incl. lice, fleas)*

> *tick repellent, acaricidal:* mites, ticks, incl. castor-bean ticks (*I. ricinus, I. pacificus*)

**Therapeutic precautions:** Lemon eucalyptus oil is a systemic cooling relaxant to most internal organ systems and is contraindicated internally in all hyposthenic/cold and hypotonic/weak conditions in general. This includes chronic poor circulation, hypotension, debility and neurasthenia with depression. It should also be used only for acute, not chronic, forms of inflammation and fever.

**Pharmacological precautions:** Lemon eucalyptus may be topically sensitizing in some because of its high aldehyde content. Like all other oils high in aldehydes, its irritant effect may be reduced or quenched with the addition of an oil high in monoterpenols, such as Lavender, Geranium, Palmarosa or Thyme ct. linalool. Avoid use in sensitive or damaged skin, and do not exceed the dilutions below.

**Preparations:**

- Diffusor: 2–4 drops in water

- Massage oil: 2–3% dilution in vegetable oil

- Liniment: 3–6% dilution in vegetable oil

- Gel cap: 2–3 drops with olive oil

## Chinese Medicine Functions and Indications

**Aroma energy:** Lemony, green

**Movement:** Dispersing, circulating

**Warmth:** Cool to cold

**Meridian tropism:** Liver, Heart, Lung, Bladder

**Five-Element affinity:** Wood, Fire, Metal

**Essential function:** To clear heat, clarify the Heart and calm the Shen

1. **Clears heat, clarifies the Heart and calms the Shen**

   - **Heart fire with Shen agitation**, with agitation, talkativeness, intense emotions, insomnia, palpitations:

     Lavender/Marjoram/Neroli/Spikenard

   - **Liver fire with Shen agitation**, with headache, red complexion, anger, possible fever:

     Lemongrass/Marjoram/Kaffir lime petitgrain

   - **Shao yang-stage heat with Shen agitation**, with alternating fever and chills:

     Lavender/Blue-gum eucalyptus/Ylang ylang no. 1

   - **Yang ming-stage heat with Shen agitation**, with fever, anxiety, restlessness, insomnia, rapid forceful pulse:

     Lemon/Lavender/Lemongrass

2. **Cools the Lung, eliminates phlegm and relieves coughing**

   - **Lung phlegm-heat** with cough, chest pain, expectoration of green-yellow sputum:

     Eucalyptus (blue gum)/Spearmint/Niaouli/Green myrtle

3. **Drains Kidney-Bladder heat and relieves pain**

   - **Kidney-Bladder heat** with acute bladder or pelvic pain, painful urination:

     Wintergreen/Lemon/Green myrtle/Niaouli

4. **Opens the meridians, dispels wind-damp-heat and relieves pain**

   - **Wind-damp-heat obstruction** with acute muscle, joint or tendon pain, swelling, redness:

     Vetiver/Wintergreen/Lime

REMARKS

A common tree in the myrtle family from tropical countries worldwide, the Lemon-scented gum or eucalyptus yields a very useful essential oil from both a physiological and psychological perspective. In some locations its leaves found traditional use for scenting linen cupboards and repelling warm-climate insects, especially cockroaches and silverfish. Its bark yields the gummy exudate Kino, an antibacterial astringent used in herbal medicine for infectious diarrhoea.

As a physiological remedy, Lemon eucalyptus is a reliable go-to oil for treating acute hot (hypersthenic) conditions. Its aromatic signature is green-lemony and its pharmacological one citronellal, a profile shared by several other oils such as

Lemongrass, Lemon myrtle, May chang and Java citronella. Its fragrance type and citronellal dominance both signal cooling, calming, pain-relieving properties for treating all conditions presenting as acute heat, inflammation and pain.

With an excellent affinity for neurovascular, respiratory and musculoskeletal functions, Lemon eucalyptus is a classic refrigerant, relaxant, sedative and analgesic remedy. It is important for acute inflammation and pain of all muscles and sinews (tendons and ligaments) in general, where topical preparations will also score. However, it does not address nerve pain or neuritis like the Camomiles, Marjoram or Tropical basil; nor is it a major spasmolytic from its lack of citral. Bronchial, colonic and pelvic inflammation will also respond to its good anti-inflammatory action. In the chest area, Lemon eucalyptus is predictably also a good expectorant, making for an important remedy in acute, hot-type bronchitis with productive cough. The oil should often be used in topical preparations for fungal skin infections, where its uplifting fragrance is a welcome plus. For those tired of Citronella, Lemon eucalyptus is here a reliable insect (including tick-) repellent, deodorant and cooling analgesic for hot weather activities – on its own or combined with Lemongrass or Geranium.

In both acute and chronic hot conditions, Lemon eucalyptus may be used as an oil for clearing systemic heat, regardless of origin, as seen in fevers, hot spells of any kind and sometimes hypertension, with usual symptoms such as a rapid pulse, red tongue body, flushed complexion and agitation. The oil is a cerebral sedative that also calms acute anxiety and insomnia. As such, it is important to avoid its use in cold conditions, which it may make worse. Lemon eucalyptus is clearly not a poor relative to the more widely known types of eucalypts, such as the blue-gum and narrow-leaf. It is a distinct remedy in its own right.

Lemon eucalyptus has more to offer as a psychological remedy when used by gentle olfaction. Sweeter than most other green, lemony oils, it is not as uplifting and mentally stimulating as high-citral oils such as Lemongrass and Lemon myrtle. Yes, it can be used for promoting an optimistic outlook on life, for improving mental focus and for creating better judgement. But where it is really needed is when the individual is weak in these areas due to emotional stagnation. Like other sweet, green oils, Lemon eucalyptus excels at aiding the emotional transformation of stuck, negative emotions and distressed feelings, especially when these result from past negative experiences. This aromatic creates emotional clarity more than cognitive or mental clarity. It can remove the emotional baggage that prevents us from thinking clearly, planning with discernment and envisioning with imagination. One might say it allows a greater two-way flow between emotions and the mind.

**Related oils:** Two oils in the verbena family (Verbenaceae) and several in the myrtle family (Myrtaceae) from Australia display similar characteristics and therapeutic uses as Lemon eucalyptus.

**Lemon verbena** (*Lippia citriodora* Ortega ex Persoon, syn. *Aloysia triphylla* Palau) in the verbena family is originally from Western South America; the oil is steam distilled in Morocco from the flowering plant tops and routinely used as an internal remedy by French-speaking practitioners. The fragrance of Lemon verbena is sweet grassy-green with sweet lemony top notes. It has a wide spectrum of constituents dominated by aldehydes 39–40% (incl. citrals neral 12%, geranial 26%), sesquiterpenes <18% (incl. β-caryophyllene, germacrene D, farnesene, curcumene) and monoterpenols <17% (incl. α-terpeneol, citronellol, geraniol, nerol), rounded off by esters 6% (incl. neryl and geranyl acetate), monoterpenes 6% (incl. limonene), sesquiterpenols <5%, oxides (1,8 cineole 3–6%, caryophyllene oxides 3%) and traces of coumarins.

Lemon verbena has mild therapeutic status with no toxicity but is a mild skin sensitizer and photosensitizer becuse of its coumarin content. The oil is systemically relaxant and cooling in acute hypertonic/tense and hypersthenic/hot conditions, especially to nervous, cardiovascular and neuromuscular functions. It is an excellent nervous sedative for states of acute anxiety, insomnia, agitation and agitated depression, especially with chronic fatigue also present. Its strong anti-inflammatory action will treat acute gastroenteritis, IBD, Crohn's disease and acute arthritic-rheumatic disorders. Lemon verbena is a good antipyretic for acute fevers with heat and agitation, including malaria. As a hypotensive vasodilatant, it will treat tachycardia with palpitations, hypertension, angina and coronaritis.

At the same time, Lemon verbena exerts a stimulant action on upper digestive functions, including the stomach, gallbadder and pancreas, thereby treating stagnant digestive functions with appetite loss and indigestion, including gastritis, cholecystitis, sludged bile ducts and gallstones. The oil has also proven helpful for psoriasis and eye fatigue and weakness. Lemon verbena is also a mild restorative to the thyroid, gonads (ovaries, testicles), pancreas and spleen and may be considered in chronic deficiencies of these organs. As such, it is sometimes given as 1 drop in a gel cap before breakfast. The oil is antibacterial and has seen success with cystitis and Staph. aureus infactions. This lemony oil is also a good insect repellent and deodorant. Use with caution on sensitive or diseased skin and avoid sun exposure after application in case coumarins are present in the oil. With internal use, Lemon verbena is contraindicated in chronic or melancholic depression and should only be used with agitated depression. It should also be avoided in hyposthenic/cold and hypotonic/weak terrain in general. Low dilutions and doses apply.

As a psychological remedy by olfaction, Lemon verbena excels at helping unproductive emotions and distressed feelings resolve. It aids the renewal of stuck emotions and accompanying negative thoughts and feelings, promoting optimism, positivity and a gentle alertness. Along with that, the oil will gently promote good judgement and insight.

**Zinziba** or Lemon bush (*Lippia javanica* [Burm. f.] Spreng.) in the verbena family is indigenous to South and East Africa. Although a well-established traditional herbal remedy, its essential oil has yet to achieve clinical importance. Its oil is distilled from the whole flowering herb, presenting an interesting complex of sweet, fruity, lemony, green notes with woody undertones. Its chemical profile is dominated by the ketones myrcenone (21–50%), trans-tagetenone (25–40%) and cis-tagetenone (11–21%) and the monoterpenes myrcene (<11%) and limonene (<5%), with very small percentages of assorted other constituents, including monoterpenols, sesquiterpenes and oxides.

Like Melissa, Zinziba as a physiological remedy has mild therapeutic status and no skin irritation or sensitization. It is essentially a relaxant and cooling oil for treating hypertonic/tense and hypersthenic/hot conditions with a good affinity for respiratory and musculoskeletal functions. A good antipyretic and anti-infective with antiviral, antibacterial and antifungal actions, Zinziba will treat a range of acute upper and lower respiratory infections with heat and fever, including flu, bronchitis, pneumonia, whooping cough and croup. It is also given in measles and malarial fever. Zinziba is specifically a fluidifying expectorant, bronchodilator and antitussive for bronchial asthma and bronchitis with dyspnoea, hard, dry phlegm and persistent chronic coughs. The oil also acts as an analgesic and anti-inflammatory in hot, irritated or painful conditions of the muscles, joints and skin (including sprains, strains and bruising). Zinziba is cooling, antipruritic, emollient and antiseptic for hot, itching skin rashes of most kinds, and insect bites. Head lice and scabies are also commonly treated with it. Zinziba has virtually no therapeutic or pharmacological precautions. Standard dilutions and doses apply.

As a psychological aromatic used by olfaction, Zinziba has much the same indications as Lemon verbena.

**Lemon-scented ironbark** (*Eucalyptus staigeriana*): see profile under Eucalyptus, Volume 1.

**Lemon myrtle** (*Backhousia citriodora*), also known as Lemon ironwood, from the coastal rainforests of Queensland, Australia, has an intense fresh lemony, somewhat green fragrance from its extremely high citral levels (90–98%, composed of the aldehydes geranial and neral). Minor constituents include myrcene, methyl heptenone, linalool, citronellal and cyclocitral. Lemon myrtle enjoys mild therapeutic status with no cumulative toxicity. Its uses reflect other oils high in citral, such as Lemongrass, May chang and Lemon verbena. Relaxant and cooling, the oil physiologically essentially treats acute tense and hot conditions with spasms, pain and inflammation, including agitation, insomnia, palpitations, irritable bowel syndrome, muscle cramps and pain, hot spells and fevers. It has also shown good antibacterial, antiviral and antifungal actions, including for flu, colds and bronchitis. Like other high-citral oils, Lemon myrtle has shown an excellent antitumoural action. Topical use should not exceed 0.7% in a carrier oil as it is a skin irritant and sensitizer, and should be avoided with hypersensitive or damaged skin. Its sensitizing effect may be reduced or quenched with the addition of an oil high in monoterpenols, such as Lavender, Geranium or Palmarosa. It is contraindicated in infants under 2, and should be used with caution in pregnancy and with diabetes medication.

Psychological applications of Lemon myrtle by olfaction are emotionally uplifting and optimizing, indicating use for helping resolve pathogenic, stuck emotions, especially with pessimism and negative thoughts. The gently inhaled oil is also mentally stimulating in cases of minor depression, mental fog, loss of concentration, distraction and possibly ADD.

**Lemon-scented tea tree** (*Leptospermum petersonii*) from Northeast Australia has typical pungent-lemony notes from the high levels of both the aldehydes citral (45–67%, consisting of geranial and neral) and citronellal (9–28%), with minor levels of α-pinene, geraniol, citronellol and isopulegol. Other chemotypes also exist. Based on its fragrance and pharmacognosy combined, Lemon tea tree would be expected to have a similar therapeutic status, character and application as Lemon myrtle and Lemon eucalyptus, and limited clinical experience has substantiated that. With three major aldehydes in almost equal proportion, it is a particularly strong nervous sedative, anti-inflammatory and analgesic. Topical sprays are likely to exert a tick-repellent effect, at least partly because of its citronellal content (see Lemon eucalyptus), if not because of its citral. The same topical dilutions and general precautions as for Lemon myrtle apply.

**Citronella tea tree** (*Leptospermum liversidgei*), also pragmatically called 'Mossie blocker', from coastal West Australia, shows high levels of either citral (55–80%) or citronellal (44%), depending on chemotype, imparting either a more fresh lemony or lemony green, citronella-like fragrance. Although having seen limited therapeutic use apart from repelling mosquitoes, the citral chemotype is expected to behave similarly to Lemon myrtle and Lemongrass; and the citronellal chemotype similarly to Java citronella. Both should be experimented with for a likely tick-repellent action. The same topical dilutions and general precautions and contraindications as for these oils apply.

# Lime

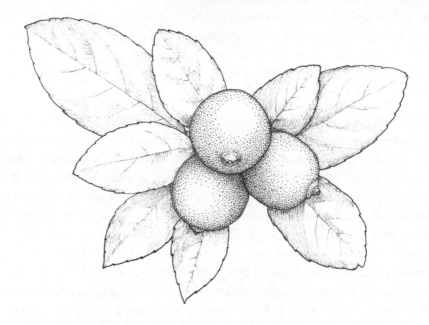

**Botanical source:** The fruit rind of *Citrus x aurantifolia* (Christm.) Swingle (Rutaceae – citrus family), a widely cultivated subtropical fruit tree

**Other names:** Key lime, West Indies lime, Mexican lime, Sour lime; Lime acide (Fr), Limette (Ge), Limetta (It), Lima (Sp), Limu (Persian), Shi hui (Mandarin)

**Appearance:** Cold-pressed lime oil is a clear or pale yellow mobile liquid with an intense fresh-fruity, somewhat sweet, green odour; the distilled oil has a much sharper, more acidic and less sweet note than the cold-pressed oil

**Perfumery status:** A head tone oil of high intensity but poor tenacity

**Extraction:** There are two distinct types of Lime essential oil: cold-pressed Lime oil and distilled Lime oil. The first type is a cold expeller pressed from the green, unripe fruit rind and is preferred for therapeutic purposes and by the perfumery industry.

The second type, more common by far, is either steam distilled from the slurry of whole ripe crushed fruits (both unripe and ripe) or is a steam distillation of the expressed lime juice. Either way, distilled lime oil is simply a by-product in the production of lime juice and is predictably also used mainly in the food and soft-drinks industries.

**1 kg yield from:** 50–100 kg (a good yield)

**Production areas:** Cuba, Central America, Florida, Italy

**Typical constituents (cold-pressed oil):** Monoterpenes <73% (incl. d-limonene 36–64%, γ-terpinene 6–18%, β-pinene 4–12%, β-myrcene <3%, α-phellandrene <3%, α-pinene <2%, α-terpinolene) • monoterpenols (incl. linalool 1–17%, α-terpineol 13–23%, β-terpineol <3%) • esters (incl. linalyl acetate <27%, terpenyl/neryl/geranyl acetate) • aldehydes <12% (incl. geranial, citronellal, decanal, perillaldehyde) • coumarins 7% (incl. limettin, sesilin, auropten, bergamottin) • aromatic p-cymene <7% • sesquiterpenes (incl. β-caryophyllene <3%, α-bisabolene 2%) • 1,8 cineole <2% • ketones (incl. piperitone)

**In the non-volatile fraction:** Flavonoids, triterpenoids, steroids, coumarins and furanocoumarins

**Chance of adulteration:** High. Cold-pressed Lime oil (i.e. Key lime) may be mixed with any of the other lime species below. Distilled Lime oil is treated the same way as Lemon oil, with removal of the coumarins and addition of various natural and synthetic fractions such as limonene and esters, as well as preservative antioxidants.

**Related oils:** Other lime oils expressed from the fruit rind include the following; these are much less commonly produced, however.

**Persian lime** (*Citrus x latifolia* Tanaka), also known as Tahiti lime and Bearss lime, is now considered a hybrid fruit of Key lime (*Citrus x aurantifolia*) and either Lemon (*Citrus limonum*) or Citron (*Citrus medica*). With a somewhat sweeter aroma than Lime oil, cold-pressed Persian lime oil is higher in aldehydes (<24%), including citral, neral and geranial, as well as having a good limonene content (<58%).

**Italian** or Sweet lime, or Limette (*Citrus limetta* Risso), is originally from South and Southeast Asia and has been cultivated in South Italy since the 9th-century Arabic era; the fruit is commonly juiced in Iran, Pakistan and India. It has sweeter notes from its combined content in linalyl acetate (<28%) and mixed coumarins and furanocoumarins. This is one of the citruses from which the bergamot orange was hybridized.

**Kaffir lime**, also known as Leech lime, Makrut or Combava (*Citrus hystrix* DC.), is cultivated throughout South and East Asia as a food flavouring; the oil is chiefly produced in Madagascar and some Mascarene islands, where it is called Combava. Its fine green, sweet lemony odour is from its c. 42% mixed content in citrals, citronellal, monoterpenols and esters, in addition to its c. 55% monoterpenes content.

While Kaffir lime oil is cold pressed from the fruit rind, the leaf oil is also sometimes produced by steam distillation and predictably called Kaffir lime petitgrain (see Petitgrain); the main producer is Indonesia.

**Citron** (*Citrus medica* L.) is one of the four original citrus fruits from which many others are now thought to have been hybridized. Originally from Southeast Asia, and possibly Burma (Myanmar), it was extensively cultivated in the Persian Gulf about

2,500 years ago and then spread around the Mediterranean with Greek and Arabic expansion. Varieties of Citron rind are to this day an important remedy in traditional Greek, Ayurvedic and Chinese medicine (Fo shou). In cooking, the depulped fruit is widely candied and used as a confection. The fruit is also extensively used in pickles and preserves in India. Citron rind oil is usually cold-pressed and has a mild lemony fragrance; it typically contains monoterpenes (incl. d-limonene, β-pinene, γ-terpinene and α-bergamotene) and aldehydes 1–20% (geranial, neral and r-citronellal), and a small amount of coumarins.

## Therapeutic Functions and Indications

### SPECIFIC SYMPTOMATOLOGY – *All applications*

Distraction, poor focus and attention span, mental fogginess, poor judgement and critical thinking, poor foresight and planning ability, discouragement, pessimism, negative thinking, procrastination, anxiety, palpitations, insomnia, hot spells, poor appetite, chronic digestive problems worse from stress, acute joint, tendon and muscle problems

### PSYCHOLOGICAL – *Aromatic diffusion, whole-body massage*

**Essential PNEI function and indication:** Stimulant in weakness conditions

**Possible brain dynamics:** Increases prefrontal cortex functioning and SNS response

**Fragrance category:** Top tone with lemony, green notes

**Indicated psychological disorders:** ADD, depression

PROMOTES EMOTIONAL RENEWAL

- All pathogenic (unproductive, stuck) emotions and distressed feelings in general, especially from past negative experiences

PROMOTES OPTIMISM AND CLARITY

- Pessimism, negativity, discouragement, depression
- Mental fogginess, poor focus and concentration, distraction, poor short-term memory

PROMOTES GOOD JUDGEMENT, INSIGHT AND FORESIGHT

- Poor judgement with loss of insight or critical thinking
- Loss of foresight, inability to envision or plan

## PHYSIOLOGICAL – *Nebulizer inhalation, gel cap, suppository, external applications*

**Therapeutic status:** Mild remedy with no cumulative toxicity

**Topical safety status:**

- Cold-pressed Lime oil: Moderately skin irritant, sensitizing and photosensitizing

- Distilled Lime oil: Non-irritant, non-sensitizing and non-photosensitizing

**Tropism:** Nervous, digestive, urinary, respiratory systems

**Essential diagnostic function:** Relaxes hypertonic/tense and cools hypersthenic/hot terrain conditions

*strong systemic nervous and vascular relaxant, SNS inhibitor, refrigerant, antipyretic:* hypertonic/tense and hypersthenic/hot conditions, esp. with agitation, spasms, inflammation, hot spells, hot flushes, fevers; acute stress-related conditions

- *cerebral sedative, hypnotic:* agitation, anxiety, insomnia

- *cardiovascular relaxant, vasodilator, hypotensive:* cardiac arrhythmia, palpitations, precordial pain, hypertension

- *gastrointestinal relaxant, anti-inflammatory, spasmolytic:* inflammatory and spasmodic gastrointestinal conditions, incl. colic, colitis, inflammatory bowel disease, IBS

- *musculoskeletal relaxant, anti-inflammatory, spasmolytic:* inflammatory rheumatic, arthritic and tendon conditions

*gastric stimulant, aperitive:* atonic indigestion, appetite loss

*diuretic*

*anticoagulant:* hyperviscous blood, thrombosis

*antiviral:* cold, flu, sore throat

### SYNERGISTIC COMBINATIONS

- Lime + Mandarin/Bergamot: nervous and cerebral sedative for acute, moderate stress-related agitation, insomnia, anxiety, headaches

- Lime + Marjoram: strong systemic nervous relaxant and spasmolytic in all hypertonic/tense conditions with spasms and pain, of smooth and striped muscles of all body systems

- Lime + Marjoram: cerebral sedative and hypnotic for agitation, acute anxiety, insomnia

COMPLEMENTARY COMBINATIONS

- Lime + Lavender/Roman camomile: anti-inflammatory, spasmolytic and analgesic in a wide range of inflammatory and spasmodic conditions, esp. gastrointestinal, neuromuscular and uterine; incl. colitis, inflammatory bowel disease, IBS, arthritis, menstrual cramps

- Lime + Lemon eucalyptus/Lemongrass: nervous, cerebral and cardiac sedative, refrigerant, hypotensive in acute tense and hot conditions with anxiety, agitation, hot spells, hot flushes, hypertension

- Lime + Ylang ylang no. 1 or extra: neurocardiac sedative for tachycardia, severe palpitations with intense anxiety, fright

- Lime + Petitgrain bigarade + Lavender: nervous, cerebral and cardiac sedative and restorative in chronic hypertonic/tense conditions with anxiety, insomnia, palpitations, cardiac dysrhythmia; nervous exhaustion or breakdown, neurasthenia

- Lime + Wintergreen: anti-inflammatory, spasmolytic and analgesic for severe acute rheumatic, arthritic and tendon inflammation

- Lime + Lavender: anticoagulant for thrombosis

## TOPICAL – *Liniment, lotion*

See 'Pharmacological precautions' below.

**Skin care:** Oily skin type (facial steam)

*anti-inflammatory:* skin, muscle and joint inflammation

*antiviral:* warts, verrucas

**Therapeutic precautions:** Lime oil is a systemic cooling relaxant to most internal organ systems and is contraindicated in all hyposthenic/cold and hypotonic/weak conditions in general. This includes chronic poor circulation, hypotension, cardiac weakness, debility and neurasthenia with depression. It should also be used only for acute, not chronic, forms of inflammation and fever.

**Pharmacological precautions:** Exercise caution with using Lime oil topically as this oil is somewhat irritant, sensitizing and photosensitizing to the skin; this applies especially to the cold-pressed oil with its higher content in coumarins. Best results are obtained when Lime oil is used topically in combination with other oils. Lime oil is best avoided on those with sensitive or damaged skin, and the doses given should not be exceeded. Exposure to sunlight should also be avoided for at least 12 hours after any topical application because of its coumarin content.

**Preparations:**

- Diffusor: 1–3 drops in water

- Massage oil: 0.5–1% dilution in vegetable oil

- Liniment: 1–2% dilution in vegetable oil after doing a patch test for sensitivity, for short-term use only and preferably in a blend

- Gel cap: 2–3 drops with olive oil. Only small doses are needed for a gastric stimulant action.

## Chinese Medicine Functions and Indications

**Aroma energy:** Lemony, green

**Movement:** Circulating, dispersing

**Warmth:** Cool to cold

**Meridian tropism:** Heart, Liver, Large Intestine

**Five-Element affinity:** Wood, Fire

**Essential function:** To clear heat, clarify the Heart, activate the Qi and calm the Shen

1. **Clears heat, clarifies the Heart and calms the Shen**

    - **Heart fire with Shen agitation,** with agitation, talkativeness, intense emotions, insomnia, palpitations:

      Lavender/Neroli/Lemongrass

    - **Liver fire with Shen agitation,** with headache, red complexion, anger, hot spells, possible fever:

      Lemongrass/Lemon eucalyptus/Marjoram

    - **Yang ming-stage heat with Shen agitation,** with fever, anxiety, restlessness, insomnia, rapid forceful pulse:

      Lemon/Lavender/Lemon eucalyptus

2. **Activates the Qi, relaxes constraint, calms the Shen and relieves pain**

    - **Qi constraint turning into heat with Shen agitation,** with irritability, restlessness, muscle tension and pain, mood swings, emotive behaviour:

      Lavender/Petitgrain bigarade/German camomile

    - **Heart and Liver Qi constraint with Shen agitation,** with restlessness, insomnia, palpitations, irritability, mood swings, anxiety:

      Mandarin/Petitgrain bigarade/Ylang ylang no. 1/Spikenard

- **Liver-Spleen disharmony** with stress, abdominal pain, cramps, flatulence, bloating:

  Peppermint/Marjoram/Roman camomile/Lavender

3. <u>**Clears heat, drains damp and relieves pain**</u>

- **Large Intestine damp-heat** with acute painful diarrhoea, colic, tenesmus:

  May chang/Vetiver/Roman camomile/Basil ct. methylchavicol

4. <u>**Opens the meridians, dispels wind-damp-heat and relieves pain**</u>

- **Wind-damp-heat obstruction** with acute muscle and joint tension, redness, swelling and pain:

  Lemon eucalyptus/Lemongrass/Wintergreen

REMARKS

Like the grapefruit, the lime too is a tropical native to the Malyasian archipelago. As with most citrus fruits, it was Arab trade networks that first introduced the fruit westwards by sea and land to the Middle East, North Africa, Sicily and Al Andalus in early medieval centuries. In the early 16th century, Spanish explorers of the West Indies then brought the lime to the Caribbean and up to the Florida Keys, from where its cultivation eventually became worldwide. Its specific name, Key lime, is a reminder of its naturalized habitat.

With its green-lemony fragrance energy, cold-pressed Lime oil as a physical remedy joins a group of oils that excel at treating acute tense, hot terrain conditions. Lime is a good cooling relaxant despite its dominance in monoterpenes – although most of its constituents are also seen in most other oils of this type, such as Lemongrass and May chang. Clearly, quantitative dominance does not always equate with dominant physiological effect and clinical indication. Regardless, Lime's relaxant action is seen in the nervous, cardiovascular and musculoskeletal systems, where it acts as a spasmolytic to both striped and smooth muscles. It is as good a sedative heat-clearing oil as any, whether involving a hot spell, a fever, or indeed heat driven by emotional agitation – as with acute elation, anxiety, anger or fear. In small doses, Lime is an effective gastric stimulant for sluggish upper digestion with appetite loss.

When gently inhaled for olfaction, cold-pressed Lime oil is preferable, being less sharp and acidic than distilled lime oil. Its fresh, fruity green fragrance makes for a nice aromatic remedy in the context of psychological applications. In a similar way as May chang, Lime has the potential for assisting emotional transformation of stagnant feelings relating to past negative experiences. In helping resolve past issues, the oil can open one up to future potentials and true change. Lime does this by supporting additional awareness, foresight and creative envisioning.

**Related lime oils:** Based on the experience of European practitioners, the following vignettes will make useful clinical distinctions among the various lime oils, which all have mild therapeutic status.

**Lime** or **Key lime** (*Citrus x aurantifolia*) (this profile) is mainly used for its good all-round nervous sedative, spasmolytic and anti-inflammatory actions, but especially when related to the gut or the heart. In functional medicine terms, it treats hypertonic/ tense and hypersthenic/hot conditions with cerebral, cardiac or gastrointestinal symptoms. See also the precautions above relating to topical use.

**Persian lime** (*Citrus x latifolia*) is used much in the same way as Lime but is not considered spasmolytic. Exercise caution with topical use as this oil is photosensitizing because of its content in coumarins; this oil is also a moderate skin irritant and sensitizer.

**Italian lime** (*Citrus limetta*) is mainly used clinically for treating painful spasmodic conditions, especially of the gut, as in IBS, colitis and IBD; the spasmolytic action arises from its high levels of linalyl acetate, which would also support use in chronic rather than acute conditions of this kind, and when presenting fatigue and neurasthenia. Exercise caution with topical use as this oil is photosensitizing because of its high content in coumarins.

**Kaffir lime** or **Combava lime** (*Citrus hystrix*) is employed differently from the other limes, and mainly as a liver-gallbladder simulant decongestant for congestive/damp conditions of these organs, including liver congestion and biliary insufficiency with sludged bile; and as a hormonal stimulant in conditions of ovarian and testicular insufficiency with amenorrhoea, loss of libido, etc. Exercise caution with topical use as Kaffir lime is photosensitizing because of its content in coumarins; it is also a moderate skin irritant and sensitizer.

**Kaffir lime petitgrain** or **Combava lime petitgrain** (*Citrus hystrix*) is often considered the most effective nervous sedative, hypnotic, analgesic and anti-inflammatory of all lime oils because of its high citronellal levels, which compare favourably with those of Citronella and Lemon eucalyptus. Like Lime oil, Kaffir lime petitgrain will treat acute tense and hot conditions with anxiety, agitation and insomnia. Like other oils high in terpenic aldehydes, moreover, it exerts a good tropism for the joints, resulting in an excellent remedy for acute, painful arthritic conditions by both topical and internal use. Exercise caution with topical use, however, as this oil is a moderate skin irritant and sensitizer, and is therefore best combined with other oils.

**Citron** (*Citrus medica*) is a refrigerant nervous sedative with mild hypnotic and spasmolytic actions and, like the Lime oils, will treat acute tense and hot conditions. Citron is also highly valued for its bitter-like gastric stimulant effect. Aperitive and carminative, it will treat upper indigestion with bloating and appetite loss, especially when related to emotional stress. Citron also has a useful wide-spectrum antibacterial action. Sun exposure should be avoided for up to 12 hours after topical use because of its coumarin content that creates photosensitization.

# Melissa

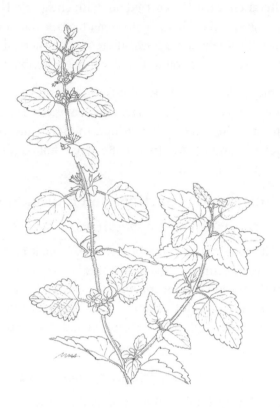

**Botanical source:** The herb of *Melissa officinalis* L. (Lamiaceae/Labiatae – lipflower/
mint family), a widespread Mediterranean and temperate herb

**Other names:** Lemon balm; Mélisse (Fr), Melisse (Ge), Melissa (It), Melisa (Sp)

**Appearance:** A clear or pale yellow mobile liquid with a citrus-sweet, herbaceous
green odour

**Perfumery status:** A head note of high intensity and medium persistence

**Extraction:** Steam distillation of the leafy herbs in the summer months

**1 kg yield from:** 6,000–7,000 kg (an extremely low yield)

**Production areas:** Bulgaria, France, USA, South Africa

**Typical constituents:** Monoterpenoid aldehydes, incl. citral 62–72% (incl. geranial 20–
37%, neral 22–35%, citronellal <10%) • Sesquiterpenes 14–17% (incl. β-caryophyllene
<18%, α-copaene <5%, germacrene D <4%, γ-cadinene, α-humulene) • ketones 5% (incl.
6-methyl-6-hepten-2-one 4%, 3-octane) • monoterpenols <5% (incl. linalool, nerol,

geraniol, citronellol, α-terpineol, terpinene-4-ol) • oxides <4% (incl. caryophyllene <4%, 1,8 cineole) • esters (geranyl/neryl/citronellyl acetate) • coumarin aesculetine

**Chance of adulteration:** Very high because of the extremely low yield and high market value. Classic adulteration is usually carried out with cheaper oils high in citral, such as Citronella, Lemongrass, May chang, Citronella tea tree, Lemon tea tree and even Lemon verbena, or with aldehyde fractions thereof. Commercial Melissa oil is up to 100% synthesized, with numerous natural and synthetic combinations possible.

**Related oils:** Botanical relatives include all oils in the large lipflower or mint family. However, Melissa is unique in its pharmacology, energetic fragrance qualities and therapeutic profile. It is the only lipflower high in aldehydes, possessing a green-lemony fragrance quality and used to treat acute, tense, hot conditions.

## Therapeutic Functions and Indications

### SPECIFIC SYMPTOMATOLOGY – *All applications*

Distraction, difficulty focusing, irritability, poor judgement and insight, depression with agitation, negative thinking, discouragement, pessimism, despair, anxiety, palpitations, insomnia, hot spells, poor appetite, chronic digestive problems worse from stress, malaise, low energy and motivation in the morning, acute allergic conditions, acute and chronic headaches, painful joint, tendon and muscle problems

### PSYCHOLOGICAL – *Aromatic diffusion, whole-body massage*

**Essential PNEI function and indication:** Stimulant in weakness conditions

**Possible brain dynamics:** Increases prefrontal cortex functioning

**Fragrance category:** Top tone with lemony, green notes

**Indicated psychological disorders:** ADD, depression

#### PROMOTES EMOTIONAL RENEWAL

- All pathogenic (unproductive, stuck) emotions and distressed feelings in general, especially from past negative experiences

#### PROMOTES OPTIMISM AND CLARITY

- Pessimism, negativity, discouragement, depression

- Mental fog, poor focus and concentration, distraction, poor short-term memory

PROMOTES GOOD JUDGEMENT, INSIGHT AND FORESIGHT

- Poor judgement or evaluation with loss of insight or critical thinking
- Loss of foresight, inability to envision or plan

## PHYSIOLOGICAL – *Nebulizer inhalation, gel cap, suppository, external applications*

**Therapeutic status:** Mild remedy with no cumulative toxicity

**Topical safety status:** Somewhat skin irritant, possibly sensitizing

**Tropism:** Nervous, cardiovascular, hepatobiliary, gastrointestinal systems

**Essential diagnostic function:** Relaxes hypertonic/tense conditions and cools hypersthenic/hot terrain conditions

PRIMARILY RELAXANT AND COOLING:

*strong systemic nervous and vascular relaxant, SNS inhibitor, vagotonic, refrigerant, antipyretic:* hypertonic/tense and hypersthenic/hot conditions, esp. with severe nervous tension, spasms, inflammation, hot spells, hot flushes, fevers; acute stress-related conditions in general

*strong spasmolytic and anti-inflammatory, analgesic:* a large range of acute spasmodic and inflammatory conditions of all types, esp. of smooth muscles; incl. tension and vascular headaches

- *strong cerebral sedative, hypnotic:* anxiety, agitation, insomnia, agitated or nervous depression, mania, psychosis, phobia, vertigo

- *strong cardiovascular relaxant, vasodilator, hypotensive, analgesic:* palpitations, tachycardia, arrhythmia, precordial pain, neurogenic angina; migraine headache, hypertension

- *muscle relaxant, spasmolytic, anti-inflammatory, analgesic:* muscle and sinew tension, spasm and pain; acute arthritic, rheumatic and tendon inflammation and pain; tendinitis, headache

- *gastrointestinal relaxant, spasmolytic, anti-inflammatory, carminative:* nervous indigestion, stomach cramps, colitis, inflammatory bowel disease, IBS

- *respiratory relaxant, broncho-spasmolytic/-dilator, antitussive:* asthma (all types), all spasmodic and nervous dyspnoea and coughs, spasmodic dysphonia, viral croup

- *uterine relaxant:* spasmodic dysmenorrhoea, severe cramps

- *urinary relaxant:* strangury, neurogenic bladder with spasmodic dysuria

- *anti-inflammatory, antiallergic, antipruritic:* type-I allergies, esp. acute dermatitis with itching, atopic asthma, colitis, cholecystitis, duodenitis, gastritis, cystitis

- *pituitary and thyroidal inhibitor:* hyperthyroid syndrome

PRIMARILY DECONGESTANT:

*strong hepatobiliary decongestant, cholagogue, choleretic, antilithic:* liver congestion with biliary insufficiency, gastric indigestion with bloating; sludged bile, bile stones

*antiemetic:* acute nausea, morning sickness

*antioxidant, antitumoural:* cancer (prevention and treatment)

ANTIMICROBIAL ACTIONS:

*antiviral:* HSV-1 (Herpes simplex) with cold sores; influenza, mumps, croup

*antifungal:* fungal infections

SYNERGISTIC COMBINATIONS

- Melissa + Lemongrass/May chang: strong systemic nervous relaxant, refrigerant, spasmolytic, anti-inflammatory and analgesic in all tense-hot conditions with smooth and striped muscle spasms, inflammation, pain, fever

- Melissa + Lemon eucalyptus: strong refrigerant, antipyretic in all acute hot spells, hot flushes and fevers

- Melissa + Lemon eucalyptus: strong nervous and cerebral sedative, hypnotic in acute agitation, anxiety, mania

COMPLEMENTARY COMBINATIONS

- Melissa + Marjoram: strong systemic nervous relaxant, cerebral sedative and hypnotic in all acute hypertonic/tense conditions with severe nervous tension, anxiety, agitation, nervous breakdown

- Melissa + Roman camomile/Basil ct. methylchavicol: strong systemic smooth-muscle relaxant and spasmolytic in a wide range of spasmodic conditions of all smooth-muscle organs, respiratory, digestive, urinary and reproductive

- Melissa + Ylang ylang no. 1/Tarragon: strong cardiovascular relaxant and cerebral sedative for severe tachycardia, neurogenic angina, hypertension, migraine, anxiety, insomnia

- Melissa + Tea tree/Yarrow: strong anti-inflammatory and antiallergic in type-I allergies, incl. pruritic dermatitis, gastritis, colitis, cystitis, cholecystitis

- Melissa + Lemon: hepatobiliary decongestant and antilithic for liver congestion with biliary insufficiency, sludged bile, bile stones

- Melissa + Frankincense: antitumoural in cancerous conditions in general

## TOPICAL – *Liniment, lotion*

See 'Pharmacological precautions' below.

**Skin care:** Oily skin type

*antioxidant:* acne, oily skin

*anti-inflammatory, antiallergic, antipruritic:* skin rashes, eczema, itching

*vasodilator:* broken capillaries

**Therapeutic precautions:** Melissa oil is a strong systemic cooling relaxant to most internal organ systems and is contraindicated in all hyposthenic/cold and hypotonic/weak conditions in general. This includes chronic poor circulation, hypotension, cardiac weakness, debility and neurasthenia with depression. Unlike the whole herb, e.g. in tincture form, Melissa oil should only be used for agitated or nervous depression, i.e. depression in the context of tension and heat, not for other types of depression seen in weak or cold conditions.

This oil should also be used only for acute, not chronic, forms of inflammation and fever, and is best avoided in hypothyroid syndrome because of its antithyroidal action.

**Pharmacological precautions:** As it is a moderate skin irritant, Melissa should not be used on damaged or sensitive skin. Although it may be used for inflammatory skin conditions, sensitization may occur in some individuals and a patch test should be done in all cases. In the case of adulterated Melissa oil (see above), the chance of skin irritation and sensitization is increased. To prevent possible skin irritation, it is best combined with oils high in monoterpenols, such as Geranium, Palmarosa or Thyme ct. linalool.

Melissa is also generally contraindicated during pregnancy as a teratogenic potential exists, depending on how much oil is absorbed. Internal use should be avoided with those on diabetic medication.

**Preparations:**

- Diffusor: 2–3 drops in water
- Massage oil: 0.5–1% dilution in vegetable oil, preferably in a blend
- Liniment: 1–1.5% dilution in vegetable oil, preferably in a blend, for short-term use
- Gel cap: 1–2 drops with olive oil

## Chinese Medicine Functions and Indications

**Aroma energy:** Lemony, green

**Movement:** Circulating, dispersing

**Warmth:** Cool to cold

**Meridian tropism:** Heart, Liver, Lung

**Five-Element affinity:** Wood, Fire, Metal

**Essential function:** To clear heat, clarify the Heart, activate the Qi and calm the Shen

1. <u>**Clears heat, clarifies the Heart and calms the Shen**</u>

   - **Heart Yin deficiency/Heart fire with Shen agitation**, with anxiety, overstimulation, agitation, insomnia, palpitations, hot spells:
   
     Lemon eucalyptus/May chang/Lime/Spikenard

   - **Shao yang-stage heat with Shen agitation**, with alternating fever and chills:
   
     Basil ct. methylchavicol/Blue-gum eucalyptus/Ylang ylang no. 1

   - **Yang ming-stage heat with Shen agitation**, with fever, anxiety, restlessness, insomnia, rapid forceful pulse:
   
     Lavender/Lemon eucalyptus/Lemongrass

2. <u>**Activates the Qi, relaxes constraint, calms the Shen and relieves pain**</u>

   - **Qi constraint turning into heat with Shen agitation**, with tension, irritability, restlessness, muscle tension, mood swings, emotive behaviour:
   
     Petitgrain bigarade/German camomile/Blue tansy/Ylang ylang no. 1

   - **Liver and Heart Qi constraint with Shen agitation**, with tension, palpitations, chest pains, anxiety, irritability, mood swings, insomnia:
   
     Mandarin/German camomile/Ylang ylang no. 1

   - **Liver-Stomach/Spleen disharmony** with stress, abdominal pain, cramps, flatulence, bloating:
   
     Fennel/Peppermint/Roman camomile

- **Bladder Qi constraint** with irritated, difficult, painful, dripping urination:
  Fennel/Carrot seed/Cypress

- **Liver and Uterus Qi constraint** with severe menstrual cramps, anxiety, irritability, PMS:
  Lavender/Marjoram/Ylang ylang no. 1

3. **Circulates and descends Lung Qi, and relieves wheezing and coughing**

- **Lung Qi accumulation** with wheeze, cough, chest distension or pain:
  Basil ct. chavicol/Siberian fir/Fennel/Cypress

- **Cough in all Lung heat and wind-heat syndromes**:
  Hyssop

4. **Clears heat and drains damp, and relieves pain**

- **Large Intestine damp-heat** with acute painful diarrhoea, colic, tenesmus:
  May chang/Lemongrass/Marjoram

5. **Dispels wind-damp-heat from the skin and meridians, and relieves pain**

- **Wind-damp-heat in the skin** with red, itchy, painful eruptions:
  Lavender/German camomile/Lemon eucalyptus

- **Wind-damp-heat obstruction** with red, swollen painful joints, rheumatic pains:
  Vetiver/Wintergreen/Lemon eucalyptus

REMARKS

The use of Melissa essential oil puts the modern practitioner in a unique predicament. Firstly, there is the challenge of obtaining the genuine and unadulterated oil, as Melissa is the most adulterated and chemically redesigned oil on the market, along with Rose oil. It probably always was. Gildemeister (1899) in the early days of synthetic perfumery already noted that commercial Melissa oil was always a co-distillation of lemon rind and melissa herb, as pure Melissa oil would otherwise have been too expensive – a classic example of good old-fashioned classic adulteration. Then there is Melissa's prohibitive cost, due to the plant's extremely low yield of oil. It could logically be argued that there are several other oils that among them would quite adequately cover all of Melissa's functions and uses. Certainly, there is no denying this: on paper there is nothing that Melissa does that other oils cannot do.

And last but not least is the sheer weight of Melissa's hoary legacy as a premier remedy for the heart and for promoting longevity in Western herbal medicine. The herb is already mentioned in Theophrastus of Ephesus' *Historia Plantarum* of 300 BC, and Melissa aromatic water is known to have been prepared since earliest days. Around the year 1100 saw Hildegard of Bingen growing the plant in her physick garden and distilling its water. The alchemist Paracelsus in the 16th century based his elixir of longevity on Melissa; this was probably an alchemical combination of the alcohol and essential oil extract of the herbs in his formula. By that time, the simple Melissa water itself had become extremely popular and was widely produced both in pharmacies and domiciles throughout Europe.

The original Eau des Carmes, or Carmelite Water, first appeared in 1374 France in the hands of the Carmelite monks of Saint-Juste monastery. Its main ingredient Melissa was co-distilled with various other herbs, typically lemon rind, clove, nutmeg, coriander, cinnamon and angelica root; these were all first infused in spring water and then co-distilled with white wine and wine spirit. This compound Melissa remedy was known as the original 'cordial' or remedy for the heart (*cor* is Latin for 'heart'). It soon became desirable as an any-time aromatic pick-me-up and eventually even doubled as a perfume for its refreshing, uplifting scent. The Eau de Melisse des Carmes was later adopted by official pharmacopeias in various countries and renamed Spiritus Melissae Compositus. The history of the commercialization and numerous renaming of this formula is more complicated and duplicitous than even that of Eau de Cologne.

Melissa oil itself is first on record as having been produced in 1550 by apothecaries in Frankfurt. It was only in the 20th century that Melissa oil reinvented itself as a serious clinical remedy among French practitioners. The problem now for the practitioner is precisely the remedy's thick patina of historical uses: how relevant are they today for the clinical use of the pure essential oil?

And yet, despite these challenges to its use, Melissa the internal remedy continues to hold its place securely in the materia aromatica, especially among European practitioners. The focus of its relaxant/sedative physiological actions is the nervous, cerebral and cardiovascular systems. Acute anxiety, severe insomnia, agitation, agitated depression, mania and other psychiatric states, tachycardia and migraines are just some of its asterisk indications. Note that, unlike the tincture, Melissa oil is not a cerebral restorative for neurasthenia, chronic depression, etc. Melissa is a wide-ranging relaxant remedy with excellent spasmolytic, anti-inflammatory and analgesic actions that include both smooth and striped muscles. Its essential indication is acute tense and hot conditions, and as such is less often given as a more long-term remedy for rebalancing the terrain. Melissa also notably exerts a powerful choleretic and cholagogue action on the gallbladder. For herpes and other viruses, the oil has also shown an excellent antiviral action.

Perhaps the key to unravelling the allure of Melissa is a new appreciation of its fragrance. It shows an intense yet seamless mix of high-intensity sweet-herbaceous notes with a lemony twist that translate as stimulating and clarifying on the emotional level especially. Certainly, its historical use as an internal remedy and aromatic perfume rolled into one, as a supreme cordial or heart remedy, shows respect for more than just its physiological actions on the heart and spirit. It also respects its profound olfactory impact.

As an olfactory remedy in the context of psychological applications, Melissa potentially assists the transformation of stagnant feelings and emotions, especially when these involve pessimism and loss of hope. Melissa is for loss of heart courage, for discouragement from past emotional setback and betrayal, often resulting in long-term emotional isolation with excessive introversion. By providing emotional clarity, this oil can help resolve and uplift chronic negativity and disorientation. Dupont (2002) insightfully adds that 'Elle favorise le sens discriminatif en relation avec le moi profond…et évite à sombrer dans l'indifférence, la tristesse et la dépression' – 'Melissa favours the discriminative faculty as regards the inner self…preventing one from sinking into indifference, sorrow and depression.' Interestingly, he attributes this syndrome to a malfunctioning of the pineal gland.

# Myrrh

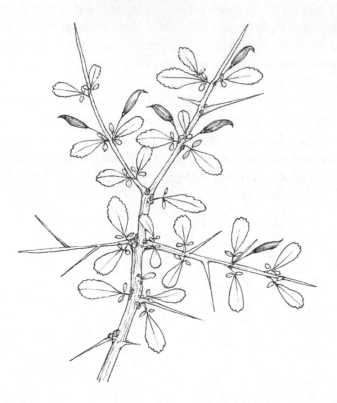

**Botanical source:** The resin of *Commiphora myrrha* (Nees) Engler (syn. *Commiphora molmol* Engler) (Burseraceae – torchwood or incense-tree family), a hardy tree of the East African and Saudi Arabian deserts

**Other names:** Somali/African myrrh, Hirabol myrrh; Myrrhe douce (Fr), Myrrhe (Ge), Molmol (Somali), Murr (Ar), Mirra (It, Sp), Mo yao (Mandarin)

**Appearance:** An extremely viscous, pale yellow to amber liquid with a deep, warm, balsamic, woody and slightly fresh-spicy odour

**Perfumery status:** A base note of medium intensity and excellent persistence

**Extraction:** Steam distillation of the ruddy-brown resin or 'tears' that form naturally or that result from incisions made on the tree trunk. Freshly broken fragments of high-quality resin are always sticky and are said to yield the most essential oil. Very often the first distillation water is redistilled with hexane and the resultant oil added to the steam-distilled oil. An absolute or resinoid is also extracted from myrrh resin by solvent extraction.

**1 kg oil yield from:** 12–15 kg of the resin (an excellent yield)

**Production areas:** Somalia, Ethiopia, North Kenya, Yemen, Oman. Myrrh is native to both East Africa and the Arabian peninsula.

**Typical constituents:** Sesquiterpenes <70% (incl. δ-elemene 28%, α-copaene 11%, β-elemene 7%, α-bergamotene 5%, bourbonene 4%, lindestrene 4–12%, muurolene, cadinene, curzerene, heerabolene, α-caryophyllene) • monoterpenes <48% (incl. furanoeudesma-1,3-diene 13–34%, furanodiene 19%, cis-ocimene 2%, p-cymene, trans-ocimene, α-thujene, myrcene, limonene, dipentene, pinene) • ketones (incl. curzerenone 12%, methylisobutyl ketone 6%, 3 meth-oxy-10-dihydrofuranodien-6-one 1.5%, 1,10 furanodiene-6-one 1%, dihydropyrocurzerenone 1%, 3 meth-oxy-10-methylenefuranogermacra-1-en-6-one 1%, furanodiene-6-one, 6-methyl-5-hepten-2-one) • aldehydes (incl. 5-methylfurfural 1.7%, furfural 1.5%, benzaldehyde, cinnamaldehyde, cuminaldehyde) • phenols eugenol and m-cresol • misc. other constituents

**Chance of adulteration:** Very high. True Myrrh oil is very often either stretched with other species of myrrh of inferior odour qualities, e.g. with *Commiphora agallocha, C. stocksiana, C. roxburghii* or with other species such as the ones listed below. Worse, Myrrh oil is often distilled or extracted from any number of different *Commiphora* species in the c. 150 species-rich genus: in the areas of collection, unfortunately most species are usually all considered to be fair sources of myrrh without discrimination and are wrongly assumed to possess similar if not identical properties and uses to Myrrh. Adulteration and botanical misidentification then may both contribute to an oil of somewhat variable constituents and unreliable therapeutic actions.

Myrrh absolute (resinoid) is sometimes used as starting material for the oil, which is decolourized and solvent-diluted, and then sold as the essential oil (Lis-Balchin 2006).

**Related oils:** In addition to the inferior types of myrrh above, other types of myrrh often extracted from the prolific *Commiphora* genus include the following.

- Yemen/Arabian/Abyssinian myrrh (*C. habessinica* [O. Berg] Engl.) from Northeast Africa and the Arabian peninsula

- Balsam of Mecca or Balsam of Gilead (*C. gileadensis* C. Chr., syn. *C. opobalsamum*)

- Bisabol myrrh or Opopanax (*Opopanax guidotti* Chiov.) from Iran, west through Somalia, available in both resinoid form by solvent extraction, and in essential oil form by steam distillation. *Bissa bol* in Hindi means 'scented myrrh', in contrast to *heera bol*, 'bitter myrrh'.

- East Indian myrrh (*C. erythraea*), the original source of Opopanax resin for the perfume industry until the 1950s

- African opopanax (*Commiphora kataf* [Forssk.] Engler)

- Guggul or Mukul myrrh (*C. wightii* [Arn.] Bhandari) from North India and Central Africa. This resin is a traditional Ayurvedic remedy, whose tree is now officially listed as an endangered species.

Bdellium is the semi-transparent resin extracted from *Commiphora roxburgii* and *C. africana*. Bdellium was burnt for its incense by ancient cultures, especially by Bactrians in Central Asia and Nubians in present-day Somalia.

The fragrant potherb cicely or sweet cicely, *Myrrhis odorata*, is also known as myrrh, but bears no botanical relation; a distilled oil is not available.

## Therapeutic Functions and Indications

### SPECIFIC SYMPTOMATOLOGY – *All applications*

Insecurity, vulnerability, loss of safety, emotional and psychic burnout, spaciness, euphoria, delusions, worry, obsession, fearfulness, anxiety, cold hands and feet, chest congestion, difficult or copious expectoration of foetid sputum, painful cough, wheezing, chronic loose mucousy stool, indigestion, abdominal pain and bloating, chronic vaginal and urinary discharges, cloudy or mucousy urine, urinary dribbling, painful scanty or stopped periods

### PSYCHOLOGICAL – *Aromatic diffusion, whole-body massage*

**Essential PNEI function and indication:** Relaxant in overstimulation conditions
**Possible brain dynamics:** Reduces basal ganglia and cingulate system hyperfunctioning
**Fragrance category:** Base tone with woody note
**Indicated psychological disorders:** ADHD, dissociative disorder

#### STABILIZES THE MIND AND PROMOTES INTEGRATION

- Dissociation, scatteredness, spaciness, oversensitivity

- Euphoria, delusion, paranoia, agitation

#### PROMOTES STABILITY AND STRENGTH

- Emotional instability with anxiety, fearfulness

- Insecurity, vulnerability, burnout

- Disowning, disempowerment

PROMOTES COGNITIVE FLEXIBILITY

- Worry, obsession, compulsivity

- Repetitive thinking, inability to let go

PHYSIOLOGICAL – *Intense inhalation, gel cap, suppository, external applications*

**Therapeutic status:** Mild remedy with no cumulative toxicity

**Topical safety status:** Non-irritant, moderately sensitizing

**Tropism:** Reproductive, urinary, digestive, respiratory, cardiovascular, nervous systems

**Essential diagnostic function:** Restores hypotonic/weak conditions and dries congestive/damp terrain conditions

PRIMARILY RESTORATIVE AND DECONGESTANT:

*strong astringent mucosal restorative and decongestant, mucostatic, antiseptic, mild spasmolytic:* chronic and acute mucous membrane weakness with mucus congestion, overproduction and discharges, simple or infectious; esp. respiratory, gastrointestinal, genital and urinary, incl.:

- – bronchitis with foetid sputum

- – diarrhoea, mucousy stool, colic; chronic gastroenteritis, gastric and peptic ulcers, dysentery, mucous colitis-type IBS

- – vaginitis with leucorrhoea; gonorrhoea, urethritis with gleet, blennorrhoea, spermatorrhoea, prostatitis, seminal emissions

- – mucous cystitis, blennuria

*gastrointestinal restorative and detoxicant, anti-inflammatory, antiallergic, tissue-regenerative:* intestinal dysbiosis and hyperpermeability with food allergies/sensitivities, allergic colitis/gastritis/duodenitis, microbial toxicosis

*cardiac restorative:* heart weakness

*antisclerotic:* arteriosclerosis

PRIMARILY STIMULANT:

*stimulant expectorant, mucolytic, anti-inflammatory, antiseptic:* congestive catarrhal respiratory conditions, esp. chronic; incl. chronic bronchitis with copious sputum, congestive dyspnoea, painful cough with sputum *arterial circulatory stimulant:* poor circulation with cold, chills

*uterine stimulant/emmenagogue:* atonic amenorrhoea, oligomenorrhoea, dysmenorrhoea

*oxytocic parturient, analgesic:* painful, difficult labour (hypotonic uterine dystocia), failure to progress, retained placenta

*immunostimulant, leukocytogenic:* misc. infections (see below)

PRIMARILY CALMING:

*anti-inflammatory, analgesic:* a wide range of acute and chronic inflammatory conditions with pain:

- hyperhistamine syndrome

- gastrointestinal: gastritis, enteritis (incl. allergic type)

- respiratory: bronchitis, atopic asthma

- throat and mouth: laryngitis, stomatitis, tonsillitis; voice loss, sore throat, hoarseness, aphonia

- reproductive and urinary: vaginitis, cervicitis, prostatitis (incl. allergic type), cystitis (incl. allergic type)

- musculoskeletal: arthritis

*antipyretic:* fevers, esp. intermittent fever

*mild nervous sedative:* mild anxiety, insomnia, mental hyperactivity, ADHD, PMS

*sexual sedative, anaphrodisiac:* sexual overstimulation (nymphomania, satyriasis), premature ejaculation

*thyroid/thyroxine inhibitor:* hyperthyroid syndrome

*antioxidant*

*antitumoural(?), anticancer(?)*

ANTIMICROBIAL ACTIONS:

*anti-infectious, immunostimulant, anti-inflammatory:*

- *antibacterial:* bacterial infections, esp. with Staph. aureus, E. coli and other gram-positive bacteria; esp. with chronic inflammation, sepsis or putrefaction; esp. respiratory, urinary, gastrointestinal, dermal; incl. bronchitis, common cold, intestinal dysbiosis, gastroenteritis, periodontitis, stomatitis, vaginitis

- *antifungal:* common fungal infections, incl. with Candida albicans, incl. intestinal dysbiosis, thrush, athlete's foot, ringworm/tinea, intestinal dysbiosis, candidiasis, lung TB

- *antiviral:* misc. viral infections

- *antiparasitic, insecticidal:* intestinal parasites, incl. Schistosoma mansoni in schistosomiasis; fascioliasis; fowl tic, mosquito larvae

SYNERGISTIC COMBINATIONS

- Myrrh + Patchouli/Yarrow: mucostatic, antibacterial, anti-inflammatory and tissue-regenerative for chronic intestinal dysbiosis and hyperpermeability with food sensitivities, or chronic gastroenteritis; with diarrhoea, mucousy stool, mucous colitis

- Myrrh + Atlas cedarwood/Sandalwood: strong mucostatic mucosal restorative for chronic discharges of most kinds, incl. leucorrhoea, blennorrhoea, mucous cystitis, mucus in stool, gonorrhoea, spermatorrhoea

COMPLEMENTARY COMBINATIONS

- Myrrh + Geranium/Green myrtle: mucostatic astringent for chronic leucorrhoea, vaginitis, blennuria

- Myrrh + Green myrtle: strong mucostatic mucosal restorative for chronic gastroenteritis, mucous colitis, chronic hyperpermeability, diarrhoea

- Myrrh + Tea tree: antifungal, antibacterial in a variety of chronic gastrointestinal infections, incl. intestinal dysbiosis and hyperpermeability

- Myrrh + Palmarosa: cardiac restorative for chronic heart weakness

- Myrrh + Cypress: antitussive, expectorant for chronic painful, difficult cough and dyspnoea

- Myrrh + Spearmint/Green myrtle: antiseptic mucolytic expectorant for chronic bronchitis with painful, difficult productive cough and congestive dyspnoea

- Myrrh + Roman camomile/Geranium: strong vulnerary and antiseptic for tissue injuries of all kinds (also topically)

- Myrrh + Sage: astringent, anti-inflammatory, antiseptic, analgesic for gum/periodontal disease, spongy gums, mouth and throat ulcers, sore throat, hoarseness (gargle)

TOPICAL – *Liniment, ointment, cream, compress and other cosmetic preparations*

**Skin care:** Mixed and mature skin type; also for wrinkles, scars

*astringent, antiseptic:* gum/periodontal disease, spongy gums with loose teeth, haemorrhoids, rectal prolapse

*vulnerary, astringent, skin regenerator, analgesic, antiseptic:* wounds, abrasions, sores, aphthous ulcers (incl. mouth ulcers), abscesses, cracks, fissures, scars; esp. with pain, swelling, purulence/putrefaction/gangrene

*anticontusion, detumescent:* contusions

*anti-inflammatory:* weeping eczema, dermatitis, gingivitis, psoriasis, boils, carbuncles, pruritus

**Therapeutic precautions:** Myrrh oil is a dry astringent and is contraindicated in all types of dry conditions, especially dry respiratory conditions with dry, unproductive cough and dry form of constipation. It is also contraindicated during pregnancy and breastfeeding, and with menorrhagia present as it is a uterine stimulant and possibly teratogenic.

**Pharmacological precautions:** Topical applications of Myrrh singly should be short term, as the oil and the resin are both somewhat cumulatively sensitizing to the skin (Anderson *et al.* 2000). Myrrh should therefore always be combined with other oils when used topically.

**Preparations:**

- Diffusor: 3–4 drops in water
- Massage oil: 2–4% dilution in vegetable oil
- Liniment: 5–10% dilution in a vegetable oil
- Mouthwashes, gargles, syrups, gum rub: 2–3 drops in water
- Vaginal sponge: 1.5% dilution in vegetable oil
- Gel cap: 1–2 drops with olive oil

## Chinese Medicine Functions and Indications

**Aroma energy:** Woody, pungent
**Movement:** Stabilizing
**Warmth:** Neutral to warm

**Meridian tropism:** Lung, Spleen, Large Intestine, Kidney, Bladder, Triple Heater

**Five-Element affinity:** Water, Earth, Metal

**Essential function:** To astringe fluids, resolve damp and stop leakage and discharge

1. **Astringes the Lung, resolves and expels phlegm, dries damp and relieves coughing**

   - **Lung phlegm-damp** with difficult expectoration of copious sputum, difficult or painful cough, chest congestion with pain, fatigue:

     Cypress/Siberian fir/Hyssop/Spearmint

2. **Braces the Kidney and resolves damp; astringes fluids, secures sperm, and stops leakage and discharge**

   - **Kidney-Bladder Qi deficiency with Lower Warmer turbid-damp**, with chronic vaginal or urinary discharges, cloudy or mucousy urine, urinary dribbling, dysmenorrhoea:

     Atlas cedarwood/Geranium/Green myrtle/Niaouli

   - **Kidney Qi deficiency** with seminal emissions, spermatorrhoea:

     Cypress/Niaouli/Sandalwood

   - **Large Intestine damp-cold** with chronic mucousy diarrhoea, indigestion, weakness:

     Black pepper/Nutmeg/Black spruce

3. **Strengthens the Spleen, resolves toxic-damp and stops discharge**

   - **Spleen Qi deficiency with toxic-damp**, with indigestion, loose stool, abdominal bloating and flatulence, appetite loss, fatigue:

     Green myrtle/Niaouli/Cardamom

4. **Activates the Lower Warmer, reduces stagnation and promotes menstruation**

   - **Lower Warmer Blood and Qi stagnation with damp**, with scanty or stopped periods, painful periods, vaginal discharges:

     Juniper berry/Rosemary/Ginger

REMARKS

Myrrh trees and shrubs are native to the desert Red Sea basin that includes Somalia, Djibouti, East Ethiopia, and Oman and Yemen in the Arabian Peninsula. In this harsh, ultra-dry climate they secrete the valuable resin that native peoples have been collecting from the tree trunk since prehistory. The tree was first described by a Western traveller in 1822 in the Tehama region of Oman; tehama means 'hell', in reference to the extreme harshness of this region. Myrrh's name derives from the Greek *Myrra*, originally *Mor* in Somali and Arabic. An old Greek myth tells the story of the princess Myrra who was seen to rival Aphrodite in her beauty: forced to flee south to the barren land of Saba, she was turned into a myrrh tree and wept tears of resin from grief.

It would be hard to overestimate the esteem in which myrrh was held in the ancient world. Successive cultures from Sumeria, Assyria, Babylon and Egypt to the Hebraic Levant prized myrrh as one of the three sacred aromatics, alongside spikenard and frankincense. Above all, myrrh was the premier sacred incense. It was used variously by censing, burning or anointing for purification, protection and contemplation, and served to stage sacred space for numerous ceremonies. At the same time, its sobering, widely recognizable odour also served to create a unified smellscape for important social events. Myrrh's trade value was often higher than its weight in gold. Ancient Egyptians traded gemstones for this resin, which they considered a powerful stone, importing huge quantities of it as far back as 3000 BC. Their sacred incense Kyphi contained myrrh, of course. We can now appreciate the high value and spiritual potency of myrrh as one of the three gifts of the Magi to the newborn Jesus.

In Hebraic culture of the Levant, myrrh became the main ingredient of the Holy Anointing Oil of the Torah and Old Testament, as well as the incense Ketoret of the Temple. Here it was combined with frankincense, according to tradition. The Orthodox Christian Church carried on this tradition of anointing with chrism or Holy Oil for performing the sacraments of unction and chrismation with myrrh as the chief ingredient; to this day the anointing ceremony is called 'receiving the myrrh'. In the Roman Catholic Church, myrrh and frankincense are also standard incense aromatics for liturgical celebrations of most kinds, including morning matins and evening vespers. But Christianity originally developed a deep symbology around these ancient aromatics that, by the early Middle Ages, became a part of popular culture. Long associated with the sacrifice and embalming of Christ, and with doing penance, Myrrh became the emblem of the preservation of the flesh and the purifying power of incense. In counterpoint, Frankincense was associated with Christ's Epiphany and so represented the transcendence of the body and its ability to commune with divinity (Dugan 2011).

In most ancient cultures, the resin was an equally important ingredient in perfume making. Women herbalist-perfumers working in a royal palace or as a guild were usually in charge of preparing sacred incense and secular perfume. They routinely used myrrh in their formulations, alongside a large range of other natural ingredients prepared as vegetable oil infusion, aromatic water and high-alcohol wine. No incense or perfume was without it.

Finally, Myrrh also played a significant role as medicine. Early Sumerian inscriptions describe its use for treating intestinal worms and topically teeth and gum problems. The famous Egyptian Ebers papyrus of about 1500 BC describes the use of Myrrh and Frankincense resin for treating wounds and skin sores, as well as for preparing an embalming ointment for the mummification process itself. The Greek doctor Dioscorides in his herbal manual prescribes Myrrh for coughs, and for infections of the eyes, teeth and mouth. In Rome, where the resin commanded five times the price of frankincense, Mendesium was a popular, fragrant liniment for relief of muscle aches, and Murra, a myrrh-based perfume equally valued, apparently, as a hair tonic and skin cleanser. Most aromatic preparations in those days (and right up to the 19th century) actually did double duty for both life enhancement – usually as a perfume – and for hygiene and treatment of particular complaints. After the invention of spirit alcohol, Myrrh soon became a herbal medicine staple as a strong antiseptic astringent and stimulant expectorant.

The modern use of Myrrh in essential oil form upholds and refines its traditional use as an outstanding topical and internal remedy. Whether used topically or internally, Myrrh is one of the finest astringents for weak, loose or boggy tissues, with a robust ability to create and preserve physiological form and structure through the skin and mucosa. Myrrh is a prime choice for topical conditions when reduction of inflammation and relief of pain and swelling are also required. The archetypal image of Myrrh, like that of the other resins Mastic and Cistus, is that of a healing, strengthening, protecting bandage – the same functions performed by the resinous tears when the tree bark is cracked. Myrrh's traditional use for mouth, gum and throat problems is clearly vindicated. These actions in concert also make Myrrh a foremost vulnerary for tissue injury of any kind, with the big advantage of being able to prevent or treat any possible infection. Myrrh clearly belongs to the group of premier topical and first-aid oils of the materia aromatica, alongside the likes of Geranium, Lavender and Helichrysum.

Myrrh as an internal remedy impacts the mucous membrane especially. Strongly astringent, restorative, calming and mucostatic to this internal skin, it excels in cases of chronic mucus overproduction with discharges – a sign of chronically weak and damp terrain. Genital, urinary and intestinal discharges, whether from infection or not, are its prime indications. In the gut, Myrrh displays expanded uses as a good astringent, tissue-healing and anti-inflammatory agent for spongy, leaky, inflammatory conditions, including those of allergic origin. Conditions involving microfloral dysbiosis and microbial toxicosis will also benefit from the resin's considerable antimicrobial action. Myrrh's rich, predominantly Yin, cooling constituents may be seen to be instrumental here.

Although primarily with a 'heavy' tropism for the organs below the diphragm, Myrrh nevertheless has just enough pungent monoterpenes to make for a good stimulant expectorant for bronchial congestion. With its predictable mucosal restorative effect, Myrrh is specifically mucolytic for excessive phlegm production. Likewise, working in stimulant mode, the remedy is a time-tested uterine stimulant and parturient for delayed, scanty or absent periods, and for failure to progress during labour.

Like Yarrow and other highly complex and versatile aromatic remedies, Myrrh may also be selected for its good general cooling, calming and pain-relieving effect for conditions beyond those involving the skin and mucosa. Myrrh is for treating a system that is hyper-reactive, hypersensitive and hyperinflammatory. The hyperhistamine, ADHD and hyperthyroid syndromes are notable systemic indications here, as well as some chonic pain conditions.

Myrrh's bracing woody, balsamic fragrance is key to its psychological effects when used purely by olfaction. With its centring, stabilizing and calming effect, the fragrance can provide inner strength, security and protection, and support calm perseverance in the face of severe challenges. It can evoke the inner resources needed in cases of emotional and psychic burnout and vulnerability. These psychological qualities were no doubt an integral, if unspoken, aspect of Myrrh's value as the premier sacred aromatic.

Myrrh is also generally useful for those prone to worry, overthinking and obsessing, especially when these are connected to acute emotions such as fear, anxiety and sorrow. By settling and slowing down the mind, the fragrance is also for those who tend to disconnect and dissociate. For all these reasons, it comes as no surprise that Myrrh, like Cypress, is a sacred aromatic also appropriate for supporting many of life's important stages of radical transition, such as birth, coming of age and death.

**Related oils:** The following oils are also extracted from an oleoresin and possess similar therapeutic properties to Myrrh.

**Copaiba** or Copahu oleoresin (*Copaifera officinalis* and spp.) is extracted by incision to the bark of various leguminous shrubs and trees in Brazil, Venezuela, Guyana and Colombia. It is a traditional remedy among indigenous peoples of these areas, who shared its uses as both topical and internal medicine to the earliest European settlers. By the early 1500s, the tincture and distilled oil of Copaiba resin had become major remedies in European apothecaries. Copaiba's use is well documented, for instance, in King's *American Dispensatory* of 1898, being the treatment of urogenital infections with discharges, and chronic wounds and ulcers.

Copaiba oil has a mild odour with sweet amber, caramel, vanilla and slight peppery notes. Its chemical profile shows dominant sesquiterpenes 72–90%, including β-caryophyllene <53%, α-copaene <16%, trans-α-bergamotene <10%, cubebene and cadinene; diterpenes are also present (copalic/carenoic/hardwickic acids). The tincture of the oleoresin also contains these constituents but in alcoholic dilution. Copaiba has mild therapeutic status with no cumulative toxicity and is non-irritant and non-sensitizing to the skin.

Like Myrrh, Copaiba is valued clinically as a strong mucostatic astringent with antiseptic and anti-inflammatory actions in the context of treating a damp terrain. Its main indication is chronic mucous membrane overproduction causing discharges, simple or infectious. Copaiba is highly effective for chronic urethritis with gleet, itching or burning, mucous cystitis with blennuria, vaginitis with leucorrhoea, and gonorrhoea. Its topical emollient, soothing effect treats bladder irritation with painful, urgent or dripping urination. Likewise, in the chest it treats congestive bronchial conditions such as chronic bronchitis with copious foetid sputum, acting as an antiseptic mucolytic expectorant. Copaiba will also astringe and calm the gut mucosa, benefiting chronic mucousy stool or diarrhoea, mucous colitis, chronic gastroenteritis with ulcers, dysentery and haemorrhoids. For these conditions, gel cap and suppository administration is preferred. The gel cap dose is 5–10 drops.

Copaiba became equally famed, especially among French doctors relying on colonial supplies from Guyana, for its strong vulnerary, anti-inflammatory and antiseptic action when treating non-healing injuries. This experience arose from its use in tropical areas where high humidity prevents proper wound healing. Today Copaiba is still valued for treating non-healing wounds, ulcers, fistulas, boils, furuncles, infected eczema and cysts, and fungal skin infections. When applied topically to painful swollen joints, sore nipples, chilblains, sprains and scaly skin disorders, including psoriasis, Copaiba proves analgesic and detumescent as well as anti-inflammatory. Generous standard dilutions and doses apply and no precautions are known.

**Elemi** (*Canarium luzonicum* [Miq.] A. Gray) is the oleoresin of a tropical tree in the torchwood (Burseraceae) family native to the Philippines and Molucca islands. The resin, essential oil and tincture have been in use in herbal medicine and pharmacy since the 16th century and are consistently listed in pharmacopeias and dispensatories under wound-healing ointments and balm formulas. Elemi oil displays a complex odour of mild fresh, pungent, lemony and balsamic notes. Main constituents include limonene (26–65%), monoterpenes (with α- and β-phellandrenes <24%), elemicin (2–10%) and sesquiterpenes and their alcohols. It has mild therapeutic status with no cumulative toxicity and is non-irritant and non-sensitizing to the skin.

Elemi finds use in French medicine as a gastrointestinal stimulant with analgesic, spasmolytic actions given for digestive stagnation with colic and diarrhoea, and secondarily as a stimulant expectorant in bronchitis. An antiamoebic action is also reported with amoebiasis. Like Copaiba, Elemi has proven especially effective as a vulnerary and tissue regenerator for atonic, non-healing wounds, ulcers, varicose ulcers, furuncles and scar tissue. Topical application may be associated with green clay. The only possible concern with its use may be its low levels of methyleugenol (0.2–0.3%); these should not cause any problems with topical use, however, nor with internal use at moderate standard therapeutic doses.

**Benzoin** (*Styrax benzoin* Dryand, *S. paralleloneuris* Perkins, *S. tonkinensis* Pierre) is the gummy brown oleoresin collected from the trunk bark of various species of tropical tree in the silver bells (Styracaceae) family native to humid tropical Southeast Asia. The first two species yield Sumatra benzoin, produced in the islands of Java, Sumatra and Malaysia; the third species, Siam benzoin, is produced in Laos, Cambodia, Vietnam and South China. While both types of Benzoin have a warm, sweet caramel scent,

Sumatra benzoin has a fine, powdery vanilla note; Siam benzoin has more balsamic, chocolate notes.

Benzoin is a mild, non-toxic remedy in herbal medicine and pharmacy since antiquity. Its name derives from the Andalusian and Catalan *benjui*, itself derived from the Arabic *luban jawi*, the 'incense from Java'. In East Asia, Benzoin has always been an important ingredient in Hindu and Buddhist temples, and was much favoured by monks in their solitary practices as well as for their often arduous physical journeys. In early Levant cultures, Benzoin was usually mixed with another resin, Labdanum, for domestic, ceremonial and religious fragrancing by censing. Practitioners in the European Middle Ages used Benzoin in the form of a powder or tincture.

In modern times, an absolute extract or resinoid is also available – a sticky, solid dark brown mass with an odour very similar to the mother resin. In turn, the resinoid is usually diluted with benzyl alcohol or benzyl benzoate, both of them non-toxic, to make it pourable for practice. The main volatile constituents of all *Styrax* species are benzyl benzoate (40–51%) and benzyl alcohol (39–43%), as well as trace amounts of the aromatic aldehyde vanillin; with small variations of minor constituents such as benzoic acid among the three species. Note, however, that minor chemical adulterants to improve the aroma may be added, including benzoic acid, benzyl cinnamate and vanillin.

Apart from serving as a vehicle in various pharmaceutical preparations such as pills and ointments, and as a perfumery ingredient, Benzoin is also a valuable remedy for respiratory, urogenital and skin conditions, especially by topical applications. It is a mucolytic expectorant with antiseptic, anti-inflamatory actions for congestive bronchitis with copious sputum and chronic cough. In addition to chest and upper back liniments, Benzoin is also traditionally used by steam inhalation for these conditions, like Turpentine, as well as for suppurative middle-ear infections (otitis) with discharges. Soothing liniments applied to the throat and upper chest for sore throat (regardless of cause) and voice loss are highly effective. As a warming arterial and capillary stimulant, the remedy will treat cold, painful rheumatic-arthritic conditions, and its mucostatic and diuretic actions are useful for controlling discharges such as leucorrhoea, mucous cystitis and gleet.

When used topically for skin conditions, Benzoin is an excellent tissue regenerator and astringent vulnerary. Its main indications are skin irritation and wounding of any kind, including bruises, scrapes, sore nipples, chapped or itching skin, wounds, sores, ulcers and scars; it is also used alone or in compound liniments, etc., for pruritic eczema, psoriasis, pityriasis, acne, minor burns, chilblains and gangrene. Benzoin is non-irritant and non-sensitizing to the skin. However, it is contraindicated for use on sensitive or damaged skin, as permanent skin sensitization may result. Topical dilutions should therefore not exceed 2% to be safe. Benzoin should be avoided in babies and infants.

With its sweet, warming fragrance, the aroma of Benzoin has a particularly penetrating emotional effect that feels deeply soothing, comforting and nurturing. Its warm balsamic embrace allows inner relaxation, especially with tension, anxiety or depression felt around issues of love, need and emotional support. Benzoin can be supportive for those who feel not only emotionally deprived or bereaved, but also wounded by past negative experiences. The fragrance is very effective with emotional wounds from childhood, especially those relating to loss of or separation from a mother's love and its important consequences.

# Neroli

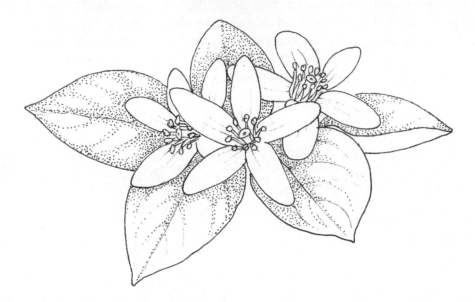

**Botanical source:** The flower of *Citrus aurantium* L. subsp. amara (syn. *Citrus aurantium* L. cv. group Bouquetier, *Citrus bigaradia* Risso), the bitter orange (Rutaceae – rue family), a widely cultivated fruit tree of most warm climates

**Other names:** Bitter/Seville/sour/bigarade orange flower, Bouquetier; Néroli bigarade (Fr), Bouquetier (Fr, Ge), Pomeranzenbluete, Orangenbluete (Ge), Zhi shi (Mandarin)

**Appearance:** A very pale yellow liquid with an intense light, sweet-floral, citrus-like fragrance with hints of floral green, honeysuckle and lily of the valley; the colour turns to amber as the oil ages

**Perfumery status:** A head note of high intensity but poor persistence

**Extraction:** Water distillation of the fresh flowers during April and May

**1 kg oil yield from:** 700–1,400 kg of the blossoms (a very poor yield)

**Production areas:** Tunisia, Morocco, Sicily, Egypt, France, China, Comoros, Haiti, Guinea. The flowers have to be hand-picked in the early-morning hours, like rose and jasmine flowers. Neroli production began on the French Riviera from the most fragrant Bouquetier cultivars as far back as the early 16th century; with French colonial expansion its production spread to the Maghreb in the 19th century.

**Typical constituents:** Monoterpenols 39–66% (incl. l-linalool 30–55%, geraniol 2%, nerol <2%, α-terpineol 6%) • monoterpenes 35–40% (including pinenes <18%, d-limonene 6–16%, sabinene, myrcene 2%, ocimene, β-ocimene 5%) • sesquiterpenols

6% (incl. transnerolidol 3–4%, farnesols I and II 3%) • esters <18% (incl. linalyl acetate 4–12%, neryl acetate 2%, geranyl acetate 3%) • aldehydes dimethylvinylhexenal, benzaldehyde, decanal • ketone jasmone • methyl anthranilate, indole • linalool oxide

**Chance of adulteration:** Very high, because of its very low yield and high price. Common adulterants would be Neroli Portugal oil (see below), Petitgrain bigarade oil (often saponified and deterpenated), Orange flower absolute, fragrance chemicals such as synthetic linalool and limonene, and citrus oil fractions such as terpenes, linalyl acetate, nerol, nerolidol and farnesol (Lis-Balchin 2006; Franchomme 2015).

**Related oils:** The flower, leaf and rind of various Bouquetier cultivars of the bitter orange tree are all extracted for different aromatic products:

**Petitgrain bigarade oil**, or Petitgrain oil for short, is distilled from the leaf of the bitter orange tree (see separate profile).

**Bitter orange oil** from the rind of this fruit, with a fragrance similar but inferior to Sweet orange (see the Sweet orange profile).

**Orange flower absolute**, the solvent extraction of the flowers; this is an orange to brown thick liquid with a warm, rich, sweet-citrus floral fragrance. It may be used topically in the same way as Neroli oil for skin care. As a psychological remedy with lemony-sweet notes, Orange flower absolute by olfaction is an excellent regulating aromatic for promoting emotional stability in states of instability and conflict. It may also help promote optimism, along with some euphoria, and is indicated for negative and distressed emotions, depression with anxiety, and states of sorrow and discouragement.

**Neroli water** or hydrosol, or Bitter orange flower water, is also obtained by water distillation of the fresh flowers but is usually produced separately from the distillation of the oil. Distilled in Arabic countries since ancient times (along with rosewater), it was traditionally known as Aqua Naphae by apothecaries in Europe. Neroli water has a sweet-floral fragrance with top notes of fruit and honeysuckle. Uplifting, clearing and euphoric by olfaction, it has a long and important history of domestic, therapeutic, perfumery and culinary use second only to Rosewater. It was a favourite among pastrychefs in southern and central Europe for over 500 years; in the 1920s it became popular again among French manufacturers to add crispness to biscuits.

Neroli water is excellent on its own or as a base for domestic preparations such as lotions, misters, mouth rinses (for gum problems) and various deodorant products; it is one of the most hydrating floral waters to the skin, especially for dry, delicate or sensitive skin. This floral water is especially welcome for babies and infants, in a diffusor or humidifier, in a carrier oil for infant massage, in the bath water and – in about a teaspoonful dose – in the baby's feeding bottle. Here it carries the same uplifting and calming actions as Neroli oil itself, but on a very much gentler scale.

**Orange flower water absolute** is obtained by solvent extraction; it is orange to brown with a dry-floral, rooty-herbaceous fragrance similar to Mandarin petitgrain oil.

**Neroli Portugal** or Neroli petalae oil is distilled from the flowers of the sweet orange tree, the Portugal orange (*Citrus x sinensis*). Neroli citronnier is similarly distilled from lemon flowers (*Citrus limonum*). Both of these have a weaker, less desirable fragrance and are mainly used in perfumery and flavouring; they are generally not used in a therapeutic context.

**Petitgrain sur fleur neroli** is an oil resulting from the co-distillation, i.e. simultaneous distillation, of the bitter orange leaves with a certain proportion of the blossoms; its fragrance profile depends on the proportion of blossoms to leaves used, being either more floral, Neroli-like or more musty, Petitgrain-like.

Note that so-called Chinese neroli oil is distilled from a different citrus flower, *Poncirus trifoliata* Rafin., the trifoliate, hardy or Chinese bitter orange.

## Therapeutic Functions and Indications

### SPECIFIC SYMPTOMATOLOGY – *All applications*

Emotional disposition, mood swings, excitability with much talk and laughter, irritability, frustration, anger, nervous tension, worry, anxiety with depression, pessimism, listlessness, negative feelings, despair, chronic depression with anxiety or agitation; anxiety around sexual performance, stress-related insomnia, palpitations, indigestion or diarrhoea; chest pain and stuffiness, upper abdominal pain and bloating after meals, varicose veins, sexual disinterest

### PSYCHOLOGICAL – *Aromatic diffusion, whole-body massage*

**Essential PNEI function and indication:** Regulating in dysregulation conditions; euphoric in acute dysregulation conditions

**Possible brain dynamics:** Reduces deep limbic system hyperfunctioning

**Fragrance category:** Middle tone with sweet and lemony notes

**Indicated psychological disorders:** Bipolar disorder, ADHD, minor depression

#### PROMOTES EMOTIONAL STABILITY

- Emotional instability with conflict and negative or distressed feelings
- Irritability, moodiness, mood swings
- Feeling/thinking conflict

PROMOTES OPTIMISM AND INSIGHT

- Pessimism, discouragement, despair

- Depression with anxiety or agitation

- Poor judgement with loss of insight or foresight

PROMOTES EUPHORIA AND RESOLVES SHOCK AND TRAUMA
For short-term use in acute conditions.

- All acute pathogenic emotions, incl. fear, anger, sorrow

- Fixation, worry, obsession, apprehension, panic

- Acute shock from trauma (mental/emotional/physical)

COMPLEMENTARY COMBINATIONS
For olfaction and topical applications.

- Neroli + Jasmine/Sambac jasmine: euphoric, stabilizing and antidepressant for severe emotional instability with conflict, depression, pessimism, despair

- Neroli + Rose: euphoric and stabilizing for emotional wounding with loss of self-esteem, shame, depression, distressed emotions with instability

- Neroli + Ylang ylang no. 1: euphoric, aphrodisiac for acute anger, acute depression, severe emotional shock; shame, low self-esteem and loss of libido from sexual trauma

## PHYSIOLOGICAL – *Nebulizer inhalation, gel cap, suppository, external applications*

**Therapeutic status:** Mild remedy with no chronic cumulative toxicity
**Topical safety status:** Non-irritant, somewhat sensitizing

**Tropism:** Neuroendocrine, circulatory, digestive, reproductive systems

**Essential diagnostic function:** Regulates dysregulation, restores hyptonic/weak and relaxes hypertonic/tense terrain conditions

PRIMARILY REGULATING:

*autonomic nervous (PNS/SNS) regulator:* ANS dysregulation with digestive, mood and temperature disorders; alternating constipation and diarrhoea, menopausal syndrome with hot flushes, PMS, hyperthyroid syndrome

PRIMARILY RESTORATIVE AND STIMULANT:

*systemic nervous trophorestorative, cerebral restorative, antidepressant:* nervous exhaustion, burnout or breakdown, incl. with anxiety, insomnia; chronic depression (any type, incl. postpartum), neurasthenia; chronic fatigue from chronic stress or disease; convalescence

*biliary/gastric/pancreatic stimulant, cholagogue, carminative, apperitive:* biliary/gastric/pancreatic deficiency with indigestion, appetite loss, epigastric pain, flatulence

*venous restorative:* venous deficiency/congestion with varicose veins, incl. haemorrhoids

*mild aphrodisiac:* loss of libido

PRIMARILY RELAXANT:

*systemic nervous relaxant, SNS inhibitor, vagotonic:* a large variety of acute and chronic hypertonic (tense) and spasmodic conditions:

- *nervous and cerebral sedative, hypnotic:* nervous tension, anxiety, insomnia, PMS, agitated depression, performance anxiety, ADHD; tension and vascular headaches; other chronic stress-related conditions

- *cardiovascular relaxant, spasmolytic, analgesic, hypotensive:* palpitations, tachycardia, precordial pain, cardiac spasms, Prinzmetal's/neurogenic angina; neurocardiac syndrome with chronic nervous depression; hypertension, electrolyte imbalance

- *gastrointestinal relaxant, spasmolytic, analgesic:* stress diarrhoea, colic, IBS

- *analeptic:* seizures

ANTIMICROBIAL ACTIONS:

*antibacterial, antimycobacterial:* bacterial and mycobacterial infections, incl. gastroenteritis, bronchitis, pleurisy, lung TB, incl. with E. coli

*antifungal:* fungal infections, incl. candidiasis, aspergillosis, incl. with Candida spp., Aspergillus niger/ochraceus, Fusarium

*antiparasitic (anthelmintic, antiprotozoal):* intestinal parasites (hookworm, giardiasis)

SYNERGISTIC COMBINATIONS

- Neroli + Petitgrain bigarade: nervous relaxant and restorative for chronic stress-related conditions with fatigue, burnout, chronic anxiety, insomnia, palpitations, agitated depression

- Neroli + Petitgrain bigarade + Bergamot: strong ANS regulator for severe digestive, mood and temperature disorders, incl. irregular stool, menopausal syndrome, PMS, hyperthyroid syndrome

COMPLEMENTARY COMBINATIONS

- Neroli + Marjoram/Roman camomile: strong systemic relaxant, SNS inhibitor and spasmolytic in a large range of hypertonic/tense conditions with pain, anxiety, spasms, emotional shock or trauma, esp. of cardiovascular and digestive systems

- Neroli + Lavender: cardiac spasmolytic and analgesic, hypotensive for neurogenic angina, anxiety, palpitations, hypertension

- Neroli + Ylang ylang no. 1/Tarragon: cardiovascular relaxant and hypotensive for severe tachycardia, cardiac spasms, neurogenic angina, headaches, hypertension

- Neroli + Clary sage: nervous restorative and sedative, antidepressant for chronic neurasthenia, stress-related conditions and depression, esp. in women

- Neroli + Palmarosa/Nutmeg: nervous and cardiac restorative for chronic neurasthenia with fatigue, weak heart, debility; in convalescence from chronic illness

- Neroli + Basil ct. chavicol/Tarragon: gastrointestinal relaxant, spasmolytic, analgesic for severe stress diarrhoea, colic, spasmodic IBS

- Neroli + Ylang ylang no. 1/extra: relaxant aphrodisiac in tense-type loss of libido

## TOPICAL – *Liniment, ointment, cream, compress and other cosmetic preparations*

**Skin care:** All skin types in general, but especially the dry, sensitive and thin or fragile types

> *skin regenerator (enhances skin cell metabolism), capillary stimulant(?):* broken capillaries and veins

*anti-inflammatory, mild emollient:* sensitive, irritated or inflamed skin (e.g. mature/ageing skin)

**Therapeutic precautions:** None

**Pharmacological precautions:** None

**Preparations:**

- **Diffusor:** 1–3 drops in water

- **Massage oil:** 2–3% dilution in vegetable oil

- **Liniment:** 5% dilution in vegetable oil

- **Gel cap:** 1–3 drops with olive oil

## Chinese Medicine Functions and Indications

**Aroma energy:** Sweet, lemony

**Movement:** Circulating

**Warmth:** Neutral to cool

**Meridian tropism:** Heart, Pericardium, Liver, Lung

**Five-Element Affinity:** Fire, Wood

**Essential function:** To regulate the Qi, settle the Heart and harmonize the Shen

1. **Regulates the Qi, relaxes constraint, settles the Heart, harmonizes the Shen**

   - **Heart and Liver Qi constraint with Shen dysregulation**, with depression and anxiety, mood swings, intense emotions, chronic headaches, chest pains, insomnia:

     Petitgrain/Bergamot/Mandarin/Ylang ylang no. 1

   - **Liver-Stomach/Spleen disharmony** with chronic stress, epigastric bloating, appetite loss, abdominal cramps, diarrhoea:

     Lavender/Bergamot/Fennel/Peppermint

2. **Settles and clarifies the Heart, and calms the Shen**

   - **Heart fire with Shen agitation**, with insomnia, agitation, excessive talk and laughter:

     May chang/Lime/Marjoram

   - **Heart Yin deficiency with Shen agitation**, with anxiety, worry, insomnia, restless or agitated depression:

     Lavender/Patchouli/Petitgrain bigarade

3. **Nourishes and animates the Heart, strengthens the Shen and relieves depression**

- **Heart Blood deficiency with Shen weakness**, with mental fatigue, anxious depression, discouragement, insomnia, easily startled:

    Palmarosa/Nutmeg/Cardamom

- **Heart Qi deficiency** with palpitations, fatigue, dyspnoea on exertion (esp. running):

    Rosemary/Palmarosa/Tea tree/Nutmeg

4. **Invigorates the Blood in the lower limbs and relieves varicosis**

- **Blood stagnation in the lower limbs** with varicose veins, tired legs, ankle oedema:

    Geranium/Yarrow/Cypress

REMARKS

Like several other citrus fruits, the bitter orange has seen a rich cultural and commercial history from its very origins in Southwest China (Yunnan) and North Vietnam. This is reflected in its Arabic name Naranj, which derives from the Sanskrit Nagranja. When Arab traders in their fast dhows finally made the first successful sailing trip to Guangzhou in 807, they returned to Siran or Basra laden with tree cuttings and its fruit, along with silk, spices and chinaware. With the expansion of their territories, they moved the bitter orange overland to Syria, Palestine, Egypt and westward to North African Mediterranean countries. In 1002 the bitter orange tree was noted in Sicily, gracing the first European botanical garden in Palermo long before the arrival of the sweet or Portugal orange. In the 10th century Arab settlers then developed the first lemon and orange plantations in Mediterranean Tunisia, Sicily, Malta, Calabria and Al Andalus; these were laid out with excellent irrigation systems, some of which survive to this day. By the 13th century, the prized fruit was enjoyed at courts from Andalusian Seville to Italian Padua and Venice for its beautiful colour and versatile culinary uses. Moreover, the tree was also widely cultivated in Italy for its brilliant white flowers, which were also distilled both at court and in private homes for their refreshing floral water. Today, the bitter orange is still widely cultivated in Tunisia, Sicily and Morocco, where the essential oil and floral waters are also distilled and exported.

The essential oil of the bitter orange flowers, called Neroli today, was only produced by apothecaries in the early 1500s in the South of France. Along with rose oil, jasmine and many other aromatics, it was routinely used by the gantiers-parfumeurs in Grasse for fragrancing fine leather gloves. However, it took a French princess, Anne Marie de La Tremoille, who married into the Italian Nerola family near Rome, to make a real fashion statement of this oil with her aromatic gloves. Lavishly, extravagantly dousing her gloves and other garments with the heady, floral notes of bitter-orange oil, she set an unstoppable trend in the 1680s that lasted well into the heady 1780s. In the process, the oil itself was renamed 'oil of Neroli'. The patronage of Madame de Pompadour in the late 1740s in turn supported the production of Neroli-scented gloves. As the king's leading mistress possessing 'exquisite and unerring taste', she delighted in promoting the revival of many small arts and crafts. This notably included perfumery; her patronage stimulated the development of French natural perfumery to new heights of sophistication before its collapse with the Revolution.

Although first described by Della Porta in 1563, the pharmacognosy of Neroli oil was first investigated by French researchers Bonastre in 1825 and Von Boullay in 1828. With a very complex and balanced chemistry that is polarized between monoterpenols and monoterpenes, the oil has the potential to both relax and restore the whole system – with the net result of an excellent regulating effect on the autonomic nervous system. Although in French medicine Neroli is often compared to Petitgrain bigarade (the twig and leaf oil of the bitter orange), their emphasis is somewhat different. While Petitgrain with its prominence of esters and monoterpenols is more relaxant than restorative, Neroli with dominant monoterpenols and monoterpenes is more restorative than relaxant, as well as somewhat stimulant.

Neroli's essential indication for both symptom relief and as a terrain oil is chronic weak and tense conditions involving the cardiac, vascular and digestive systems. The oil exerts a strong trophorestorative effect on the brain and whole nervous system, making nervous exhaustion, chronic depression and chronic fatigue important indications. As an inhibitor of sympathetic nervous activity, Neroli is also a good spasmolytic and analgesic for virtually any acute or chronic cardiovascular event, especially with emotional trauma present in the case history. Because of its superb regulating effect on the autonomic nervous system, Neroli is one of the best aromatics for autonomic dysregulation and stronger than Petitgrain in this respect. It should again be considered when either cardiac or emotional pathology is involved. Less used but equally useful are Neroli's stimulant action on all the organs of upper digestion, including the pancreas and gallbladder. Its sesquiterpenols nerolidol and farnesol have been found to possess anticancer properties (Bowles 2003).

It is no accident that Neroli oil, like the floral water, became a perennial favourite of women at Italian and French courts from the Renaissance onwards. The pure white orange flowers with their intoxicating indolic fragrance have always been linked to one or other aspect of woman, of the feminine principle. Although in the West the flowers are a traditional emblem of female purity, chastity and even virginity (similarly to the lily), they also imply the presence of female passion. Their scent manages to be at once uplifting and divine, and an aphrodisiac. In the South of France there is an interesting tradition of using orange blossoms as bridal decoration – in the bridal wreath, for instance. The significance here is purity of both physical and spiritual love mingled with heartfelt joy. In short, Neroli is an emblem of heartfelt feminine love and passion as an integrated, non-dual expression.

With its refined, uplifting sweet-floral fragrance, Neroli as an aromatic remedy also represents refinement and purification. It evokes the theme of elevating physical love into spiritual love, redeeming sexual desire by a longing for true intimacy, and transforming pathological emotions into pure feelings. Certainly, practitioners often value Neroli for helping resolve distressed emotions such as anger, bitterness, jealousy and resentment; it is also one of the key oils for treating unresolved sexual trauma and its sticky residue of shame. Here Neroli's well-established euphoric, mood-elevating effect creates a true enlightening effect, lightening the emotional darkness and intensity, and promoting hope and true optimism.

However, as a result of supporting this process of transformation, Neroli ends up being truly integrating and harmonizing at all levels. Integrating body and soul, Neroli expresses the potential for a refined sensuality and a unified, non-dual love; and for the lyrical yet embodied expression of emotion. No less than other sweet, citrusy oils, Neroli is highly effective for re-establishing emotional balance and stability, regardless of the types of conflict present and the original causes of imbalance. The oil's physiological action on the heart as the supreme regulating organ – restoring, regulating and calming, as needed – is a physical expression of this harmonizing effect.

# Niaouli

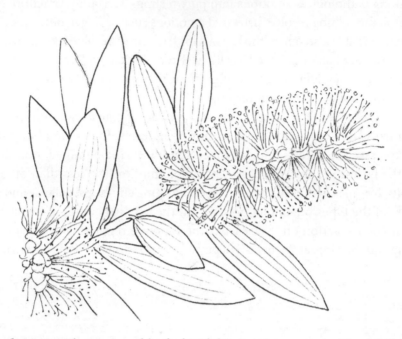

**Botanical source:** The stem and leaf of *Melaleuca quinquenervia* (Cav.) S.T. Blake ct. cineole (syn. *M. maidenii, M. smithii*) (Myrtaceae – myrtle family), a tropical tree of the humid Pacific region

**Other names:** Broad-leaf/Five-vein paperbark, Paperbark/Broad-leaf tea tree, Punk tree, Gomen oil; Niaouli (Fr), Niauli (Ge)

**Appearance:** A mobile clear or very pale yellow-green fluid with a fresh-camphoraceous, somewhat sweet odour with mild lemony top notes and musty-earthy base notes

**Perfumery status:** A head note of medium intensity and poor persistence

**Extraction:** Steam distillation of the leaves and stems all year round. Like Blue-gum eucalyptus, Niaouli oil is often rectified to remove the harsh aldehydes.

**1 kg oil yield from:** 35–100 kg of the leaves and stems (a very good yield)

**Production areas:** Mainly the Pacific region: New Caledonia, East Australia, southern Papua New Guinea, Tasmania; also Madagascar

**Typical constituents:** Oxide 1,8 cineole 38–68% • monoterpenes 5–23% (incl. α-pinene 3–16%, limonene 4–9%, β-pinene <3%, myrcene, terpinene, terpinolene) • sesquiterpenols 12–20% (incl. viridiflorol 3–15%, trans-nerolidol <7%, epi-globulol 1%, ledol) • monoterpenols 9–16% (incl. α-terpineol 7–14%, terpinene-4-ol 1–2%, l-linalool) • sesquiterpenes 9% (incl. β-caryophyllene 2%, aromadendrenes 1%, viridiflorene 4%, α-humulene 1%, δ-cadinene 1%) • benzaldehyde, isovaleraldehyde

**Chance of adulteration or misidentification:** Fair, as *M. quinquenervia* ct. viridiflorol, Madagascar Niaouli, is sometimes sold as Niaouli oil. Niaouli can also be reconstituted from a cineole-rich Eucalyptus and traces of other compounds; a cineole content above 70% would clearly indicate a reconstitution. Conversely, Niaouli oil is frequently misidentified and labelled as *M. viridiflora* Sol. ex Gaertner, the Broad-leaf tea tree, which is not the source of Niaouli as was once thought. This species from the tip of Northwest Australia is no longer or rarely distilled (Guenther 1972; Webb 2000). This commercial misidentification merely increases the confusion surrounding the botanical identity of Niaouli oil.

**Related oils:** Other species of *Melaleuca* are detailed in the Tea tree profile in Volume 1. Niaouli oil itself has several chemotypes. In addition to Niaouli, which is the chemotype cineole, the two other most commonly seen Niaouli chemotypes are:

- **Nerolina** (*Melaleuca quinquenervia* ct. nerolidol/linalool) from Australia, with its higher nerolidol (48–65%) and/or linalool (25–45%) content and a sweeter, rounder aroma (see below)

- **Madagascar niaouli** (*Melaleuca quinquenervia* ct. viridiflorol) from Vohibola in Northwest Madagascar, with a viridiflorol content of c. 30–66% and a much lower 1,8 cineole content (c. 13%).

## Therapeutic Functions and Indications

### SPECIFIC SYMPTOMATOLOGY – *All applications*

Vulnerability, feelings of low self-esteem, feelings of being overwhelmed, apathy, low self-confidence, pessimism, listlessness, depression, chronic habitual routine, low vitality, chronic tiredness, debility, mental fog, lethargy, low energy and motivation in the morning, poor stamina, chronic allergies and inflammations, chronic or recurrent infections, sinus problems, chronic cough with some expectoration, swollen glands, varicose veins, muscle and joint aches and pains, chronic menstrual problems, including scanty or absent periods, irregular cycles; infertility, low sex drive

### PSYCHOLOGICAL – *Aromatic diffusion, whole-body massage*

**Essential PNEI function and indication:** Stimulant in weakness conditions
**Possible brain dynamics:** Increases prefrontal cortex and basal ganglia functioning
**Fragrance category:** Top tone with pungent, lemony notes
**Indicated psychological disorders:** Minor depression, ADD

- Lethargy, drowsiness, stupor

- Mental confusion, poor concentration, poor short-term memory

PROMOTES SELF-CONFIDENCE AND MOTIVATION

- Low self-confidence and self-esteem, vulnerability, pessimism, depression

- Loss of motivation, procrastination, self-neglect


## PHYSIOLOGICAL – *Nebulizer inhalation, gel cap, suppository, external applications*

**Therapeutic status:** Mild remedy with no cumulative toxicity

**Topical safety status:** Non-irritant, possibly sensitizing in some people

**Tropism:** Neuroendocrine, respiratory, digestive, urinary, reproductive systems

**Essential diagnostic function:** Decongests damp/congestive and restores hypotonic/weak terrain conditions

PRIMARILY STIMULANT AND DECONGESTANT:

*arterial circulatory stimulant:* asthenic (cold) and congestive conditions with poor circulation, cold extremities

*respiratory decongestant, mucolytic expectorant, antitussive:* chronic congestive bronchial infections with cough, sputum, dyspnoea, incl. bronchitis, emphysema

*nasal decongestant:* sinusitis, rhinitis (incl. allergic forms)

*venous and lymphatic decongestant:* venous and lymphatic congestion with varicose veins, esp. haemorrhoids; lymphedema

*pelvic and uterine decongestant:* pelvic congestion with congestive dysmenorrhoea, prostate congestion (BPH)

*liver decongestant and restorative, liver-cell stimulant, antilithic:* liver and portal congestion, liver disease in general, gallstones

PRIMARILY RESTORATIVE:

*nervous and cerebral restorative:* hypotonic (weak) conditions with cerebral deficiency, mental and physical fatigue, debility, memory or concentration loss, somnolence; neurasthenia, CFS, postviral depression, MS and other neurodegenerative disorders *pituitary-adrenal restorative and regulator, adaptogenic:* adrenal dysregulation or fatigue with low stamina; HPA axis deficiency; chronic inflammation and allergies

*pituitary-gonadal (ovarian) restorative and regulator (oestrogenic/progesteronic/testosteronic):* HPG axis deficiency with hormonal dysregulation and oestrogen/progesterone/testosterone deficiency, incl. amenorrhoea, oligomenorrhoea, irregular cycles, frigidity, impotence; menopausal syndrome

*immune restorative:* chronic immune deficiency with recurrent infections

*anti-inflammatory, antiallergic, antihistamine:* type-I allergy conditions, incl. rhinitis, atopic dermatitis and asthma, prostatitis, colitis, duodenitis, gastritis, cystitis

*anti-inflammatory, analgesic:* prostatitis and cystitis with dysuria, tonsillitis and most of the infections below; rheumatic pain, myalgia, rheumatoid arthritis; labour pains

MISCELLANEOUS ACTIONS:

*hypotensive:* hypertension

*antitumoural:* non-hormonal breast cancer, rectal cancer, fibroma

ANTIMICROBIAL ACTIONS:

*broad-spectrum anti-infective, antimicrobial, detoxicant, immunostimulant, antipyretic, anti-inflammatory:* a large range of infections, incl. with fever; esp. ear-nose-throat, respiratory, gastrointestinal, urogenital

- *strong antiviral:* viral infections, incl. influenza, adenovirus, rhinovirus, HPV, HSV-1 and -2, incl. flu, common cold, acute bronchitis/pneumonia, croup, pleurisy, cold sores, herpes zoster/shingles, genital herpes, condyloma, cervical dysplasia, viral hepatitis

- *strong antibacterial:* bacterial infections, esp. gram-positive, incl. with Staph. aureus, Strep. pneum. and pyogenes, Enterococcus, Mycobacterium spp., incl. common cold, bronchitis, tuberculosis, whooping cough, intestinal dysbiosis, gastroenteritis, gastric and duodenal ulcers, urinary tract infections (cystitis, urethritis, nephritis), vaginitis, MRSA, septicaemia, leprosy

- *strong antifungal:* fungal infections with Aspergillus niger, incl. aspergillosis, chronic sinusitis

- *antiparasitic, anthelmintic:* amoebiasis, taeniasis, Plasmodium (blood-flukes), lice

### Synergistic combinations

- Niaouli + Cajeput/Narrow-leaf eucalyptus/Ravintsara: strong antiviral, immunostimulant, anti-inflammatory and analgesic for acute upper respiratory infections and flu, esp. with fatigue, neurasthenia, recurrent infections

- Niaouli + Ravintsara: nervous, cerebral and immune restorative: for mental and physical fatigue, postviral depression, recurrent infections

- Niaouli + Ravintsara + Thyme ct. thymol: strong immune restorative and anti-infective in chronic immune deficiency with recurrent or chronic infections, debility, poor circulation

- Niaouli + Rosemary ct. cineole/camphor: analgesic, antirheumatic, arterial stimulant in rheumatic-arthritic conditions, cold skin and extremities (also topically)

### Complementary combinations

- Niaouli + Thyme ct. thymol: strong broad-spectrum anti-infective, anti-inflammatory and detoxicant in a wide variety of acute and chronic infections of all body systems in adults (short-term use)

- Niaouli + Thyme ct. linalool: broad-spectrum anti-infective, anti-inflammatory, detoxicant in a wide variety of acute and chronic infections in children, esp. respiratory

- Niaouli + Tea tree: broad-spectrum anti-infective and antipyretic in a wide variety of infections, esp. chronic, with weakness, debility, fever

- Niaouli + Winter savoury/Oregano: strong anti-infective and immunostimulant in acute and chronic urinary and genital infections (short-term use)

- Niaouli + Blue tansy/Tea tree: anti-inflammatory and antiallergic for type-I allergies, incl. with infection, incl. sinusitis, rhinitis, dermatitis, asthma, asthmatic bronchitis, cystitis, colitis

- Niaouli + Black spruce/Hemlock spruce: stimulant expectorant, antitussive in congestive lower respiratory infections with chronic productive cough and dyspnoea

- Niaouli + Cypress: venous restorative and decongestant for venous congestion with varicose veins, ankle oedema, haemorrhoids

- Niaouli + Lemon + Carrot seed: liver trophorestorative for liver congestion, liver disease

- Niaouli + Geranium + Atlas cedarwood: pelvic and venous decongestant for pelvic and venous congestion with dysmenorrhoea, haemorrhoids, varicose veins, phlebitis

- Niaouli + Black spruce + Basil ct. methylchavicol: prostate decongestant, anti-inflammatory for prostate congestion (BPH), prostatitis, esp. with immune deficiency, fatigue, dysuria

- Niaouli + Coriander seed: pituitary-gonadal (ovarian) restorative, oestrogenic, progesteronic for hypo-oestrogen or hypo-progesterone syndrome with PMS, amenorrhoea, dysmenorrhoea, low libido, depression

- Niaouli + Scotch pine + Winter savoury: strong reproductive restorative/pituitary-gonadal stimulant for severe sexual debility, loss of libido, amenorrhoea

## TOPICAL – *Liminent, ointment, cream, compress and other cosmetic preparations*

**Skin care:** Oily skin type

*antiseptic, decongestant:* congested skin; acne, boils, furuncles, seborrhoea

*antimicrobial, antifungal:* fungal skin infections, incl. athlete's foot; psoriasis, leprosy, lichen plana, lice

*vulnerary, skin-regenerative:* wounds (esp. infected, pus-filled), ulcers, eczema, cuts

*anti-inflammatory, analgesic:* rheumatic aches and pains; insect bites, burns

*radiation protectant:* radiation exposure, radiation treatment with burns (x-ray, y-ray, 5G mobile phones)

**Therapeutic precautions:** Niaouli is somewhat warming, drying and stimulating, and as such is best avoided in hypersthenic/hot and dry conditions.

**Pharmacological precautions:** Because of its high cineole content, Niaouli is contraindicated in babies and infants, and should be avoided in young children, and during pregnancy and lactation. For topical use, a patch test should ideally be done first as its content in aldehydes may be skin-sensitizing to some individuals.

**Preparations:**

- Diffusor: 2–4 drops in water

- Massage oil: 2–4% dilution in a vegetable oil

- Liniment: 5–20% dilution in a vegetable carrier oil

- Gel cap: 2–4 drops with some olive oil

## Chinese Medicine Functions and Indications

**Aroma energy:** Pungent, lemony

**Movement:** Rising, dispersing

**Warmth:** Neutral to warm

**Meridian tropism:** Lung, Bladder, Triple Heater, Kidney

**Five-Element affinity:** Metal, Water

**Essential function:** To tonify and raise the Qi, nourish Blood and Essence, and strengthen the Shen

1. **Tonifies the Qi, raises the clear Yang, strengthens the Shen and relieves fatigue and depression**

    - **Qi and protective Qi deficiency with Shen weakness**, with chronic physical and mental fatigue, chronic or recurring infections, cold extremities, grief:
    Rosemary/Ravintsara/Black spruce

    - **Clear Yang Qi deficiency with Shen weakness**, with mental confusion and fog, poor focus, depression, headaches:
    Cajeput/Peppermint/Ravintsara

2. **Nourishes the Blood and Essence, tonifies Chong and Ren Mai, and regulates menstruation**

    - **Blood deficiency** with irregular periods, scanty or absent periods, fatigue:
    Geranium/Clary sage/Rose

    - **Chong and Ren Mai Essence deficiency** with loss of sex drive, frigidity, impotence, sterility in both sexes:
    Black spruce/Sage/Rose

3. **Warms the Lung, expels phlegm, diffuses Lung Qi and relieves coughing**

    - **Lung phlegm cold/damp** with sputum expectoration, chronic cough, fatigue, cold extremities:
    Rosemary/Hyssop/Cypress/Thyme ct. thymol

4.  **Warms and releases the exterior, dispels wind, opens the sinuses and relieves pain and congestion; boosts the protective Qi**

    -   **External wind-cold with Qi or Yang deficiency**, with sneezing, sinus congestion and pain, muscle aches and pains, fatigue, possible fever:

        Cajeput/Ravintsara/Laurel

    -   **Lung wind-cold** with chills, sore throat, cough with slight expectoration, possible fever:

        Grand fir/Siberian fir/Ravintsara

5.  **Warms and opens the meridians, dispels wind-damp-cold, and relieves pain**

    -   **Wind-damp-cold obstruction** with chronic rheumatic aches and pains:

        Juniper berry/Rosemary/Black pepper

REMARKS

The paperbark tree that is distilled for its Niaouli oil comes from the same Pacific region as Cajeput. Its leaves are still decocted in New Caledonia for treating fever and diarrhoea, and pain with topical rubs. It is one of several *Melaleuca* oils used mainly in physical medicine today, although it also presents a fascinating psychological profile. The oil was first shipped to France from its overseas territory, New Caledonia, as early as the 18th century and has been adopted by a growing number of French medical practitioners ever since.

From the therapeutic perspective, Niaouli presents two completely different yet clinically equally important images. The first is a stimulant and decongestant remedy with a strong tropism for respiratory and pelvic organ functions. The second is a deeply restorative remedy for most neuroendocrine functions. Besides, its outstanding anti-infective actions make many practitioners think of Niaouli first and foremost as a premier remedy for infections. Certainly, they cannot be contradicted: among all the antimicrobial oils available, Niouli is probably able to catch the widest spectrum of microbes. It is also one of the very few oils that has shown success with septicaemia in its ability to reach to the deepest level of infection, the blood level.

Still, the delivery method and the oil's other actions and innate tropism must be considered here as always, making Niaouli a classic for respiratory infections of most kinds. Its decongestant, expectorant and antitussive actions clearly contribute much to its use for bronchial infections. Although Niaouli is often used for urogenital infections of all kinds – courtesy of its strong, broad-spectrum antibacterial and antiviral actions – it is also an excellent decongestant woman's remedy for venous and lymphatic congestion from the pelvis down. It is complex and adaptive enough to combine well here with the likes of Geranium and Cypress. Its decongestant action actually includes the liver, gallbladder and portal vein, where it has shown a cell-regenerative effect. In the telling words of André Bitsas (2009), 'La complexité interne de cette huile essentielle est garante, tout a la fois, d'indications multiples, d'une grande efficacité et d'une tolérance exceptionelle' – 'The internal chemical complexity of this oil ensures, all at the same time, numerous indications, great efficacity and exceptional tolerance.'

Unlike most other remedies that treat infections, Niaouli has a neuroendocrine restorative action that is very similar to Scotch pine and Black spruce, and qualifies it for an adaptogen. Working along the HPA and HPG axis, it is a good regulator of most female reproductive hormones and can be considered a good long-term uterine tonic. It should be used in formulas for menstrual and menopausal conditions of many kinds arising from a chronic weak terrain. Chronic adrenocortical dysregulation and exhaustion is also part of its systemic restorative effect, as is its cerebral, nervous and immune restoration in treating chronic weak conditions of all kinds. These typically present fatigue, nervous exhaustion or debility, and chronic or recurring infections.

Last but not least, Niaouli is not only an important anti-inflammatory and analgesic for rheumatic conditions, but also specifically antihistamine in most type-I allergies. The list of these allergies has grown over the last decade and includes allergic cystitis, prostatitis and gut inflammations, in addition to the more familar dermatitis and rhinitis.

Niaouli is equally valuable as a psychological remedy by olfaction. Its fresh, pungent fragrance qualities resonate with other similar leaf oils that stimulate the lungs, promote deep breathing and tend to relax the diaphragm, such as Cajeput and Ravintsara; it has both similar and distinctive uses. A boost to the psyche, the oil promotes internal strength and feelings of security while allowing one to remain open and transparent to others. It can promote personal protection from negative influences while allowing one to remain connected to the external world. Niaouli is for those who feel weak and run down, vulnerable and lacking all self-assurance. Unable to cope with much stress, they feel overwhelmed, raw and over-exposed to the demands of life, and often lacking in a personal life. This predisposes them to listlessness, depression and apathy as they lose motivation. At the same time, they may be struggling against their own inner demons – a struggle that usually proves ineffective and further increases their feelings of deep vulnerability. Like a wise, ever-available guardian, Niaouli offers this individual a strong boost to his or her inner fortitude, while reinforcing the protective energies of their body and psyche.

**Related oils:** The following types of *Melaleuca* and other related oils also have interesting clinical uses.

**Nerolina** (*Melaleuca quinquenervia* ct. nerolidol/linalool) from northern New South Wales on Australia's East coast has gentle fresh lemony and sweet floral notes that reflect high levels of nerolidol (30–60%) and linalool (30–50%); trace–3% of 1,8 cineole and very small amounts of sesquiterpenes (incl. β-caryophyllene, aromadendrene, α-humulene and δ-cadinene) complete the major constituents. Nerolina has mild therapeutic status with no cumulative toxicity. It shows much promise as an important aromatic remedy for internal use for treating insufficiency of the hypothalamic-pituitary-adrenocortical (HPA) and hypothalamic-pituitary-gonadal (HPG) axes, and for restoring and balancing the central nervous system. As a nervous and endocrine restorative, the oil will treat chronic weak terrain presenting fatigue, loss of stamina, neurasthenia and loss of sex drive. Nerolina's tonic action also extends to digestive functions, indicating upper gastric indigestion, liver congestion and pancreatic deficiency. The oil is also hypotensive in hypertension and anti-inflammatory in respiratory, urinary, reproductive and arthritic inflammation. Topically Nerolina treats burns and wounds. Its anti-infective actions, although reported as variable in strength (Pénoel and Franchomme 1990), include antifungal, antiviral, antibacterial and antiparasitic effects; tapeworms, protozoa and amoebas respond to it, as will malaria and possibly other tropical fevers. The constituent nerolidol in isolation has shown to be antitumoural in experimental lab rats with cancerous intestinal tumours, an action that may extend to human tissue (Webb 2000). Nerolina's other major constituent, linalool, is also considered potentially antitumoural. As Nerolina is non-toxic, non-irritant and non-skin sensitizing, there are no precautions to its use and standard dilutions and doses apply.

With its fresh-lemony, sweet fragrance qualities, Nerolina by olfaction will promote emotional clarity, stability and balance. This aromatic remedy can help re-establish emotional sensitivity and integrate thinking and feeling. It can support individuals presenting conflict, confusion or negativity, as well as treat mood swings and irritability. Gently promoting mental focus, Nerolina can aid distractibility and mild states of depression.

**Rosalina** or Lavender tea tree (*Melaleuca ericifolia* Smith) from Tasmania and coastal Southeast Australia has mild rosy-sweet and fresh notes with linalool dominant (35–55%), followed by 1,8 cineole (15–35%) and monoterpenes (<16% with major α-pinene). Therapeutically, Rosalina is a milder version of Niaouli with linalool as the dominant monoterpenol that provides a sweeter fragrance. It is completely mild and non-toxic. Its general character is relaxant with a nervous sedative action useful in stress-related disorders, insomnia, mild anxiety, etc., i.e. tense/hypertonic conditions. By inhalation and chest rub, Rosalina is a gentle but an effective stimulant expectorant and respiratory decongestant for congestive conditions of the upper and lower respiratory tract, including colds, sinusitis and bronchitis. Like all other *Melaleucas*, it is a good anti-infective and antiseptic in general. It is particularly useful in children's congestive infections when the child presents irritability, sleeping problems and anxiety. Topical use of Rosalina includes the treatment of boils, acne, herpes and tinea, as well as insect bites for its analgesic action. Rosalina is non-irritant and non-skin sensitizing and therefore carries no precautions or contraindiactions to its use. Standard dilutions and doses apply.

**Manuka** or Manuka myrtle (*Leptospermum scoparium* J.R. Forster & G. Forster), also in the myrtle family, from Australia and New Zealand, has sweet, herbaceous green and mild camphoraceous notes. Dominant constituents are sesquiterpenes (<17%) and triketones (<31%), with small amounts of monoterpenols and monoterpenes. Decoctions of the leaves have been traditionally prepared for numerous complaints by the Maori people of New Zealand. Manuka oil is completely mild and non-toxic. Its main use is as an antibacterial and antifungal in a wide range of infections by topical and internal administration and works especially well on Gram-positive bacteria. It has also shown to be a good antiviral against HSV-1.

The oil also shows antipruritic, anti-inflammatory and possibly skin-regenerative actions, and is much used for topical conditions ranging from skin infections, acne and boils to acute (allergic) eczema with redness and itching, burns, ulcers, scars and insect bites. Rheumatic and arthritic disorders with pain and stiffness will also benefit from its analgesic and stimulant actions. Manuka is non-irritant and non-skin sensitizing and therefore carries no precautions or contraindications to its therapeutic use. Standard dilutions and doses apply.

**Kunzea** (*Kunzea ambigua* [Smith] Druce), also in the myrtle family and known as Tick bush and White kunzea, originates in Tasmania and Southeast Australia, like Rosalina. The pale yellow oil has a fresh-pungent, somewhat sweet and green fragrance. Kunzea's major constituents are α-pinene (30–48%), 1,8 cineole (9–17%), globulol (7–13%), viridiflorol (6–12%), germacrene (4–6%) and α-terpineol (1–3%). Kunzea is a mild remedy with no cumulative toxicity and is valued for its reliable anti-infective, immune stimulant, analgesic and anti-inflammatory actions that have been compared to those of Niaouli. Its broad-spectrum antibacterial action has shown high activity against Staph. aureus, Pseudomonas aer. and E. coli; its good antifungal action includes tinea (athlete's foot, nail fungus, etc.) and Candida; its antiviral action is excellent in influenza and shingles. Kunzea is used in a large variety of infectious conditions presenting with pain, inflammation and nervous tension, including respiratory, digestive and dermal (dermatitis, eczema) infections. Painful rheumatic and arthritic conditions with muscle and tissue tension also respond well to its relaxant analgesic action. Kunzea is also known to regenerate weak mucous membranes. A mild nervous relaxant, the oil is useful for mild to moderate stress-related conditions, including insomnia and mild anxiety.

Topically, Kunzea is an excellent vulnerary with skin-regenerative, analgesic and antiseptic actions that finds use for soft tissue injuries such as sprains and strains, wounds, scars, ulcers, cuts, abrasions, insect bites, acne, minor burns and chilblains. It has also been found useful in allergic dermatitis with itching. In a diffuser, Kunzea is a good environmental antiseptic, deodorant and insect repellent. Although generally non-toxic, non-irritant and non-skin sensitizing, those with sensitive skin should use this oil with some caution because of its cineole content. Standard dilutions and doses apply.

As a psychological remedy for olfaction, Kunzea acts as a gentle stimulant with fresh-pungent qualities in hypotonic/weak conditions with mental fatigue with loss of concentration, lethargy, low self-confidence and loss of motivation.

**Fragonia** (*Agonis fragrans* J.R. Wheeler & N.G. Marchant) (Myrtaceae) is distilled in small batches in southwest Western Australia from the fresh leafy twigs of a tall shrub in the myrtle family. Its botanical name *Agonis* derives from *agon* in Greek, meaning 'gathered', referring to its tight flower clusters. The oil has a complex odour that combines a fresh, pungent top note with sweet, herbaceous and balsamic woody notes. Its pharmacognosy is dominant in three main constituents: 1,8 cineole (26–33%), α-pinene (21–27%) and linalool (11–12%), supported by small percentages of miscellaneous other monoterpenes and monoterpenols (including d-limonene 2.5%, α-terpineol 5–8%, terpinen-4-ol <4%, myrtenol <4% and geraniol).

Fragonia is essentially a stimulant with a secondary restorative effect, acting mainly on the nervous and respiratory systems. It treats acute and chronic weak conditions such as neurasthenia with low energy, mental and physical fatigue, and depression; and upper and lower respiratory infections with mucous congestion (as an antiseptic mucolytic expectorant). Based on its constituent profile, anti-inflammatory and somewhat analgesic actions are also present, which are also engaged in topical liniments for painful rheumatic-arthritic conditions. Fragonia has also been found helpful for regulating disturbed sleep-wake cycles caused by shift work or jet lag; it is thought to possibly regulate the circadian rhythm. The oil may also be useful in PMS and dysmenorrhoea, again through unknown mechanisms of action. Fragonia is mild and non-toxic, and non-irritant and non-sensitizing to the skin, although those with sensitive skin should use this oil with some caution because of its cineole content – and especially if an oxidized oil is used. Fragonia carries no other known precautions or contraindications to its therapeutic use. Standard dilutions and doses apply.

As a psychological remedy, Fragonia has been found useful for helping resolve distressed feelings in general and promote renewed emotional balance. The fragrance will support relieving the emotional stagnation stemming from grief in particular, allowing the individual to process and move on.

# Nutmeg

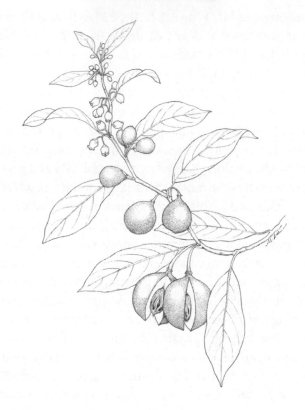

**Botanical source:** The seed of *Myristica fragrans* Houtt. (Myristicaceae – nutmeg family), a cultivated evergreen tree of the wet tropics

**Other names:** Noix de Muscade (Fr), Muskatnuss (Ge), Pala, Jebugarung (Indonesian), Rou dou kou (Mandarin), Nuez moscada (Sp)

**Appearance:** A mobile clear or pale-yellow fluid with a deep, warm sweet-spicy, somewhat fresh, odour

**Perfumery status:** A base note of high intensity and good persistence

**Extraction:** Steam distillation of the dried, coarsely powdered seeds throughout most of the year; only the defective, worm-eaten seeds are chosen for distillation, as these are suitably devoid of fat, protein and carbohydrate and will yield their oil more easily

**1 kg oil yield from:** 10–14 kg of the seeds (an excellent yield)

**Production areas:** Moluccas, Indonesia (native), Java, Sumatra, Grenada, Jamaica, Sri Lanka; the important Grenadan production began in 1843

**Typical constituents:** Monoterpenes 70–82% (incl. α-pinene 16–24%, β-pinene 10–15%, α- and γ-terpinenes 4–12%, sabinene 15–50%, limonene 3%, dipentene, camphene, p-cymene, terpinolene) • phenolic ethers (incl. myristicin 3–11%, safrole, elemicin, eugenol, methyleugenol) • monoterpenols (incl. terpinen-4-ol 4–10%, α-terpineol <1.4%) • 1,8 cineole 2–3% • sesquiterpene β-caryophyllene 0–1% • trans/cis-sabinene hydrate

**Note:** The above ranges include Nutmeg oil from different countries. The Jamaican oil, for instance, has shown to be lowest in myristicin, which is considered a neurotoxin.

**Chance of adulteration:** Moderate, usually with synthetic components, e.g. pinenes, sabinene, terpinenes; sometimes with Tea tree oil. Another possibility includes classic adulteration with the oils of other, undesirable species of *Myristica*, such as the high-safrole Macassar or Papua nutmeg (*M. argentea* Warb.) from Irian Jaya and Papua New Guinea, the Halmahera nutmeg (*M. Succedanea* Blume) from the hilly North Moluccas, and Bombay or Malabar nutmeg (*M. malabrica* Lamk.) from coastal Southwest India.

**Related oils:** The rarer Mace oil, which is distilled from the orange-coloured aril or husk that envelops the nutmeg seed; the oil is higher in myristicin but otherwise very similar in constituent profile. Mace oil's therapeutic functions and indications are exactly the same as those of Nutmeg. Nutmeg and Mace absolute or oleoresin are also extracted for the perfumery industry.

## Therapeutic Functions and Indications

### SPECIFIC SYMPTOMATOLOGY – *All applications*

Apathy, discouragement, listlessness, depression, poor motivation, insecurity, loss of self-confidence, timidity, fearfulness, apprehension, vulnerability, phobias and fears, mental and physical tiredness, poor concentration and memory, chronic headaches, dizzy and fainting spells, cold hands and feet, poor appetite, digestive problems with flatulence, irregular or loose stool, muscle/nerve/joint pains, scanty or stopped periods, low sex drive

### PSYCHOLOGICAL – *Aromatic diffusion, whole-body massage*

**Essential PNEI function and indication:** Stimulant in deficiency conditions; mild euphoric in depressed conditions

**Possible brain dynamics:** Increases basal ganglia functioning

**Fragrance category:** Base tone with rooty, pungent notes

**Indicated psychological disorders:** Depression, ADD

<small>PROMOTES COURAGE AND SELF-CONFIDENCE</small>

- Apathy, discouragement, listlessness, depression
- Low self-esteem and self-confidence, self-neglect

<small>PROMOTES GROUNDING AND STRENGTH</small>

- Insecurity, vulnerability, fearfulness
- Mental and emotional burnout

## PHYSIOLOGICAL – *Nebulizer inhalation, gel cap, suppository, external applications*

**Therapeutic status:** Medium-strength remedy with some cumulative toxicity

**Topical safety status:** Non-irritant, non-sensitizing

**Tropism:** Nervous, cardiovascular, digestive, musculoskeletal, reproductive systems

**Essential diagnostic function:** Warms asthenic/cold, stimulates hypotonic/weak and decongests congestive/damp terrain conditions

<small>PRIMARILY STIMULANT AND WARMING:</small>

*strong central and diffusive arterial circulatory stimulant:* a wide range of asthenic (cold) and hypotonic (weak) conditions with poor circulation, cold skin

- *neurocardiac restorative/stimulant:* neurasthenia with fatigue, nervous and heart weakness, debility

- *cerebral stimulant, antidepressant:* dizziness, vertigo, fainting, somnolence, headaches, memory loss, hypochondria, agoraphobia; depression; motion sickness

- *musculoskeletal stimulant:* chronic rheumatic conditions, incl. chronic fibromyalgia, arthritis, esp. with cold skin and joints, stiffness

- *digestive stimulant, gastrointestinal and pancreatic stimulant, aperitive, carminative:* atonic digestive conditions with indigestion, appetite loss, flatulence, constipation or diarrhoea; chronic gastroenteritis, pancreatitis

- *uterine stimulant, emmenagogue, oxytocic partus preparator:* amenorrhoea, oligomenorrhoea; to prepare the uterus for delivery; uterine dystocia

- *reproductive/sexual stimulant:* loss of libido (frigidity, impotence)

PRIMARILY RELAXANT:

*musculoskeletal relaxant, strong analgesic, spasmolytic:* acute painful rheumatic and arthritic conditions with pain, cramping; neuralgia, incl. sciatica

*gastrointestinal relaxant, spasmolytic, analgesic, antiseptic, anti-inflammatory, antidiarrhoeal:* spasmodic digestive conditions with diarrhoea, incl. enteritis and colitis with painful colic, Crohn's disease; bacterial intestinal dysbiosis, intestinal fermentation; food poisoning, halitosis

*anti-inflammatory, antihistamine, immune regulator(?):* allergic and autoimmune disorders, incl. Crohn's disease

*antiemetic:* vomiting, travel and altitude sickness, morning sickness

*antioxidant*

*anticoagulant:* thrombosis

*antilipaemic:* hyperlipidaemia

ANTIMICROBIAL ACTIONS:

*antibacterial:* acute bacterial infections, esp. gastrointestinal and urinary, incl. with Staph. aureus, E. coli, incl. gastritis, enteritis, food poisoning, microbial toxicosis; cystitis

*antiparasitic:* intestinal parasites; amoebiasis with dysentery

*antifungal:* with Aspergillus niger and ochraeus, Fusarium culmorum

SYNERGISTIC COMBINATIONS

- Nutmeg + Rosemary/Cajeput: strong arterial stimulant, analgesic for circulatory deficiency with cold skin and extremities, chronic rheumatic-arthritic pain

- Nutmeg + Niaouli/Cajeput: strong neuromuscular stimulant and analgesic in most rheumatic, arthritic and neuralgic conditions with pain, cold skin, stiffness

- Nutmeg + Black pepper: cerebral nervous stimulant for mental, cognitive and visual impairment

- Nutmeg + Juniper berry: emmenagogue uterine stimulant for amenorrhoea, oligomenorrhoea

- Nutmeg + Niaouli: antimicrobial for bacterial dysbiosis with chronic digestive symptoms, esp. with food sensitivities

- Nutmeg + Black pepper: antibacterial, spasmolytic, analgesic and antidiarrhoeal for food poisoning, enteritis, colitis, dysentery

- Nutmeg + Black spruce: antiparasitic for intestinal parasites

COMPLEMENTARY COMBINATIONS

- Nutmeg + Palmarosa: neurocardiac restorative for chronic nervous and heart weakness with depression, debility, palpitations

- Nutmeg + Peppermint: cerebral stimulant for mental fatigue, headaches, dizziness, fainting, cerebral/mental deficiency with depression, cognitive impairment, neurasthenia

- Nutmeg + Marjoram: strong neuromuscular relaxant, analgesic, spasmolytic for all acute rheumatic and arthritic conditions, with pain and cramping

- Nutmeg + Ginger: strong digestive stimulant, antiemetic in atonic digestive conditions with appetite loss, bloating, flatulence, nausea, vomiting, travel sickness

- Nutmeg + Roman camomile/Fennel: gastrointestinal relaxant in spasmodic digestive conditions with painful colic and diarrhoea

- Nutmeg + Marjoram/Basil ct. chavicol: strong gastrointestinal relaxant, anti-inflammatory, analgesic in a wide range of hyperactive/tense and spasmodic digestive conditions with pain, anxiety, insomnia

- Nutmeg + Clove/Cinnamon: antiparasitic for intestinal parasites, esp. amoebiasis with dysentery

## TOPICAL – *Liniment, ointment, cream, compress and other cosmetic preparations*

**Skin care:** Oily skin type

*analgesic:* muscle aches, pains and cramps, neuralgias, paralysis; hair loss; to warm and tone muscles before and after sports

*rubefacient:* sprains, strains, toothache, painful lesions, sores

*antiseptic, larvicidal, antiparasitic:* skin parasites

**Caution:** Avoid use of this rubefacient oil on sensitive skin.

**Therapeutic precautions:** Nutmeg is a strong, warming stimulant to nervous and most internal organ functions and is therefore contraindicated in all hypersthenic/hot, hypertonic/tense and dry conditions, especially with high fever, acute inflammation, hypertension, agitation or insomnia present. Because of this, and because it is a uterine stimulant, Nutmeg is also contraindicated during pregnancy and breastfeeding, as well as generally in babies, infants and sensitive individuals.

Dosage should be strictly followed for all preparations: when taken internally in much larger quantities, Nutmeg becomes sedative and narcotic because of its moderate cumulative toxicity. Absorption through the skin is generally low, however, and as usual will primarily treat topical (i.e. skin, muscle, tendon and joint) conditions.

**Pharmacological precautions:** Nutmeg oil carries cumulative toxicity because of its myristicin content that can cause potential neurotoxicity. This implies avoiding continuous internal use, especially on its own. Nutmeg is noted to contain very small levels of carcinogenic constituents which, however, are balanced by anticarcinogenic constituents such as limonene. It may be advisable to avoid internal use in cancerous conditions. Intake of spinach, high in phenethylamines, should also be avoided as it may cause hypertension (Franchomme 2015).

**Preparations:**

- Diffusor: 3–4 drops in water

- Massage oil: 1–3% dilution in a lotion or vegetable oil

- Liniment: 4–8% dilution in a vegetable carrier oil

- Gel cap: 1–2 drops per day maximum with some olive oil for short-term use only, e.g. a course of seven days and best used in a formula rather than on its own

## Chinese Medicine Functions and Indications

**Aroma energy:** Pungent

**Movement:** Rising

**Warmth:** Warm to hot

**Meridian tropism:** Kidney, Spleen, Stomach, Heart, Bladder

**Five-Element affinity:** Water, Fire, Earth

**Essential function:** To tonify and raise the Yang, warm the interior and strengthen the Shen

1.  **Tonifies the Yang and warms the Kidney; raises the clear Yang, animates the Heart and strengthens the Shen and libido**

    - **Kidney Yang deficiency with Shen weakness**, with chronic fatigue, exhaustion, lumbar pain, cold extremities, loss of sex drive, apathy, discouragement:
      Ginger/Black spruce/Black pepper

    - **Clear Yang Qi deficiency with Shen weakness**, with light-headedness, headaches, mental fog, poor focus, apathy, depression:
      Rosemary/Ravintsara/Peppermint

2.  **Warms and harmonizes the Middle Warmer, resolves damp and relieves pain and distension**

    - **Stomach-Spleen empty cold** (Spleen Yang deficiency with cold) with epigastric or abdominal pain, odourless loose stool, morning diarrhoea:
      Pimenta berry/Black pepper/Clove

    - **Stomach-Spleen damp-cold or toxic-damp** with chronic indigestion, abdominal bloating, diarrhoea:
      Patchouli/Niaouli/Thyme ct. thymol

    - **Stomach-Spleen Qi stagnation** with indigestion, epigastric bloating and pain, nausea, belching:
      Fennel/Peppermint/Cardamom

3.  **Harmonizes the Stomach, descends rebellious Qi and relieves vomiting**

    - **Stomach cold with Qi rebellion**, with nausea, hiccups, vomiting, travel sickness:
      Fennel/Ginger/Clove

4.  **Warms and activates the Lower Warmer, breaks up stagnation, promotes menstruation and relieves pain**

    - **Lower Warmer Blood and Qi stagnation with cold**, with painful, late, scanty or absent periods, painful periods, loss of sex drive:
      Ginger/Juniper berry/Fennel

5.  **Warms and opens the meridians, dispels wind-damp-cold, relaxes the tendons and relieves pain**

    - **Wind-damp-cold obstruction** with muscle aches, pains, cramping, joint stiffness:
      Rosemary/Niaouli/Frankincense

Remarks

A native of the Banda islands in the southern tip of the Maluku archipelago (the Moluccas) in East Indonesia, Nutmeg saw widespread distribution from earliest times. This was largely courtesy of enterprising Arabic seafaring traders who in the medieval period developed a vast maritime trade network from Egypt to India, on to Indonesia and up to Northeast China. Nutmeg is on record as having also been imported from Arabic traders into the port of Constantinople as far back as 540 and the Italian port of Genoa by the 11th century; the spice is documented as a deodorant aromatic for environmental smudging in 1158 by the city's spice merchants, the aromatarii, in emulation of traditional Roman practice. With its unique warm, musty aroma, Nutmeg in Europe soon became a valuable, expensive spice, like black pepper. Joining the ranks of other medicinal spices, it saw use in many a traditional European apothecary preparation, including the famous Carmelite Melissa Water, the Garrus Elixir, Paracelsus Elixir and many others.

The ruthless colonial Portuguese monopoly of the valuable nutmeg trade in the early 1500s was followed in later centuries by a calculating Dutch monopoly. It involved not only the forcible destruction of all trees save for those on the two islands of Banda and Amboina in 1650 (as with clove trees), but also the burning of 570,000 kg of surplus nutmegs in Amsterdam itself (1735). Eventually, a cunning French trader, Pierre Poivre, succeeded in absconding some priceless nuts to the equally colonial Indian Ocean island of Mauritius in 1772. In a domino effect, 1798 saw the British happily laying out nutmeg plantations in Sumatra and the island of Penang (where patchouli was also to become a major oil crop in the 1830s).

Nutmeg now yields a useful oil today that is produced in locations as different and as far apart as Java and Grenada – the latter now known as the 'nutmeg isle'. Used by internal methods of delivery, Nutmeg is essentially a strongly warming, stimulant remedy, like the majority of other tropical spice oils. Its basic indication is cold, weak and damp conditions, whether systemic or local, and especially when presenting as chronic terrain. Without going quite as far as the endocrine level, its systemic stimulant action is due to combined neurological and arterial circulatory engagement. The brain is therefore a major beneficiary of Nutmeg's cerebral stimulant action, with a list of very interesting indications that include hypochondria, agoraphobia, vertigo and depression in addition to the more common dizziness, fainting, somnolence, and so on found with similar oils. For depression, it has shown specifically to be an MAO inhibitor (Faucon 2015).

The next area in which Nutmeg excels is in the management of both acute and chronic painful rheumatic, arthritic and neuralgic conditions. Here a strong analgesic action is coupled with an anti-inflammatory one, the result of prostaglandin synthesis inhibition. We should not forget Nutmeg's circulatory stimulant action here too, with its net detoxicant effect in what energetic medicine calls damp conditions. For these, topical and internal delivery methods combined can be highly effective here.

At the level of the gut, Nutmeg acts as both a stimulant and relaxant, like Fennel and Laurel: the oil is reputed to be one of the most effective remedies for digestive and intestinal conditions in general. As a digestive/gastrointestinal stimulant, it addresses atonic conditions of the whole gut, from the stomach to the colon. As a digestive/gastrointestinal relaxant, its indications range from spasmodic, inflammatory gut disorders such as colitis and inflammatory bowel disease, to intestinal dysbiosis and fermentation, to bacterial enteritis with its production of toxins. Nutmeg sustains a good antibacterial effect throughout these conditions and is particularly valued by practitioners for altering gut dysbiosis and eliminating intestinal toxins. In energetic medicine this again is covered under the concept of damp, in this case intestinal toxic-damp. Interestingly, the key symptom that this oil treats in all of these instances is diarrhoea. In terms of symptom relief, this makes Nutmeg probably the finest remedy for treating diarrhoea.

When used by olfaction, Nutmeg as a psychological remedy again works deeply into the gut region, the physical seat of everything that is unknown to us – the unconscious. Its warm, spicy, sweet fragrance feels strengthening, supportive and protective. Nutmeg essentially encourages us to connect to our inner power and express it without fear of the consequences. It enables us to connect to our gut feelings and instincts in a safe, secure space, devoid of fear of the unknown. The fragrance is for those who feel weak, vulnerable, unprotected and easily hurt by others, and prone to lack of timidity, apprehension and discouragement. Just as the nutmeg seed protects itself with two layers of aril and rind, so it may help create firm personal boundaries as an expression of a grounded ego-self. It can provide the inner strength to say no to over-accommodate from fear of repercussions in the face of external demands. By promoting a self-assured, fearless expression of who we are deep down, Nutmeg is invaluable for helping develop a gut-felt sense of our true self-worth.

# Oregano

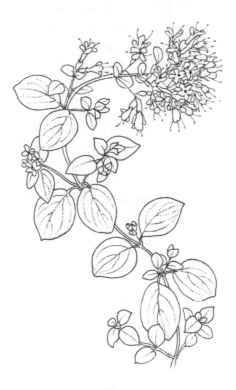

**Botanical source:** The herb of *Origanum vulgare* L. (Lamiaceae/Labiatae – lipflower/mint family), a widespread herb of West Asia and the Eastern Mediterranean

**Other names:** Common oregano, Wild oregano; Origan (Fr), Oregano (Ge, Sp), Origanon (Gr), Zatar (Arabic)

**Appearance:** A mobile brown-yellow liquid with a strong warm, spicy, herbaceous odour with some dry, acrid bottom notes

**Perfumery status:** A heart note of high intensity and poor persistence

**Extraction:** Steam distillation of the dried herb in flower, usually in August

**1 kg oil yield from:** 100–200 kg of the herb (a good yield)

**Production areas:** Turkey, Greece, Bulgaria, Bosnia-Herzegovina, Spain, Morocco

**Typical constituents:** Phenols 50–91% (incl. carvacrol 30–87%, thymol trace–6%) • monoterpenes <14% (incl. p-cymene 2–9%, α-pinene, α-thujene, α- and β-phellandrene, α-terpinene, γ-terpinene) • monoterpenols (incl. linalool 1–2%, borneol, terpinen-4-ol) • sesquiterpenes (incl. β-bisabolene, β-caryophyllene, aromadendrene, γ- and δ-cadinene) • sesquiterpenol spathulenol • caryophyllene oxide • adamantane

**Chance of adulteration:** Fairly good, as much commercial oregano oil is actually extracted from Capitate or Cretan thyme (*Thymus capitatus*) (see the Thyme ct. thymol profile), as well as from any one or several of the oregano species below

**Related oils:** The main species of *Origanum* distilled include the following. All of these oils except for Marjoram and Lavender oregano are chemically dominant in the phenol carvacrol. They may be used fairly interchangeably, like most of the acrid-herbaceous thyme oils that are also dominant in phenols. Like Oregano, they focus on treating acute symptoms rather than the chronic systemic condition or terrain and are also strongly skin irritant and sensitizing.

- Compact oregano (*Origanum compactum* Bentham) from Morocco and North Africa, with carvacrol levels of 30–70%, monoterpenes c. 25% and monoterpenols <10%

- Greek or Green oregano (*Origanum heracleoticum* L. ct. carvacrol) from Greece, with carvacrol levels of 50–75%, monoterpenes c. 15%

- Cretan oregano or Rigani (*Origanum onites* L. ct. carvacrol), from Greece, Turkey and Sicily, with carvacrol levels of 60–70%

- Moroccan oregano (*Origanum vulgare* L. subsp. *virens* Hoffmanns. & Link)

- Wavering oregano (*Origanum dubium* Boiss. ct. carvacrol), with carvacrol levels of 65–74%

- Lavender oregano (*Origanum dubium* Boiss. ct. linalool, syn. *Origanum smyrnaeum* L.), exceptionally with a lower carvacrol content of c. 23% and a high content of l-linalool c. 67%. This oregano chemotype was already reported by Gildemeister (1899) and was then called Smyrna oregano after its port of shipment (Smyrna is now Izmir)

- Marjoram (*Origanum maiorana* L.) with no or only traces of carvacrol and high levels of assorted monoterpenols (<50%) instead (see separate profile)

Because of their major dominance in the phenol carvacrol, and with their stimulating, heating nature, all of the above Oregano oils (if available) except for Lavender oregano and Marjoram have essentially the same functions, indications and cautions as the Common oregano. They all treat hypotonic/weak and asthenic/cold conditions with their typical physiological and psychological profiles.

Other essential oils dominant in carvacrol and with similar uses as the Oregano oils include Thyme ct. carvacrol and Winter savoury. Other oils with high levels of phenols in general include Thyme ct. thymol (see the profiles for Capitate thyme, Wild thyme and Moroccan thyme), as well as the eugenol-rich oils of Clove and Pimenta berry. High-phenol oils share a commonality but also show significant differences among them.

# Therapeutic Functions and Indications

## Specific symptomatology – *All applications*

Apathy, discouragement, self-neglect, flat affect, low self-esteem and self-confidence, pessimism, lethargy, drowsiness, stupor, mental confusion, poor focus, afternoon fatigue, low stamina, cold hands and feet, recurrent infections, coughing and wheezing with expectoration, chest distension, low sex drive, scanty or absent menstrual flow, painful periods, appetite loss, chronic diarrhoea, irregular bowel movement, epigastric or abdominal pain

## Psychological – *Aromatic diffusion*

**Essential PNEI function and indication:** Stimulant in weakness conditions
**Possible brain dynamics:** Increases basal ganglia and prefrontal cortex functioning
**Fragrance category:** Middle tone with green and pungent notes
**Indicated psychological disorders:** ADD, minor depression

### Promotes willpower, courage and self-confidence

- Low willpower or strength, indecision
- Discouragement with apathy, loss of motivation, self-neglect
- Low self-confidence and self-esteem, pessimism, depression

### Stimulates the mind and promotes alertness

- Lethargy, drowsiness, stupor
- Mental confusion, disorientation, poor concentration
- Mental and emotional burnout

## Physiological – *Suppository, gel cap, external applications*

Use with caution.
**Therapeutic status:** Mild remedy with no cumulative toxicity
**Topical safety status:** A strong skin irritant and sensitizer
**Tropism:** Nervous, respiratory, digestive, urogenital systems
**Essential diagnostic function:** Stimulates hypotonic/weak and warms asthenic/cold terrain conditions

PRIMARILY STIMULANT AND WARMING:

*strong systemic nervous and central arterial circulatory stimulant, SNS stimulant:* a wide range of asthenic (cold) and chronic hypotonic (weak) conditions with circulatory deficiency, chronic debility and fatigue; incl. convalescence, CFS

- *adrenal stimulant, hypertensive:* adrenal fatigue syndrome (esp. with afternoon or evening fatigue), hypotension

- *reproductive stimulant, aphrodisiac:* sexual debility, loss of libido (impotence, frigidity)

*diuretic*

PRIMARILY STIMULANT AND RELAXANT:

*bronchial stimulant and relaxant, expectorant, mucolytic, spasmolytic, bronchodilator, antitussive:* congestive and spasmodic lower respiratory conditions with dyspnoea and cough, incl. chronic bronchitis, emphysema, asthma, croup, whooping cough

*gastrointestinal stimulant and relaxant, aperitive, stomachic, carminative, spasmolytic, analgesic:* asthenic (cold) digestive conditions with indigestion, appetite loss, flatulence, diarrhoea; gastroenteritis, colitis, colic, IBS, abdominal pain in general

*neuromuscular stimulant and relaxant, analgesic, spasmolytic, anti-inflammatory:* chronic rheumatic and arthritic conditions with pain, cramps, stiffness

*strong antioxidant*

ANTIMICROBIAL ACTIONS:

*broad-spectrum anti-infective, antimicrobial, immunostimulant, detoxicant, diuretic:* a wide range of severe infections, esp. gastrointestinal, respiratory, urogenital, haematological, lymphatic; esp. acute

- *strong antibacterial:* bacterial infections both gram-positive and gram-negative, esp. with Staph. aureus, E. coli, Strep. pneumoniae, Pseudomonas, Salmonella, Mycobacterium, incl. gastroenteritis, colitis, dysentery, food poisoning, microbial toxicosis; bronchitis, whooping-cough, pharyngitis, rhinitis, adenitis; cystitis, nephritis; bacteraemia, malaria

- *antiviral:* misc. viral infections, esp. gastrointestinal, respiratory, urogenital, neurological, incl. viraemia, HSV-1, shingles, cold sores, viral bronchitis, pleurisy

- *strong antifungal:* fungal infections, incl. Candida spp.

- *strong anthelmintic, antiamoebic:* amoebic dysentery, amoebiasis

SYNERGISTIC COMBINATIONS

All for short-term use only: see 'Therapeutic precautions' below.

- Oregano + Thyme ct. thymol: strong anti-infective, immunostimulant and detoxicant for a wide range of severe viral, bacterial, fungal and parasitic infections of all body systems, esp. with weak, cold terrain (for short-term use)

- Oregano + Cinnamon bark: strong anthelmintic, antiamoebic, haemostatic for amoebic dysentery and a wide range of other intestinal parasites (for short-term use)

COMPLEMENTARY COMBINATIONS

All for short-term use only: see 'Therapeutic precautions' below.

- Oregano + Niaouli: strong anti-infective and immunostimulant for a wide range of acute viral, bacterial, fungal infections of all body systems (for short-term use)

- Oregano + Black spruce: strong anthelmintic for a wide range of intestinal parasites (for short-term use)

- Oregano + Rosemary: strong arterial, nervous and adrenal stimulant and hypertensive for chronic asthenia in cold, weak terrain, with cold limbs, fatigue or debility, loss of stamina, hypotension (for short-term use)

- Oregano + Lemongrass: strong digestive stimulant, aperitive, carminative in acute atonic digestive conditions with appetite loss, bloating (for short-term use)

- Oregano + Basil ct. methylchavicol: strong antiseptic expectorant, bronchodilator and antitussive in all spasmodic bronchial conditions with severe dyspnoea, apnoea, asthma, cough; spasmodic dysphonia (for short-term use)

- Oregano + Angelica root/Juniper berry: strong emmenagogue for chronic amenorrhoea, esp. from exposure to cold (for short-term use)

## TOPICAL – *Liniment, lotion*

See 'Pharmacological precautions' below.

**Lotion:** See 'Pharmacological precautions' below.

> *rubefacient, analgesic:* cold, lifeless, devitalized skin; rheumatic and neuralgic conditions in general; cellulite; sprains, strains

> *strong antiseptic:* infected cuts and wounds, acne, eczema, impetigo, psoriasis, leprosy

> *antiparasitic:* skin parasites, lice, fleas

**Therapeutic precautions:** Oregano oil is a strongly warming stimulant to nervous, circulatory and adrenal functions, and is therefore contraindicated in all hypersthenic/hot, hypertonic/tense and dry conditions or terrain, which may include high fever, acute inflammation, hypertension, agitation and insomnia. It should also be avoided in dry conditions. Because of this, and because it is a uterine stimulant, Oregano is also generally contraindicated during pregnancy and breastfeeding, as well as in babies, infants, young children and sensitive individuals in general.

Internal use should be limited to a single eight-day course, and then always within a formula rather than on its own, as with all high-phenol oils (see below). Long-term internal use may cause liver damage and inhibit the healthy microflora; this should be prevented with the adjunctive use of liver restorative oils and/or herbs, and prebiotic foods, supplements or oils. Inhalation with an essential oil nebulizer is not recommended to avoid serious irritation to the mucous membrane.

**Pharmacological precautions:** Because Oregano oil is highly dermocaustic (skin irritant), only very low dilutions should be used topically and clearly avoided in all damaged or diseased skin. Internally, carvacrol and thymol may interfere with blood clotting, making Oregano oil contraindicated in bleeding disorders or with concurrent intake of anticoagulant or diabetic medication.

**Preparations:**

- Diffusor: Not used

- Massage oil: Up to 1% dilution in vegetable oil after first doing a patch test

- Liniment: Up to 1% in a formula

- Gel cap: 1–2 drops with some olive oil for short-term use, e.g. an eight-day course; and usually as part of a formula; the maximum daily dose is 6 drops. Like all phenolic oils, Oregano should always be combined with other oils to soften its intensity and enhance treatment results; especially with sweet, monoterpenol-rich oils such as Palmarosa, Lavender, Tea tree or Thyme ct. linalool.

# Chinese Medicine Functions and Indications

**Aroma energy:** Pungent, green

**Movement:** Rising

**Warmth:** Warm to hot

**Meridian tropism:** Kidney, Lung, Spleen, Stomach

**Five-Element affinity:** Metal, Earth

**Essential function:** To tonify the Yang, warm the interior and strengthen the Shen

1. **Tonifies the Yang, warms the Kidney and strengthens the Shen and libido**

   - **Yang deficiency with Shen weakness**, with fatigue, apathy, cold hands and feet, loss of sex drive, recurrent infections:

     Pimenta berry/Black spruce/Clove

2. **Warms the Lung, circulates and descends Lung Qi, expels phlegm and relieves coughing and wheezing**

   - **Lung phlegm-cold with Qi accumulation**, with coughing, wheezing, sputum expectoration, chest distension, cold extremities:

     Grand fir/Hyssop/Green myrtle

   - **Lung Qi accumulation in other patterns**, with wheezing, chest distension and pain, coughing:

     Siberian fir/Cypress/Basil ct. methylchavicol

3. **Warms and harmonizes the Middle Warmer, resolves damp and relieves pain**

   - **Stomach-Spleen empty cold** (Spleen Yang deficiency with cold) with epigastric or abdominal pain, appetite loss, chronic diarrhoea, irregular bowel movement:

     Juniper berry/Ginger/Nutmeg

   - **Stomach-Spleen damp-cold** with chronic diarrhoea, undigested food in stool, cold limbs, debility, poor appetite:

     Patchouli/Nutmeg/Black pepper

4. **Warms and activates the Lower Warmer, breaks up stagnation and promotes menstruation**

   - **Lower Warmer Blood and Qi stagnation with internal cold**, with scanty or absent periods, painful periods, loss of sex drive:

     Rosemary/Niaouli/Juniper berry

REMARKS

Oregano is one of many classic herbal remedies of traditional Greek medicine with hundreds of years of empirical use by healers and doctors behind it. The herb was widely valued as a versatile cough and respiratory remedy, a fact confirmed by the Elder Pliny in his encyclopaedic *Historia Naturalis*. Its Greek name *Origanon* means 'joy of the mountains' and originates in the eastern Mediterranean, including Cyprus and southeast Turkey.

Oregano essential oil found early distillation and chemical investigation in Europe. Medical botanist Joseph Roques in 1837 was already able to report that 'L'huile volatile est très énergétique; on la prend par gouttes sur un morceau de sucre. On en fait des bains aromatiques, des fumigations, des lotions stimulantes' – 'The volatile oil is very energetic; it is taken by drops on a piece of sugar. It is used for making aromatic baths, fumigations and stimulating lotions.' This quote also confirms that in those days essential oils were widely used and prescribed in a variety of different delivery forms. Apparently, there was no shying away from the topical use of highly irritant oils either.

Today Oregano is highly valued for its broad antimicrobial potency, a use rationalized by its dominance in the phenolic compound carvacrol. However, it would be a severe fallacy to think of the oil as a mere substitute for antibiotics. When used as an internal remedy, each oil has a specific tropism or affinity for particular organs and tissues, not to mention energy meridians and acupuncture points. Each oil also possesses functional therapeutic properties that doctors of traditional Greek medicine have empirically developed for over 2,000 years. In short, therapeutic considerations will inform an oil's indications for use as much as, if sometimes not more than, its experimental activity against microbes and its pharmacognosy. This is no less true of Oregano, today's much popularized 'antibiotic' oil. To fully understand this aromatic remedy, we clearly need to move beyond seeing it through the 19th-century lens of microbial warfare – a simplistic, retrograde, reductionistic paradigm that is unfortunately still touted in allopathic medicine and its pharma-driven commercialization today.

Warm, herbaceous and acridly pungent, Oregano is another example of a strong general stimulant, especially to nervous, arterial circulatory and adrenal functions. With an equal affinity for the organs above and below the diaphragm, the oil addresses weak and/or cold respiratory, digestive and urogenital conditions. It is a good stimulant expectorant, digestive stimulant and neuromuscular stimulant. Within this broad therapeutic profile, Oregano has a built-in spasmolytic action on both smooth and striped muscles. Spasmodic respiratory conditions – as asthma, croup and spasmodic cough and dysphonia are – are thereby well served by it. In the gut, Oregano achieves a very comprehensive action on a range of atonic, cold and spasmodic symptoms. When any of these conditions involve an infectious component, this oil will manage it with ease.

Oregano's pharmacology, fragrance quality and therapeutic functions are very similar to those of Winter savoury. However, many practitioners claim that Oregano has more of an affinity for the respiratory tract and Winter savoury a greater affinity for the urogenital organs. Nevertheless, Oregano in Greece was as much valued among women doctors for its stimulant effect on sluggish or absent menstrual and sexual functioning as for respiratory functions.

As a psychological remedy by olfaction, Oregano plays a very similar role to Thyme ct. thymol from the same geographic region. The oil's warm, spicy-herbaceous fragrance enters deeply into the solar plexus region, stirring up issues of our sense of personal power, self-esteem and courage. Oregano is for the weak-willed individual who is easily manipulated, for poor self-discipline and courage leading to self-neglect and poor follow-through, and for low self-esteem leading to lack of self-confidence and pessimism. With insufficient mental and emotional energy, this person often presents mental fog, confusion and loss of focus, and often comes off as emotionally cold, withdrawn and unexpressive. Oregano can here be a valuable guide to the development of true self-empowerment, to becoming a free autonomous individual by the intentional exercise of choice and will.

# Petitgrain Bigarade

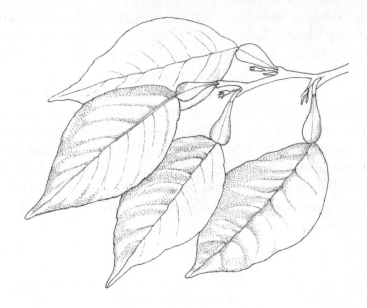

**Botanical source:** The twig and leaf of *Citrus aurantium* L. subsp. *amara*, the bitter orange (Rutaceae – citrus family), a widely cultivated fruit tree of warm climates

**Other names:** Bitter orange petitgrain, Bitter orange leaf; Petit grain bigarade (Fr)

**Appearance:** A mobile amber-yellow liquid with a fruity-sweet, warm-spicy odour with mild earthy-rooty base notes

**Perfumery status:** A heart note of medium intensity and poor persistence

**Extraction:** Steam distillation of the leaves, twigs and small branches in March, April or May when the harvest of the flowers for Neroli oil is over and the trees are pruned; also in October after the fruits appear. Until the 1950s, Petitgrain bigarade oil was a co-distillation of the bitter orange leaves, twigs and small, green unripe fruits, as its name implies. Since then, the tendency has been to distil only the leafy parts of the tree.

**1 kg oil yield from:** 150–200 kg of the leafy twigs (a good yield)

**Production areas:** Paraguay, Uruguay, South Italy, Morocco, Haiti. Petigrain distillation was brought from South France to Paraguay by French botanist Benjamin Balansa in the 1870s; Paraguay eventually became the main production area.

**Typical constituents:** Esters 50–75% (incl. linalyl acetate 46–70%, geranyl acetate <4%, neryl acetate <2%, terpenyl acetate) • monoterpenols 30–42% (incl. l-linalool 19–29%, α-terpineol 5–8%, geraniol 2–4%, nerol 1–2%, terpinen-4-ol 1%, citronellol) • monoterpenes 10% (incl. myrcene 1–6%, d-limonene <8%, cis/trans-β-cymenes 3–5%, p-cymene 1–4%, pinene, sabinene, γ-terpinene, trans-ocimene, terpinene, terpinolene) • methyl anthranilate (trace) • thymol (trace) • aldehydes (traces) • jasmone (trace)

**Chance of adulteration:** Fairly good, with both natural and synthetic materials. Many of the other petitgrain oils below are used to stretch Petitgrain bigarade, as well as Lemon and Lemongrass oil, and isolates such as citral, linalool, methyl anthranilate and others (Lis Balchin 2006). Sometimes Petitgrain bigarade is distilled from a variety or mix of leafy citrus twigs in the first place, including mandarin, clementine, sweet orange and bitter orange.

**Related oils:** The bitter orange tree that provides Petitgrain oil also yields Bitter orange oil (from the fruit rind) and Neroli oil (from the flower) (see the profiles for these oils). There are various other Petitgrain oils, each extracted from the leafy twigs of different citrus trees. Very few of these are used clinically, however.

- Bergamot petitgrain from *Citrus x bergamia*, with its fresh lemony fragrance and high levels of the aldehyde citral (45%), is a cooling, calming remedy with anti-inflammatory and nervous sedative actions.

- Mandarin petitgrain from *Citrus reticulata* var. *mandarine*, with a deep earthy-musty spicy aroma, contains c. 50% levels of the ester N-methyl anthranilate; it is used as a strong nervous sedative with spasmolytic and analgesic actions for acute anxiety, agitation and insomnia, especially with spasms or pain present.

- Kaffir or Combava lime petitgrain from *Citrus hystrix* from Indonesia and Madagascar, with its fine-powdery lime-citrus top notes, is a cooling, calming remedy with good anti-inflammatory, nervous sedative and analgesic actions. The dominant constituent is the aldehyde citronellal (45–85%) with <9% of mixed monoterpenols. Like the similar Lemon eucalyptus, it is particularly indicated in conditions of acute musculoskeletal pain and inflammation.

- Sweet orange petitgrain from *Citrus x sinensis* shows a fresh-fruity and earthy aroma, and an olive-green to green-orange colour.

- Clementine petitgrain from *Citrus x reticulata* var. *clementine* has a deep earthy-musty spicy aroma; clementine is a hybrid between the bitter orange and the mandarin.

- Lemon petitgrain from *Citrus limonum*.

Very occasionally a producer will distil a Petitgrain oil in the original, traditional manner, namely a codistillation of the leafy end-twigs and the unripe green fruits. The result is a much sweeter oil with a fuller, rounder middle note.

The aromatic water or hydrosol remaining after Petitgrain distillation is called Eau de brout, from which an absolute extract is also made by solvent extraction for perfumery purposes.

# Therapeutic Functions and Indications

## SPECIFIC SYMPTOMATOLOGY – *All applications*

Irritability, frustration, mood swings, distraction, emotional confusion, nervous tension, chronic anxiety, fearfulness, chronic sleeping problems, chronic fatigue, disconnection, spaciness, euphoria, delusion, palpitations, rapid heart beats, digestive problems worse with stress, irregular stool

## PSYCHOLOGICAL – *Aromatic diffusion, whole-body massage*

**Essential PNEI function and indication:** Regulating in dysregulation conditions; relaxant in overstimulation conditions

**Possible brain dynamics:** Reduces deep limbic and cingulate system hyperfunctioning

**Fragrance category:** Middle tone with sweet, rooty notes

**Indicated psychological disorders:** Bipolar disorder, minor depression anxiety states

### PROMOTES EMOTIONAL STABILITY AND STRENGTH

- Emotional instability with conflict, with mood swings, worry, fearfulness

- Negativity, frustration, irritability

- Loss of emotional security and strength, burnout

- Anxiety with depression

## PHYSIOLOGICAL – *Nebulizer inhalation, gel cap, suppository, external applications*

**Therapeutic status:** Mild remedy with no cumulative toxicity

**Topical safety status:** Non-irritant, non-sensitizing (including non-photosensitizing unless the oil has been adulterated with a citrus rind oil, e.g. Sweet orange oil, which contains photosensitizing coumarins)

**Tropism:** Nervous, cardiovascular, digestive, respiratory systems

**Essential diagnostic function:** Relaxes hypertonic/tense and regulates dysregulated terrain conditions

### PRIMARILY RELAXANT:

*systemic nervous relaxant, SNS inhibitor, vagotonic:* a large variety of acute and chronic hypertonic (tense) and spasmodic conditions; stress-related conditions in general

- *mild cerebral sedative, mild hypnotic:* agitation, mild anxiety, insomnia, vertigo, ADHD

- *gastrointestinal relaxant, spasmolytic, carminative:* upper digestive indigestion, epigastric cramps and colic, flatulence, IBS

- *neurocardiac relaxant and regulator:* cardiac neurosis and dysrhythmia (nervous heart), palpitations, tachycardia

- *respiratory relaxant and regulator:* spasmodic dyspnoea, cough and dysphonia; asthma, irregular breathing patterns

- *uterine relaxant:* spasmodic dysmenorrhoea

- *anti-inflammatory:* chronic arthritis, rheumatic conditions

PRIMARILY REGULATING:

*autonomic nervous (PNS/SNS) regulator:* ANS dysregulation with mood, respiratory, digestive and temperature disorders, especially stress- and trauma-related; alternating constipation and diarrhoea, menopausal syndrome with hot flushes, hyperthyroid syndrome

PRIMARILY RESTORATIVE:

*nervous trophorestorative and cerebral restorative:* nervous exhaustion, burnout or breakdown, esp. emotional; neurasthenia; with chronic insomnia, anxious depression, anxiety; convalescence, incl. postpartum; tinnitus

*liver decongestant:* liver congestion, chronic hepatitis

ANTIMICROBIAL ACTIONS:

*antifungal:* fungal infections with Candida spp., Microsporum spp., Aspergillus spp., incl. tinea/ringworm, candidiasis

*mild antibacterial, anti-inflammatory:* respiratory infections, incl. bronchitis; infected boils, furuncles

SYNERGISTIC COMBINATIONS

- Petitgrain + Lavender: nervous relaxant and spasmolytic in many stress-related and/or spasmodic conditions, incl. neurogenic digestive conditions, asthma, 'nervous heart', tachycardia, insomnia

- Petitgrain + Mandarin/Bergamot: nervous relaxant, sedative and regulator for mood swings, nervous tension, anxiety, insomnia, stress- or mood-related digestive problems

- Petitgrain + Siberian fir/Fennel: bronchial and gastrointestinal regulator and relaxant: spasmodic dyspnoea and cough; asthma, whooping cough; all spasmodic digestive symptoms

- Petitgrain + Clary sage: nervous sedative and restorative in chronic tense-weak conditions with fatigue, insomnia, chronic stress; neurasthenia with fatigue, burnout, exhaustion (incl. postpartum, convalescence)

- Petitgrain + Coriander seed: nervous trophorestorative and antidepressant for nervous exhaustion or breakdown, chronic depression, insomnia or anxiety

- Petitgrain + Bergamot/Cardamom: ANS regulator for dysregulated respiratory, digestive, mood and temperature disorders; menopausal syndrome, hyperthyroid syndrome

COMPLEMENTARY COMBINATIONS

- Petitgrain + Ravintsara: nervous restorative and sedative for neurasthenia with fatigue, burnout, depression, chronic insomnia, anxiety

- Petitgrain + Angelica root: cerebral sedative and nervous restorative for ADD, ADHD, chronic neurasthenia, nervous burnout or breakdown, convalescence

- Petitgrain + Ylang ylang no. 1: nervous and systemic relaxant in severe stress-related conditions, e.g. asthma, tachycardia, hypertension, colic, IBS

- Petitgrain + Cypress/Marjoram: bronchial relaxant and antitussive for asthma, spasmodic cough and dyspnoea, whooping cough

TOPICAL – *Liniment, ointment, cream, compress and other cosmetic preparations*

**Skin care:** Combination and oily skin types

*skin detoxicant, cellular regenerator:* skin impurities, devitalized skin, scars

*antibacterial and antifungal antiseptic:* acne, boils, furuncles, rosacea; fungal infections

*lipolytic:* oily skin, scalp and hair, seborrhoea

*astringent:* excessive perspiration

*deodorant:* environmental use

**Therapeutic precautions:** None

**Pharmacological precautions:** None

**Preparations:**

- Diffusor: 3–5 drops in water

- Massage oil: 2–5% dilution in a lotion or vegetable oil

- Liniment: 5–10% dilution in a vegetable carrier oil

- Gel cap: 2–3 drops with some olive oil

## Chinese Medicine Functions and Indications

**Aroma energy:** Sweet, rooty

**Movement:** Circulating

**Warmth:** Neutral

**Meridian tropism:** Heart, Liver, Lung

**Five-Element affinity:** Wood, Fire

**Essential function:** To regulate the Qi, settle the Heart and harmonize the Shen

1. **Regulates the Qi, relaxes constraint, settles the Heart and harmonizes the Shen**

   - **Heart and Liver Qi constraint with Shen dysregulation**, with insomnia, palpitations, mood swings, irritability, anxiety with possible depression:

     Lavender/Marjoram/German camomile/Ylang ylang

   - **Liver-Stomach/Spleen disharmony** with indigestion, mood swings, bloating, poor appetite, colic, digestive symptoms worse from stress feelings:

     Lemongrass/Peppermint/Basil ct. methylchavicol

2. **Nourishes Heart Blood, settles the Heart and harmonizes the Shen**

   - **Heart Blood deficiency with Shen dysregulation**, with insomnia, restlessness, anxiety, papitations:

     Palmarosa/Cardamom/Clary sage

3. **Circulates and descends Lung Qi, and relieves wheezing and coughing**

   - **Lung Qi accumulation** with irregular breathing, chest distension, wheezing, coughing, feelings of stress:

     Fennel/Cypress/Basil ct. methylchavicol

REMARKS

The name 'petit grain bigarade' in French literally means 'small grains of the bitter orange'. 'Bigarade' refers to the French word for the bitter orange tree, *bigaradier*, which derives from the Provencal *bigarrado*, meaning 'mottled'. The name of this oil originates from the earliest days – probably the 17th century, when natural perfumery really began to flourish – when the oil was distilled only from the small, green unripe bitter oranges, usually the size of large cherries. Over the years, Petitgrain bigarade oil has seen a gradual transformation. At first, the pure green bitter orange fruit oil came to include leaves and twigs, a co-distillation that was practised well into the 1950s. Since then, the tendency has been to only distil the leafy parts of the tree without any fruits. Although now a misnomer, the name 'petitgrain' has stuck. Regardless, this is a valuable and much-used remedy of the materia aromatica.

As a physiological remedy, Petitgrain bigarade belongs to an elite group of oils that combine regulating, relaxant and restorative actions on the nervous system. These actions are also evident in its pharmacology, with dominant calming esters and restorative monoterpenols enhanced with a garnish of bracing monoterpenes. As a prime balancing oil, Petitgrain essentially treats dysregulation of the organs above the diaphragm, when these swing in alternation from tension to weakness. The oil works equally to relax and balance cardiac, respiratory and upper gastrointestinal functions. As a cardiac relaxant, it can be seen as a gentler, more practical version of Neroli for nervous heart conditions, palpitations and tachycardia. As a bronchial relaxant, Petitgrain will treat both spasmodic coughs and asthmatic conditions in general. As a gastrointestinal relaxant, it will relieve most symptoms of nervous indigestion. French practitioners think of this oil whenever these conditions are caused by an emotional disturbance; when the individual symptom picture includes prominent emotional distress.

Moreover, Petitgrain is especially indicated when these forms of spasmodic tension become chronic, causing underlying weakness. This oil is especially useful for a terrain of chronic tension and weakness, resulting in nervous system depletion. Petitgrain is particularly high in linalyl acetate, a well-established nervous restorative constituent also found in Lavender. The oil exerts a good nervous trophorestorative effect that will serve chronic neurasthenic, exhausted conditions of the above organ functions. Any chronic condition needing additional nervous support – a common situation – will also benefit from the inclusion of Petitgrain in a formula.

When used purely by olfaction, Petitgrain bigarade exerts a good calming and grounding effect on the psyche, embodied in its sweet and rooty fragrance energies. Just as it regulates tension on a physiological level, so it also has the ability to regulate emotional tone and harmonize mood. Petitgrain bigarade has become a classic among practitioners for promoting emotional stability and relieving mood swings with its retinue of symptoms – frustration, irritability and negativity on one hand and worry, anxiety and depression on the other.

The gently inhaled oil is also specific for treating emotional burnout and its consequences – worry, anxiety, sleepless nights and anxious depression. Here Petitgrain bigarade can help the individual let go of repetitive thinking, fretting about past mistakes and poor decisions made, and support connecting with his or her gut feelings instead. In this realm of subconscious instinct, the oil can resolve individual neurosis into the pool of collective safety. It can immerse one into the security, support and comfort of the unspoken values and assumptions of one's family and ancestral heritage. By engendering feelings of deep acceptance and nurture, Petitgrain bigarade can help one relieve deep-seated feelings of insecurity, loss of safety and anxiety. In connecting one to sublimated emotions in one's personal history, the oil can also provide valuable support for coming to terms with past unresolved contradictions, of accepting and integrating the negative along with the positive.

# Pimenta Berry

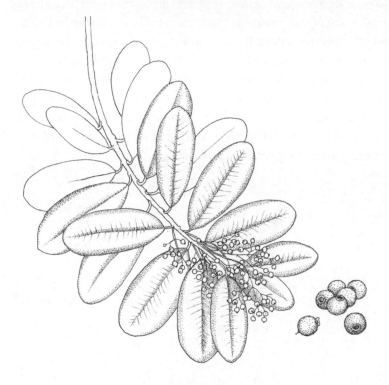

**Botanical source:** The fruit of *Pimenta dioica* (L.) Merr. (syn. *P. officinalis* Lindl.) (Myrtaceae – myrtle family), an evergreen midcanopy tree of the Caribbean tropics

**Other names:** Pimento, Allspice, Jamaica pepper, Clove pepper; Piment de la Jamaïque (Fr), Pimienta de Jamaica (Sp), Piment, Nelkenpfeffer (Ge), Bahar (Arabic)

**Appearance:** A mobile pale yellow to amber liquid with a light warm-spicy, sweet odour reminiscent of cloves and cinnamon.

The essential oil extracted by $CO_2$ has a semi-viscous intense olive-green liquid with a warm, spicy, woody odour somewhat reminiscent of Ginger $CO_2$ oil.

**Perfumery status:** A heart note of low intensity and poor tenacity; the $CO_2$ oil has better tenacity

**Extraction:** Steam distillation of the crushed, dried, unripe green berries throughout the year; cohobation is usually practised; an oil extracted by $CO_2$ technology may also be available

**1 kg oil yield from:** 30–50 kg of the dried berries (a good yield)

**Production areas:** Jamaica, Grenada, Mexico, India

**Typical constituents:** Phenols (incl. eugenol 70–94%, isoeugenol 6%, methylchavicol) • methyleugenol 3–13% • sesquiterpenes (incl. β-caryophyllene 3–7%, humulene, selinene, cadinene, calamenene) • 1,8 cineole <3% • monoterpenes (incl. limonene <4%, α-pinene, β-pinene, myrcene, phellandrene, terpinolene) • hydrocarbons (octane, undecane, dodecane) • p-cymene, ar-curcumene • alcohols terpineol, linalool, caryophyllene alcohol • caryophyllene aldehyde

**Chance of adulteration:** Moderate, especially with isolated or synthetic eugenol. Common classic adulterants are Pimenta leaf oil (itself sometimes adulterated with clove stem and leaf oils), Bay rum berry oil (*Pimenta racemosa*) and the oil of *Pimenta dioica* var. *tabasco*, a species with less aromatic berries and lower eugenol content. Confusion among local pickers between similar-looking pimento and bay rum trees is common and may also contribute to falsify the final oil; this was already noted by Gildemeister (1899).

**Related oils:** Pimenta leaf oil, a brownish yellow liquid with a warm-spicy, dry balsamic odour that lacks the sweetness of the berry oil. Bay rum berry and Bay rum leaf oils are distilled from the related species *Pimenta racemosa*, the West Indies bay rum tree (see below).

## Therapeutic Functions and Indications

### SPECIFIC SYMPTOMATOLOGY – *All applications*

Apathy, discouragement, loss of self-confidence, low self-esteem, insecurity, cold hands and feet, feels cold easily, chronic fatigue, debility, late-afternoon fatigue, low vitality, mental exhaustion, spaciness, delusions, depression for no reason, appetite loss, indigestion with bloating and pain, abdominal colic, chronic diarrhoea, undigested food in stool, loss of sex drive, scanty or stopped periods, muscle and joint aches and pains, headache

### PSYCHOLOGICAL – *Aromatic diffusion, whole-body massage*

**Essential PNEI function and indication:** Stimulant in weakness conditions

**Possible brain dynamics:** Increases basal ganglia functioning

**Fragrance category:** Middle tone with sweet, woody and pungent notes

**Indicated psychological disorders:** ADD, depression, dissociative disorder, psychotic and schizoid conditions

PROMOTES MOTIVATION AND SELF-CONFIDENCE

- Loss of motivation, discouragement
- Low self-confidence and self-esteem, depression, self-neglect

PROMOTES GROUNDING, STABILITY AND STRENGTH

- Insecurity, vulnerability
- Mental and emotional instability, anxiety, fearfulness
- Disconnection, oversensitivity, delusion, paranoia, dissociation
- Mental and emotional burnout

PHYSIOLOGICAL – *Nebulizer inhalation, gel cap, suppository, external applications*

**Therapeutic status:** Mild remedy with no cumulative toxicity

**Topical safety status:** Non-irritant, possibly moderately sensitizing

**Tropism:** Nervous, respiratory, digestive, urogenital systems

**Essential diagnostic function:** Warms asthenic/cold and stimulates hypotonic/weak terrain conditions

PRIMARILY STIMULANT AND WARMING:

*systemic nervous and central arterial circulatory stimulant, SNS stimulant:* a wide range of asthenic (cold) and chronic hypotonic (weak) conditions with circulatory deficiency, chronic debility and fatigue; incl. convalescence, CFS

- *adrenal stimulant, hypertensive:* adrenal fatigue syndrome (esp. with afternoon or evening fatigue), hypotension

- *thyroid/thyroxine stimulant:* hypothyroid syndrome (thyroxine resistance), with cold, fatigue, depression

- *uterine stimulant, emmenagogue, parturient:* amenorrhoea, oligomenorrhoea, stalled labour (uterine dystocia)

- *mild reproductive stimulant, aphrodisiac:* sexual debility, loss of libido

- *gastrointestinal stimulant, carminative, antifermentative/anti-putrifactive:* atonic lower gastrointestinal indigestion with bloating, pain, appetite loss; intestinal fermentation, dysbiosis, esp. bacterial

- *strong antioxidant*

PRIMARILY RELAXANT:

*spasmolytic, anti-inflammatory, analgesic:* acute spasmodic and inflammatory conditions with pain, esp. local, intestinal and musculoskeletal, incl. toothache, headache, intestinal colic, spasmodic IBS, dysmenorrhoea, neuralgia, rheumatic and arthritic conditions

*anti-oestrogenic:* oestrogen accumulation syndrome

ANTIMICROBIAL ACTIONS:

***broad-spectrum anti-infective, immunostimulant, anti-inflammatory, deep lymphatic stimulant:*** a wide range of infections, esp. neurological, gastrointestinal, urinary

- *strong antiviral:* shingles, viral neuritis, polio, enteritis, enterocolitis, viral hepatitis, influenza, dengue fever

- *strong broad-spectrum antibacterial:* both gram-positive and gram-negative bacteria, incl. mucous colitis, cholera, amoebic dysentery; bronchitis, sinusitis, cystitis, nephritis, salpingitis, abscesses; malaria

- *broad-spectrum antifungal:* fungal infections, incl. candidiasis, athlete's foot, nail-bed fungus, tinea/ringworm, jock itch

- *anthelmintic:* intestinal parasites

SYNERGISTIC COMBINATIONS

- Pimenta berry + Thyme ct. thymol: strong broad-spectrum anti-infective, immunostimulant, antiviral, antibacterial, antifungal and antiparasitic in a wide range of acute infections; esp. in weak, cold terrain, with chronic physical and mental fatigue, cold, recurring infections (for short-term use)

- Pimenta berry + Winter savoury: strong antibacterial and antiviral for urinary infections, incl. cystitis, urethritis, nephritis (for short-term use)

- Pimenta berry + Clove bud: thyroid restorative/stimulant in many hypothyroid and thyroxine resistance syndromes, esp. with fatigue, cold, depression (for short-term use)

COMPLEMENTARY COMBINATIONS

- Pimenta berry + Rosemary: nervous, circulatory and adrenal stimulant in a wide range of cold and weak conditions with fatigue, loss of stamina, chronic debility; hypotension, adrenal fatigue syndrome

- Pimenta berry + Carrot seed/Green myrtle: thyroid restorative/stimulant in many hypothyroid and thyroxine resistance syndromes, esp. with fatigue, depression

- Pimenta berry + Black pepper: strong analgesic and anti-inflammatory for acute local pain, esp. rheumatic, arthritic and neuralgic (also topically)

- Pimenta berry + Niaouli: strong broad-spectrum anti-infective, antimicrobial, immunostimulant, esp. antiviral and antibacterial in a wide range of acute and chronic infections; esp. with chronic physical and mental fatigue, cold, recurring infections

- Pimenta berry + Juniper berry/Laurel: gastrointestinal stimulant, carminative, analgesic and antifermentative for chronic indigestion, intestinal dysbiosis or food poisoning with bloating, flatulence, colic, diarrhoea

- Pimenta berry + Cinnamon/Nutmeg: antiparasitic for intestinal and other parasites, incl. amoebiasis, amoebic dysentery

- Pimenta berry + Fennel/Juniper berry: uterine stimulant, emmenagogue, analgesic for oligomenorrhoea, amenorrhoea, dysmenorrhoea; long cycles

## TOPICAL – *Liniment, ointment, cream, compress and other cosmetic preparations*

**Skin care:** Oily skin

*vulnerary, antispetic:* chronic infected wounds, ulcers, boils; furuncles, abscesses (incl. dental), gum infection, infected acne

*antifungal:* fungal skin conditions, incl. athlete's foot

*analgesic, rubefacient, counterirritant:* toothache, insect bites, arthritic/rheumatic pain; weak spongy gums; hair loss; for sports warm-up

*insect repellent, moderate tick-repellent, larvicidal:* mosquitoes, moths, flies, mites, ticks

*deodorant*

**Hair and scalp care:**

*hair restorative and stimulant:* weak or oily hair, hair loss, dandruff, seborrhoea

**Therapeutic precautions:** Because of its systemic stimulant, warming nature, Pimenta berry is contraindicated in hypersthenic/hot, hypertonic/tense conditions, including with acute inflammation, high fever, agitation, hypertension, and hyperadrenal and hyperthyroid syndromes. It should also be avoided with symptoms of dryness present, and in babies, infants, sensitive individuals and nursing mothers. Being a mild uterine stimulant, internal use of Pimenta berry is also contraindicated throughout pregnancy.

Internal use should be limited to ten-day courses, and then usually within a formula rather than on their own, as with all high-phenol oils. Long-term internal use may cause liver damage and inhibit the healthy microflora; this should be prevented with the concomitant use of liver restoratives and prebiotic foods, supplements or oils.

**Pharmacological precautions:** Pimenta berry oil is essentially non-irritant to the skin when used in proper dilution. Still, care should be taken to avoid any potential long-term sensitization in some people because of its eugenol content; the oil is clearly contraindicated in all forms of dermatitis.

Pimenta berry is contraindicated in those taking anticoagulant medication as the oil's eugenol content may inhibit blood clotting. Although there is a theoretical risk of Pimenta berry's methyleugenol content acting as a carcinogenic, its dominant constituent eugenol is anticarcinogenic and is likely to quench the former's carcinogenic potential. Its constituents, limonene and caryophyllene, would also inhibit such activity. In addition, no record of a carcinogenic risk is recorded in French medicine, and no related prohibition exists in French pharmacy regulations.

**Preparations:**

- Diffusor: 2–4 drops in water, also to deodorize or disinfect

- Massage oil: 2–4% dilution in vegetable oil

- Counterirritant liniment: 5–10% dilution in vegetable oil for short-term use

- Spot application: 1 drop on tooth or gums for toothache, tooth abscess, gum disease; 2 drops on a boil, furuncle or abscess to promote maturation

- Gel cap: 1–3 drops with olive oil for short-term use, e.g. an eight-day course; and usually as part of a formula; the maximum daily dose is 8 drops. Like all phenolic oils, Pimenta berry should always be combined with other oils to soften its intensity and enhance treatment results; especially with sweet, monoterpenol-rich oils such as Palmarosa, Lavender, Tea tree or Thyme ct. linalool.

## Chinese Medicine Functions and Indications

**Aroma energy:** Pungent, sweet, woody

**Movement:** Stabilizing

**Warmth:** Warm to hot

**Meridian tropism:** Kidney, Spleen, Stomach

**Five-Element affinity:** Water, Earth

**Essential function:** To tonify the Yang, warm the interior and strengthen the Shen

1. **Tonifies the Yang, warms the Kidney and strengthens the Shen**

   - **Kidney Yang deficiency with Shen weakness**, with fatigue, cold extremities, apathy, loss of self-confidence, low sex drive:

     Rosemary/Ginger/Black spruce/Clove

2. **Warms and harmonizes the Stomach, resolves accumulation and relieves pain**

   - **Stomach cold with food stagnation**, with indigestion, appetite loss, epigastric and/or abdominal bloating, nausea, belching:

     Juniper berry/Cypress/Fennel/Black pepper

   - **Stomach cold with shan qi**, with sharp or colicky abdominal pain:

     Fennel/Peppermint/Nutmeg

3. **Warms and harmonizes the Middle Warmer, resolves damp and relieves pain**

   - **Stomach-Spleen damp-cold** with chronic diarrhoea, undigested food in stool, cold limbs:

     Patchouli/Nutmeg/Black pepper

   - **Stomach-Spleen empty cold** (Spleen Yang deficiency with cold) with nausea, vomiting, epigastric or abdominal pain, chronic loose stool:

     Juniper berry/Ginger/Nutmeg/Basil (all cts.)

4. **Warms and activates the Lower Warmer, breaks up stagnation and promotes menstruation**

   - **Lower Warmer Blood and Qi stagnation with cold**, with scanty or absent periods:

     Rosemary/Juniper berry/Thyme ct. thymol

REMARKS

The pimento is an elegant tropical midcanopy tree whose berries are distilled to produce Pimenta berry oil. Thriving in hot, humid climates, the coastal tree is native to Cuba, Jamaica and the necklace of islands of the Greater Antilles in the Caribbean and extends over the Yucatan peninsula in Mexico and southward into Central America. The small, seedlike berries were much used by native Caribs and Mayans for flavouring chocolate beverages, a tradition that is still alive in Mexico today. On his second voyage to the West Indies, Christopher Columbus noted the trees on Jamaica in 1494; sailors made regular use of the berries' antiseptic preservative effect to prevent fish from spoiling on their long transatlantic voyages. Sephardic Jews, diaspora refugees from Andalusia in Iberia living in Santiago de la Vega (now Spanish Town) in Jamaica, were the original exporters of the exotic berries to hungry Old World ports such as Genoa, Venice, London, Amsterdam and Constantinople (Nabhan 2014).

It was apparently the English who in the late 16th century finally renamed pimento berries 'allspice', which soon became *piment quatres épices* in French. The chewed berry really does kick off with a sharp taste of pepper, rapidly followed by zings of clove, cinnamon and nutmeg – courtesy of the chemical synergy of eugenol, methyleugenol and beta-caryophyllene. The popular berry is now found extensively not only in Caribbean but also in numerous Middle Eastern dishes.

It should be noted that, because of the similar appearance and treatment use of Pimento and Bay rum berries and leaves, there is some confusion as to the therapeutic poperties of each remedy. This confusion exists not only in the Caribbean itself, but also in the French literature on essential oils. Sadly, even relatively modern research papers are known to confuse or conflate various species of Pimenta. Although the use of *P. dioica* and *P. racemosa* is similar, and varies between the berry and the leaf, each has particular therapeutic emphases (see below).

Pimenta berry's taste is a giveaway to its therapeutic nature and applications. The oil is very much in the league of other spicy, sweet, warming stimulant oils. It would be no exaggeration to say that Pimenta berry is only a slightly milder version of Clove oil, possessing the same functions and indications, but in an easier-to-use and safer package. Like Clove, this oil is a systemic warming stimulant working through the arterial circulation, sympathetic nervous system and adrenal and thyroid glands, essentially addressing cold and weak terrain. In the first phase of labour, it is also a good uterine stimulant for both amenorrhoea and situations of stalled labour. Its relaxant actions may not be quite as strong as Clove's, but it is still widely valued for treating the same acute painful spasmodic and inflammatory conditions.

Again thanks to its high but safe levels of eugenol, Pimenta berry is an excellent all-round anti-infective remedy with potent action against viral, bacterial, fungal and parasitic infections. It is notably a deep lymphatic stimulant here and is especially indicated in chronic infections arising from cold, weak terrain. When used in topical preparations, Pimenta berry acts very much like the tincture with a good combination of actions for treating chronic wounds, especially infected ones. As a non-irritant rubefacient and analgesic, the oil is also indicated for any kind of soft tissue pain. In short, Pimenta berry does everything we wish we could do with Clove oil but usually cannot because of its skin irritation.

The olfactory use of Pimenta berry for aromatic therapy brings us face to face with issues related to our true power. Its warm, pungent and somewhat woody fragrance allows us to connect with our inner resources, thereby loosening the long-held grip of deeply rooted cultural conditioning around them. Unblocking emotional obstruction, the inhaled oil will help release bound-up, long-held distressed emotions that we are barely aware of any more. It especially targets distressed emotions associated with loss of freedom and imagination, and loss of childhood creativity resulting from power issues in upbringing. Pimenta berry can generally help us let go of suppressed, uncomfortable feelings that we may still cling to for sheer safety. As a result, the oil can be a valuable ally for those who are discouraged, lack motivation and self-confidence, and are incapable of genuine emotional responses. For these individuals, through releasing emotional stuckness, Pimenta berry will support the potential for their own authentic power to arise.

**Related oils:** Several other related oils should be considered separately from Pimenta berry oil, even though the eugenol chemotype of Bay rum has a very similar therapeutic profile.

**Pimenta leaf oil** is a brownish-yellow, dry-woody, warm spicy liquid that is only produced in Jamaica. It carries virtually the same functions and indications as Pimenta berry oil. However, because it is somewhat more fresh-pungent and less sweet in aroma, by olfaction it provides a good uplifting effect on mental functions and is invigorating in states of loss of self-confidence, optimism and motivation. Its chemical profile is also almost identical, with eugenol at 65–96%, methyleugenol 1–4% and sesquiterpenes <8%; it will essentially also treat hypotonic/weak, hyposthenic/cold conditions, especially when involving chronic infections. Pimenta leaf, like the berry oil, enjoys mild therapeutic status with no cumulative toxicity and is non-irritant or sensitizing for the skin; the same cautions and dilutions as for Pimenta berry apply.

**Bay rum leaf** (*Pimenta racemosa* var. *racemosa* [Miller] J. Moore), also known as West Indian bay and Bois d'Inde in French and French Creole, is distilled mainly in the Caribbean islands of Jamaica, Dominica and Guadeloupe for the production of bay rum liniment. The tree occurs widely in the Lesser Antilles from Antigua, St. Thomas and Barbados in the north down to Trinidad and Venezuela in the south. The medicinal use of the leaves and berries in infusion and decoction goes back to indigenous Carib tribes, while the leaves are a common spice in many Creole dishes. Longuefosse (2008) traces its reported uses back to 1667, many centring around the analgesic Bay rum friction and liniment.

Bay rum has three known chemotypes, the ct. eugenol being the most common by far. Other chemotypes may well exist.

**Bay rum ct. eugenol** with its warm, clove-like aroma shows the phenol eugenol dominant at 40–75% but also contains methylchavicol 10–22% and methyleugenol; monoterpenes including myrcene <32%; monoterpenols including linalool <3%; and the aldehydes citral, citronellal, neral and geranial. This oil is a mild remedy with no cumulative toxicity but mildly skin irritant, with the same dilutions and precautions as for Pimenta berry. It is very similar in character and uses to Pimenta berry. The main clinical difference between the two oils is that Bay rum is more often used for its analgesic action with rheumatic and arthritic pains, etc., while Pimenta berry is noted especially for its restorative and stimulant actions in cold, weak conditions with hypofunctioning circulation, thyroid, adrenals and nervous system. Pimenta berry and leaf oils are also more commonly selected for treating infectious conditions.

**Bay rum ct. citral**, or Lemon-scented bay rum, is high in citral (<80%) and very low in eugenol. This suggests uses similar to May chang, Lemongrass and Melissa in respect to both physiological and psychological applications. The same therapeutic and topical safety status, cautions and dilutions apply as with these three oils.

**Bay rum ct. methylchavicol**, with its aniseed-like aroma, is high in methyleugenol (<44%) and methylchavicol (<32%) and also very low in eugenol; this implies uses similar to Basil ct. methylchavicol and Tarragon. The same therapeutic and topical safety status, cautions and dilutions apply as with these two oils.

# Rose

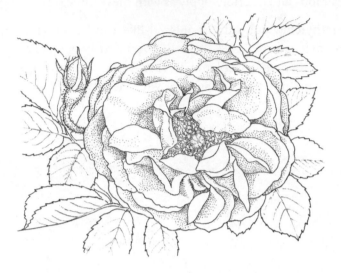

**Botanical source:** The flower of *Rosa x damascena* P. Mill. (Rosaceae – rose family), an inland cultivated shrub of mild to warm Mediterranean climates. Several Damask rose cultivars supply production of rose essential oil worldwide; e.g. in Bulgaria the Kazanlak damask rose is used: *R. x damascena* var. *trigintipetala* (Dieck) Koehne. According to modern genetic tests, the Damask rose originated in Central Asia as a hybrid of Rosa moschata and Rosa gallica crossed with the pollen of Rosa fedtschenkoana (Iwata *et al.* 2000).

**Other names:** Damask rose, Rose otto; Rose de damas (Fr), Damaskus Rose (Ge), Rosa (Bulgarian), Rosa di Damasco (It), Gül fidani, Murr gülü (Turkish), Ward (Arabic), Lord (Berber), Suri (Persian). The traditional term 'rose otto' comes from *attar*, meaning essence or perfume in Arabic. The Damask rose is so called after the Syrian town of Damascus which during the 13th century became an important distillation centre for crude, first-distillation rosewater.

**Appearance:** A semiviscous pale yellow fluid with an intense, warm rosy-sweet-floral odour with sweet-honey notes and very faint spicy-fruity overtones

**Perfumery status:** A heart note of extremely high intensity and fair persistence, mainly used in the production of high-quality perfumes and cosmetics

**Extraction:** Distillation of the fresh flowers by hot water injected with hot steam, i.e. a type of hydrodistillation. Distillation occupies most of May and June in all major production centres, and only the fresh flowers are (or should be) used in the production of Rose oil and Rosewater (see below). The distillation process of rose flowers is remarkably unique and complex, with the aim of maximizing the essential oil yield of an extremely low-yield but highly desirable plant. The key technique employed is a two-stage process called cohobation. This process basically involves distilling the oil-rich aromatic water left over from the first distillation a second time (and often a third time) and adding that second distilled oil to the first distillation (called the decant or first oil). A separate cohobation column is used for this purpose. However, the actual techniques for cohobating the oil are complex and in addition vary greatly among all the major production centres in Bulgaria, Turkey, Morocco and Iran.

**1 kg oil yield from:** 3,000–5,500 kg of the fresh flowers (an extremely poor yield). By contrast, only about 300 kg are needed to make 1 kg of the Rose absolute extract and only 1 kg to make fresh Rosewater. This extremely low yield of the oil, combined with the time- and cost-intensive cultivation and collection of this rose species, and the extreme desirability of its fragrance, conspire to make Damask rose oil one of the costliest essential oils available. Like other soft flowers, the dewy rose flowers must be hand-picked in the early morning hours before the sun's heat reduces their oil content. They must be distilled within 24 hours to prevent spoilage and an off-note in the oil.

**Production areas:** Bulgaria (Kazanlak), Turkey (Isparta), Morocco (South of the High Atlas), Iran (Shiraz, Kashan), India (Uttar Pradesh), Saudi Arabia (Taif), Russia and China. Production in Iran and Saudi Arabia was well-established by the 16th century. Bulgarian production of Rose oil began in the early 1600s under Ottoman rule (in 1610 in Kazanlak, according to some sources), while production in Anatolian Turkey began in 1892, the rose plant having been brought back by Bulgarian immigrants in 1870 (Yilmaz 2011). Moroccan production of Rose oil began only in 1945, although south of the Atlas Mountains Rosewater has been popularly produced in domestic circles since the 10th Century (see Rosewater below). In Morocco, rose bushes also serve as hedgerows among wheat fields. Arab traders brought the Damask rose to the Maghreb in the 10th or 11th century, as well as to Iberian Al Andalus.

**Typical constituents:** Monoterpenols 48–93% (incl. l-citronellol 18–55%, geraniol 14–32%, nerol <5%, linalool 1.5–3%) • stearoptene 16–22% • nonadecane and nonadecene 2–15% • terpenoid esters 2–6% (incl. neryl/geranyl/citronellyl acetate) • sesquiterpenols (incl. farnesol <2%) • phenyl ethyl alcohols 1–3% • phenols and their methylesters 1–3% (incl. eugenol and its esters) • rose oxyde <0.3–10% • methyleugenol 1–3% • ketone damascenone, β-ionone <1% • rosefuran <1% • numerous trace components, many unidentifable

**Chance of adulteration:** Extremely high, with similar natural and many synthetic compounds. Historical adulteration practices of Rose oil include classic stretching with the oils of Sandalwood and especially Palmarosa (Gildemeister 1899). Rose oil is extremely desirable in the perfume industry and commands an ever-increasing price. Natural reconstitutions and additives of Rose oil include blended oils from other rose species or varieties (see below), Geranium, Ho wood and Lemon essential oils, as well as fractions of similar-scented oils such as Palmarosa, Geranium (esp. rhodinol) and Guaiac wood. Synthetic adulterants include phenyl-ethyl alcohols, diethylphthalate, l-citronellol (rhodinol), geraniol, isoeugenol, eugenol, heliotropine, cyclamal, as well as the acetates of neryl, geranyl and citronellyl. In addition, gross diluents such as stearin and terpenic alcohol are also known adulterants. The completely synthetically reconstructed oil is also available. Rose absolute, although more affordable, also sees adulteration with natural or synthetic fractions of Palmarosa, Clovebud and Peru balsam (Lis-Balchin 2006; Franchomme 2015).

**Related oils:** Very small quantities of the oil and the absolute are sometimes extracted from other rose species and varieties such as the May or Cabbage rose, or Rose de mai (*Rosa centifolia* L.) (France), Gallic rose (*Rosa gallica* L.) (Egypt, Russia), White rose (*Rosa damascena* P. Mill. var. *alba*) (Bulgaria), Musk rose (*Rosa moschata* (Herrm.) (Bulgaria), Japanese rose (*Rosa rugosa* Thunb. ex Murray) (China) and Moonseason rose (*R. chinensis* Jacquet) (China). Nice as many of these are from the fragrance perspective, they cannot, however, replace Damask rose in terms of therapeutic applications, their essential oil will not perform in the same way. These other rose species have different, if slightly overlapping, traditional uses; and then not in the oil form, but in herbal preparations such as infusions.

**Related products:** Producers of Rose essential oil also routinely produce Rosewater and Rose absolute during the busy production season. Historically however, infused Rose oil was also an important aromatic product, especially before the appearance of the distilled oil.

**Rosewater**, or Rose hydrosol as it is also called, is also extensively produced in most rose production areas, and again mainly from the Damask rose. Like many traditional aromatic waters, Rosewater is always produced separately from the production of essential oil, thereby ensuring optimal quality. This sets Rosewater apart from aromatic waters that are often simply by-products of essential oil distillation. As in Rose oil production, only the freshly picked flowers are used, and the process is a mixed hot water and steam distillation without any cohobation. In other words, Rosewater is simply the basic rose distillate using the optimal ratio of flowers to water, which ranges between 0.75:1 and 1:1.

Rosewater is the oldest plant perfume and medicine known, dating back to Assyrian and Babylonian cultures in West Asia. Water-distilled cohobated Rosewater was recorded in the 850s in the Persian (Iranian) province of Sabur and later perfected in the 11th century in the Shiraz area (Forbes 1970).

With its extraordinarily stable shelf life, the prized Persian rosewater of the Damask rose was widely exported to both East and West until the mid-18th century (Gildemeister 1899). Still, it appears that China had developed the skill of making 'rose dew' or rosewater long before the 958 arrival of the famous Persian missions that brought Persian rosewater to the Later Chou court (Schafer 1963). Persian immigrants in the early 900s brought rosewater extraction technology to Southwest China, where its production using native roses has been carried out ever since (Needham 1980).

Persian rosewater also enjoyed a long history of use in the West, especially during the European Middle Ages, the whole Ottoman period in the Middle East from the 1570s on, the Tudor era in England (where the rose became a dynastic symbol), and during the height of natural perfumery in early 18th-century France. Meanwhile, with the Western spread of Arabian caliphates to the Maghreb and Iberia in the 10th century, the production of rosewater from the Damask rose also became established in Tunisia, Algeria, Morocco and Al Andalus (Forbes (1970). Moved by Spanish traders, precious Moroccan rosewater even found its way to England right up to the 16th century – at which time the Damask rosebush itself became established and its aromatic water eagerly distilled (Dugan 2011). The 1850s then saw the industrial production of Rosewater in France, using the flowers of the may or cabbage rose. In several Mediterranean countries, notably in Cyprus, Turkey, Lebanon, Algeria and Morocco, Rosewater from the damask rose to this day is still sometimes distilled domestically in regions where the Damask rose grows; while a generation ago it was still much more common. Today's main commercial producer of Rosewater is Bulgaria.

Apart from its use in Western perfumery since the 1650s, the versatile Rosewater has served a large number of cosmetic and treatment preparations that include creams, ointments, tinctures, elixirs and so on; as well as culinary preparations such as drinks, pastries, biscuits, jams, honeys, nougat and other sweets such as Turkish delight. Like Rose oil and Rose absolute, Rosewater today is again seeing increased use in high-quality cosmetic and food products, as well as for therapeutic applications.

Rose absolute in most production centres, and especially in Bulgaria is extracted from the dried Damask rose flowers, Turkey and Morocco. The extraction requires chemical solvents such as hexane and in the first stage results in rose concrete, which is used in perfumery. After the solvent is boiled off with high-temperature alcohol, what remains is the pure Rose absolute. This is a viscous liquid with a deep amber to reddish orange colour and a deep, complex rosy-sweet-floral odour, that is much truer to the fragrance of an actual Damask rose flower than the distilled oil. This is partly from the higher levels of phenyl ethyl alcohols present. Because of its higher yield – about six times that of the essential oil, even with repeated cohobation – the absolute is much more cost effective; about one-third that of Rose oil. This, together with its desirable rosy fragrance, makes Rose absolute often preferred over the oil in perfumes, cosmetics and other fragrance and flavour applications.

# Therapeutic Functions and Indications

## SPECIFIC SYMPTOMATOLOGY – *All applications*

Emotional depravation and injury, discouragement, sorrow, low self-esteem, insecurity, emotional disconnection, thoughts of suicide, mood swings, anxiety, fear of the unknown, depression with anxiety or agitation, shame feelings, jealousy, embitterment, restless sleep, nightmares, emotional/mental/physical exhaustion, long or irregular menstrual cycles, scanty or flooding menstruation, PMS, sexual disinterest, vaginal irritation and dryness

## PSYCHOLOGICAL – *Rose oil or absolute for aromatic diffusion, whole-body massage*

**Essential PNEI function and indication:** Regulating in dysregulation conditions; euphoric in acute overstimulation conditions

**Possible brain dynamics:** Reduces deep limbic system hyperfunctioning

**Fragrance category:** Middle tone with sweet note

**Indicated psychological disorders:** Addiction disorders, including food addictions, codependency; bipolar disorder, minor depression

### PROMOTES EMOTIONAL SECURITY AND STRENGTH

- Loss of emotional security and safety; grief, anxiety

- Emotional withdrawal, discouragement, pessimism, disconnection

- Emotional wounding or shock, including loss, betrayal, deprivation

### PROMOTES EMOTIONAL STABILITY AND INTEGRATION

- Emotional instability with distressed feelings (including shame, jealousy, envy, embitterment, despair, self-destructiveness, suicidal tendency)

- Irritability, mood swings, frustration

- Thinking/feeling conflict with rigidity, inability to change

### PROMOTES EUPHORIA AND OPTIMISM (FOR SHORT-TERM USE)

- Intense acute emotions, incl. sorrow/anxiety/anger/fear (especially fear of the unknown, instinctive fear, nightmares)

- Severe anxious or agitated depression

COMPLEMENTARY COMBINATIONS – OLFACTION AND TOPICAL APPLICATIONS

- Rose + Jasmine: nurturing, stabilizing, euphoric for emotional wounding with loss of self-esteem; severe shame, emotional instability, negative or distressed emotions, suicidal tendencies

- Rose + Neroli: euphoric and stabilizing for emotional wounding with loss of self-esteem, guilt and shame, depression; for distressed emotions with instability

## PHYSIOLOGICAL – *Rose oil for nebulizer inhalation, gel cap, suppository, pessary, vaginal sponge, external applications*

**Therapeutic status:** Mild remedy with no cumulative toxicity

**Topical safety status:** Non-irritant, non-sensitizing

**Tropism:** Neuroendocrine, reproductive, cardiovascular, digestive systems

**Essential diagnostic function:** Balances dysregulated and relaxes hypertonic/tense terrain conditions

### PRIMARILY RESTORATIVE AND REGULATIVE:

*strong reproductive and hormonal regulator, progesteronic/oestrogenic:* hormonal disorders from progesterone or oestrogen deficiency, incl. PMS, dysmenorrhoea, amenorrhoea, menopausal syndrome, postpartum depression, post-hysterectomy syndrome; vaginal dryness; infertility, incompetent sperm, low sperm count

*aphrodisiac: loss of libido (frigidity, impotence)*

### PRIMARILY RELAXANT:

*nervous relaxant, cerebral sedative, SNS inhibitor, analgesic:* neurasthenia, esp. stress- or disease-related, esp. in women; with insomnia, anxiety, palpitations, pain; PMS; headaches, incl. migraine

*refrigerant, antipyretic:* hot spells, menopausal hot flushes, fevers (many kinds)

*vasodilator, hypotensive, anticonvulsant:* hypertension; seizures

*bronchodilator, anti-inflammatory:* spasmodic cough, asthma

PRIMARILY DECONGESTANT:

*liver stimulant, decongestant and detoxicant, cholagogue, anti-inflammatory:* liver and biliary congestion with toxicosis, headache; metabolic toxicosis, cholecystitis

*pelvic and uterine decongestant:* pelvic and uterine congestion with congestive dysmenorrhoea, menorrhagia

*haemostatic, astringent:* intermenstrual bleeding, menorrhagia, haemorrhage in general

*antioxidant, antitumoural:* cancer

ANTIMICROBIAL ACTIONS:

*moderate antibacterial:* mild bacterial infections, esp. with Staph. aureus, E. coli, P. acnes, incl. colitis, enteritis, cholecystitis, cholangitis, bronchitis, laryngitis, cystitis, lung TB

SYNERGISTIC COMBINATIONS

- Rose + Geranium: strong hormonal regulator in chronic progesterone or oestrogen deficiencies with PMS, dysmenorrhoea, menopausal syndrome, vaginal dryness, frigidity, infertility

- Rose + Geranium: pelvic and uterine decongestant for pelvic and uterine congestion with congestive dysmenorrhoea, menorrhagia

- Rose + Geranium: liver decongestant and detoxicant, cholagogue for chronic hepatobiliary congestion with toxicosis; metabolic toxicosis, cholecystitis

COMPLEMENTARY COMBINATIONS

- Rose + Clary sage + Scotch pine: hormonal regulator and restorative in progesterone or oestrogen deficiencies with chronic PMS, dysmenorrhoea, amenorrhoea, menopausal syndrome, vaginal dryness, frigidity, infertility

- Rose + Niaouli + Cypress: strong pelvic decongestant for severe pelvic congestion with menorrhagia or congestive dysmenorrhoea

- Rose + Scotch pine/Black spruce: reproductive and sexual restorative for impotence, low sperm count

- Rose + Petitgrain bigarade/Lavender: nervous relaxant in chronic stress- or trauma-related conditions of all kinds, esp. with palpitations, insomnia, anxiety

**TOPICAL** – *Rose oil or absolute for liniment, cream, other cosmetic preparations*

**Skin care:** Dry, sensitive or mature skin types

*emollient:* dry, dehydrated, irritated or inflamed skin

*skin regenerator, capillary stimulant:* rosacea, broken capillaries, wrinkles, stretch marks after pregnancy

*vulnerary, anti-inflammatory, astringent, antiseptic:* wounds, ulcers, sores, mouth ulcers, sprains, strains; herpes, shingles, gingivitis, acne

**Therapeutic precautions:** Rose oil is best avoided in hypotonic/weak conditions, including with chronic fatigue, debility and hypotension.

**Pharmacological precautions:** Adulterated or reconstituted Rose oils, especially with topical use, are very likely to cause side effects. Although there is a theoretical risk of Rose oil's methyleugenol acting as a carcinogenic, its dominant constituent geraniol is anticarcinogenic and is likely to quench the former's carcinogenic potential. No record of a carcinogenic risk is recorded in French medicine and no related prohibition exists in French pharmacy regulations.

**Preparations:**

- Diffusor: 1–2 drops in water
- Massage oil: 1–2% dilution in vegetable oil
- Liniment: 2–4% dilution in vegetable oil
- Vaginal sponge: 1.5% dilution in vegetable oil
- Gel cap: 1 drop with olive oil

## Chinese Medicine Functions and Indications

**Aroma energy:** Sweet

**Movement:** Circulating

**Warmth:** Neutral

**Meridian tropism:** Heart, Pericardium, Liver, Gallbladder, Triple Heater, Lung, Chong, Ren

**Five-Element affinity:** Fire, Wood

**Essential function:** To nourish Blood, Yin and Essence, and harmonizes the Heart and Shen

1.  **Nourishes the Blood and Essence, harmonizes the Shen, regulates menstruation and menopause, and moistens dryness**

    - **Blood deficiency with Shen dysregulation**, with scanty or absent periods, long or irregular cycles, dysmenorrhoea, PMS:

      Geranium/Clary sage

    - **Blood deficiency with Shen dysregulation in perimenopause**, with hot flushes, irritability, depression, dryness:

      Vetiver/Geranium/Clary sage

    - **Uterus Blood deficiency/Chong and Ren Mai Essence deficiency with internal dryness**, with vaginal dryness, loss of sex drive, infertility, sterility in both sexes:

      Jasmine/Niaouli/Vetiver

2.  **Nourishes Heart and Liver Blood, animates the Heart and strengthens the Shen**

    - **Heart Blood deficiency with Shen weakness**, with mental and emotional fatigue, discouragement, worry, grief, insomnia:

      Palmarosa/Petitgrain bigarade/Ylang ylang/Jasmine

    - **Liver Blood deficiency with Shen weakness**, with low self-esteem, sadness, depression, chronic anger with depression, insomnia:

      Grapefruit/Ylang ylang/Blue tansy

3.  **Nourishes Heart and Liver Yin, settles the Heart and calms the Shen**

    - **Heart Yin deficiency with Shen agitation**, with anxiety, fearfulness, worry at night, mental restlessness, dejection, insomnia:

      Atlas cedarwood/Vetiver/Lime/Neroli

    - **Liver Yin deficiency with Shen agitation**, with irritability, agitated depression, frustration, anger, restless sleep, nightmares:

      Clary sage/Helichrysum/Blue tansy/Sambac jasmine

4.  **Regulates Heart Qi and harmonizes the Shen, suspends emotions and relieves depression**

    - **Heart Qi constraint with Shen dysregulation**, with moodiness, irritability, agitated depression, anxious depression:

      Petitgrain bigarade/Fennel/Sweet orange/Lavender

    - **Acute emotions**, incl. acute grief, anxiety, anger, fear:

      Jasmine/Sandalwood/Neroli

- **Deep depression, despair, loss of self-esteem:**

  Ylang ylang/Jasmine

REMARKS

A perennial shrub originating in Central Asia, the rose has long trailed across continents, evolved over 300 species and enjoyed unparalleled cultivation. More than three millennia ago, however, the hybrid Damask rose in particlar achieved unique prominence for its iconic floral fragrance – a hybrid that has now been genetically proven to originate in Central Asia. Not ony that, but the flower has also achieved an emblematic value that goes far beyond its cultural cradle in the foothills of the Western Himalayas.

The Cosmic Tree or Tree of Life and Immortality of Central Asian cultures was actually an emblematic rose bush. The rose embodied the female wellspring of all life on earth – the source of nature's power to support all living beings through its power of endless regeneration. It symbolised the Great Mother, who through her unconditional cosmic love generated the continuous cycles of life that always promise transformation for another rebirth, for new growth and fruition. According to past Persian Sufi poets, spiritual seekers have long cherished the rose as symbol of the Beloved Divine. The aromatic rosewater then in common use in Central Asia since earliest times must also have been a reassuring reminder of that fundamental life blessing.

The deep sweet, rosy fragrance of rosewater was long ferried along the Silk Road networks East towards Beijing, South towards Saudi Arabia and West towards Byzantium (Constantinople or Istanbul). The rose as cosmic emblem of the Divine Feminine was quickly – and gratefully – adopted by other cultures and gradually personalised to represent various aspects of the human feminine, such as love, beauty, sexuality and compassion; it was embodied by the ancient matriarchal goddesses. The Chinese goddess of compassion Guan Yin in the Tang dynasty assumed the rose as her symbol. Cyprian goddess of love, beauty and procreation, Aphrodite adopted the rose as her symbol in early Greece. As Venus she was celebrated on the feast of Rosalia and whenever her fragrant rose petals bedecked Roman nuptial beds. Ancient Rome eventually developed a truly insatiable appetite for roses and rosewater, strewing untold tons of the pink petals in villas during banquets and throughout the streets during various festivals. Emperor Nero is credited with running rosewater through many of Rome's countless fountains.

In mediaeval Europe the Virgin Mary assumed the rose emblem, becoming the Mystic Rose, the Rose Garland. Gothic cathedrals were her temples where, goddess-like Queen of Heaven, she was worshipped. Sanctioned by its association with the cult of Mary, Persian rosewater from the Middle Ages onward found universal acceptance in the home, the bakery, the apothecary, and at times even the Church.

It is hard to ascertain with any certainty whether the Damsak rose was ever discretely distilled for its essential oil rather than for its aromatic water before the discovery of distilled alcohol in the 12th century. Certainly, it is known that rose's prized essence was always considered to be embodied in its whole aromatic water, not in its content of essential oil. The first reliable documentation of rose oil distillation is found in Saladini di Asculi's *Compendium Aromatariorum* of 1488 Italy, after which the oil finds increasing mention in European distillation manuals, herbals and pharmacopeias.

It is interesting that the applications of rose oil for medicinal, beauty-care and psychological purposes fall right in line with the emblematic and mythical values of the rose flower. Rose oil has always been a prime woman's remedy, a uterine tonic, as it still remains today. Today it enjoys well documented physiological effects that reflect its traditional herbal medicine use in hydrosol and tincture form as a major internal remedy for weak, congestive conditions of the uterus, liver and heart. Rose's strong restorative and regulating effect on reproductive functions are confirmed by theevidence of clinical experience, although apparently not by current research. The exceptionally wide range of gynecological disorders that Rose adresses suggests a bivalent hormonal effect with progesterone and oestrogen, possibly by regulation of the hypothalamus-pituitary-gonadal axis. If used for nothing else as a physiological remedy, Rose oil should be considered top choice for several major patterns of endocrine imbalance, especially progesterone deficiency, oestrogen deficiency, infertility and menopausal syndrome. In all these conditions it also shines at relieving key symptoms such as loss of libido, vaginal dryness, chronic miscarriage and postpartum depression. At the same time, Rose will relieve the mental-emotional aspects of these syndromes, notably withdrawal, depression and anxiety, as seen in hormone-deficiency PMS and postpartum depression.

Rose's systemic hormonal support is enhanced by a good astringent uterine and pelvic decongestant action with a haemostatic effect in the case of actual bleeding. With a somewhat similar fragrance and chemistry profile as Geranium, Rose may be seen as a stronger version of that oil for treating gynecological conditions. One of its key constituents, geraniol, has shown liver detoxicant and anticancer properties: Rose is very much a liver decongestant. Moreover, rose oil is also able to successfully treat male reproductive problems, including low sperm count and deficient quality sperm.

Many of Rose's traditional actions on the heart are now subsumed under its systemic sedative effect on the nervous system. Even when given in single drop quantities, Rose is effective for chronic tense-weak terrain presenting fatigue, anxiety, insomnia and palpitations. It is even more indicated if some of the mental-emotional symptomatology is present – especially depression, emotional withdrawal and a history of past trauma.

Few practitioners will use Rose oil today purely for its physiological actions – especially considering its superb performance as a medicine for the soul. Rose is one of the few remedies whose psychological indications follow seamlessly from its uses as a physiological remedy. More than any other remedy perhaps, it will serve the totality of a woman's condition – body, mind and soul – by internal and/or olfactory delivery. Sweet, soft, warm and floral, the fragrance of the rose essentially exudes calm, nurture and harmony. At the root of its mythic, hyperbolic status as the Essential Feminine in both divine and human form lies its iconic scent.

When gently inhaled to create olfaction, the basic theme of the rose archetype of female cyclic nurture and regeneration carries right though to Rose oil's psychological applications. No other aromatic remedy is so closely connected with providing emotional support of the most intimate kind. Like a mermaid, its floral fragrance can lure us into the fluid realm of feeling, softening us up to seeing and accepting our true feelings. In the individual who is ready, signalled by a person's instinctive attraction for the fragrance, Rose can quickly reveal the pure inner feminine of the soul in its many aspects – and reveal it with unconditional love and presence. It can assist us in healing the tender, vulnerable layers of our emotional wounds, helping us truly come to terms with obscure sources of our hurt and anger. A deep, compassionate healer to the true heart, Rose is for those burdened by emotional injuries inflicted by past deprivation or trauma that have resulted in either withdrawal or instability – wounds such as heartbreak, emotional loss, broken trust and violated feelings in general. Emotional withdrawal with loss of self-esteem, pessimism, unresolved grief and shame with feelings of deep insecurity, is the prime psychological terrain of Rose. This terrain often progresses to depression, including the anxious and bipolar types of depression. Again this may be seen in hormone-deficiency PMS, pospartum depression, menopausal syndrome, and so on.

Rose is also a powerful emotional stabiliser and integrator. By olfaction it can strongly stabilise mood swings and help the individual resolve chronic cycles of distressed feelings such as stuck shame, anger, jealousy, embitterment and despair. Here Rose's ultimate function is to promote emotional regeneration and transformation, as with liver functions and the menstrual cycle. This aromatic remedy is especially effective when the individual is not only out of touch with her (or his) inner woman and lacking feminine self image and self esteem, but also cut off from her healthy cycles of ongoing emotional renewal. Because cultural conditioning makes it is easier for women to stay in touch with their feelings than men, Rose will be especially effective in women. Nevertheless, it should clearly be considered for anyone in a state of emotional disconnection, showing coldness and harshness towards themselves and others. Here the bitter fruits of childhood traumas and lack of parental love once again emerge.

**Related oils:** Apart from its use as a psychological and topical remedy, Rose absolute should be considered a separate aromatic remedy from Rose oil, and Rosewood oil shares many of the latter's properties.

**Rose absolute** from *Rosa x damascena*. Being a chemical extract rather than a steam-distilled oil, it is valued mainly for its psychological applications by olfaction for its uses in energetic medicine and for topical applications. Its chemical profile is largely dominant in phenylethanol, with smaller amounts of citronellol, geraniol, nerol, eugenol and farnesol. The fragrance of Rose absolute is a rich rosy-sweet one with some mild woody notes. The Bulgarian absolute tends to present deep, rounded honey-sweet notes, while the Turkish absolute is typically lined with tart citrusy notes. The Moroccan absolute is similar to the Bulgarian but often brighter and lighter. The dilution for topical use of Rose absolute is 1–3% in a carrier excipient.

Whereas Rose oil has a regulating and circulating effect on a person's energy, the absolute has a regulating, centring and sinking effect; on the whole it acts more like the sweet-woody oils Sandalwood and Rosewood. The final action is harmonizing, restoring and stabilizing. Rose absolute is very useful for promoting emotional stability, security and inner strength, like the oil. Its main indications are emotional instability and insecurity of any kind, especially when vulnerability and loss of safety are involved. Again, like other sweet-wood oils, Rose absolute helps promote cognitive flexibility in individuals prone to worry, compulsions and repetitive thinking.

**Rosewood**, or *Bois de rose* in French, is steam distilled from the heartwood of a tropical tree, *Aniba rosaeodora* Ducke, in the laurel (Lauraceae) family native to the Amazon basin. In the past, rosewood was used for building, carving and French cabinet making, e.g. in French Guiana. The tree has now been on the international endangered species list for several years because of logging and deforestation. Most rosewood now still goes to make chopsticks and only small amounts of genuine rosewood remain. Clearly, only the oil from a guaranteed ethical source should be used. In an effort to maintain populations, currently the leaves of this tree are also extracted – Rosewood leaf oil.

Note that the general term 'rosewood' actually applies to a large number of various trees and shrubs in the *Dalbergia* genus from India and Southeast Asia, as well as the *Aniba* genus from Brazil, Peru and French Guiana, all of which are valued for furniture making. In the past, Rosewood oil was also commonly extracted from *Convulvulus scoparius* and spp. in the Canary Islands. However, only the above species of *Aniba* is considered to yield true Rosewood oil.

Rosewood oil is a colourless to pale yellow liquid with a light rosy-sweet, somewhat dry woody odour with a hint of a spicy note. Its main constituents are monoterpenols with dominant linalool 82–95% and some α-terpineol 3–5%; the remaining percentages are made up of oxides 3–5% (incl. 1,8 cineole <2%, cis- and trans-linalool oxide 3%), less than 1% each of monoterpenes, sesquiterpenes (incl. α-selinene and β-elemene), the ester geranyl acetate, the ketone methyl heptenone and the aldehydes neral, geranial and benzaldehyde. The chances of Rosewood being adulterated are high, as it is often reconstituted from synthetic linalool and other synthetic components such as terpineol; it may also be cut with Ho leaf oil, and various fractions of Pine oil. Ironically, the endangered status of the source tree also promotes stretching and reconstituting of this valuable oil.

True Rosewood oil is a mild remedy with no toxicity and is non-irritant for the skin, nor is it sensitizing. With rosy, sweet, woody middle tone fragrance notes and energies, its main use is by olfaction for psychological purposes. Like Rose absolute, Rosewood is essentially harmonizing and restoring (sweet), as well as centring and stabilizing (woody). Working mainly on the emotional body, it has the bivalent potential to either calm or stimulate mood and feelings, with a net balancing effect. Mood swings and emotional lability and insecurity are the keynote indications here. Rosewood can also soften rigid or repetitive thinking causing chronic worry and compulsions.

As a physiological remedy, Rosewood is sometimes employed in skin care preparations for combination and sensitive type of skin – as a skin regenerator and connective tissue stimulant for chronic skin conditions such as rosacea, broken capillaries, scars, stretch marks and wrinkles, and as a vulnerary, tissue repairer, astringent and antiseptic for wounds, sores, ulcers and eczema. In the past, French doctors prescribed (and may still prescribe today) Rosewood internally as a mild nervous restorative and sedative for infants and children with neurasthenia, physical and mental fatigue, depression, nervous breakdown, anxiety and insomnia. Its antifungal, antibacterial, antiviral and anti-inflammatory actions are occasionally engaged for children's oral infections of the mouth, throat, bronchi and urinary tract. Standard doses apply. However, considering Rosewood's endangered condition and the high chance of it being adulterated, it clearly makes more sense to look to any number of other oils – rosy, sweet and monoterpenol-rich – that will fulfil the very same functions.

**Ho leaf** (*Cinnamomum camphora* Siebold var. *glavescens* Hayata) is the oil steam distilled from the leaves of a tropical tree in the laurel family related to the various types of camphor trees. Unfortunately, in commerce the oil is often erroneously called 'Ho wood'. Its fragrance is rosy-sweet, somewhat woody and similar to Rosewood. The oil consists largely of linalool (80–95%) with small amounts of terpinene-4-ol, citronellol, tagetonol, linalyl acetate and traces of geraniol, limonene and various terpenes. Ho leaf oil generally has a relaxant and spasmolytic effect and is therefore useful in tense (hypertonic) conditions. Like Rosewood, however, it also acts a nervous restorative for weak conditions with fatigue. It is clinically also used for treating respiratory, intestinal and genital infections: its good anti-infective action is equally antibacterial, antiviral and antifungal. Standard precautions and doses apply.

# Rosemary ct. Verbenone

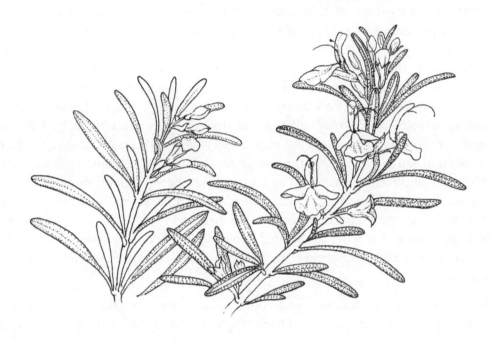

**Botanical source:** The herb of *Rosmarinus officinalis* L. ct. verbenone (Lamiaceae/ Labiatae – lipflower/mint family), a widespread woody Mediterranean herb or small shrub also naturalized in temperate biomes

**Other names:** Romarin à verbénone, Romarin abv (Fr)

**Appearance:** A mobile clear fluid with a warm, sweet-green herbaceous odour with a mild to moderate fresh-camphoraceous top note

**Perfumery status:** A head note of moderate intensity and poor persistence

**Extraction:** Steam distillation of the fresh herb in flower, in May and June

**1 kg oil yield from:** 50–100 kg of the herb (a good yield)

**Production areas:** France (incl. Corsica), Spain, Italy, Egypt, South Africa

**Typical constituents:** Monoterpenes <59% (incl. α-pinene 2.5–34%, camphene 2–11%, β-myrcene 2%, p-cymene 2–6%, limonene 0–7%, terpinolene, α-terpinene) • monoterpene ketones 11–57% (incl. verbenone 8–40%, camphor 1–15%) • monoterpenols 8–20% (incl. borneol 1–6%, linalool 2–7%, α-terpineol 3–5%, α-terpinenol) • 1,8 cineole (0–20%) • ester bornyl acetate 2–10% • sesquiterpenes <5% (incl. β-caryophyllene <3%) • caryophyllene oxide <1.3%

**Note:** There are large variations of constituent percentages within this chemotype, depending on the oil's country of origin. The same is true for all Rosemary oils in general.

**Chance of adulteration:** Moderate, and possibly reconstituted from rectified Rosemary ct. camphor

**Related oils:** See the Rosemary profile in Volume 1 for a discussion of Rosemary chemotypes and constituent variations

## Therapeutic Functions and Indications

SPECIFIC SYMPTOMATOLOGY – *All applications*

Depression with anxiety, emotional confusion, despondency, low or excessive self-confidence, irritability, negative thoughts, distraction, chronic physical and mental fatigue, lethargy, sluggishness in the morning, chronic headaches, malaise, palpitations, chronic cough with sputum, indigestion soon after eating, right subcostal or flank pain, irregular periods, long cycles, vaginal dryness, low sex drive, recurring infections

PSYCHOLOGICAL – *Aromatic diffusion, whole-body massage*

**Essential PNEI function and indication:** Regulating in dysregulated conditions; stimulant in weakness conditions

**Possible brain dynamics:** Reduces deep limbic system hyperfunctioning

**Fragrance category:** Middle tone with sweet, green and mild pungent notes

**Indicated psychological disorders:** Bipolar disorder

PROMOTES EMOTIONAL RENEWAL, STABILITY AND INSIGHT

- All pathogenic (stuck) emotions and distressed emotions in general
- Irritability, moodiness, negative feelings, incl. shame
- Emotional conflict or instability, shame

PROMOTES MENTAL STABILITY

- Mental confusion, distraction
- Negative thoughts, pessimism, cynicism, repetitive thinking

PHYSIOLOGICAL – *Nebulizer inhalation, gel cap, suppository, external applications*

**Therapeutic status:** Medium-strength remedy with some cumulative neurotoxicity

**Topical safety status:** Non-irritant, non-sensitizing

**Tropism:** Neuroendocrine, respiratory, cardiovascular, digestive systems

**Essential diagnostic function:** Restores hypotonic/weak terrain conditions

PRIMARILY RESTORATIVE:

*endocrine restorative and regulator, pituitary-gonadal stimulant, progesteronic:* hypotonic (weak) conditions involving pituitary-gonadal (HPG) imbalance, incl. progesterone or testosterone deficiency with menstrual and reproductive dysfunctions; incl. PMS, dysmenorrhoea, vaginal dryness, loss of libido, habitual miscarriage, menopausal syndrome

*nervous and cerebral restorative, antidepressant:* neurasthenia with physical and mental fatigue, depression (incl. postnatal), headaches, CFS

*immune restorative/enhancer:* chronic immune deficient conditions, incl. from toxicosis (all types), with recurring infections, hidden virus syndrome, depression, chronic fatigue

*hepatobiliary trophorestorative and detoxicant, diuretic:* chronic liver congestion in any condition; metabolic toxicosis, liver disease, incl. hepatitis; drug poisoning

PRIMARILY STIMULANT:

*strong hepatobiliary stimulant, decongestant and regulator, choleretic, cholagogue:* liver and gallbladder congestion with upper indigestion, right subcostal or flank pain, morning fatigue

*respiratory stimulant, mucolytic expectorant, antiseptic, anti-inflammatory, antitussive:* congestive lower and upper respiratory conditions, esp. chronic bronchitis with cough, dyspnoea; emphysema, sinusitis, rhinitis

*neurocardiac relaxant/regulator, spasmolytic:* arrhythmia, tachycardia, spasmodic angina

*intestinal spasmolytic:* spasmodic intestinal conditions, incl. colic, IBS

*antilipaemic:* high blood cholesterol, hyperlipidaemia

*mucostatic astringent:* vaginitis with leucorrhoea

ANTIMICROBIAL ACTIONS:

*immunostimulant, antimicrobial*

*antiviral:* viral infections, incl. viral colitis, enteritis, hepatitis

*moderate antibacterial:* bacterial infections, incl. with several Staph. and Strep. species, incl. sinusitis, bronchitis, vaginitis with leucorrhoea; cholera

*antifungal:* fungal infections, esp. candidiasis

SYNERGISTIC COMBINATIONS

- Rosemary ct. verbenone + Petitgrain bigarade/Hyssop/Coriander seed: cerebral restorative and antidepressant in neurasthenia, depression, burnout

- Rosemary ct. verbenone + Scotch pine/Black spruce: systemic neuroendocrine-immune restorative and regulator for chronic hormonal HPG deficiency or dysregulation; for chronic immune deficiency with recurrent infections (for intermittent use only)

COMPLEMENTARY COMBINATIONS

- Rosemary ct. verbenone + Clary sage: nervous and endocrine restorative for chronic neurasthenia in women, with fatigue, depression, hormonal deficiency/imbalance

- Rosemary ct. verbenone + Ravintsara: nervous and immune restorative for chronic neurasthenia, esp. in men, with mental and physical fatigue, irregular energy, recurring infections

- Rosemary ct. verbenone + Niaouli: pituitary-gonadal regulator in chronic female hormonal imbalance, incl. with PMS, dysmenorrhoea, menopausal syndrome

- Rosemary ct. verbenone + Coriander seed: progesteronic in progesterone-deficiency PMS, vaginal dryness, dysmenorrhoea, repeated miscarriage

- Rosemary ct. verbenone + Carrot seed/Thyme ct. thujanol: liver trophorestorative and detoxicant for chronic liver congestion and all liver disease

- Rosemary ct. verbenone + Peppermint: strong hepatobiliary stimulant-decongestant, choleretic, cholagogue for liver-gallbladder congestion, esp. with upper indigestion, subcostal pain, fat intolerance, gallbladder or gallstone colic

- Rosemary ct. verbenone + Green myrtle/Niaouli: mucolytic expectorant and nasal decongestant for congestive bronchitis, esp. chronic; rhinitis, sinusitis, postnasal drip

- Rosemary ct. verbenone + Sage: mucostatic astringent for vaginitis with leucorrhoea

- Rosemary ct. verbenone + Lavender: neurocardiac regulator for arrhythmia, palpitations, hypertension, esp. with fatigue or nervous exhaustion

- Rosemary ct. verbenone + Peppermint/Niaouli: antiviral for viral infections in general

## TOPICAL – *Liminent, ointment, cream, compress and other cosmetic preparations*

**Skin care:** Dry, sensitive and combination skin type

*skin regenerator, tissue repairer, vulnerary:* wounds, scars, eczema, chafes, burns, acne; couperose, broken veins, rosacea, age spots, wrinkles

**Hair and scalp care:**

*hair restorative:* chronic devitalized or dry scalp and hair, seborrhoea, dandruff

**Therapeutic precautions:** Rosemary ct. verbenone is best used in combination, i.e. formulas, and never over two weeks at a time. The oil is useful here as a liver protective against high-phenol oils when acute infections are being treated. Caution is advised in hypertension.

**Pharmacological precautions:** Avoid using Rosemary ct. verbenone on sensitive or damaged skin, as it is an untested oil. Its ketone verbenone possesses moderate neurotoxicity and is a mild uterine stimulant. For both these reasons this oil is contraindicated during pregnancy and nursing, and generally avoided in babies, infants and children.

**Preparations:**

- Diffusor: 2–4 drops in water

- Massage oil: 2–5% dilution in vegetable oil

- Liniment: 2–10% dilution in vegetable oil

- Gel cap: 1–2 drops with olive oil; not for extensive use without breaks

# Chinese Medicine Functions and Indications

**Aroma energy:** Green, sweet

**Movement:** Circulating

**Warmth:** Neutral to warm

**Meridian tropism:** Lung, Kidney, Heart, Spleen

**Five-Element affinity:** Metal, Fire, Earth

**Essential function:** To tonify Qi and Blood, and strengthen the Shen

1. <u>**Tonifies Qi and Blood, regulates menstruation, strengthens the Shen and relieves depression**</u>

   - **Qi deficiency with Shen weakness**, with physical and mental fatigue, lethargy, headaches, low self-confidence, depression:

     Ravintsara/Grand fir/Cardamom

   - **Uterus Blood deficiency with Shen weakness**, with irregular or long cycles, painful periods, vaginal dryness, fatigue, PMS with withdrawal, low sex drive, depression:

     Coriander seed/Niaouli/Vetiver

2. <u>**Tonifies Heart and Lung Qi, regulates the Heart and harmonizes the Shen**</u>

   - **Heart and Lung Qi deficiency with Shen weakness**, with sadness, grief, insecurity, anxiety, nervous depression:

     Rosemary/Niaouli/Saro

   - **Heart Qi constraint with Shen disharmony**, with distraction, restlessness, worry, anxiety, palpitations, irregular or rapid heartbeats:

     Petitgrain bigarade/Lavender/Fennel

3. <u>**Harmonizes the Middle Warmer, reduces stagnation and relieves distension**</u>

   - **Stomach-Spleen Qi stagnation** with indigestion, fullness on eating, right subcostal pain, epigastric bloating:

     Spearmint/Fennel/Lemon

4. <u>**Expels phlegm, dries damp and relieves coughing**</u>

   - **Lung phlegm-damp** with cough, sputum expectoration, chronic tiredness:

     Hyssop/Green myrtle/Sage

## Remarks

The verbenone chemotype of Rosemary oil has long enjoyed a special therapeutic reputation among practitioners. While its pharmacognosy profile is essentially the same as that of the two cineole and camphor chemotypes, its high levels of the ketone verbenone, as well as its additional content in bornyl acetate, make it distinctive. Rosemary verbenone as a physical remedy is consequently valued for two main effects – firstly, its comprehensive restorative, stimulant and detoxicant action on the liver and gallbladder; secondly, its neuroendocrine restorative action, especially as applied to gynaecology. We should think of Rosemary verbenone essentially as a key oil for weak, hypotonic terrain involving the neuroendocrine, immune, hepatobiliary and lower respiratory organs.

As a prime liver-gallbladder remedy, Rosemary verbenone operates on one hand as a stimulant to sluggish hepatobiliary functions with acute symptoms of upper digestive distress. On the other hand, the oil is one of the few true trophorestoratives on these organs, like Carrot seed oil, Milkthistle seed and Schisandra berry, indicated for a chronically tired, sludged, toxic and chemically abused liver. Like these other herbs, Rosemary verbenone can be a good component of detoxification courses, especially in those with toxicosis and its resultant immune deficiency. This also explains the common practice of adding Rosemary verbenone to a formula containing phenolic oils: by increasing the liver clearance time of hepatotoxic phenols, it is able to moderate their toxicity and enhance their absorption. Rosemary verbenone routinely finds use for regulating addictions and reducing chemical dependency, including anorexia, bulimia, food addictions, and 'pleasure' drug addictions from nicotine, alcohol and most others.

Rosemary verbenone also enjoys quite a reputation for its action on the pituitary gland. As a systemic regulator and restorative of neuroendocrine and immune functions, the oil has become a classic not only for neurasthenic conditions involving chronic fatigue and depression, but also for chronic immune impairment with recurring or hidden infections. The implications in gynaecology are many: Rosemary verbenone has been found useful in low progesterone and low testosterone syndromes, especially with the resulting menstrual and reproductive dysfunctions, such as vaginal dryness, introverted-type PMS and as a preventative for habitual miscarriage.

Like the other Rosemary chemotypes, this oil too is a reliable stimulant expectorant – with the emphasis on lower respiratory congestion, infective or otherwise, given the special presence of bornyl acetate. Its neurocardiac relaxant action also proves reliable for symptoms and disorders of a tense or dysregulated cardiovascular system.

By gentle inhalation, the sober, elegant fragrance of this Rosemary transforms into an effective psychological remedy. Sweet, green, warm and herbaceous instead of fresh, pungent and sweet like the cineole and camphor chemotypes, it moves and circulates rather than raises up energy; and turns the gaze inward rather than to the outside world. Rosemary verbenone invites a gentle, self-accepting look at ourselves as autonomous individuals. The oil has much potential for helping resolve negative feelings and thoughts, with humility and compassion, into radiant positivity. Rosemary verbenone may particularly help those suffering from issues of shame and fear arising from deeply unsettling past childhood experiences involving emotional manipulation or authoritarianism. In so doing, the fragrance is able to realign the self operating in the world with its true inner identity. Supporting the individual in going beyond emotional conflict, the need to always stay in control and have the last word, Rosemary verbenone has the potential for promoting inner transformation to a more positive, forgiving, secure self that always remains connected to a deeper, more authentic self-identity.

# Sage

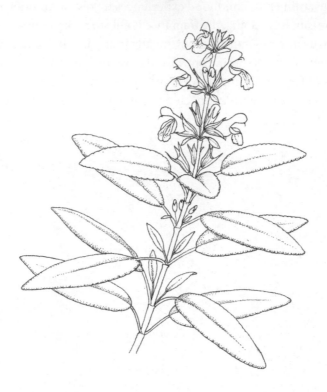

**Botanical source:** The herb of *Salvia officinalis* L. (Lamiaceae/Labiatae – lipflower/ mint family), a widespread herb or small woody shrub of the Mediterranean and West Asia

**Other names:** Dalmatian sage, Garden or common sage; Sauge (Fr), Salbei (Ge), Salvia (It, Sp)

**Appearance:** A mobile pale yellow liquid with a dry tea-leaf herbaceous, somewhat sweet odour topped with fresh-pungent notes

**Perfumery status:** A head note of medium intensity and fair persistence

**Extraction:** Steam distillation of the dried herb tops (mostly leaves), usually in May to June and again in September to October

**1 kg oil yield from:** 50–100 kg of the fresh herb (a good yield)

**Production areas:** Dalmatia (Croatia, Herzegovina, Albania, native), Bosnia, Bulgaria, Ukraine, Hungary, Italy, France, Spain

**Typical constituents:** Monoterpenone ketones 20–70% (incl. α-thujone 7–50%, β-thujone 2–33%, camphor <26%, fenchone) • monoterpenols 3–40% (incl. borneol <14%, linalool <12%, terpinen-4-ol, salviol, trace trans-sabinol) • monoterpenes 3–15% (incl. α- and β-pinene, camphene, myrcene, limonene, p-cymene, terpinolene, salvene, phellandrene, sabinene) • oxides (incl. 1,8 cineole 5–15%, caryophyllene oxide) • sesquiterpenes (incl. β-caryophyllene 1–7%, aromadendrene, humulene, cadinene, copaene) • sesquiterpenol viridiflorol 8% • esters (incl. linalyl/bornyl/sabinyl acetate, linalyl and methyl-isovalerates) • methylchavicol

**Note:** The α-thujone level varies significantly with the time of harvest: in the spring the content is low, 25–30%, while in autumn it rises to 50–60%.

**Chance of adulteration:** Moderate, often with Greek sage (*Salvia fruticosa*; see below), with its tell-tale high cineole (40–65%) and low α-thujone (1–5%) content. In this case, other sources of thujone may be added, e.g. from Thuja oil (*Thuja occidentalis*), to balance the profile of constituents, making the adulteration hard to detect.

**Related oils:** Of the almost 1,000 species of *Salvia* known, many are used in herbal medicine throughout Southern Europe, North Africa and North America. Only the following are distilled for their essential oil in any commercial quantities, the main ones by far being Dalmatian sage and Clary sage. These can usefully be divided by their chemical dominance into three groups. Note that sage oils rarely express a singular chemical dominance, and instead usually a plural dominance of two main constituents; these express a variety of creative combinations among the key constituents noted below, e.g. the sweet-herbaceous sage oils contain both linalool and linalyl acetate.

1. **Pungent-sweet-herbaceous sage oil with thujone dominant**

   • **Dalmatian sage** (this oil profile)

2. **Sweet-herbaceous sage oils with high linalool and linalyl acetate content**

   These two sage oils tend to be more restorative and often selected in chronic conditions.

   • **Clary sage** (*Salvia sclarea* L.), a sweet-herbaceous green oil from Eastern Europe with very high levels of linalyl acetate and a good linalool content (see separate profile)

   • **Lavender Sage** or Spanish sage (*Salvia lavandulifolia* Vahl), native to the Western Mediterranean, with its floral sweet-green notes from a high linalool content (28%) as well as fresh-pungent notes from a variable but good 1,8 cineole content (10–32%) and up to 30% content in various monoterpenes. Lavender sage displays a nice balance among its linalool, cineole and monoterpene constituents.

### 3. Fresh-camphoraceous sage oils with 1,8 cineole and camphor dominant

These constituents impart a good revitalizing and analgesic action.

- **Greek sage** or Lebanese sage (*Salvia fruticosa* Miller, syn. *S. triloba* L., *S. libanotica* Boiss. and Gaill.) from the Eastern Mediterranean, with strong fresh-pungent notes from its high cineole levels (34–64%); other constituents include camphor (15%), thujone (67%), terpineol and borneol (7%) and pinenes (6%)

- **White sage** or Bee sage (*Salvia apiana* Jeps.) from the American Southwest, with fresh-pungent top notes and sweet heart notes; the level of 1,8 cineole varies between 34 and 61%, the camphor 2–22%; white sage is one of the plants used by Native Americans for making smudging sticks

- **Black sage** or Honeybutton sage (*Salvia mellifera* Greene), native to California, is sweeter than Dalmatian sage but with deep rooty, musty base notes; the 1,8 cineole level is around 40%, the camphor 12%

Many other sage species are occasionally distilled in small quantities, and many more have potential for distillation. Among these, it is worth noting:

- **Hummingbird sage** or Pitcher sage (*Salvia spathacea* Greene), native to California, with a sweet-green fragrance

- **Algerian sage** (*Salvia algeriensis* Desf.), abundant in northwest Algeria and northeast Morocco, with its pleasant light, fresh-herbaceous aroma

- **Somalian sage** (*Salvia somalensis*), with its content in bornyl acetate and absence of thujones

## Therapeutic Functions and Indications

### Specific symptomatology – *All applications*

Loss of courage and motivation, apathy, low self-esteem, despondency, low vitality, mental and physical fatigue, poor stamina, exhaustion, mental confusion or instability, depression, distraction, spaciness, poor concentration, poor resistance with recurring infections, cold dry skin and extremities, day or night sweats, sluggish digestion with bloating, scanty urination, menstrual disorders, especially scanty or stopped periods, severe menstrual cramps, hot flushes, muscle aches and pains, vaginal discharges

### Psychological – *Aromatic diffusion, whole-body massage*

**Essential PNEI function and indication:** Stimulant in weakness conditions; regulating in dysregulation conditions

**Possible brain dynamics:** Increases basal ganglia functioning and reduces deep limbic system hyperfunctioning

**Fragrance category:** Middle tone with green, sweet, pungent notes

**Indicated psychological disorders:** ADD, depression, bipolar disorder

PROMOTES COURAGE, SELF-CONFIDENCE AND ALERTNESS

- Discouragement with apathy, loss of motivation

- Low self-confidence and self-esteem, pessimism, depression

- Poor concentration, poor short-term memory, drowsiness

PROMOTES EMOTIONAL RENEWAL AND CLARITY

- All pathogenic (stuck) emotions and distressed feelings in general

- Emotional confusion and illusion with conflict; emotivity

## PHYSIOLOGICAL – *Gel cap, pessary, suppository, external applications*

All to be used with caution.

**Therapeutic category:** Medium-strength remedy with some cumulative toxicity

**Topical safety status:** Non-irritant, non-sensitizing

**Tropism:** Neuroendocrine-immune, respiratory, digestive, urinary, reproductive systems

**Essential diagnostic function:** Restores hypotonic/weak and warms hyposthenic/cold terrain conditions

PRIMARILY RESTORATIVE AND REGULATIVE:

*strong systemic neuroendocrine-immune restorative and regulator, adaptogenic:* chronic hypotonic (weak) conditions involving functional endocrine-immune deficiencies and dysregulation; esp. with chronic fatigue, ANS dysregulation, hormonal imbalance, menstrual disorders, debility, poor circulation; esp. weakness from constitution, chronic disease of any kind, convalescence

- *cerebral restorative:* cerebral deficiency with cognition or memory impairment (disease or age related), premature senility, neurasthenia, depression, MS and other neurodegenerative disorders

- *immune enhancer:* immune impairment with chronic or recurring infections; all immunodeficiency disorders, incl. CFS, FM, AIDS

- *pituitary-gonadal/reproductive restorative and regulator, oestrogenic:* HPG axis deficiency with hormonal dysregulation and oestrogen deficiency (and progesterone deficiency?), incl. dysmenorrhoea, amenorrheoa, PMS, menopausal syndrome with night sweats, hot flushes; frigidity, infertility

- *pituitary-adrenal and -thyroid restorative, hypertensive, antidepressant:* HPA axis deficiency with adrenal fatigue or exhaustion, hypotension; hypothyroid syndrome (thyroxine resistance) with depression

- *hypoglycaemiant:* hyperglycaemia, prediabetic conditions

- *anaphrodisiac:* sexual overstimulation

PRIMARILY STIMULANT:

*strong uterine stimulant-relaxant, emmenagogue, spasmolytic, analgesic:* amenorrhoea, oligomenorrhoea, spasmodic dysmenorrhoea, uterine dystocia or failure to progress during labour

*diffusive arterial and capillary circulatory stimulant, analgesic:* asthenic (cold) conditions with poor circulation, with cold, dry skin and extremities; rheumatic-arthritic conditions

*respiratory stimulant, mucolytic expectorant:* congestive dyspnoea and bronchitis

*gastrointestinal stimulant, detoxicant, carminative, aperitive:* gastric indigestion, appetite loss, bloating; enteritis, mucous colitis, intestinal fermentation and dysbiosis

*hepatobiliary stimulant, choleretic, cholagogue:* biliary deficiency with gastric indigestion

*renal stimulant, detoxicant, diuretic, analgesic:* oliguria, dysuria, cystitis; metabolic toxicosis

MISCELLANEOUS ACTIONS:

*antipyretic:* remittent or low tidal fevers from infection, esp. with debility

*anti-inflammatory, detoxicant:* acute arthritic and rheumatic conditions, esp. with pain

*mucostatic astringent:* mucous colitis, vaginitis, leucorrhoea, spermatorrhoea

*anhydrotic:* excessive sweating (day/night)

*agalactic:* excessive lactation, for weaning

*antilipaemic:* hyperlipidaemia

*antioxidant, liver protective, antitumoural, anticancer:* cancer

ANTIMICROBIAL ACTIONS:

*broad-spectrum anti-infective:* a wide range of infections, esp. upper and lower respiratory, urogenital

- *strong antiviral:* flu, sinusitis, rhinitis, laryngitis, bronchitis, aphthous sores, genital and labial herpes, HPV, condyloma, enteritis, neuritis, meningitis

- *strong antibacterial:* esp. with gram-positive bacteria (Strep., Staph.) and Klebsiella, Neisseria men.; incl. sinusitis, rhinitis, laryngitis, tonsillitis, bronchitis, gingivitis; cystitis, urethritis; meningitis

- *antifungal:* fungal infections with Candida spp., incl. thrush, candidiasis

SYNERGISTIC COMBINATIONS
Usually for short-term use: see 'Therapeutic precautions' below.

- Sage + Rosemary ct. verbenone: strong systemic neuroendocrine-immune restorative and regulator for chronic fatigue syndrome with debility; for cognitive impairment, chronic immune deficiency with chronic or recurrent infections (for short-term use)

- Sage + Hyssop: arterial circulatory stimulant, hypertensive for poor circulation with cold skin and extremities, hypotension (for short-term use)

- Sage + Spearmint: antibacterial anti-infective, mucolytic expectorant for chronic upper and lower respiratory infections with discharge, esp. sinusitis, laryngitis, bronchitis

- Sage + Peppermint: biliary and gastrointestinal stimulant for atonic indigestion with bloating, upper abdominal pain, appetite loss

COMPLEMENTARY COMBINATIONS
Usually for short-term use: see 'Therapeutic precautions' below.

- Sage + Ravintsara/Niaouli: strong nervous, cerebral and immune restorative for chronic mental and physical debility or fatigue, esp. with recurring infections

- Sage + Clary sage: strong uterine/ovarian hormonal restorative for gonadal (oestrogen/progesterone) deficiency with amenorrhoea, dysmenorrhoea, PMS with fatigue; menopausal syndrome, loss of libido, infertility

- Sage + Rosemary/Juniper berry: strong uterine stimulant, analgesic for amenorrhoea, oligomenorrhoea, dysmenorrhoea, uterine dystocia; esp. in cold terrain

- Sage + Pimenta berry/Clove: strong thyroid restorative/stimulant in chronic hypothyroid syndromes, thyroxine resistance, esp. with symptoms of cold

- Sage + Niaouli/Ravintsara: strong antiviral anti-infective in acute or chronic viral infections of all kinds, esp. with debility (also topically)

- Sage + Eucalyptus (blue-gum): strong antibacterial anti-infective and mucolytic expectorant in congestive upper and lower respiratory infections, with cough, dyspnoea, expectoration

- Sage + Green myrtle/Myrrh: mucostatic astringent for chonic vaginitis with leucorrhoea, blennuria, mucous colitis, spermatorrhoea

- Sage + Cypress: anhydrotic for spontaneous sweating, night sweats

- Sage + Spike lavender: anti-inflammatory, detoxicant and analgesic in acute, painful arthritic and rheumatic conditions (also topically)

- Sage + Tea tree/Sandalwood: antipyretic for late-stage fevers with debility, night sweats

- Sage + Lemon + Cypress: antilipaemic for hyperlipidaemia with high cholesterol

## TOPICAL – *Liminent, ointment, cream, compress and other cosmetic preparations*

**Skin care:** Oily or mature skin types

*capillary stimulant:* cold, devitalized, overhydrated, damp skin; hair loss, scar tissue, weak spongy gums

*vulnerary, antiseptic:* infected wounds, sores and ulcers (incl. bedsores; of mouth and throat); acne, periodontal disease, laryngitis, pharyngitis

*lipolytic, anticellulite:* cellulite

*analgesic:* toothache, throat pain, muscle and joint aches, neuralgic pains, insect bites antiperspirant, deodorant

**Therapeutic precautions:** Sage is a strong restorative, warming and drying stimulant to most organ and endocrine functions, and is therefore generally contraindicated in hypertonic/tense, hypersthenic/hot and dry conditions. This includes high fever, hypertension, excessive blood volume, hyperadrenal and hyperthyroid syndromes, and dry conditions presenting e.g. thirst, dry cough and constipation. Internal use is limited to short-term use at the dosages below; frequent five-day breaks are advisable. Sage is one of several oils that clinically should always be taken in blends and formulas rather than on its own.

**Pharmacological precautions:** Sage oil presents some cumulative toxicity as its ketone thujone is an oral neurotoxin; for safety reasons the oil distilled in spring with its moderate levels of thujone is therefore preferred. Avoid any overdosing, regardless of the preparation used. For the same reason and because of its 1,8 acineole content, internal use of Sage is contraindicated by air-pump or ultrasound nebulization during pregnancy and breastfeeding, and in babies, infants and children. The oil is also contraindicated in those with a tendency to epileptic seizures, including migraine headaches (which are considered mini-seizures).

**Preparations:**
For Spring sage oil with maximum 30% α-thujone content.

- Diffusor: 2–3 drops in water
- Steam inhalation: 1–2 drops maximum in hot water for short-term use
- Massage oil: 1–2% dilution in vegetable oil for occasional use
- Liniment: 1–4% dilution in vegetable oil for short-term use
- Foot bath: 2–3 drops with some sea salt for fatigue, excessive sweating, cold sweaty feet – for short-term use
- Gel cap: 1 drop with some olive oil once per day only, for a maximum of ten days; or twice a day for a maximum of five days only. For more long-term use in 7–10-day courses, Sage oil should be combined with other oils in a formula at no more than 10% of the whole formula.

## Chinese Medicine Functions and Indications

**Aroma energy:** Pungent, green, sweet

**Movement:** Rising, circulating

**Warmth:** Neutral to warm

**Meridian tropism:** Lung, Bladder, Triple Heater, Spleen, Heart, Kidney

**Five-Element affinity:** Metal, Earth, Water

**Essential function:** To tonify the Qi, nourish Blood and Essence, resolve damp and strengthen the Shen

1.  **Tonifies the Qi, strengthens the Shen and relieves fatigue and depression; consolidates the exterior and stops sweating**

    - **Qi deficiency with Shen weakness**, with chronic fatigue, debility, low stamina, low resistance with chronic or recurring infections, poor concentration, depression, excessive daytime sweating:

      Ravintsara/Niaouli/Frankincense

    - **Day or night-sweats from Qi or Yin deficiency**:

      Cypress/Tea tree

2.  **Nourishes Blood and Essence, tonifies Chong and Ren Mai, and regulates menstruation and menopause**

    - **Blood deficiency with scanty/absent periods and cramps** with flow, dry skin, dry shins, fatigue:

      Geranium/Clary sage/Rose

    - **Blood deficiency with menopausal syndrome**, with fatigue, loss of sex drive, night sweats, hot flushes:

      Vetiver/Geranium/Rose

    - **Uterus Blood deficiency/Chong and Ren Mai Essence deficiency**, with vaginal dryness, loss of sex drive, impotence, sterility:

      Black spruce/Vetiver/Rose

3.  **Strengthens the Spleen, resolves damp and stops discharge**

    - **Spleen toxic-damp** with indigestion, abdominal bloating and pain, appetite loss, fatigue, mucousy stool:

      Patchouli/Black pepper/Niaouli

    - **Lower Warmer damp-cold** with chronic vaginal discharges, fatigue, scanty urine, cold low-back and abdomen:

      Green myrtle/Juniper berry/Silver fir

4.  **Resolves and expels phlegm, diffuses Lung Qi, relaxes the chest and relieves coughing and wheezing**

    - **Lung phlegm-damp with Qi accumulation**, with expectoration of copious sputum, coughing, chest distension, sternum pain, wheezing:

      Siberian fir/Hyssop/Thyme ct. linalool/Fennel

5. **Warms and releases the exterior, dispels wind-cold, opens the sinuses and relieves pain and congestion; boosts the protective Qi**

- **External wind-cold with Qi deficiency**, with sneezing, sinus congestion, sore throat, aches and pains, fatigue:

  Narrow-leaf Eucalyptus/Ravintsara/Ginger

- **External wind-cold with Middle Warmer damp**, with chills, fever, nausea, bloating:

  Patchouli/Thyme ct. linalool/Niaouli

- **Lung wind-cold** with sore throat, cough, sinus congestion, fatigue:

  Cajeput/Niaouli/Saro/Ravintsara

6. **Warms and opens the meridians, dispels wind-damp-cold and relieves pain**

- **Wind-damp-cold obstruction** with rheumatic aches and pains, cold joints and muscles:

  Rosemary/Juniper berry/Nutmeg

7. **Clears empty heat and reduces fever**

- **Empty heat in late-stage fevers** with rcmittent (tidal) low-grade afternoon or evening fever, night sweats, debility, thirst:

  Niaouli/Tea tree/Blue tansy/Sandalwood

REMARKS

It is hard to overestimate the esteem that sage, the humble shrubby East Mediterranean lipflower, has enjoyed since ancient times. Recognizing its effectiveness and wide range of uses, Greek and Roman practitioners considered this herb a supreme panacea, like Angelica root. In praise they dubbed the remedy *Salvus*, *Salvia salvatrix*, *Herba sacra* and many other epithets – the root words *salvia* and *salvus* mean 'healthy', 'safe', 'to save'. In the Middle Ages, sage was commonly grown in the physick or herb gardens of monasteries and nunneries, and figured prominently in the longevity elixirs produced there. Since those specialized days of monastic medicine, practitioners of all kinds have continued to experiment with and eulogize the herb until the present day (Holmes 2007). Today it would not be misleading to think of this remedy as Europe's answer to the supertonic herbs of East Asia – Asian ginseng and Rhodiola in particular. Like them, Sage has turned out to possess adaptogenic properties as a result of its comprehensive restorative and normalizing effect on human physiology.

The essential oil's first recorded production is in Germany in about 1550, although it is very likely that the oil was distilled long before that, like its related lipflowers rosemary, lavender and spike lavender. German chemists began analysing the oil's composition in 1829 and, with continued medical use by herbalists, pharmacists and doctors, it eventually became clear that the remedy was a systemic restorative and regulator of the nervous, endocrine and immune systems (Duraffourd *et al.* 1988). Sage oil has a complex and very complete chemistry, as well as an exceptionally wide range of applications. It harnesses the tonifying power of the ketone alpha-thujone in a buffering, supportive basket of other constituents both stimulating and relaxing – this is the key to its many uses, as well as key to its safe use with accurate administration.

Working deeply into the neuroendocrine-immune core of human physiology, Sage is essentially restorative and regulative to the brain, hypothalamus, pituitary, thyroid, adrenal cortex and gonads. A superb terrain oil for chonic weak, cold and, to some extent, damp conditions, it systemically restores their neuroendocrine control and stimulates their organ functions involved – with an emphasis on circulatory, respiratory, digestive, renal and uterine stimulation. As Sage is indicated for most chronic disorders presenting as weak and cold with mucosal discharge, it combines well with most other oils, which in any case will be less strong. Like Scotch pine and Black spruce, Sage is a classic for convalescence, chronic fatigue syndrome, chronic or recurring infections, adrenocortical exhaustion, mucous discharges, spermatorrhoea and a large range of gynaecological conditions. French practitioners consider the oil also a prime detoxicant working on both the liver and kidney end of detoxification, much like Dandelion root. Sage is a considerable antimicrobial: the leaves were traditionally infused in bowls of boiling hot water in French hospitals for sanitization; bacterial and especially a range of viral infections will respond well to the oil, where thujone again is considered active.

In ancient Greece, Sage was particularly associated with the Amazonian moon goddess Artemis, the eternal virgin and protectress of wildlife; the herb was freely censed at her sacred temples. At her temple in Ephesos, her image shows her torso completely covered in breasts: known as the 'many-breasted', she 'was always a patroness of nurture, fertility and birth' (Walker 1983). A more apt emblem for Sage as a woman's remedy is hard to imagine, especially as Artemis's psycho-spiritual character closely resembles that of Sage.

Artemis represents another important aspect of this multifaceted remedy, one that many practitioners throughout Europe actually consider primary: a supreme woman's ally (Mailhebiau 2002). Here the oil is prescribed as a systemic regulator of endocrine functions, acting on the hypothalamic-pituitary-gonadal axis to normalize hormonal cycles and hormone production (whether oestrogen or progesterone) – hormonal dysregulation, for short. Not only menstrual but also disorders associated with libido, fertility and menopause will benefit as a result. In tandem, Sage also exerts a direct uterine stimulant action that tips the scale in favour of absent, late or scanty periods, and with its analgesic effect provides reliable relief of cramping before or during the flow.

The fragrance of Sage is a vital, clear herbaceaous-green with complements of sweet and fresh-pungent notes. By olfaction, this oil will turn the gaze inward with a firm hand, leaving no room for ambiguity or evasion. Unmasking superficial feelings and illusions by inviting clear, fresh insight and discernment, the fragrance may confront us to take an honest, sober look at ourselves and see ourselves as we really are – not as we wish or idealize ourselves to be. In the process, Sage may act as a powerful dispeller of emotions that are stagnant and outworn, helping to cut off negative feelings that act as a drain on physical and mental energy.

Sage is for the individual burdened with feeling unmotivated, discouraged and depressed that their life is 'going nowhere' but lacking the braveness to come to terms with his or her malaise and despairing of ever being able to make a difference in the real world. Here the oil can help summon the necessary courage needed to overcome internal resistance. Without fail it will encourage an honest expression of what is emotionally completely real and true – including emotions that are less socially acceptable, such as righteous anger and grief. Sage thereby supports pure, fresh emotions to arise from a deeper, more authentic wellspring within the self – a vital renewal, a rebirth.

**Related oils:** Among the various species of Sage oil available, the following are more often available; they should be carefully differentiated.

**Lavender sage** (Spanish sage) (*Salvia lavandulifolia*) is a restorative and stimulant oil for treating weak, cold conditions, like Sage, but with differences – its sweet-floral linalool note and absence of the 'bitter' thujone note found in Sage. This oil is a mild remedy with no cumulative toxicity and no skin irritation or sensitization. Lavender sage presents a moderate, balanced restorative character that is particularly effective for treating chronic hypotonic/weak terrain conditions. It is a cerebral and arterial stimulant, a mucolytic stimulant expectorant, digestive stimulant and uterine stimulant (emmenagogue). Lavender sage is the actual species that was used in *in vivo* research that confirmed Sage's effect in preventing and treating senile dementia, e.g. Alzheimer's disease (Mills and Bone 2000). Topical use will benefit from its analgesic and muscle-relaxant actions in liniments up to 12% dilution. Taken internally, Lavender sage is abortifacient and therefore contraindicated during pregnancy. Use is also contraindicated in babies and infants. Standard dilutions and doses apply.

The psychological effect of Lavender sage is the inverse of Sage oil: mainly an emotional balancer, especially for irritability, mood swings, emotional confusion and distressed emotions. This is complemented with a gentle secondary uplifting and confidence-promoting effect.

**Greek sage** (*Salvia fruticosa*) may in general be used interchangeably with Sage oil, except that it is generally milder and its regulating actions on endocrine glands is largely missing. Although less neurotoxic than Sage because of its lower thujone content, it is still contraindicated during pregnancy and breastfeeding, and in babies and infants. Very moderate dilutions and doses apply.

# Sambac Jasmine

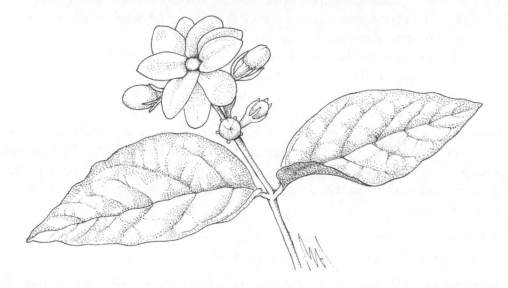

**Botanical source:** *Jasminum sambac* (L.) Aiton (Oleaceae – olive family), an evergreen shrub or woody vine from the humid Asian and Pacific subtropics; also adapted to a Mediterranean climate

**Other names:** Arabian jasmine; Pikake (Hawaiian), Sampaguita (Filipino), Melati putih (Indonesian), Mo li hua (Mandarin), Mali (Thai), Motia (Punjabi), Beli (Bengali), Moghra (Hindi, Marathi), Sumana, Yesmana (Arabic), Xamelera (Catalan)

**Appearance:** A viscous pale olive-green fluid with an intense sweet-green-floral odour with oily, leafy-green notes

**Perfumery status:** A heart note of high intensity and good persistence

**Extraction:** Solvent extraction by hexane of the fresh flowers, usually March to July; the first extract produces the concrete, which is washed with ethanol to produce the absolute extract

**1 kg oil yield from:** 1,000 kg (a very low yield)

**Production areas:** China, India

**Main constituents:** Esters 19–28% (incl. methyl anthranilate 6–14%, benzyl acetate <5%, methyl benzoate 3%, hexen-1-yl benzoate 2%, methyl palmitate 2%) • sesquiterpene α-farnesene 18% • monoterpenols (incl. d-linalool <15%) • azoturic indole <14% • phenylethanol <3% • benzyl alcohol 1%

**Chance of adulteration:** High, including with synthetic indole, benzyl acetate and other components. The quality of Jasmine absolute depends not only on lack of adulteration, but also in the first place on how well the solvent hexane has been removed from the concrete extract (see 'Extraction' above).

**Related absolutes:** Mainly Jasmine (see the separate profile)

## Therapeutic Functions and Indications

SPECIFIC SYMPTOMATOLOGY – *All applications*

Irritability, mood swings, frustration, anger, resentment, negativity, pessimism, cynicism, anxiety, shame, despair, self-sabotaging tendencies, depression with agitation, restlessness, nervous tension, impulsivity, worry, obsessing

PSYCHOLOGICAL – *Aromatic diffusion, whole-body massage*

**Essential PNEI function and indication:** Regulating in dysregulation conditions; euphoric in acute overstimulation conditions

**Possible brain dynamics:** Reduces deep limbic and cingulate system hyperfunctioning; resolves temporal lobe dysregulation

**Fragrance category:** Middle tone with sweet, green notes

**Indicated psychological disorders:** Bipolar disorder, minor depression, PMS, phobias, OCD, panic attacks, PTSD, shock

PROMOTES EMOTIONAL STABILITY, FLEXIBILITY AND RENEWAL

- Emotional instability with distressed feelings (including pessimism, cynicism, jealousy, resentment)

- Irritability, mood swings, anger management issues

- Feeling/thinking conflict with rigidity, enmeshment, inability to change

CALMS THE MIND AND PROMOTES COGNITIVE FLEXIBILITY

- Nervous tension, restlessness, anxiety

- Agitated depression, especially with anxiety, anger, hostility

- Worry, impulsivity, obsessions, compulsions

PROMOTES EUPHORIA AND RESOLVES SHOCK AND TRAUMA
For short-term use in acute conditions.

- Severe shame, recrimination, cynicism, despair, self-destructiveness

- Acute shock from trauma (mental/emotional/physical)

For olfaction and topical applications.

- Sambac jasmine + Lavender/German camomile: emotional stabilizer and sedative for emotional instability, incl. mood swings, frustration, anger, negativity, anxiety and all persistent distressed emotions in general

- Sambac jasmine + Ylang ylang no. 1 or extra: strong emotional stabilizer and sedative for severe emotional instability, incl. severe agitation, overstimulation, anger, hostility and other intense distressed emotions

- Sambac jasmine + Ylang ylang no. 1 or extra: strong euphoric for acute shock from trauma of any kind

COMPLEMENTARY COMBINATIONS

For olfaction and topical applications.

- Sambac jasmine + Jasmine: strong euphoric for severe acute shock from trauma; for severe shame and depression

- Sambac jasmine + Neroli: strong stabilizer, sedative and antidepressant for severe emotional instability with agitated depression, anger, worry, obsession and other distressed emotions

- Sambac jasmine + Neroli: strong euphoric for acute shock from intense trauma

- Sambac jasmine + Rose: stabilizing, euphoric for emotional instability, negative or distressed emotions, severe shame, depression, suicidal tendencies

## PHYSIOLOGICAL – *External applications only*

**Therapeutic status:** Mild remedy with no cumulative toxicity

**Topical safety status:** Non-irritant, non-sensitizing

**Tropism:** Digestive, nervous systems

**Essential diagnostic function:** Cools hypersthenic/hot terrain conditions

*refrigerant, antipyretic:* hot spells, fevers

*anti-inflammatory:* skin inflammations, dermatitis

*diuretic*

## TOPICAL – *Liniment, lotion*

See 'Pharmacological precautions' below.

**Skin care:**

*anti-inflammatory, astringent:* skin inflammations, ulcers

**Therapeutic precautions:** All use of Sambac jasmine absolute is contraindicated in babies, infants and young children. Internal absorption is contraindicated during pregnancy as it may be a uterine stimulant.

**Pharmacological precautions:** An allergic reaction is very occasionally seen with topical use of Sambac jasmine absolute, most likely from a poor quality product, i.e. one that is chemically adulterated or simply poorly produced with measurable remnants of hexane from production of the concrete. For both these reasons, internal use is discouraged and should only be considered with a high-quality absolute.

**Preparations:**

- Diffusor: 1 drop in water
- Massage oil: 0.5–3% dilution in vegetable oil
- Liniment: 3–4% dilution in vegetable oil

## Chinese Medicine Functions and Indications

**Aroma energy:** Sweet, green
**Movement:** Circulating
**Warmth:** Neutral to cool
**Meridian tropism:** Heart, Pericardium, Liver, Triple Heater
**Five-Element affinity:** Fire, Wood
**Essential function:** To regulate the Qi, settle the Heart and calm the Shen

1. **Regulates the Qi, relaxes constraint, settles the Heart and harmonizes the Shen**

   - **Qi constraint turning into heat with Shen dysregulation**, with irritability, mood swings, restlessness, emotional behaviour:
   Mandarin/Petitgrain/Lavender/Ylang ylang no. 1

   - **Heart and Liver Qi constraint with Shen agitation**, with tension, irritability, restlessness, anxiety:
   Lavender/Marjoram/Vetiver

2. **Nourishes Heart and Liver Yin, settles the Heart and calms the Shen**

   - **Heart Yin deficiency with Shen agitation,** with anxiety, worry at night, restlessness, fearfulness, insomnia, palpitations:
   Lavender/Neroli/Blue tansy

- **Liver Yin deficiency with Shen agitation**, with restlessness, irritability, agitated depression, anger, resentment, restless sleep, insomnia, nightmares: Vetiver/Patchouli/Helichrysum

3. <u>Glosses the Shen and suspends emotions</u>

- **Shock, acute trauma, acute emotions**:
  Jasmine/Rose/Lavender

- **Depression in general** (symptom relief for all types of depression):
  Jasmine/Neroli/Ylang ylang

REMARKS

The sambac species of jasmine is native to the humid subtropics of Southeast Asia and/or the eastern Himalayas and is widely naturalized in the Indian Ocean islands, the Upper Antilles and Central America. The national flower of Indonesia and the Philippines, Sambac jasmine is a common ornamental throughout Southeast Asia and Polynesia. The delicate starburst flowers release their full floral fragrance only at night but are widely enjoyed and commonly strung into aromatic garlands for different occasions. For personal use, sambac flowers are placed in the hair for adornment as well as infused in coconut oil for making sweet perfumes and body oils. In Hawaii, the popular flowers are known as Pikake, meaning 'peacock'; they often occur in Hawaiian songs and are sometimes strung up for a special floral lei. In South China, the dried flowers of Mo li hua have for millennia been used to create a floral tea with green or oolong tea leaves – the classic jasmine tea. The process is similar to the enfleurage with which jasmine, neroli and rose absolutes used to be produced in the South of France, but without the fat.

Sambac jasmine's other name, 'Arabian jasmine', is a historical misnomer: botanist William Aiton coined the name in 1789, having only seen its widespread cultivation in Persia and Arabia. The plant's species name *sambac* comes from the late medieval Latin *sambacus* and *zambacca*, in turn from the medieval Arabic *zanbaq*, in turn again from the Filipino root word *sampaguita*. In Arabic culture, *zanbaq* also referred to the infused oil of these flowers (and most likely of other species of jasmine flowers too). One of the plant's many Indian names translates as 'moonlight of the grove' – an interesting image in view of its psychological properties.

William Salmon (1691) reported that Persian physicians such as Mesue and Serapio considered the infused oil of *zanbaq* flowers warm in the second degree, stating that it 'is good against cold rheums [and]…good to be anointed after baths, in those bodies that have need to be suppled and warmed'. However, it is likely that these authors were actually referring to Royal jasmine rather than Sambac jasmine, known as it is for these warming types of applications. With its high levels of indole and green, floral-sweet fragrance, Sambac jasmine has a cooling rather than a warming effect. Its action on the nervous system by olfaction is essentially relaxing and euphoric – in contrast to the more restoring euphoric effect of Royal jasmine. The flowers and leaves of Sambac jasmine are still used medicinally in South China for their cooling, diaphoretic effect in colds with fever – external wind-heat onset in Chinese medicine – and for their astringent, anti-inflammatory actions for diarrhoea and dysentery, as well as topically for skin ulcers, eye inflammations, including styes and conjunctivitis, and tumours.

With production of the absolute extract in China and India, Sambac jasmine becomes a star aromatic psychological remedy by olfaction. Its intensely sweet, green notes signal a cooling effect on an emotional level that parallels its cooling effect physiologically. This fragrance excels at resolving intense distressed emotions, especially those revolving around issues of desire, pleasure, sexuality and emotional dependency. Its cooling, soothing, softening and lightening qualities can assist hot-headed individuals in coming to terms with negative emotional experiences from the past and then letting go of suppressed residual distressed feelings, such as anger, resentment and jealousy. In this way, Sambac jasmine is able to refine intense autonomic emotional reactions connected with the ego-self into more subtle feelings connected to the inner self.

Euphoric and calming, Sambac jasmine is highly effective in resolving and uplifting an agitated type of depression, especially with anxiety or persistent, repetitive emotions present. Here Sambac jasmine truly carries the potential for creating a lightness of being.

# Sandalwood

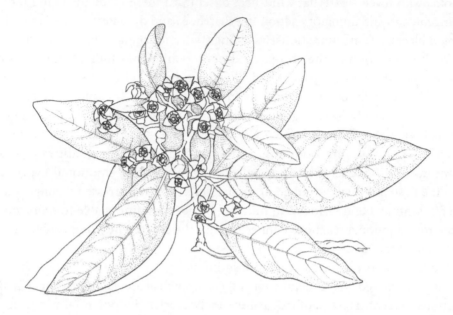

**Botanical source:** The heartwood of *Santalum album* L. (Santalaceae – sandalwood family), a small evergreen tree of the tropics of South India, Malaysia and Indonesia

**Other names:** East Indian sandalwood, White sandalwood, Mysore sandalwood; Bois de santal (Fr), Sandelholz (Ge), Chandan (Hindi), Chendana (Malaysian), Kayu cendana (Indonesian), Tan xiang (Mandarin)

**Appearance:** A viscous pale yellow fluid with a soft, sweet-woody, animal-balsamic odour

**Perfumery status:** A base note of low intensity and excellent persistence

**Extraction:** Steam distillation in March and November of the dried and chipped or coarsely ground heartwood, ideally once the trees reach maturity after 15 years

**1 kg oil yield from:** 20–30 kg of the wood (a very good yield)

**Production areas:** South India (Mysore province) and Sri Lanka, although this and related sandalwood species have been introduced and cultivated in various Southeast Asian locations for over 1,600 years, including Indonesia (Java, Sumatra, Timor, Sumba), Malaysia, Taiwan and the South China province Guangdong (see also below). Despite this extensive propagation, high demand and insufficient supply of East Indian sandalwood oil have since the 1980s turned this and all other sandalwoods into threatened species. It has also severely increased the adulteration of all Sandalwood oils, despite continued plantation programmes of some sandalwoods.

**Typical constituents:** Sesquiterpenols <75% (α-santalol 45–60%, β-santalol 17–30%, epi-β-santalol 5%, trans-β-santalol 1–2%, iso-α-santalol, iso-β-santalol, cis-lanceol) • sesquiterpenes <6% (α-santalene 5–7%, β-santalene, iso-β-santalene) • sesquiterpenals (incl. teresantalal) • 2,5% carboxylic acid (mainly nortricycloekasantalic acid)

**Chance of adulteration:** Extremely high, because of the very small production of this oil, its extremely high cost and great desirability in perfumery and 'aromatherapy'. Fragrance chemicals are common adulterants, as well as other whole or fractions of other oils such as the less expensive sandalwood oils (see below), Amyris (*Amyris balsamifera*) (see below), Araucaria (*Neocallitropsis pancheri*), Indian bastard sandal (*Erythroxylum monogynum*), Himalaya cedarwood (*Cedrus deodora*), bleached Copaiba (*Copaifera* spp.) and extenders such as castor oil, coconut oil and polyethylene glycol (Oyen and Dung 1999).

**Related oils:** Various other sandalwood species are cultivated and distilled for their oils throughout Southeast Asia and parts of Australia. Their availability is often poor and all are under pressure of unsustainable production. These sandalwoods have a similar but usually not as desirable a fragrance as the Indian sandalwood, missing the full creamy sweetness that the latter alone usually possesses from its high santalene content. The main species distilled are the following.

**Australian sandalwood** (*Santalum spicatum* (R. Br.) DC. (syn. *Eucarya spicata* (R. Br.) Sprague & Summerh.), from West Australia, is the most common sandalwood oil available today; it has seen a recent welcome increase in plantation production. It contains lower levels of the santalols, and higher amounts of nuciferols, bisabolols, farnesols and curcumenols. Based on both organoleptic and chemical analysis, the Australian type of sandalwood oil is considered fairly interchangeable with the East Indian type, although not all of its medical applications have yet been explored or documented. The exact clinical differences, if any, between the two remedies have yet to be established, therefore. *Santalum lanceolatum* is a less-available species also cultivated for its essential oil in North Queensland, Australia.

**Hawaiian sandalwood** or Iliahi alo'e (*Santalum ellipticum*) is plantation grown today but despite that still suffers from sustainability issues (Leopold 2017). The tree once widely populated the Sandwich Islands – as the Hawaiian islands were originally called – but its wood was overexploited just short of extinction and the essential oil never extracted. Hawaii sandalwood oil is another strong contender for replicating the therapeutic effects of East India sandalwood oil, although again any clinical differences between the two types still remain to be established.

**New Caledonian sandalwood** (*Santalum austrocaledonicum* Vieill.) from Vanuatu and New Caledonia.

**New Guinean sandalwood** (*Santalum mcgregori* F. Mueller) from Papua New Guinea and East Indonesia.

For the sake of disambiguation, several other woods and their distilled essential oils have been historically, and still are today, sometimes called sandalwood, despite being botanically and therapeutically unrelated.

- **Amyris** or Balsam torchwood (*Amyris balsamifera* L.) in the citrus family from Haiti is misleadingly also called 'West Indian sandalwood' in commerce (see profile below).

- **Muhuhu** (*Brachyleana hutchinsii*), a shrub in the carrot family from Tanzania and Kenya, is also confusingly called 'African sandalwood'; the oil is a deep red with a smoky, dry woody odour that bears little resemblance to any of the Sandalwood oils above. The tree is also reported to be endangered from overexploitation.

- **Red sandalwood** or red sanders (*Pterocarpus santalinus*) in the legume family from South India does not yield an oil, although the wood is an astringent, haemostatic and diuretic South Indian remedy; the red wood is also used for the manufacture of furniture and musical instruments. This was one of the 'three sandalwoods' used in Western herbal medicine since earliest days.

- **The wood of the bead tree**, red sandalwood or false wiliwili (*Adenanthera pavonina* L.) in the legume family from Sri Lanka and Southeast Asia is sometimes substituted for genuine sandalwood in making wooden objects only; its round red seeds are highly valued for making jewellery.

## Therapeutic Functions and Indications

SPECIFIC SYMPTOMATOLOGY – *All applications*

Anxiety, worry, compulsions, hidden fears, shame, low emotional affect and responsiveness, coldness, moralizing, insecurity, masked vulnerability, low self-esteem, scattered thoughts, low sex drive, easily fatigued from exercise, exhaustion, nervous tension, dry skin with rashes, chronic dry cough, chronic mucus discharges, swollen ankles, varicose veins, haemorrhoids, urinary and prostate congestion with dribbling urination, swollen glands, food allergies, chronic urogenital infections with foetid discharges, bedwetting, seminal emissions

PSYCHOLOGICAL – *Aromatic diffusion, whole-body massage*

**Essential PNEI function and indication:** Sensory integrating in sensory-emotional deficiency

**Possible brain dynamics:** Reduces cingulate system hyperfunctioning

**Fragrance category:** Middle tone with sweet, woody notes

**Indicated psychological disorders:** Obsessive-compulsive disorder, dissociative disorder, sensory integration disorder

PROMOTES COGNITIVE FLEXIBILITY

- Worry, obsessions, compulsions
- Repetitive or scattered thinking

PROMOTES INTEGRATION AND DISINHIBITION

- Sensing/feeling disconnection, dissociation
- Sensory deprivation and disintegration, euphoria, delusion
- Emotional, sensual and sexual inhibition; loss of libido

PROMOTES STRENGTH AND STABILITY

- Insecurity, vulnerability, loss of safety
- Disowning, disempowerment, loss of self-esteem
- Mental and emotional instability with anxiety, fearfulness

## PHYSIOLOGICAL – *Nebulizer inhalation, gel cap, suppository, external applications*

**Therapeutic status:** Mild remedy with no cumulative toxicity

**Topical safety status:** Non-irritant, non-sensitizing

**Tropism:** Nervous, reproductive, respiratory, venous and lymphatic circulatory, digestive and cardiovascular systems

**Essential diagnostic function:** Decongests congested/damp and restores hypotonic/weak terrain conditions

PRIMARILY RESTORATIVE:

*nervous (tropho)restorative and analgesic sedative:* chronic hypotonic (weak) and hypertonic (tense) conditions, incl. stress-related ones, incl.:

- nervous fatigue, debility, burnout, nervous breakdown
- sexual debility and anxiety
- neuritis, neuralgia: all types, including sciatic, intercostal

*mild cerebral sedative, hypnotic:* mild anxiety, mental hyperactivity

*cardiac restorative:* cardiac weakness, chronic stress-related heart disorders

*reproductive restorative:* impotence, frigidity

*mild antipyretic:* fevers, esp. with thirst

*antitumoural, antiproliferative:* cancer

PRIMARILY RESTORATIVE AND DECONGESTANT:

*mucosal restorative and decongestant, mucostatic, antiseptic:* chronic and subacute mucous membrane weakness with congestion and discharges, simple or infectious; esp. genital, urinary, intestinal, respiratory, incl.:

- vaginitis with leucorrhoea, gonorrhoea, urethritis with gleet, blennorrhoea, cystitis

- spermatorrhoea, seminal emissions

- mucousy diarrhoea

- bronchitis with foetid sputum

PRIMARILY DEMULCENT:

*respiratory demulcent, antitussive, anti-inflammatory:* bronchial conditions with dry, irritating cough (especially chronic), incl. bronchitis, atopic asthma, lung TB

*intestinal demulcent, anti-inflammatory, antiallergic:* chronic intestinal inflammation or enteritis, allergic colitis and duodenitis, IBD, allergic cystitis and prostatitis, food allergies; atopic eczema/dermatitis

PRIMARILY DECONGESTANT:

*venous, pelvic and lymphatic decongestant:* venous and lymphatic congestion with varicose veins, phlebitis; pelvic congestion with haemorrhoids; ankle oedema, swollen glands, lymphadenitis

*urinary and prostatic decongestant, diuretic:* chronic urinary congestion and infection, prostate congestion with hyperplasia (BPH), enuresis

ANTIMICROBIAL ACTIONS:

*antibacterial, anti-inflammatory:* bacterial infections, esp. chronic, with discharges; esp. urinary, genital, bronchial, throat; with E. coli, N. gonorrhoeae, Staph. aureus, incl. cystitis, urethritis, pyelitis, interstitial cystitis, prostatitis,

Aromatica

vaginitis, gonorrhoea; bronchitis, pharyngitis, laryngitis with sore throat and irritation; enteritis, dysentery; MRSA

*antifungal:* fungal infections, esp. with Candida albicans, C. neoformans, Trichophyton, Microsporum, incl. vaginitis, thrush, candidiasis, ringworm

*antiviral:* viral infections, esp. with Herpes simplex, HSV-1, HSV-2, incl. cold sores, genital herpes

**Note:** The East Indian and Australian sandalwoods have both shown most of the above antimicrobial actions.

### SYNERGISTIC COMBINATIONS

- Sandalwood + Atlas cedarwood/Patchouli: nervous restorative-sedative in chronic stress-related conditions with nervous exhaustion, insomnia, worry, burnout

- Sandalwood + Patchouli/Atlas cedarwood: venous restorative and decongestant for pelvic congestion, varicose veins, phlebitis

- Sandalwood + Myrrh/Copaiba: mucostatic mucosal restorative in chronic discharges, incl. leucorrhoea, gonorrhoea, blennorrhoea, mucous cystitis, mucousy diarrhoea, bronchial sputum, spermatorrhoea

- Sandalwood + Vetiver/Ginger: hormonal reproductive restorative for loss of libido, incl. sexual anxiety, impotence

- Sandalwood + Patchouli: anti-inflammatory, antiallergic, antipruritic for eczema (dermatitis), pruritus

### COMPLEMENTARY COMBINATIONS

- Sandalwood + Palmarosa + Nutmeg: cardiac restorative for chronic heart weakness

- Sandalwood + Scotch pine: reproductive restorative for loss of libido

- Sandalwood + Hyssop + Niaouli: antitussive for chronic dry cough

- Sandalwood + Green myrtle: mucostatic for chronic vaginitis with discharges/ leucorrhoea, chronic mucous cystitis, blennuria

- Sandalwood + Niaouli: urinary and prostatic decongestant for chronic urinary and prostate congestion and infection, prostatitis, enuresis

- Sandalwood + Geranium: venous restorative and pelvic decongestant for varicose veins, ankle oedema, pelvic congestion with haemorrhoids, dysmenorrhoea

TOPICAL – *Liminent, ointment, cream, compress
and other cosmetic preparations*

**Skin care:** Dry or sensitive skin types

*emollient, antipruritic:* dry, dehydrated, irritated, inflamed skin; acute dermatitis with pruritus and redness; skin chaps and cracks

*anti-inflammatory, antiallergic, antiseptic, mild astringent:* acute eczema/dermatitis and other skin inflammations, incl. prickly heat, with itching; stings, insect bites, scabies, acne, boils, wounds, MRSA

*antitumoural, anticancer:* skin cancers

**Therapeutic precautions:** None, although Eclectic doctors considered Sandalwood contraindicated for acute conditions and should be reserved for chronic conditions only. Certainly, the remedy is most effective for chronic weak and damp/congestive terrain (see 'Remarks' below).

**Pharmacological precautions:** None

**Preparations:**

- Diffusor: 2–6 drops in water

- Massage oil: 2–5% dilution in vegetable oil

- Liniment: 3–10% dilution in vegetable oil

- Gel cap: 5 drops with some olive oil; traditional use is 5–10 drops

## Chinese Medicine Functions and Indications

**Aroma energy:** Woody, sweet

**Movement:** Stabilizing

**Warmth:** Neutral to cool

**Meridian tropism:** Heart, Kidney, Lung, Large Intestine

**Five-Element affinity:** Fire, Metal

**Essential function:** To nourish the Yin, resolve damp and calm the Shen

1. **Nourishes the Yin, settles the Heart, calms the Shen and relieves debility**

   - **Heart and Kidney Yin deficiency with Shen agitation**, with exhaustion, restlessness, anxiety, palpitations, burnout:

     Patchouli/Atlas cedarwood/Clary sage

- **Yin deficiency with empty heat in late-stage fevers**, with remittent or hectic fever, thirst, weakness, debility:

Vetiver/Tea tree/Lavender

2. <u>Nourishes Lung Yin, moistens dryness and relieves coughing</u>

- **Lung Yin deficiency with dryness**, with chronic dry cough, dry throat, thirst, dry skin:

Copaiba/Niaouli/Hyssop

3. <u>Braces the Kidney and resolves damp; astringes fluids, secures sperm and stops leakage and discharge</u>

- **Kidney-Bladder Qi deficiency with Lower Warmer turbid-damp**, with frequent scanty urination, chronic vaginal and urinary discharges, dysuria, fatigue:

Silver fir/Green myrtle/Myrrh/Sage

- **Kidney Qi deficiency** with seminal emissions, spermatorrhoea, enuresis:

Cypress/Myrrh/Niaouli

4. <u>Clears heat, dries damp, astringes fluids and stops discharge</u>

- **Lower Warmer damp-heat** with irritated or painful urination, vaginal/seminal discharges:

Tea tree/Thyme ct. linalool/Blue-gum eucalyptus

- **Large Intestine damp-heat** with foetid diarrhoea, bloody stool:

Tea tree/Myrrh/Cistus

5. <u>Invigorates the Blood in the lower limbs and Lower Warmer, reduces stagnation and relieves varicosis</u>

- **Blood stagnation in the lower limbs**, with varicose veins, swollen ankles:

Geranium/Atlas cedarwood/Rosemary

- **Lower Warmer Blood stagnation** with pelvic weight or dragging sensation; haemorrhoids, dribbling urination:

Geranium/Yarrow/Cypress

6. <u>Tonifies Heart Qi and Blood, reduces stagnation and harmonizes the Shen</u>

- **Heart Qi and Blood deficiency with stagnation**, with chronic physical and mental fatigue, chest discomfort, breathlessness, mild anxiety or depression:

Palmarosa/Neroli/Rosemary

416

REMARKS

Sandalwood is a small parasitic tree that originates in South India, Sri Lanka, Malaysia and Indonesia. Cultivated since prehistory, its fragrant heartwood has seen more wide use for religious and therapeutic purposes than any other Asian plant. Hindu ceremonies have relied on it for millennia and Ayurvedic medical texts of the fifth century BC already discuss the wood's therapeutic properties. The original meaning of the name of Vientiane, the capital of Laos, is 'sandalwood city'. The Lesser Sunda Islands (Nusa Tenggara) of East Indonesia, Sumba and Timor, have always been known as the 'sandalwood islands'; they have seen sandalwood production since antiquity, exporting the wood as Makassar sandalwood from Sulawesi (Celebes). John King notes in his 1898 *American Dispensatory* that 'In Chinese markets the darker-colored wood is most valued (that from the root being the best quality). Three grades are known: South Sea Island, Timor and Malabar (the most expensive).' The islands of Hawaii too were once abundant in a species of sandalwood and were long called the 'Sandwich Islands'; although mundanely named by Captain James Cook after the Earl of Sandwich, this by synchronicity is also a subtle reference to sandalwood.

Despite being mainly valued today for its essential oil, historically sandalwood was used far more in the form of the actual wood. The fine, pale yellow, close-grained wood lends itself well to the creation of high-quality carved objects. It is also fragrant, long-lasting and termite resistant, thanks to the high content of essential oil, making sandalwood artefacts highly desirable. Like the more common Asian rosewood and sanderswood, this smooth, expensive 'botanical ivory' was shaped into special utilitarian objects throughout Southeast Asia, such as trinkets, jewellery boxes and fragrant fans. In Ming-dynasty China the expanding ribs of quality folding fans were always made of sandalwood, complete with the same fine cut-out work found in ivory artefacts. More lavishly, sandalwood was occasionally used by joiners and woodcraftsmen during the Tang period for screens, small windows and lattice-work grilles, and for special insets in designer furniture. Tang emperor Xuanzong's famous oversize couches generously appliquéd in sandalwood are outstanding examples.

Sandalwood objects were also highly desirable for fragrancing domestic and religious environments, especially Buddhist temples. This 'divinely sweet' wood naturally lent itself to the creation of statues and images of spiritual beings. Statues large and small of various Bodhisattvas, and of Avalokitesvara in particular, survive to this day. The three-foot tall image of Shakyamuni Buddha in the Kaiyuan temple in Quanzhou, Southeast China, is another example. Wherever Buddhist monks spread the teachings from India eastward to China, Korea and Japan, sandalwood followed to create an integral psycho-spiritual smellscape, thereby adding potent aromatic imprints to its hoary religious associations. The burning of joss sticks made of finely ground sandalwood in Buddhist temples is perhaps the purest example of sandalwood as the aromatic foundation for Buddhist practice. Here sandalwood is the psycho-aromatic equivalent to aloeswood in Daoism (which in Daoist temples was also burned in the form of precious joss sticks), cedarwood in the Ancient Levant (with which Solomon raised his temple and the Egyptians built their mummy cases), and myrrh and frankincense in the Levant (the main aromatics of Hebraic and Islamic cultures).

Sandalwood has always played a key role in perfumery and cosmetics as well. After the development of steam distillation, the extracted essential oil itself came into use during the 19th century both in the West and in South India. All traditional Indian attars (perfumes) originally used sandalwood oil as a fixative base for the distillation of flowers such as jasmine, champaca and tuberose; today this expensive, time-consuming process has virtually disappeared. In the West, perfumery has relied on sandalwood oil as an excellent base-note fragrance ever since the aromatic explosion of the Napoleonic era. In the early 1800s in France, sandalwood oil was being applied to fans, for example, turning those often-dowdy objects into especially potent weapons of seduction. The oil is a common blender-fixative in numerous perfume types, including chypre, fougère, carnation and Oriental types. Woody, balsamic and sweet with just a hint of rosiness, sandalwood provides a smooth patina of ageless elegance to most fragrance blends, much like the pale verdigris that ennobles copper church domes. The fragrance thereby evokes a refined simplicity, a time-worn sublimity. For cosmetic use, the oil is highly valued for its soothing, cooling and moisturizing effect on the skin, with chief application for dry skin conditions, as well as skin irritation and inflammation in general.

Ayurvedic, Malaysian and Chinese medicine have all included Sandalwood in their materia medica from earliest times. Originally, its fragrance was believed capable of removing the evil spirits or winds that caused disease. Whether applied to the body directly in paste form or decocted along with other herbs, Sandalwood provided gentle yet effective demulcent and mucostatic properties in diarrhoea and urinary and venereal discharges, and a relaxant effect for intestinal colic. Raw sandalwood chips are still a Chinese herbal remedy today, just one of several xiang or aromatic remedies. The use of Tan xiang, the 'Sandalwood aromatic', closely parallels that of Jiang xiang or Rosewood, Chen xiang or Aloeswood, and Ru xiang or Frankincense. The majority of these aromatics are used in formulas for treating pain from tissue trauma or intestinal colic. Li Shi Zhen's encyclopaedic 17th-century herbal, the *Ben Cao Gang Mu*, actually lists over 30 different xiang remedies in use in Chinese medicine at the time.

In Europe, Sandalwood took about 800 years to turn from an obscure Ayurvedic remedy into an established medicinal herb. First brokered by Arab sea merchants for the long maritime trade arms of Venice and Genoa, Sandalwood first found its way into medieval Europe as an exotic aromatic wood and soon became a minor remedy in Galenic medicine. Florentine apothecaries in 15th-century Renaissance Italy were probably the first to create formulas that included South Indian Sandalwood. Saladin of Ascoli's important *Compendium Aromatorium* of 1488 describes white, yellow and red types of Sandalwood, the yellow being the true Sandalwood. He also discusses Sandalwood oil distillation, as do later botanists such as Conrad Gesner (1555) and Friedrich Hoffmann (1722). Sandalwood's therapeutic uses in the West again continued to follow Ayurvedic medicine closely. In the words of Nadkarni (1954), 'Dr. Henderson of Glasgow was the first to direct the attention of the European physicians to the use of the oil as a remedy for gonorrhoea…it is preferable to Copaiba as it does not communicate an unpleasant odour to the urine, nor does it so readily produce untoward effects.' By the turn of the 20th century, both French and Eclectic physicians were making extensive use of Sandalwood for treating urinary and venereal infections with discharges. Researchers had then already established its specific tropism for the microbes colibacillus (Escherichia coli) and gonococci (Neisseria gonorrhoeae). Since then, French practitioners have continued to expand its medical applications to what is known today.

Sandalwood oil is one of the few true demulcents with restorative and mucostatic properties in the materia aromatica. It embodies the paradox of a cool, moist restorative remedy that is also mucostatic and decongestant for reducing discharges and fluid congestion. It would be a mistake to consider it a dry astringent. In treating essentially weak and damp terrain, Sandalwood excels firstly as a nervous (tropho)restorative, addressing chronic debility and burnout, especially when seen with resultant tension, e.g. anxiety or neuralgia, or with loss of libido. Secondly, the oil is an excellent mucosal restorative for chronic congestive (damp) mucus discharges, whether infectious or not, like Myrrh but without the astringency. Its decongestant action focuses on the Blood, relieving blood and lymph congestion (another type of damp) in the lower limbs and pelvis, including urinary congestion and benign prostate hyperplasia. The oil's high content in sesquiterpene alcohols is significant here.

As a demulcent restorative in the bronchi and the gut, Sandalwood is cooling and calming to all irritated, hyperactive conditions with dryness and inflammation, including allergic inflammation. Sandalwood here shows good resonances with other sweet, woody oils such as Patchouli and Atlas cedarwood. However, in contrast to Patchouli, which is mainly antifungal, Sandalwood has good antibacterial as well as antifungal and antiviral actions that serve it well when managing various types of infectious.

As an iconic sweet, woody type of fragrance, Sandalwood exerts a centring, stabilizing and harmonizing effect on one's energy that is physical, palpable and sensuous. Connecting our emotions with our senses, the fragrance allows us to come calmly but firmly to our embodied centre – a sensuous, heart-centred affirmation of our embodied self.

Sandalwood's historic connection to Buddhism is no accident when seen from the larger perspective of the oil's fragrance effect through olfaction. Like a gentle, supportive Bodhisattva guide, Sandalwood's compassionate presence may help us to accept ourselves just as we are now, without judgement, and with unconditional benevolence and presence of being. In so doing, it may help us to let go of insecurity, past regrets and future anxieties, as well as relieve worries, obsessions and repetitive thinking.

By helping us gently relax into our true centre, our essential being, the oil may ultimately connect us to the true source of our power, our intrinsic wisdom.

**Amyris** oil (*Amyris balsamifera*) has a sweet, woody, dry, almost 'bitter' note that is uncharacteristic of the *Santalum* oils. Its name is derived from the Greek *amyron*, 'strong-scented'. The wood is often used for torches and firewood, and both the essential oil and its resin are widely used in varnishes, cosmetics and perfumery. The oil is high in sesquiterpenols (<70%, incl. valerianol, eudesmol, elemol); sesquiterpenes are also reported. Although not a true sandalwood, Amyris shares two main properties in common with Sandalwood oil. Firstly, a good venous, pelvic and lymphatic decongestant action useful in congestive conditions of the lower and pelvic circulation, including varicose veins and haemorrhoids. Secondly, a cardiac restorative action for heart weakness, chronic stress-related heart disorders, and in all chronic conditions where heart support is needed. This action is reportedly milder than that of Sandalwood.

For psychological application based on olfaction techniques, Amyris is also useful for promoting cognitive flexibility and sensory integration, although again it is not as effective as Sandalwood.

# Saro

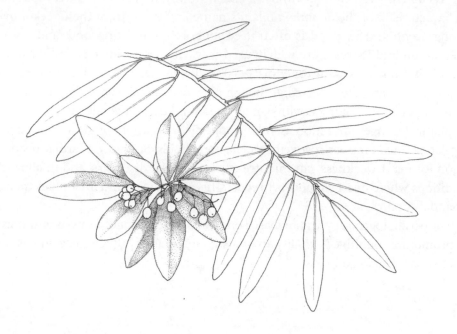

**Botanical source:** The leaves and twigs of *Cinnamosma fragrans* Baillon ct. cineole (Canellaceae – wild cinnamon family), a small tree from the wet tropical forests of West Madagascar

**Other names:** Mandravasarotra, Fanalamangidy (Malagasy)

**Appearance:** A mobile clear to pale yellow liquid with a fresh-pungent, sweet odour with faint lemony and spicy notes

**Perfumery status:** A head note of low intensity and medium persistence

**Extraction:** Steam distillation of the fresh leaves and sometimes twigs

**1 kg oil yield from:** 40–80 kg of the leaves (an excellent yield)

**Production areas:** Madagascar

**Typical constituents:** Oxide 1,8 cineole 37–60%, trace caryophyllene epoxyde • monoterpenes 27–49% (incl. sabinene 9–17%, α-pinene 4–7%, β-pinene 5–8%, δ-limonene 2–9%, β-myrcene 2–3%, γ-terpinene 1–2%, cis-β-ocimene 1%, terpinolene <1%, α-terpinene 1%) • monoterpenols 18–20% (incl. linalool 2–11%, α-terpineol 2–5%, terpinen-4-ol 2–6%) • sesquiterpenes (β-caryophyllene 1–2%, α-humulene 0.5%, traces cadinene, germacrene D) • ester terpenyl acetate <4%, traces misc. others • aldehyde geranial 1.4%

**Chance of adulteration:** Minimal while this oil is still relatively unknown, but progressively greater if it ever became popular, possibly with the similar oil Ravintsara (*Cinnamomum camphora* ct. cineole) but more likely with cheaper cineolic oils such as Cajeput (*Melaleuca cajuputi*), Niaouli (*Melaleuca quinquenervia* ct. cineole) and Eucalyptus species

**Related oils:** A second chemotype exists, *Cinnamosma fragrans* ct. limonene, with limonene levels 30–71% and traces of linalool

## Therapeutic Functions and Indications

### SPECIFIC SYMPTOMATOLOGY – *All applications*

Low vitality, chronic mental and physical fatigue, mental fog, debility, loss of enthusiasm, depression, low self-confidence, insecurity, withdrawal, difficulty with making decisions, grief, mild anxiety, daytime drowsiness, cold hands and feet, weak muscles, joint and muscle aches, low-back ache, swollen glands, chronic or recurrent infections

### PSYCHOLOGICAL – *Aromatic diffusion, whole-body massage*

**Essential PNEI function and indication:** Stimulant in weakness conditions
**Possible brain dynamics:** Increases prefrontal cortex and basal ganglia functioning
**Fragrance category:** High tone with fresh-pungent and sweet notes
**Indicated psychological disorders:** ADD, depression

#### STIMULATES THE MIND AND PROMOTES ALERTNESS

- Lethargy, drowsiness, stupor
- Mental confusion, poor concentration, poor short-term memory

#### PROMOTES SELF-CONFIDENCE AND MOTIVATION

- Low self-confidence and self-esteem, pessimism, depression
- Loss of motivation, self-neglect

### PHYSIOLOGICAL – *Nebulizer inhalation, gel cap, suppository, external applications*

**Therapeutic status:** Mild remedy with no cumulative toxicity
**Topical safety status:** Non-irritant, non-sensitizing

**Tropism:** Nervous, respiratory, urinary, reproductive, musculoskeletal systems

**Essential diagnostic function:** Restores hypotonic/weak and warms asthenic/cold terrain conditions

PRIMARILY RESTORATIVE:

*nervous and cerebral restorative:* hypotonic (weak) conditions with cerebral deficiency, mental and physical fatigue, debility, burnout, depression, memory or concentration loss, somnolence; neurasthenia, CFS, postviral depression, convalescence

*mild nervous sedative:* insomnia, mild anxiety, esp. with chronic mental and physical fatigue; nervous or anxious depression

*analgesic:* pain conditions, incl. spasmodic; incl. colic, headache, neuromuscular and arthritic pain, dysuria

*urogenital mucosal restorative (anticatarrhal), antibacterial:* chronic vaginitis with discharges/leucorrhoea, chronic mucous cystitis, blennuria

PRIMARILY STIMULANT:

*arterial circulatory stimulant:* a wide range of asthenic (cold) conditions with poor circulation, cold skin

*respiratory stimulant, mucolytic and fluidifying expectorant, antiseptic, antitussive:* acute and chronic congestive respiratory conditions (upper and lower) with cough and dyspnoea, incl. bronchitis, emphysema

*musculoskeletal stimulant, antirheumatic, anti-inflammatory, analgesic:* rheumatic and arthritic pain and inflammation; fibromyalgia, headaches

*antioxidant*

ANTIMICROBIAL ACTIONS:

*anti-infective, immunostimulant, anti-inflammatory, analgesic:* a large range of infections with resultant painful inflammation; esp. acute, viral or epidemic infections, esp. respiratory, gastrointestinal, urinary and genital

– *strong antiviral:* colds and flu, rhinitis, sinusitis, otitis, gingivitis, aphthous sores; bronchitis, gastroenteritis, viral croup, viral enteritis, viral hepatitis, infectious mononucleosis/glandular fever, chickenpox, herpes zoster/ shingles, dendritis, herpes simplex/genital herpes, cold sores, cervical dysplasia/HPV, EBV

- **broad-spectrum antibacterial:** gram-positive and gram-negative bacterial infections, incl. common cold, sinusitis, rhinitis, chronic bronchitis, pneumonia, whooping cough; gastroenteritis, dysentery, food poisoning, typhoid; skin infections; septicaemia; endo- and pericarditis; gonorrhoea

*antifungal:* misc. fungal infections, incl. skin, nails, vaginal

*antiparasitic:* amoebiasis

SYNERGISTIC COMBINATIONS

- Saro + Rosemary/Ravintsara: nervous restorative and circulatory stimulant for neurasthenia or burnout with fatigue, depression, cold extremities

- Saro + Ravintsara/Niaouli: strong antiviral, anti-inflammatory, analgesic for the onset of upper respiratory infections, influenza, esp. with fatigue, low immunity

- Saro + Cajeput/Green myrtle: strong arterial and bronchial stimulant, expectorant, antibacterial for bacterial bronchitis with cough, sputum, dyspnoea, esp. with poor circulation

- Saro + Niaouli/Ravintsara: immune restorative and stimulant, antiviral in chronic immune deficiency with recurrent, chronic or dormant infections, fatigue, systemic toxicosis

- Saro + Green myrtle: anticatarrhal mucosal restorative, antibacterial for chronic vaginitis with leucorrhoea, chronic mucous cystitis

- Saro + Cypress/Siberian fir: strong antitussive for a wide range of chronic coughs and dyspnoea

- Saro + Nutmeg/Black pepper: antiparasitic for amoebiasis

COMPLEMENTARY COMBINATIONS

- Saro + Tea tree/Niaouli: strong antiviral in a wide range of viral infections

- Saro + Spearmint: mucolytic stimulant expectorant for congestive bronchial infections with copious sputum, esp. purulent

- Saro + Lemongrass/May chang: anti-inflammatory, analgesic in rheumatic and arthritic conditions

- Saro + Lavender/Petitgrain bigarade: nervous sedative-restorative for chronic mental and physical fatigue with insomnia, anxiety, anxious depression

- Saro + Atlas cedarwood: anticatarrhal mucosal restorative, antibacterial and analgesic for chronic vaginitis with leucorrhoea, chronic mucous cystitis with dysuria

## TOPICAL – *Liniment, ointment, cream, compress and other cosmetic preparations*

**Skin care:** Not used

> ***vulnerary, antiseptic, analgesic:*** cuts, wounds, infections; boils, abscesses

> ***antiviral, antibacterial, antifungal:*** herpes, shingles, acne and other local infections

**Therapeutic precautions:** As Saro oil is essentially a warming, drying stimulant, internal use is best avoided in those presenting with hypersthenic/hot and dry conditions. It should be used with caution during pregnancy. Saro is suitable for treating both acute and chronic forms of inflammation.

**Pharmacological precautions:** Saro should be avoided in babies and infants because of its 1,8 cineole content. It is otherwise well tolerated in children and adults. It has no carcinogenic potential.

**Preparations:**

- Diffusor: 3–4 drops in water
- Massage oil: 2–5% dilution in vegetable oil
- Liniment: 5–10% dilution in vegetable oil
- Gel cap: 2–3 drops with olive oil

## Chinese Medicine Functions and Indications

**Aroma energy:** Pungent, sweet

**Movement:** Rising

**Warmth:** Neutral to warm

**Meridian tropism:** Lung, Bladder, Spleen, Stomach

**Five-Element affinity:** Metal, Earth

**Essential function:** To tonify the Qi and Yang, raise the Yang and strengthen the Shen

1. **Tonifies the Qi, raises the clear Yang, animates the Heart, strengthens the Shen and relieves depression**

   - **Qi deficiency with Shen weakness**, with fatigue, poor focus and memory, apathy, depression, recurring infections:

     Rosemary/Niaouli/Ravintsara

   - **Clear Yang Qi deficiency with Shen weakness**, with mental fog, poor focus, confusion, slow response, dizziness:

     Peppermint/Grand fir/Rosemary

2. **Warms the Middle Warmer, dries damp and relieves pain and distension**

   - **Stomach-Spleen empty cold** (Spleen Yang deficiency) with epigastric or abdominal pain, nausea, appetite loss, odourless loose stool:

     Ginger/Juniper berry/Pimenta berry

   - **Stomach-Spleen damp-cold** with indigestion, flatulence, nausea, abdominal bloating, chronic diarrhoea:

     Nutmeg/Clove/Ginger

3. **Warms the Lung, expels phlegm and relieves coughing**

   - **Lung phlegm-cold** with sputum expectoration, chronic cough, cold extremities:

     Cardamom/Grand fir/Laurel

   - **Lung phlegm-heat-dryness** with dry cough, thirst, fever, fatigue, expectoration of scanty, sticky sputum:

     Lemon eucalyptus/Lavender/Spearmint/Tea tree

4. **Warms and releases the exterior, dispels wind-cold, opens the sinuses and relieves pain and congestion; boosts the protective Qi**

   - **External wind-cold with Qi or Yang deficiency**, with aches and pains, sneezing, sinus congestion, cough, fatigue, cold extremities, frequent infections:

     Eucalyptus, narrow-leaf/Ravintsara/Niaouli

   - **Lung wind-cold** with coughing, chest congestion and pain:

     Grand fir/Niaouli/Cypress

5. **Warms and opens the meridians, dispels wind-damp-cold and relieves pain**

   - **Wind-damp-cold obstruction** with rheumatic aches and pains, cold joints and muscles:

     Rosemary/Juniper berry/Black pepper

REMARKS

The Saro tree is a Malagasy representative of a small botanical family, the wild-cinnamon or Canellaceae family, that counts various aromatic tropical trees and shrubs in East Africa and in Florida down to the chain of the Greater Antilles. With their thick, large aromatic leaves, trees of the *Cinnamosma* genus are found only in the dry, dense forests of Western Madagascar. The tree's local Malagasy name of Mandravasarotra means 'which overcomes all challenges' or 'which fights off illness'. The decocted leaves are considered a virtual panacea and are drunk freely to build energy, as well as to treat infections such as colds, flus and food poisoning. It seems that an enterprising French distiller during the late 20th century was the first to extract the essential oil, which he quickly renamed Saro. This aromatic remedy has definitely become more prominent among European practitioners since the turn of this century.

With its fresh-pungent, yet sweet and somewhat spicy fragrance, Saro oil can easily be mistaken for Ravintsara or Niaouli, but its note is rounder and gentler, yet deeper. Nevertheless, its physiological effects are as profound as these other two. Not surprisingly, they are also remarkably similar. The pharmacognosical footprints of these three oils are quite similar, with a nice balance of more Yang, stimulating constituents and more Yin, calming ones.

In terms of clinical usage, it is best to think of Saro as a good nervous restorative on one hand, and a good respiratory stimulant on the other. However, it is only fair to point out that, in allopathic medical circles, Saro is seen as simply another antiviral agent, alongside many others. But even in this reductionistic theatre, it is admitted that Saro really excels at treating chronic and dormant viral infections. This is considered its asterisk indication, despite widespread use in formulas for a wide range of microbial conditions in general.

Like Ravintsara, Saro specifically exerts a twin action on the nervous system, both restorative and mildly sedative. As such, the oil is perfect for chronic signs of weakness, such as fatigue, debility, burnout and convalescence, but especially when accompanied by some mental or psychic tension, causing insomnia, mild but chronic anxiety, nervous depression and pain. Stated another way, Saro treats weak and somewhat tense terrain. Its analgesic effect, combined with its circulatory stimulant action, also makes for a useful ingredient in formulas targeting chronic cold, painful rheumatic-arthritic disorders. Saro's secondary action of toning the mucous membrane may also be a useful addition in patients with additional damp-type discharges of the bladder or reproductive organs. Like Ravintsara again, Saro is essentially a gentle remedy, but an effective one nonetheless, despite the absence of acrid, aggressive phenols.

Like most other fresh-pungent oils rich in 1,8 cineole, Saro exerts an excellent expectorant action that has been noted as both drying and fluidifying to the respiratory mucosa. The oil shines in all types of congestive respiratory conditions, including infectious ones. Its local antiseptic and systemic immunostimulant actions will also engage here. Upper respiratory infections, especially with painful sinus congestion, will also benefit from steam inhalations, nebulizer sessions and such like.

Saro can also serve as a welcome psychological remedy when used by olfaction. Embodying fresh, pungent fragrance energy with considerable sweetness, the oil is gently uplifting for states of combined mental and emotional lethargy, inability to fully focus and emotional apathy arising from discouragement. Saro can be a gentle but persistent ally for those whose loss of self-confidence and low self-esteem is connected to their inability to see and think clearly, to think for oneself. At the same time, the fragrance opens a dialogue between the self and the world based on trust and integrity. Like the breath itself, Saro has the ability to transform this exchange, the receiving and giving between individual and universal life energy, from a disconnected, difficult process to an easy, smooth and fluid exchange.

# Scotch Pine

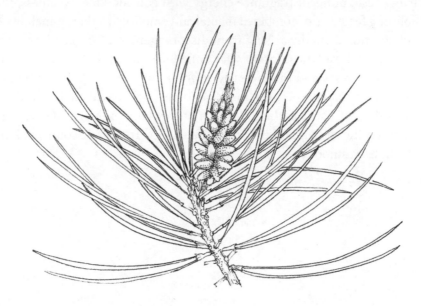

**Botanical source:** The twig and needle of *Pinus sylvestris* L. (Coniferae/Pinaceae – pine family), an evergreen coniferous tree from temperate boreal forests

**Other names:** Scots pine, Forest/Norway pine; Pin sylvestre (Fr), Kiefer (Ge), Bor bijeli (Serbian, Croatian), Pino scozzese (It), Pino escocés (Sp)

**Appearance:** A mobile clear or yellow-greenish liquid with a fresh-conifer pungent-green odour with balsamic, resinous or tarry base tones

**Perfumery status:** A head note of low intensity and medium persistence

**Extraction:** Steam distillation of the fresh needles and branch tips, October to April

**1 kg oil yield from:** 100–200 kg of the needles (a fairly good yield)

**Production areas:** France, Switzerland, Austria, Hungary, Serbia, Sweden, Canada

**Typical constituents:** Monoterpenes 60–80% (incl. α-pinene 20–50%, β-pinene 2–35%, δ-3-carene 1–32%, l-limonene 25–30%, camphene, sabinene, ocimene, terpinene, terpinolene) • sesquiterpenes <8% (incl. β-caryophyllene 2%, longifolene, cadinene, copaene, β-guaiene, β-farnesene, muurolene, patchoulene) • monoterpenols (incl. borneol <2%, pinocarveol, terpinen-4-ol 1%, terpineol) • sesquiterpenols (incl. epi-/α-cadenol, muurolol) • esters (incl. bornyl acetate 1–6%) • citronellal, myrtenal

**Chance of adulteration:** Fairly high, as commercial pine oil is usually created from any number of different *Pinus* species (including those below), with or without synthetic additives such as camphene, pinenes, limonene and esters such as bornyl and isobornyl acetate (Lis-Balchin 2006)

**Related oils:** In addition to the other conifer tree oils such as the firs and spruces, the following species of pine are also regularly produced. Most have similar therapeutic functions, although some of them are not considered as profound as the functions of Scotch pine or have no established therapeutic functions beyond a common respiratory restorative and stimulant action.

- Sea or Maritime pine (*Pinus pinaster* Soland) from France, with fine top notes

- Black pine (*Pinus nigra* J.F. Arnold) from France and Austria, with deeper base notes

- Dwarf Swiss mountain or Dwarf mugo pine (*Pinus mugo* Turra, *P. mugo* var. *pumilio* Zenari) from Austria and Switzerland, with its salty-fresh-pungent-green notes, dominated by terpinolene

- Swiss pine (*Pinus cembra* L.) from Austria and Switzerland, with its fine sweet-green notes.

- Corsican pine (*Pinus nigra* subsp. *laricio* Poir.) from Corsica, with its sweeter fresh aroma

- Aleppo pine (*Pinus halepensis* Miller) from various Mediterranean countries

- White pine (*Pinus strobus* L.) from Northeast North America, with a soft, sweet-green, pine-like aroma

- Norway or Red pine (*Pinus resinosa* Sol. ex Aiton) from Canada, with salty, pungent green notes

- Jack pine (*Pinus banksiana* Lamb.) from Canada, with a sweeter, less tarry, pine-like aroma

- Ponderosa pine (*Pinus ponderosa* Douglas ex P. and C. Lawson) from North America

Other pine oils too numerous to mention are sometimes produced as well, although most of them are simply sources of industrial turpentine oil, extracted from the tree bark, or used for Scotch pine adulteration

## Therapeutic Functions and Indications

SPECIFIC SYMPTOMATOLOGY – *All applications*

Chronic mental and physical tiredness, burnout, exhaustion, low self-confidence, low stamina, low vitality, shallow breathing, chronic weak cough, chest congestion with expectoration, sore throat, swollen glands, muscle and nerve aches and pains, weight loss or gain, dry skin, malaise, chronic menstrual problems, early or heavy periods with pain before onset, clots in flow

## PSYCHOLOGICAL – *Aromatic diffusion, whole-body massage*

**Essential PNEI function and indication:** Stimulant in weakness conditions

**Possible brain dynamics:** Increases prefrontal cortex and basal ganglia functioning

**Fragrance category:** Base tone with pungent, woody notes

**Indicated psychological disorders:** ADD, depression, dissociative disorder, psychotic and schizoid conditions

### PROMOTES WILLPOWER AND PERSEVERANCE

- Low willpower, mental and emotional burnout

- Loss of perseverance, discouragement, self-neglect

### PROMOTES SELF-CONFIDENCE AND MOTIVATION

- Low self-confidence and self-esteem, insecurity, pessimism, depression

- Loss of motivation, self-neglect

## PHYSIOLOGICAL – *Nebulizer inhalation, gel cap, suppository, external applications*

**Therapeutic status:** Mild remedy with no cumulative toxicity

**Topical safety status:** Non-irritant, non-sensitizing. However, some skin sensitization is possible with significant δ-3-carene content, and some irritation if the oil is oxidized.

**Tropism:** Neuroendocrine, respiratory, urinary, reproductive, hepatic, musculoskeletal systems

**Essential diagnostic function:** Restores hypotonic/weak terrain conditions

### PRIMARILY RESTORATIVE AND REGULATING:

> ***strong systemic neuroendocrine and immune restorative and regulator, adaptogenic:*** chronic hypotonic (weak) conditions involving pituitary/adrenal/thyroid/thymus/gonadal (and other endocrine) deficiencies and dysregulations, with chronic inflammation, allergies, fatigue, debility, malaise

- *pituitary-adrenal restorative and regulator:* HPA axis deficiency with adrenal fatigue or exhaustion, loss of stamina, afternoon fatigue, salt cravings; anabolic and catabolic deficiencies with weight loss, weight gain, debility; metabolic disorders in general, CFS, neurasthenia, chronic asthma, MS and other neurodegenerative disorders

- *hypertensive:* hypotension

- *pituitary-gonadal (ovarian and testicular/reproductive) restorative and regulator, aphrodisiac:* HPG axis deficiency with hormonal dysregulation; oestrogen/progesterone/testosterone deficiency, incl. dysmenorrhoea, amenorrhoea, PMS, menopausal syndrome, loss of libido, low sperm count

- *pituitary-pancreatic restorative:* hypo- and hyperglycaemia; diabetes

- *respiratory restorative:* chronic weak lungs and low respiratory capacity, shallow breathing, chronic cough, any chronic lung condition

PRIMARILY DECONGESTANT:

*respiratory decongestant, mucolytic and fluidifying expectorant:* acute and chronic congestive respiratory conditions (upper and lower), incl. bronchitis, sinusitis, laryngitis, pharyngitis, colds, sore throat

*uterine, ovarian and pelvic decongestant:* congestive dysmenorrhoea, menorrhagia

*lymphatic decongestant:* lymphatic congestion with swollen glands, oedema

*metabolic detoxicant, diuretic, litholytic:* metabolic toxicosis, incl. arthritic and rheumatic conditions, gout, gallstones, chronic urinary infections, incl. cystitis

*anti-inflammatory, analgesic:* inflammatory neuromuscular, urinary and hepatobiliary conditions with pain, incl. fibromyalgia, neuralgias (incl. sciatica); urinary infections, incl. prostatitis and cystitis with dysuria, nephritis; laryngitis, cholecystitis, hepatitis

*anhydrotic:* excessive foot perspiration

ANTIMICROBIAL ACTIONS:

*mild antibacterial, antiviral, immunostimulant(?)*

SYNERGISTIC COMBINATIONS

- Scotch pine + Black spruce: strong systemic neuroendocrine restorative and adaptogenic in multiple endocrine deficiencies with neurasthenia, adrenal exhaustion, immune deficiency, chronic fatigue, loss of libido

- Scotch pine + Black spruce: strong respiratory restorative, antitussive for weak lungs or chronic respiratory conditions, with chronic cough, low vitality, fatigue

- Scotch pine + Rosemary/Green myrtle: mucolytic expectorant for chronic bronchitis with copious sputum, congestive dyspnoea

- Scotch pine + Cypress/Hyssop: strong antitussive and bronchospasmolytic for chronic spasmodic cough and dyspnoea, asthma

- Scotch pine + Juniper berry + Tea tree: urinary antiseptic and diuretic for chronic urinary infections with dysuria

- Scotch pine + Juniper berry/Yarrow: detoxicant diuretic for metabolic toxicosis with rheumatic and arthritic conditions, eczema

- Scotch pine + Cypress/Mastic: strong prostatic and lymphatic decongestant for prostate swelling, swollen glands, haemorrhoids

COMPLEMENTARY COMBINATIONS

- Scotch pine + Sage: strong systemic neuroendocrine-immune restorative in many and multiple endocrine deficiencies, incl. adrenal exhaustion, hypothyroid syndrome, chronic female hormonal imbalance, menopausal syndrome, chronic fatigue syndrome, chronic immune deficiency with recurrent or hidden infections

- Scotch pine + Geranium: strong pituitary-adrenocortical restorative for menopausal syndrome

- Scotch pine + Rose/Geranium: strong pituitary-gonadal restorative for chronic irregular periods, dysmenorrhoea, menopausal syndrome, loss of libido

- Scotch pine + Geranium: pancreatic restorative, blood-sugar regulator for hyper- and hypo-glycaemia, diabetes

- Scotch pine + Niaouli: anti-infective respiratory and immune restorative in chronic or recurring respiratory infections with weak lungs

- Scotch pine + Sage: anti-inflammatory, analgesic and antiseptic for chronic sore throat, hoarseness, aphonia, spasmodic dysphonia

- Scotch pine + Geranium: uterine and pelvic decongestant for pelvic congestion with menorrhagia, haemorrhoids

- Scotch pine + Black pepper/Spike lavender/Cajeput: strong antirheumatic and analgesic in painful, cold rheumatic-arthritic conditions

- Scotch pine + Lemon eucalyptus/Wintergreen: anti-inflammatory, analgesic and antiseptic in acute painful inflammatory urinary conditions with dysuria, incl. cystitis, interstitial cystitis, urethritis, nephritis, kidney stone with colic

## TOPICAL – *Liniment, ointment, cream, compress and other cosmetic preparations*

**Skin care:** Not used

*analgesic, anti-inflammatory, mild rubefacient, antiseptic:* rheumatic-arthritic and neuralgic conditions; sinus pain, toothache

*vulnerary:* injuries, wounds

*insect repellent, insecticidal:* incl. mosquitoes

*deodorant*

**Therapeutic precautions:** Scotch pine oil is best used in chronic, not acute, asthma, and in between, not during, attacks; this is partly because of a theoretical risk of causing bronchospasm.

**Pharmacological precautions:** Some skin sensitization with rashes is possible if Scotch pine oil is high in δ-carene or is somewhat oxidized from age; it should therefore be avoided in those with sensitive skin. For all topical use, only Pine oil that is relatively fresh (i.e. non-oxidized) should be used.

**Preparations:**

- Diffusor: 3–5 drops in water
- Massage oil: 2–5% dilution in vegetable oil
- Liniment: 5–10% dilution in vegetable oil
- Footbath: 3–6 drops in hot water for tired or sweaty feet
- Gel cap: 2–3 drops with some olive oil

## Chinese Medicine Functions and Indications

**Aroma energy:** Pungent, woody

**Movement:** Stabilizing, rising

**Warmth:** Neutral to warm

**Meridian tropism:** Lung, Kidney, Bladder

**Five Element affinity:** Metal, Water

**Essential function:** To tonify the Qi and Yang, and strengthen the Lung and Shen

1. **Tonifies the Qi, strengthens the Lung, lifts the Shen and relieves fatigue**

   - **Qi deficiency with Shen weakness**, with fatigue, low endurance, frequent infections, chronic sore throat, disconnection, slow emotional response:
     Rosemary/Ravintsara/Niaouli/Sage

   - **Lung Qi deficiency with Shen weakness**, with mental and physical fatigue, chronic cough, shallow breathing, sadness, withdrawal:
     Rosemary/Grand fir/Eucalyptus/Frankincense

2. **Tonifies the Lung and Kidney, fortifies the Yang, diffuses Lung Qi and relieves coughing and wheezing**

   - **Lung and Kidney Yang deficiency** with chronic cough, wheeze, chest tightness:
     Black spruce/Thyme ct. thymol/Cypress

   - **Kidney Yang deficiency with Shen weakness**, with low stamina, mental and physical fatigue, loss of sex drive, backache, weak knees and legs, fearfulness:
     Ginger/Black spruce/Clove/Cinnamon

3. **Resolves and expels phlegm, dries damp, diffuses Lung Qi and relieves pain and coughing**

   - **Lung phlegm-damp** with cough, expectoration of copious loose sputum, wheezing, chest pain and congestion, fatigue:
     Atlas cedarwood/Hyssop/Grand fir/Green myrtle

4. **Warms and opens the meridians, dispels wind-damp, relaxes the tendons and relieves pain**

   - **Wind-damp-cold obstruction** with rheumatic pain (esp. in the upper parts), joint cramping:
     Spike lavender/Ginger/Frankincense/Juniper berry

REMARKS

Along with spruce and larch, the pine is a member of the world's largest land biome, the taiga or boreal conifer forests of the northern hemisphere that wrap around the planet westward from the Russian Far East through to Scandinavia, Canada and Alaska. The Scotch pine in particular has been distilled for its essential oil since the Middle Ages, especially in Sweden, Germany and, of course, the Scottish Highlands.

As a traditional herbal remedy, the pine is already mentioned in the Greek medicine writings of Hippocrates and Theophrastus. However, it was not until the emergence of naturopathic treatments in 18th-century Europe (themselves Hippocratic hygienic revivals) that Scotch pine oil really found its niche. Its fresh, balsamic, invigorating scent made its way into Turkish or hot steam baths, respiratory steam inhalations and whole-body water irrigation. By the mid-19th century, Scotch pine had become iconic in the steamy smellscape of spas, hot springs and sanatoriums from Yalta in Crimea to Baden-Baden in Germany; from Bath and Harrogate in England to Berkeley Springs and other tony watering holes in the Eastern United States.

As to this day, Pine oil was considered revitalizing, detoxifying and decongesting to the lungs. In addition, it was found extremely effective for treating throat conditions and became an official remedy in the 1872 Pharmacopoeia of the Hospital for Diseases of the Throat housed in Golden Square, London. Pine was one of several essential oils (including Myrtle, Thyme, Benzoin, Cajeput, Juniper berry and Sandalwood) used for hot steam inhalations for treating various throat conditions. Since Victorian days, European practitioners and therapists of all kinds have kept Pine at the top of their aromatic arsenal for deep revitalization, respiratory tonification and decongestion, and general detoxification. On the spirit and psychological level too, Pine in various textbooks to this day still inspires eulogies on its deeply restorative effects.

In terms of its tropism, Scotch pine works very much on the chest-pelvis axis, linking respiratory and urogenital functions, including the significant throat-genitals polarity. In both these areas the oil boosts and strengthens functions on one hand and decongests and detoxifies on the other. Scotch pine is one of the few true oxygenating respiratory restoratives for any chronic weak lung condition with poor oxygenation, fatigue and chronic weak cough. In the pelvic region, the oil is likewise a comprehensive reproductive restorative with a strong endocrine influence along the pituitary-gonadal (HPG) axis. Most reproductive hormonal dysregulations will benefit here, especially as Scotch pine also acts as a systemic neuroendocrine restorative along the pituitary-adrenal cortex (HPA) axis. In short, Scotch pine is an adaptogen useful in all those presenting a chronic weak terrain with one or more endocrine deficiencies. Success with these chronic conditions includes not only adrenal fatigue, chronic fatigue syndrome, chronic dysmenorrhoea and loss of libido, but also a pancreatic restorative and regulative action for blood-sugar dysregulations, much like Geranium.

As an important decongestant remedy, Scotch pine again spans the lung-reproductive axis. Congestive upper and respiratory conditions, as well as throat congestion, are the beneficiaries from its gentle stimulant and good mucolytic action. For the pelvic organs, Scotch pine is a detoxicant decongestant that acts equally on fluid, lymph and blood circulation. Chronic conditions of uterine, ovarian, pelvic and lower venous congestion will stand to benefit here. Its detoxicant diuretic action, like that of Juniper berry, addresses conditions of metabolic toxicosis with resultant rheumatic and arthritic disorders. Built into this broad action are good analgesic and anti-inflammatory actions that have also been applied to conditions as different as gout, cystitis, laryngitis and cholecystitis – not to mention use for topical preparations.

Like Sage, Scotch pine is a good anhydrotic, detoxicant and restorative when used in warm footbaths.

With its exceptional longevity and vertical thrust to heaven despite rude climes, the pine tree in many cultures worldwide is an iconic emblem of the will to live, persevere and survive with complete uprightness in the face of adversity. Pine is all about perennial presence, longevity and timeless grace. As an olfactory remedy with deep pungent, woody notes that remind us of Black spruce, Pine oil also can evoke the faculties of honesty, courage and willpower in the individual. Pine is for the person whose soul strength has been crushed by severe hardships or harsh circumstances. The oil may help create enough soul presence and honesty to kindle a spark of courage and motivation to continue on life's journey, despite all odds and opposition. Pine may revive the will to start over again, taking one day at a time, being content to just be alive, to exist.

**Related oils:** Turpentine oil, or térébenthine in French, sometimes known as Pine resin oil, was much used in the past both in France (since the Middle Ages) and the US (since the 18th century). The oil is steam distilled from the oleoresin secreted by the wood and trunk of any number of different pine, fir and larch species. Eclectic and regular doctors in North America made extensive use of its warming, circulatory stimulant, diuretic, mucostatic and somewhat haemostatic actions for congestive, mucousy conditions of the pelvic organs (urinary, reproductive and intestinal) with chronic discharges. It was used both internally and in topical preparations. Topical applications made extensive use of its rubefacient, counterirritant, analgesic and moderate anti-inflammatory actions.

The source of **Turpentine oil** in France is *Pinus pinaster*; its dominant constituents are monoterpenes (<90%), with small amounts of monoterpenols (2%), sesquiterpenes (5%), the ketones pinocarvone and piperitone (3%) and the ester bornyl acetate (0.5%). French practitioners utilize the oil only for steam inhalations and in various topical preparations but contraindicate internal use. Indications for Turpentine oil include urinary infections with bleeding or gleet, andropause, respiratory infections with copious phlegm (as a fluidifying and antiseptic expectorant), and chronic, cold arthritic and neuralgic disorders. Caution is advised with topical use as it may be allergenic in some individuals.

**Terebine** is a distilled monoterpenic remedy prepared by the action of sulphuric acid on raw Turpentine. It was formerly valued for treating the same and further respiratory conditions as Turpentine (King, Felter and Lloyd 1898).

# Spikenard

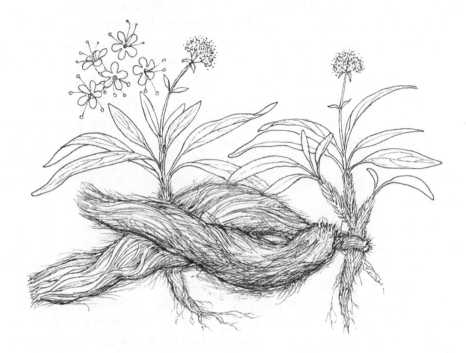

**Botanical source:** The root of *Nardostachys jatamansi* DC. (syn. *N. grandiflora* DC.) and *N. chinensis* Batalin (Valerianaceae – valerian family). The two species that furnish Spikenard oil occur wild in the Himalayan region that spans Nepal to Yunnan in East China in high alpine meadows at 3,200 to 5,000 feet in elevation.

**Other names:** *N. jatamansi*: Nepalese spikenard, Indian nard; Nard indien (Fr), Jatamansi (Nepalese, Hindi, Bengali), Nardus (It), Nardus indica (Lat)

*N. chinensis:* Chinese spikenard; Gan song, Gan Song xiang (Mandarin), Gam chung (Cantonese)

**Appearance:** *N. jatamansi*: A mobile green or olive liquid with a fresh earthy-musty-rooty odour with faint, delicate mossy green and sweet-wood notes

*N. chinensis:* A thick dark amber to dark brown liquid with a deep rooty, earthy-musty and somewhat sweet-woody odour

**Perfumery status:** A base note of medium intensity and good persistence

**Extraction:** Steam distillation of the dried crushed roots throughout the year, as needed; collection of both species is in October

**1 kg oil yield from:** 75–90 kg of the root (a good yield)

**Production areas:** Nepal (Nepal spikenard), Tibet/East China (Chinese spikenard)

**Typical constituents** *(N. jatamansi)*: Sesquiterpenes 35–60% (incl. patchoulenes <29%, β-gurjunene 8%, guaiadiene 9%, α-selinene 2–9%, germacrene-D 3%, aristolene, seychellene, maaliene, dihydroazulenes, calamenene, hexadecene, β-caryophyllene) • sesquiterpenols (incl. nardol <10%, patchouli alcohols 6%, calarenol, valerianol, cubebol, nerolidol) • sesquiterpenones (incl. valeranone 5–20%, hydroxyaristolenone 6%, nardostachone, aristolenone, ionone) • aldehydes, incl. sesquiterpenal valerianal 7% • esters (incl. bornyl acetate, isobornyl valerianate, terpenyl valerianate, methylcarvacylester) • coumarins • jatamansinic acid • monoterpenes

**Chance of adulteration:** Moderate, and possibly with sesquiterpene and sesquiterpenol-rich Patchouli oil. However, it is common practice to mix or blend the two types of Spikenard oils, the Nepalese and the Chinese, in various proportions, all depending on availability and need. As the two oils are distinct in both colour and fragrance, it should be possible to estimate the approximate proportion of each in a blended Spikenard oil.

**Related oils:** Spikenard belongs to the large and widespread valerian family that includes the herbal remedy Valerian root (*Valeriana officinalis*). Note that there are two plant sources for Spikenard oil, the Nepalese and the Chinese spikenard, which are commonly confused both at the production end and in the literature. Each oil has a somewhat different profile of fragrance and constituents, but any clinical differences of use have yet to be established. The Nepalese spikenard oil is more commonly available.

An essential oil is also distilled from the Indian valerian or Tagar (*Valeriana wallichii* DC.), a close relative with somewhat different properties. In the past, Hardwick's valerian (*V. hardwickii* Wall.), also from the Himalayas, was also distilled for its oil.

Spikenard should not be confused with American spikenard (*Aralia racemosa*), which is not an aromatic plant (although highly medicinal), nor with Muskroot (*Ferula sumbul, F. moschata*) from Central Asia and Tibet, an aromatic plant historically used as a musk substitute, especially in Russia.

## Therapeutic Functions and Indications

### SPECIFIC SYMPTOMATOLOGY – *All applications*

Fears, anxieties for no known reason, emotionally sensitive, feelings of insecurity, mental delusions, flights of fancy, irrational speech, restlessness, agitation with depression, intense dreams and nightmares with no recollection on waking, palpitations with chest pains, headaches, aches and pains that come and go for no reason, skin allergies, hot spells, ticks and tremors, painful or stopped periods, sluggish energy, irregular bowel movement, heavy tired legs

## PSYCHOLOGICAL – *Aromatic diffusion, whole-body massage*

**Essential PNEI function and indication:** Relaxant in overstimulation conditions

**Possible brain dynamics:** Reduces basal ganglia and anterior cingulate gyrus hyperfunctioning, resolves temporal lobes dysregulation

**Fragrance category:** Base tone with rooty, woody, sweet notes

**Indicated psychological disorders:** Dissociative disorder, psychotic and schizoid conditions, obsessive-compulsive disorder

### STABILIZES THE MIND AND PROMOTES INTEGRATION

- Disconnection, scatteredness, spaciness, oversensitivity, dissociation
- Euphoria, delusion, paranoia, agitation

### PROMOTES STABILITY AND STRENGTH

- Emotional instability with anxiety, fearfulness
- Loss of emotional security and strength

### PROMOTES COGNITIVE FLEXIBILITY

- Worry, obsession, compulsivity
- Repetitive thinking, inability to let go

## PHYSIOLOGICAL – *Nebulizer inhalation, gel cap, suppository, external applications*

**Therapeutic status:** Mild remedy with no cumulative toxicity

**Topical safety status:** Non-irritant, non-sensitizing

**Tropism:** Nervous, cardiovascular, digestive, respiratory, reproductive systems

**Essential diagnostic function:** Relaxes hypertonic/tense and cools hypersthenic/hot terrain conditions

### PRIMARILY RELAXANT AND COOLING:

*strong systemic nervous and vascular relaxant, SNS inhibitor, vagotonic, refrigerant, antipyretic:* hypertonic/tense and hypersthenic/hot conditions, esp. with nervous tension, spasms, inflammation, hot spells, hot flushes, fevers; acute stress-related conditions *strong spasmolytic, anti-inflammatory, analgesic:* a large range of acute spasmodic and inflammatory conditions, esp. of smooth muscles, esp. cardiovascular, gastrointestinal and uterine

- *strong cerebral sedative, hypnotic:* anxiety, insomnia, agitation, PMS, psychosis

- *strong cardiovascular relaxant, vasodilator, hypotensive, analgesic:* palpitations, tachycardia, arrhythmia, dysrhythmia, hyperpnoea, neurogenic angina, neurocardiac syndrome (nervous heart); hypertension, incl. with headaches, migraines

- *intestinal relaxant:* intestinal colic, cramps, IBS, IBD, incl. Crohn's disease

- *uterine relaxant:* spasmodic dysmenorrhoea with cramps

- *anticonvulsant:* seizures, incl. epileptic

- *anti-inflammatory, antiallergic:* allergic skin conditions, incl. atopic eczema/dermatitis, esp. stress-related

PRIMARILY STIMULANT:

*stimulant expectorant:* bronchitis, cough

*uterine stimulant:* amenorrhoea, oligomenorrhoea

*venous restorative:* venous deficiency with varicose veins, haemorrhoids

ANTIMICROBIAL ACTIONS:

*antifungal:* fungal infections with various Aspergillus spp.

*antibacterial:* bacterial infections, incl. Staph.

*antimalarial:* malaria

SYNERGISTIC COMBINATIONS

- Spikenard + Roman camomile: strong systemic nervous relaxant, sedative, spasmolytic and anti-inflammatory for a wide range of spasmodic and inflammatory tense conditions, esp. of smooth muscle organs

- Spikenard + Ylang ylang: strong neurocardiac relaxant, vasodilator and hypotensive for moderate to severe hypertension, tachycardia, headaches and other spasmodic tense conditions

- Spikenard + Vetiver: strong refrigerant and antipyretic for hot spells with red complexion; menopausal hot flushes, fevers in general

COMPLEMENTARY COMBINATIONS

- Spikenard + Marjoram/Clary sage/Petitgrain: systemic nervous relaxant and sedative in many acute and chronic hypertonic/tense, spasmodic stress-related conditions, incl. anxiety, insomnia, palpitations, colic

- Spikenard + Lavender: hypotensive and nervous relaxant for mild to moderate hypertension, insomnia, anxiety

- Spikenard + Ylang ylang + Hyssop: strong hypotensive for severe chronic hypertension

- Spikenard + Blue tansy/Helichrysum: for chronic nightmares

- Spikenard + Tarragon/Basil ct. methylchavicol: strong uterine spasmolytic and analgesic for severe spasmodic dysmenorrhoea

- Spikenard + Patchouli + Rosemary: venous restorative for chronic varicose veins, haemorrhoids, phlebitis

## TOPICAL – *Liniment, ointment, cream, compress and other cosmetic preparations*

**Skin care:** Mature skin type

*anti-inflammatory, antiallergic, mild analgesic:* skin irritations and inflammations, allergic eczema/dermatitis, psoriasis, ulcers, boils, varicose veins, phlebitis

*antifungal:* fungal infections

*hair restorative:* hair loss, hair greying

*deodorant*

**Therapeutic precautions:** As Spikenard is a systemic cooling relaxant to all the major organ systems, internal use of any kind is contraindicated in hypotonic/weak and hyposthenic/cold conditions. Being a strong anti-inflammatory and refrigerant, it is best given for acute forms of inflammation and fever rather than chronic inflammation and low-grade fever. Likewise, Spikenard is best used for acute, not chronic, hypersthenic/tense conditions. Being a uterine stimulant, Spikenard is also contraindicated internally during pregnancy.

**Pharmacological precautions:** None for topical use. Continuous internal use of Spikenard oil, especially on its own, is discouraged (as well as unnecessary), as some practitioners claim it has mild cumulative toxicity. This oil is always best combined with others in blends and formulas.

**Preparations:**

- Diffusor: 2–4 drops in water

- Massage oil: 2–3% dilution in vegetable oil

- Gel cap: 1–2 drops with olive oil

## Chinese Medicine Functions and Indications

**Aroma energy:** Rooty, woody

**Movement:** Sinking, stabilizing

**Warmth:** Cool to cold

**Meridian tropism:** Heart, Kidney, Liver, Spleen

**Five-Element affinity:** Water, Fire, Wood

**Essential function:** To nourish the Yin, descend the Yang, clear heat and calm the Shen

1. **Nourishes the Yin, clears heat, clarifies the Heart and calms the Shen**

   - **Yin deficiency with empty heat**, with hot spells, hot flushes, restlessness, irritability, night sweats:
     Niaouli/Tea tree/Vetiver

   - **Heart and Kidney Yin deficiency with Shen agitation**, with tension, irritability, anxiety, fearfulness, insomnia, nightmares:
     Patchouli/Ylang ylang no. 1/Vetiver/Sandalwood

   - **Yin deficiency with empty heat in late-stage fevers**, with chronic low or remittent afternoon or evening fever, debility, night sweats, five centres heat:
     Lavender/Tea tree/Wintergreen

2. **Regulates Heart Qi, settles the Heart and relieves chest oppression**

   - **Heart Qi constraint** with palpitations, rapid heart beats, precordial oppression, anxiety, insomnia:
     Petitgrain bigarade/Ylang ylang/Neroli

3. **Nourishes Liver Yin, descends the Yang and calms the Shen**

   - **Liver Yin deficiency with floating Yang and Shen agitation**, with tension, agitated depression, ringing ears, dizziness, palpitations, insomnia, nightmares:
     Clary sage/Helichrysum/Vetiver/Sambac jasmine

## 4.  Calms the Liver, extinguishes wind and relieves spasms

- **Liver Yin deficiency with internal wind,** with spasms, tremors, convulsions, palpitations, low-grade fever:

Vetiver/Marjoram/Roman camomile

REMARKS

Despite little use in modern times, Himalayan spikenard has enjoyed the status of a major aromatic plant source for both medicine and perfume for untold millennia. It is one of just a handful of herbal remedies found in the materia medicas of all three of the world's extant major medical systems – Chinese medicine, Ayurvedic medicine and traditional Greek medicine (Tibb Unani). Equally, Spikenard is one of the few aromatic substances employed since prehistory the world over in traditional perfumes and cosmetics. All ancient cultures from Assyria, Babylon and Egypt to North India, Persia, Greece and Rome made use of Spikenard's unique earthy, rooty, mossy fragrance for aesthetic, therapeutic and sacred ritual purposes. Its name 'nar' is said to derive either from the suffix 'ar', meaning fragrance; or from the town of Naar near the river Euphrates in Mesopotamia. Its Nepalese name, Jatamansi or Akashamansi, significantly means 'spirit incarnate'.

Long ago, Spikenard joined the rank of none less than Myrrh and Frankincense: all three were the most sacred aromatics of antiquity, perhaps of all time. It is no accident that all three were particularly esteemed as powerful emblems of spirit and transcendent divinity. Jews and Romans made much use of Spikenard, particularly for sacred anointing balms, for instance to consecrate their priests and bless their sepulchres; the aromatic is mentioned in the Bible's Song of Solomon. Hindu and Buddhist monks made traditional use of the fragrant, smouldering root for meditation practice. During the Tang dynasty Buddhist monks travelling home from India diligently brought the sacred root back with them to the Central Kingdom. Ayurvedic doctors too have always affirmed its benefits in developing awareness and strengthening the spirit – in addition to its purely physiological properties.

As a physiological remedy, Spikenard oil shares many of the properties of Vetiver and Ylang ylang extra or no. 1; its woody, rooty, musty olfactory signature is certainly close to that of Vetiver. The scent of this root reminded John King, the famous 19th-century Eclectic physician, of the smell of Virginia snakeroot. Its pharmacological signature too profiles esters and sesquiterpenes and their variations, like those other two oils. And like them, Spikenard is a strong, systemic relaxant, cooling remedy for treating acute tense and hot conditions. Its effect is essentially calming to three major nerve plexi, the cardiac, solar (coeliac) and sacral.

Spikenard's tropism is particularly the brain and the cardiovascular system. A strong hypnotic cerebral sedative with an action similar to its close botanical cousins Indian and European valerian root (*Valeriana wallichii, V. officinalis*), Spikenard is able to go beyond treating simple anxiety, insomnia and PMS: like Melissa oil too, it can extend its use to psychotic and other extreme states, as well as seizures. As an excellent neurocardiovascular relaxant, like Ylang ylang, Spikenard is for severe palpitations, tachycardia, angina pectoris and vascular headaches, especially migraines. The connection of these conditions with a history of emotional insecurity and wounding is especially interesting and a further indication for its use. Coronary disorders are further supported by the presence of anticoagulant, sedative and spasmolytic coumarins.

Like Vetiver again, Spikenard is a supreme heat-draining or refrigerant remedy, especially when pathogenic heat needs to be pulled down from the head or upper body. Skin allergies have also responded well to its anti-inflammatory and antihistamine actions, including with topical preparations. As a hair restorative for retarding greying, Spikenard is the Ayurvedic and Western equivalent to the Chinese herb He shou wu (*Polygonum multiflorum*); the Roman hair tonic formulas, Foliatum and Regalium, both contained generous amounts of the prized root.

Using Spikenard by olfaction rather than by internal absorption is the best way to access its inner nature and to allow its psychological benefits to unfold. The oil's mysterious woody, rooty and somewhat sweet fragrance has a centring, rooting, grounding effect in the body that simultaneously involves a descent into the present moment. Individuals who tend to become oversensitive, spacey and even delusional will benefit here, as well as those prone to spells of anxiety or fearfulness, along with feelings of insecurity and vulnerability. Because the fragrance also promotes cognitive flexibility, it is a boon for patterns of constant worrying, obsessing and repetitive thinking – essentially an inability to let go of emotionally charged ideas. Likewise, Spikenard can help one let go of old wounds and resentments that are difficult to uproot and let go of.

Turning our attention inward, the fragrance also invites simple reflection on our 'essentials', on our true values, as well as evoking contemplation on the existential mystery of life itself. Spikenard's association with spiritual issues is evident here, as its name Jatamansi, 'spirit incarnate', attests. Its fragrance supports the process of turning inward and resolving our common existential fear, which often arises in times of major personal change and transition, where tension and anxiety about the future is a given. Facilitating inner transformation, Spikenard is known to smooth the passage towards the next stage of a process, while supporting the release of the old in favour of onward movement. Its perennial use as a sacred anointing balm becomes clearer, including its use to ease the transition from earthly life into spirit life. Although we cannot know for certain which type of Nard oil Mary Magdalen used to massage the feet of Jesus and pour some over his head before his death – Plinius the Elder discusses 12 types of Nard in his *Natural History* – the fact remains that her act was more about a preparation for his passing into the spirit world than a simple declaration of love. Here again, Spikenard demonstrates its important role as a grounding aromatic that helps spirit descend into the human body – the downward channel of the Rainbow Bridge – thereby becoming a channel between heaven and earth, and between life and death.

# Sweet Orange

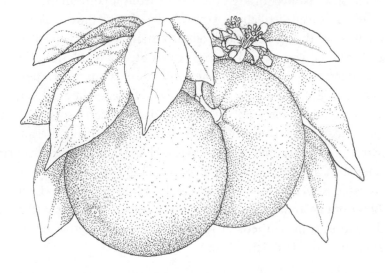

**Botanical source:** The rind of *Citrus x sinensis* [L.] Osbeck (syn. *Citrus aurantium* Osbeck var. *dulcis*) (Rutaceae – rue family), a widely cultivated shrub or small fruit tree of Mediterranean climates. The sweet orange is now considered an ancient cultivated hybrid, possibly between the pomelo (*Citrus maxima*) and the mandarin (*Citrus reticulata*), which are two of the four original, non-hybridized citrus species.

**Other names:** China/Portugal orange; Orange douce (Fr), Orange (Ge), Arancio dolce (It), Naranja dulce (Sp)

**Appearance:** A mobile orangey-yellow to dark orange fluid with a full-bodied warm, fruity-sweet odour. Machine-pressed oils are lighter in colour, while hand-pressed oils are darker (Weiss 1997). Note also that distilled Sweet orange oil (discussed below) is pale yellow and has a thinner, less rich odour than the cold-pressed oil.

**Perfumery status:** A head note of medium intensity and poor persistence

**Extraction:** Cold expression of the fresh ripe orange rinds after scarring

**1 kg oil yield from:** 80–200 kg of the fresh rind (a good yield)

**Production areas:** Italy, South Africa, Brazil, USA, Israel

**Typical constituents:** Monoterpenes <98% (incl. d-limonene 86–95%, myrcene 1–4%, α-pinene) • aldehydes 1.5% (incl. octanal, decanal, citronellal, geranial, neral, traces perillaldehyde, dodecanal, *et al.*) • monoterpenols 1% (mostly linalool) • esters <0.5% (mostly octyl and neryl acetates) • coumarins (incl. bergaptenes) • non-volatile flavonoids

**Chance of adulteration:** Very high, because of the predominant use of distilled Sweet orange oil for the soft-drink, food and perfume industry. Like most other citrus oils, commercial Sweet and Bitter orange oils are simply designer by-products of orange juice production. Distilled orange oils result from a combination of processing techniques such as: steam distillation of the caked peels after the orange juice extraction; steam distillation of the concentrated, oil-rich orange juice itself; solvent extraction of processed residual waters; and in some cases, steam distillation of virgin orange peels (Arctander 1960). In addition, the distilled oil is often deterpenated (i.e. has the terpenes removed), thereby further robbing it of therapeutic potency. Finally, any commercial citrus oil will have UV absorbers and antioxidants such as BHA and BHT added to prevent spoilage from oxidation and increase shelf-life. Because of all these processing techniques, distilled Sweet orange oil has a different profile of constituents and characteristics, and for treatment purposes should be avoided.

Cold-pressed Sweet orange oil itself can be adulterated with the distilled oil of Sweet or Bitter orange (often terpene- and sesquiterpene-free), as well as undergoing further admixtures with synthetic or natural limonene and other terpenes extracted from other citrus oils (Lis-Balchin 2006).

**Related oils:** Sweet orange is divided into three groups, the common, blood and navel orange, each with numerous cultivars; oils are extracted from all three types, with minor differences of fragrance and constituents. Bitter orange (*Citrus aurantium* L. var. *amara*) is the closest relative and has a milder, less sweet fragrance.

## Therapeutic Functions and Indications

### Specific symptomatology – *All applications*

Moodiness, mood swings, irritability, frustration, anger, nervous tension, mild anxiety, distraction, discouragement, pessimism, mild stress-related insomnia, palpitations, low energy in the morning, digestive problems all worse from stress

### Psychological – *Aromatic diffusion, whole-body massage*

**Essential PNEI function and indication:** Regulating in dysregulation conditions
**Possible brain dynamics:** Reduces deep limbic system hyperfunctioning
**Fragrance category:** Middle tone with sweet and lemony notes
**Indicated psychological disorders:** Minor depression, bipolar disorder, ADHD

PROMOTES EMOTIONAL STABILITY AND MILD EUPHORIA

- Emotional instability with irritability, moodiness, mood swings, agitation
- Distraction, emotional confusion with conflict

PROMOTES OPTIMISM AND JOY

- Pessimism, negative or distressed emotions, discouragement

- Mild depression, esp. with anxiety or grief

## PHYSIOLOGICAL – *Nebulizer inhalation, gel cap, suppository, external applications*

**Therapeutic status:** Mild remedy with no cumulative toxicity

**Topical safety status:**

- Cold-pressed oil: Mild skin irritant, moderately skin sensitizing, photo-sensitizing

- Distilled oil: Non-irritant, non-sensitizing, non-photosensitizing

**Tropism:** Nervous, cardiovascular, digestive, urinary, respiratory systems

**Essential diagnostic function:** Balances dysregulated and relaxes hypertonic/tense terrain conditions

PRIMARILY RELAXANT:

*mild nervous relaxant, mild hypnotic:* mild hypertonic (tense) stress-related conditions, esp. in children, the elderly and sensitive people; esp. with nervous tension, anxiety, insomnia, dizziness

*neurocardiac and arterial circulatory relaxant, hypotensive:* palpitations, stress-related heart conditions or 'nervous heart', hypertension

*mild digestive relaxant, spasmolytic:* nervous indigestion, colic, constipation

PRIMARILY STIMULANT:

*gastric and biliary stimulant, aperitive, stomachic, cholagogue, carminative*: atonic upper digestive indigestion with flatulence and bloating, appetite loss, constipation

*mild diuretic:* general oedema

*anti-inflammatory*

*antioxidant*

*antibacterial, mild antifungal:* bronchitis, common cold, mild fungal infections

*deodorant, environmental disinfectant:* air-borne infections

SYNERGISTIC COMBINATIONS

- Sweet orange + Mandarin/Bergamot: nervous sedative and hypnotic for nervous tension, anxiety, insomnia

- Sweet orange + Mandarin/Bergamot: neuro-digestive regulator for chronic neurogenic digestive symptoms or conditions, esp. with constipation or alternating constipation and diarrhoea

- Sweet orange + Grapefruit: lymphatic decongestant for varicose veins, swollen lymph glands; topically also as a detoxicant skin and muscle toner

COMPLEMENTARY COMBINATIONS

- Sweet orange + Geranium: nervous sedative/relaxant for nervous tension, anxiety, insomnia

- Sweet orange + Lavender: cardiac relaxant and hypotensive for palpitations, hypertension, esp. from unproductive stress

- Sweet orange + Spearmint: upper digestive stimulant for gastric or biliary indigestion with fullness after taking a few bites, belching, hiccups

- Sweet orange + Peppermint: lower digestive stimulant for intestinal indigestion with fullness, abdominal pain, colic, irregular stool

## TOPICAL – *Liment, ointment, cream, compress and other cosmetic preparations*

**Skin care:** Dry, oily and combination skin types

*skin and muscle toner, detoxicant:* tired, devitalized or congested skin with toxins; weak gums; muscle and tendon fatigue (e.g. from work, sports)

*mild antiseptic, anti-inflammatory:* acne, mouth sores/ulcers

*skin-softener:* thickened skin, callouses, chapped skin

*connective tissue and epidermal restorative, capillary stimulant, melanocyte stimulant:* wrinkles, cellulite, stretch marks, sprains, strains, poor muscle tone

**Therapeutic precautions:** None

**Pharmacological precautions:** Avoid using Sweet orange oil on sensitive or damaged skin as it may be slightly irritant. Because Orange oils, like all citrus oils, degrade and oxidize easily on contact with oxygen, it is important, in skin care especially, to use fresh, non-oxidized oils. Oxidized Orange oils may cause skin irritation and sensitization. The generally accepted shelf-life of genuine Orange oils at room temperature is 12 months, or 24 months if stored in a refrigerator (assuming no preservative has been added in the first place).

In addition, cold-pressed Orange oil (both the sweet and bitter type) has caused skin reactions due to photosensitization, arising from its content in coumarins (including bergaptenes). As a rule, therefore, as far as topical applications go, it is safest to use the cold-pressed oil for environmental and internal use; and a genuine distilled oil for topical use.

**Preparations:**

- Diffusor: 4–8 drops in water

- Massage oil: 3–5% dilution in vegetable oil

- Liniment: 5–10% dilution in vegetable oil

- Gel cap: 3–6 drops with olive oil

## Chinese Medicine Functions and Indications

**Aroma energy:** Sweet, lemony

**Movement:** Circulating

**Warmth:** Neutral

**Meridian tropism:** Liver, Heart, Stomach

**Five-Element affinity:** Wood, Fire, Earth

**Essential function:** To regulate the Qi, settle the Heart and harmonize the Shen

1. **Regulates the Qi, relaxes constraint, settles the Heart and harmonizes the Shen**

   - **Qi constraint with Shen dysregulation**, with distraction, irritability, mood swings, nervous tension, emotivity:

     Bergamot/Mandarin/Grapefruit/Lavender

   - **Heart and Liver Qi constraint with Shen dysregulation**, with restlessness, irritability, anxiety, mood swings, insomnia, palpitations:

     Petitgrain bigarade/Lavender/German camomile

2. **Regulates the Qi and harmonizes the Middle Warmer**

   - **Liver-Stomach/Spleen disharmony** with indigestion, bloating, colic, poor appetite, epigastric fullness:

     Spearmint/Peppermint/German camomile/May chang

REMARKS

The word 'orange' is derived from its Italian name *Arancio*, itself based on the Persian *Narang*. The sweet orange is a hybrid citrus that was originally cultivated over 4,000 years ago in Yunnan and Sichuan provinces of Southwest China. It is known to have travelled west to the Malaysian archipelago and India, and in 800 BC orange groves are on record in the famous hanging gardens of Babylon at Semiramide. In the 13th century, Arab maritime Silk Roads ferried the fruit (like so many other herbs, spices and chinaware) westward up the Persian Gulf to Syria and on to coastal North Africa, ending in the far West with Morocco and Al Andalus. By 1336, sweet orange trees were already cultivated ornamentals in Nice, France. Within a few decades they freely adorned the whole sun-blessed French and Ligurian riviera (Gildemeister 1899).

In the early years of the 16th century, Portuguese traders brought the sweet orange back to Portugal and the Canary Islands directly from Ceylon and China – hence its traditional Western name, Portugal orange. Soon after, the fruit enjoyed widespread cultivation in Italy. For hundreds of years the royal courts of Europe prized the Portugal orange for its fragrant flowers, building dedicated fragrant orangeries for the fully immersed enjoyment of a sweet orange aromatic environment. In the 20th century the fruit then became a worldwide favourite for both its sweet juice and for the commercial flavouring of soft drinks.

In physical medicine it is usual to think of the cold-pressed Sweet orange oil as a secondary oil, but even secondary oils have their interesting, niche uses. This oil could be stereotyped both as a child's oil and as a gentler version of Mandarin; both these tags would certainly be useful mnemonics. Its actions are moderate and ideal for conditions needing a gentle touch. Gentle relaxation of tense, stress-related nervous, cardiovascular and digestive functions, with a mild hypnotic effect; gentle but effective stimulation of biliary and gastric functions for atonic, weak forms of indigestion. Sweet orange is especially effective for, and much appreciated by, children and the elderly, as well as in mild to moderate conditions in general.

Sweet orange is also a child's oil from the psychological perspective. Used just by olfaction, Sweet orange encourages carefree, light-hearted emotions and a happy, harmonious, joyful mood – none less than those of a happy, contented child. Uplifting and mildly euphoric at the same time, its psychological functions consist of a complex yet seamless blend of promoting joy, optimism and emotional stability.

Sweet orange is actually a universal favourite with infants, children and those needing to touch the child within. The fragrance of Sweet orange is perhaps the closest of all to evoking the eidetic joy of the true, unwounded emotional heart; the joyful, selfless, spontaneously giving expression of a child's heart. Sweet orange can connect us to the innocent heart that as cultured adults we were taught to cover up out of fears and insecurities with layers of denial and pretence. It invites the heart to gently relax into its true feelings, knowing it is safe and supported by a warm, loving embrace.

Sweet orange is clearly not a secondary but a prime aromatic with the potential to support the wounded heart seeking that precious connection to its true source.

**Bitter orange** oil is very similar in fragrance, constituents, functions and indications to Sweet orange, but is allegedly somewhat stronger in its physiological effects. Practitioners often use it for its anticoagulant action because of its coumarin content that helps prevent thrombosis. Bitter orange is also a moderate venous and lymphatic decongestant that treats venous and lymphatic congestion. If used topically, exposure to sunlight should be avoided for up to 18 hours to prevent possible photosensitization.

# Tarragon

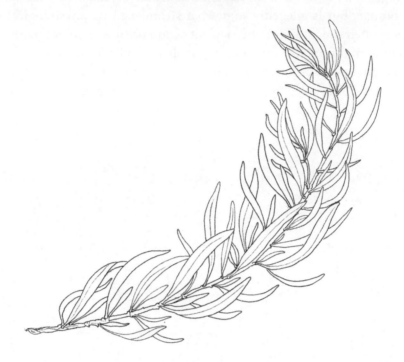

**Botanical source:** *Artemisia dracunculus* L. ct. methylchavicol (Asteraceae/Compositae – daisy family), a Mediterranean and temperate East European herb native to Central and Southwest Asia; *A. dracunculus forma redowskii* is the source in Ukraine and South Russia

**Other names:** Estragon, Russian tarragon; Estragon (Fr), Estragone (It), Estragón (Sp)

**Appearance:** A mobile colourless or pale viridian liquid that turns yellow with age; the odour is sweet-anisic with fresh green notes

**Perfumery status:** A head note of medium intensity and poor persistence

**Extraction:** Steam distillation of the fresh flowering herb

**1 kg oil yield from:** 300–500 kg of the fresh herb (a moderate yield)

**Production areas:** France, Hungary, Ukraine

**Typical constituents:** Phenolic ethers (incl. methylchavicol 60–87%, p-anol methyl ether) • monoterpenes (incl. cis- and trans-β-ocimene trace–19%, d-limonene 0–3.5%, α-pinene <2%, phellandrene, p-cymene, capillene) • coumarins (incl. esculetin, methoxycoumarins herniarine, scopoletin, scoparone) • trace–1.5% methyleugenol

**Chance of adulteration:** Almost none, as most other Artemisia oils are very different in composition and neurotoxic, but possibly with Basil ct. methylchavicol (*Ocimum basilicum* ct. methylchavicol)

**Related oils:** Between 300 and 400 aromatic species of Artemisia grow worldwide, the majority commonly known as various types of mugwort or wormwood. However, only a handful are ever regularly distilled and used for their essential oil in a therapeutic setting. The majority of those distilled end up in the hands of perfume chemists.

As a group, the Artemisias are potent remedies when given internally, as their consistent and successful historical and contemporary use in herbal medicine goes to show. The majority will treat mucousy respiratory conditions, intestinal parasites and amenorrhoea. They are used both by folk practitioners and professional herbal medicine practitioners alike throughout Europe, North Africa and the Middle East, and mainly in infusion and tincture preparations. The use of Artemisias in essential oil form is a relatively recent development within French herbal and allopathic medicine since the late 19th century.

While Tarragon oil is safe and easy to use clinically, most other Artemisia oils possess some degree of cumulative toxicity, making their safe prescribing an important therapeutic consideration. Most of their neurotoxic effects arise from their content in ketones such as thujone and other constituents. As a result, when used in the form of their extracted essential oil, the majority of Artemisias require great circumspection as regards dosage and administration method. The therapeutic status of Artemisia oils ranges from completely mild, non-toxic all the way to strong, toxic, depending on the speed and intensity of their cumulative toxicity (see the summary at the end of this profile).

Grouped by their chemical dominance and listed from the non-toxic to the most toxic within each group, the Artemisia oils include the following:

1. **Methylchavicol dominant**

   - Tarragon (*Artemisia dracunculus* ct. methylchavicol) (this profile), essentially a non-toxic remedy in the mild category, like its pharmcognosical relative Basil ct. methylchavicol

   - Russian tarragon (*Artemisia dracunculus* ct. sabinene), also a non-toxic remedy in the mild category, dominant in sabinene (c. 50%), methyleugenol (10–30%) and elemicine (5–25%)

2. **Camphor dominant**

   - White mugwort (*Artemisia alba* Turra, syn. *A. suavis*), possibly moderately toxic

### 3. Sesquiterpene lactone dominant

- White mugwort/wormwood ct. davanone (*Artemisia herba-alba* Asso ct. davanone) from Spain and Morocco, moderately neurotoxic, with davanone dominant (40–55%), chrysanthenone and cis-chrysanthenol; other chemotypes also exist (see below).

- Davana (*Artemisia pallens* Wall ex DC.), strongly neurotoxic, with davanone (25–52%), isodavanone, nordavanone and artemone

### 4. Artemisia ketone dominant

- Annual wormwood (*Artemisia annua* L.), non-toxic, with artemisia ketone (12–76%) artemisyl acetate and the antimalarial sesquiterpene lactone artemisinine

- California mugwort (*Artemisia douglasiana* Besser), non-toxic, with artemisia ketone (59%), 1,8 cineole (6%), artemisia alcohol (6%); this is a traditional medicinal herb in the Western US

- African wormwood (*Artemisia afra* Jacq.), strongly neurotoxic, with artemisia ketone (24%), α- and β-thujones (15%), 1,8 cineole (30%) and terpenols (20%, incl. artemisia and yomogi alcohol)

### 5. Thujone dominant

- Tree wormwood (*Artemisia arborescens* L.), moderately neurotoxic, with isothujone (30–45%), camphor (2–18%), chamazulene (<22%) and epoxycaryophyllene

- White mugwort ct. thujone (*Artemisia herba-alba* Asso ct. thujone), strongly neurotoxic, with α-thujone (26–72%), β-thujone (2–9%) and sesquiterpene lactones; a mixed thujone/camphor chemotype is also reported with camphor (34–55%) and α-thujone (25–37%); as well as further chemotypes

- Mugwort (*Artemisia vulgaris* L. ct. thujone/camphor), strongly neurotoxic, with thujones (12%), camphor (<21%), artemisia alcohol (15%) and β-caryophyllene (11%); an *A. vulgaris* ct. chrysanthenyl acetate is also reported

- Wormwood (*Artemisia absinthium* L. ct. thujone), strongly neurotoxic, with β-thujone (33–60%), α-thujone (2–3%), sabinyl acetate (6–32%) and monoterpenols (thujol 9%); three further chemotypes are reported, all strongly neurotoxic

Other Artemisias are often distilled in smaller quantities in the American Southwest, including White sagebrush or Silver wormwood (*Artemisia ludoviciana* Nutt.), with <60% artemisyl acetate; Big sagebrush (*Artemisia tridentata* Nutt.); and Coastal or California sagebrush (*Artemisia californica* Less.).

# Therapeutic Functions and Indications

Specific symptomatology – *All applications*

Lethargy, emotivity, mood swings, emotional outbursts, chronic chest discomfort and pains, muscle, joint and nerve pain, irregular stool, right subcostal and abdominal pain, tendency to allergies, asthmatic breathing, spasmodic cough, urinary irritation, dribbling and pain, pain from stones, cramping before or during the period

Psychological – *Aromatic diffusion, whole-body massage*

**Essential PNEI function and indication:** Regulating in dysregulated conditions; stimulant in weakness conditions

**Possible brain dynamics:** Reduces deep limbic system hyperfunctioning

**Fragrance category:** Middle tone with sweet, green, pungent notes

**Indicated psychological disorders:** Bipolar disorder, ADD

Promotes emotional renewal and clarity

- All pathogenic (stuck) emotions and distressed feelings in general, esp. anger

- Emotional confusion and illusion with conflict; emotional dependency

Stimulates the mind and promotes alertness

- Lethargy, drowsiness

- Mental illusions, confusion, disorientation

- Pessimism, depression

Physiological – *Nebulizer inhalation, gel cap, suppository, external applications*

**Therapeutic status:** Mild remedy with no cumulative toxicity

**Topical safety status:** Mild skin irritant, non-sensitizing

**Tropism:** Nervous, respiratory, digestive, urinary and musculoskeletal systems

**Essential diagnostic function:** Relaxes hypertonic/tense terrain conditions

*systemic nervous relaxant, SNS inhibitor, vagotonic:* hypertonic/tense conditions with nervous tension; acute stress-related conditions in general

*strong spasmolytic and analgesic, moderate anti-inflammatory:* a large range of acute spasmodic conditions with pain, esp. of smooth muscles; acute and chronic pain conditions, tension headaches

- *strong neuromuscular relaxant, anticonvulsant:* muscle spasms and pain, neuralgia, incl. sciatica; (fibro)myalgia, rheumatoid arthritis, gout, arteriosclerosis; seizures, dizziness, vertigo, coma

- *strong neurocardiac relaxant:* neurogenic angina with precordial pain, palpitations, tachycardia, cardiac dysrhythmia

- *gastrointestinal, biliary and pancreatic relaxant and regulator, also carminative:* spasmodic, neurogenic and inflammatory digestive conditions with pain, incl. nervous indigestion, biliary and intestinal colic, spasmodic IBS, gastritis, enteritis; gastric pain from ulcers, hyperacidity; flatulence, nausea, hiccups

- *kidney and urinary relaxant:* strangury, neurogenic bladder with spasmodic dysuria, incl. from stones; prostate congestion (BPH)

- *uterine relaxant:* spasmodic dysmenorrhoea, premenstrual cramps

- *respiratory relaxant (bronchospasmolytic):* spasmodic or nervous cough and dyspnoea; spasmodic asthma and bronchitis, whooping cough, croup

*antiallergic, antihistamine:* type-I allergies, incl. allergic rhinitis, sinusitis, asthma, dermatitis, colitis, duodenitis, gastritis, cholecystitis, prostatitis, cystitis

*diuretic*

*anticoagulant, antiplatelet:* thrombosis

ANTIMICROBIAL ACTIONS:

*strong antiviral:* viral infections, incl. shingles, herpes, neuritis, croup, pleurisy, hepatitis

*mild antibacterial, antifungal*

*anthelmintic:* intestinal parasites

SYNERGISTIC COMBINATIONS

- Tarragon + Fennel/Basil ct. methylchavicol: strong systemic nervous relaxant, spasmolytic, analgesic and antiviral in a wide range of moderate to severe acute hypertonic/tense and spasmodic conditions with pain and inflammation, incl. neuromuscular, respiratory, biliary, gastrointestinal and uterine conditions

- Tarragon + Fennel/Basil ct. methylchavicol: strong digestive relaxant, carminative for severe acute flatulence, distension, nervous indigestion, gallbladder/gallstone colic

- Tarragon + Fennel/Laurel: strong urinary relaxant for spasmodic bladder and kidney disorders with dysuria, strangury

COMPLEMENTARY COMBINATIONS

- Tarragon + Lavender: systemic nervous relaxant in a wide range of moderate spasmodic/tense conditions with pain and inflammation, incl. neuromuscular, cardiovascular, gastrointestinal and respiratory

- Tarragon + Marjoram: strong systemic nervous relaxant in a wide range of severe acute spasmodic/tense conditions with pain and inflammation, incl. neuromuscular, cardiovascular, gastrointestinal, biliary, respiratory and nephritic

- Tarragon + Lemongrass + Rosemary: strong neuromuscular spasmolytic and analgesic for severe acute muscle and tendon cramps, pain and contractions

- Tarragon + Petitgrain bigarade/Ylang ylang no. 1: neurocardiac spasmolytic for acute neurogenic angina with precordial pain, palpitations

- Tarragon + Blue tansy/Tea tree: anti-inflammatory antiallergic for type-I allergies, incl. rhinitis, sinusitis, asthma, colitis, prostatitis, cystitis

- Tarragon + Cypress/Siberian fir: strong bronchospasmolytic and antitussive for all acute spasmodic respiratory conditions, incl. asthma, croup, spasmodic cough and dyspnoea of all kinds

- Tarragon + Clary sage: strong uterine spasmolytic, analgesic for spasmodic dysmenorrhoea

## TOPICAL – *Liminent, ointment, cream, compress and other cosmetic preparations*

**Skin care:** Not used

*anti-inflammatory, antiallergic:* skin allergies, acute dermatitis

*spasmolytic, analgesic, anti-inflammatory:* painful muscle cramps and spasms, rheumatic pain; sprains, strains

**Therapeutic precautions:** Tarragon treats acute spasmodic, painful, inflammatory conditions and is best avoided in chronic hypertonic/tense conditions. The oil is best avoided internally during pregnancy because of its spasmolytic action on the uterus.

**Pharmacological precautions:** Tarragon oil is a mild skin irritant from its methylchavicol content: the dilutions below should not be exceeded. Internal use of

Tarragon should be cautious and avoided during the first trimester and only used with caution during the remainder of pregnancy and lactation. Although there is a theoretical risk of Tarragon's methyleugenol content acting as a carcinogen, its limonene content likely quenches the former's carcinogenic potential. In addition, no record of a carcinogenic risk is noted in French medicine and no related prohibition exists in French pharmacy regulations.

**Preparations:**

- Diffusor: 2–3 drops in water

- Massage oil: 0.5–1% dilution in vegetable oil

- Liniment: 1–4% dilution in vegetable oil for short-term use after doing a patch test

- Gel cap: 1–2 drops with olive oil

## Chinese Medicine Functions and Indications

**Aroma energy:** Sweet, green, pungent

**Movement:** Circulating

**Warmth:** Neutral

**Meridian tropism:** Liver, Heart, Spleen, Stomach, Lung

**Five-Element affinity:** Wood, Earth, Metal

**Essential function:** To activate the Qi, calm the Liver and harmonize the Shen

1. **Activates the Qi, relaxes constraint, harmonizes the Shen and relieves pain**

   - **Qi constraint with Shen dysregulation**, with nervous tension, restlessness, muscle tension and pain, mood swings, emotional lability:
     Lavender/Marjoram/German camomile

   - **Heart and Liver Qi constraint with Shen agitation**, with restlessness, insomnia, palpitations, irritability, anxiety:
     Mandarin/Blue tansy/Ylang ylang no. 1

   - **Liver and Uterus Qi constraint** with severe menstrual cramps, irritability:
     Roman camomile/Clary sage/Ylang ylang no. 1

   - **Bladder Qi constraint** with irritated, difficult, painful, dripping urination:
     Fennel/Carrot seed/Cypress

2. <u>**Regulates the Qi, breaks up stagnation, harmonizes the Middle Warmer and relieves pain**</u>

- **Liver-Spleen/Stomach disharmony** with severe abdominal pain and bloating, flatulence, diarrhoea, feelings of stress, mood swings:
  Peppermint/German camomile/Roman camomile

3. <u>**Circulates and descends Lung Qi, relaxes the chest and relieves wheezing and coughing**</u>

- **Lung Qi accumulation** with wheezing, coughing, chest distension and pain:
  Cypress/Siberian fir/Fennel/Hyssop

4. <u>**Calms the Liver, descends the Yang, extinguishes wind and relieves spasms**</u>

- **Liver Yang rising** with headache, tinnitus, dizziness, muscle tension:
  Clary sage/Lavender/Marjoram

- **Internal Liver wind** with tremors, muscle spasms, seizures:
  Vetiver/Roman camomile/Laurel

- **Wind-phlegm obstruction** with seizures, spasms, paralysis:
  Laurel/Ylang ylang no. 1

5. <u>**Opens the meridians, dispels wind-damp, relaxes the tendons and relieves pain**</u>

- **Wind-damp obstruction** with acute muscle pain and cramping, joint pain:
  Juniper berry/Frankincense/Nutmeg

REMARKS

Like many essential oils, Tarragon is distilled from a plant long used as both a domestic cooking herb and a medicinal remedy. Originating in Central Asia and Siberia, the herb may have been brought back to Europe by knights during the 12th or 13th-century religious crusades. Tarragon's first name of Estragon derives from the Latin *dracunculus*, meaning 'little dragon'. Small in stature but potent, the herb has an old reputation for antidoting the bites of venomous creatures and 'madde dogs', as well as enjoying various medicinal uses.

European practitioners often consider Tarragon oil an alternative to Basil ct. methylchavicol, but with greater emphasis on relaxing cardiovascular functions. Seeing that the constituents of both oils are dominated by the phenolic ether methylchavicol, they consider both oils equally strong spasmolytics and analgesics. This is their pharmacological potency. Tarragon often finds use for acute, painful smooth muscle spasms, especially digestive, menstrual and bronchial (e.g. for spasmodic asthma, croup and other spasmodic coughs). The oil is also a particularly strong neuromuscular relaxant in painful neuralgic and rheumatic disorders, both acute and chronic, and a useful anticonvulsant for seizures. Taking the functional medicine approach, Tarragon is clearly a major systemic relaxant remedy for treating acute tense conditions with pain and spasm. Its systemic effect involves an inhibition of sympathetic nervous functions.

However, what truly distinguishes Tarragon from Basil ct. methylchavicol is its anti-inflammatory effect that shines in acute type-I allergic conditions. This antihistamine action includes relief of allergic rhinitis, asthma, dermatitis, colitis, duodenitis, cholecystitis and prostatitis. Here it acts in the same way as Tree wormwood (see below), but without the inconvenience of any possible interference from the latter's moderate neurotoxicity arising from its content in thujone.

As a fresh, pungent, green psychological remedy used by olfaction, Tarragon's functions and indications are the same as those of Basil ct. methylchavicol (Tropical basil). As noted by Dupont (2002), it addresses issues relating to the solar plexus or third chakra region, which are essentially about our relationship to the world and the development of personal power.

**Related oils:** It is crucial to differentiate the therapeutic statuses among the many Artemisia oils. This should be done on the basis of their chemical dominance, regardless of particular species or chemotype; this largely determines their degree of neurotoxicity. The following summaries should be considered as a guide.

- **Mild Artemisia oils with no cumulative neurotoxicity**

    - *Tarragon* (*Artemisia dracunculus* ct. methylchavicol) (this profile)

    - *Russian tarragon* (*Artemisia dracunculus* ct. sabinene)

    - *Annual wormwood* (*Artemisia annua*) is a respiratory mucolytic for congestive bronchitis, an excellent antiparasitic for tapeworms and roundworms, an antimalarial, a tissue regenerative for painful injuries, and possibly antitumoural for certain cancers.

- **Medium-strength Artemisia oils with moderate cumulative neurotoxicity**

    **Caution:** All medium-strength Artemisia oils are contraindicated during pregnancy and breastfeeding, being considered neurotoxic, teratogenic and abortive; and are contraindicated in babies, infants and children. They should be used with the preparation guidelines for Sage oil (which also contains thujone).

    - *White mugwort ct. davanone* (*Artemisia herba-alba* ct. davanone) is a respiratory mucolytic for chronic bronchitis, and possibly antitumoural.

    - *Tree wormwood* (*Artemisia arborescens*) is an excellent antihistamine antiallergic remedy given successfully for type-I allergies, especially allergic/atopic asthma and eczema (dermatitis). It is a respiratory mucolytic for congestive bronchitis, and a choleretic for biliary deficiency with upper digestive stagnation.

- **Strong Artemisia oils with strong, rapid cumulative neurotoxicity**

  **Caution:** These strong Artemisia oils should be generally avoided for internal use. If chosen at all, their safe use would require clinical training. They are best given in infusion or tincture form. All are contraindicated during pregnancy and breastfeeding, being considered neurotoxic, teratogenic and abortive; and are contraindicated in babies, infants and children.

  - *Davana* (*Artemisia pallens*) is a respiratory mucolytic for chronic bronchitis, a nervous restorative in weak, neurasthenic conditions, and topically a good tissue regenerative for painful wound healing.

  - *African wormwood* (*Artemisia afra*) is used as a respiratory mucolytic for congestive bronchitis, a strong antiparasitic for intestinal parasites, and a specific remedy for migraine headaches.

  - *White mugwort ct. thujone* (*Artemisia herba-alba* ct. thujone) is an antiviral and antibacterial respiratory mucolytic for mucousy upper and lower respiratory infections; it is also antiviral with verrucas and warts, and will treat varicose ulcers. Its mucolytic action is also applied for leucorrhoea, and its emmenagogue action for amenorrhoea. Like many other Artemisias, it is also a strong antiparasitic for various intestinal parasites, especially pinworms (Oxyuria).

  - *Mugwort* (*Artemisia vulgaris*) is an emmenagogue for amenorrhoea, an antiparasitic for a range of intestinal parasites, and a cholagogue for upper indigestion due to biliary and gastric stagnation. The herb also has a long history of use as a spasmolytic and anticonvulsant for muscle tremors and spasms, and seizures.

  - *Wormwood* (*Artemisia absinthium*) is a strong upper digestive and liver stimulant for gastric indigestion with appetite loss, and for liver congestion with bilious headache, jaundice, etc. The oil is also a nervous restorative for depression, neurasthenia and convalescence, an emmenagogue for amenorrhoea, and a strong antiparasitic for a range of intestinal parasites.

# Thyme ct. Thymol

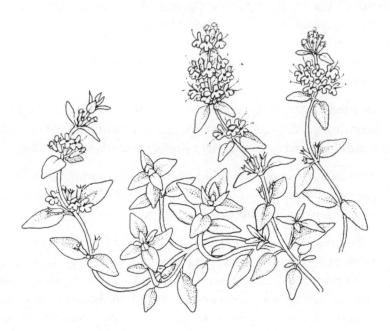

**Botanical source:** The herb of *Thymus vulgaris* L. ct. thymol or *Thymus zygis* L. ct. thymol (Lamiaceae/Labiateae – lipflower family), a widespread Mediterranean herb or small shrub

**Other names:** Thym à thymol (Fr), Thymian-thymol (Ge), Timo di thymol (It), Tomillo thymol (Sp)

- *Thymus vulgaris:* Garden/Common thyme, thymol chemotype; Narrow-leaf French thyme

- *Thymus zygis:* Spanish thyme, Spanish red thyme, Spanish sauce thyme

**Appearance:** A mobile clear, yellow or red fluid with a strong spicy-fresh herbaceous-green odour with mild acrid bottom notes; the variation in colour is a natural occurrence

**Perfumery status:** A heart note of high intensity and poor persistence

**Extraction:** Steam distillation of the fresh herb in flower, usually in May

**1 kg oil yield from:** 100–150 kg of the fresh herb (a fairly good yield)

**Production areas:** France (*Thymus vulgaris*); Spain and Portugal (*Thymus zygis*)

**Typical constituents:** Phenols 32–53% (incl. thymol 30–48%, carvacrol 0.5–6%) • monoterpenes 11–56% (incl. p-cymene 2–40%, γ-terpinene 0.3–11%, camphene 1–3%, myrcene <2.5%, terpinolene trace–2%, α-terpinene 1%, limonene 0.4–3%, α-thujene 0.5%, δ-3-carene 0.1%, sabinene 0.6%, α-phellandrene, trace β-pinene) • oxides (incl. 1,8 cineole <8%, cis-linalool, trans-linalool oxide) • ketones (incl. camphor 5–16%, α-thujone 0.3%) • sesquiterpene caryophyllene <3% • monoterpenols (incl. linalool 1–12%, α-terpineol 0.4–10%, terpinen-4-ol 0.3–10%) • sesquiterpenol nerolidol <1% • esters (incl. linalyl/terpenyl/geranyl acetate)

**Note:** The constituent profiles of *Thymus vulgaris* and *Thymus zygis* show only extremely minor variations in their percentages.

**Chance of adulteration:** Only moderate if the identity of this chemotype is firmly established with accompanying certificates of authenticity and GC analysis, as well as through direct examination of odour, colour and so on. Otherwise, many Thyme oils often contain admixtures of Oregano, Capitate thyme, Ajowan and other phenol-rich oils.

Generic commercial designations such as 'Thyme oil', 'White thyme oil' and 'Red thyme oil' are meaningless in terms of purity and chemotypes. Thyme ct. thymol is a designation for a specific natural oil, whereas 'White thyme' and 'Red thyme' are for the most part industrial types of thyme oils that have been standardized by natural or synthetic addition, or even completely reconstituted. 'Red thyme' may also be the result of distillation in iron stills, while 'White thyme' is usually rectified and highlighted Spanish or other types of thyme to eliminate their red colour; it might also be a complete reconstruction using terpineol, fractions of Pine, Rosemary, Eucalyptus, Oregano, Spanish thyme, etc., and/or synthetic pinenes, limonene, p-cymene and caryophyllene. However, note that, confusingly, the colour of pure and botanically specific thyme oils, regardless of species and chemotype, presents natural variations ranging from clear to yellow and even red – making organoleptic identification through colour alone extremely unreliable (Mailhebiau 1995; Lis-Balchin 2006).

**Related oils:** The thyme genus is extremely polymorphic, producing about 350 species and a variety of different chemical types and cultivars. Below is a summary of the main types and chemotypes of Thyme oil encountered. These are produced either in the Far West Mediterranean (France, Spain, Portugal and Morocco) or the Far East Mediterranean (Turkey, Cyprus and Greece).

- **Sweet-herbaceous thyme oils with monoterpenols dominant**

  These three chemotypes of Thyme oil alone are non-irritant to the skin and so are more widely useful and versatile in practice than the other chemotypes (see profiles below).

- *Thyme ct. linalool* (*Thymus vulgaris* L. ct. linalool, *T. zygis* L. ct. linalool) from the South of France and Spain, with its sweet-green-herbaceous fragrance and linalool levels <80%

- *Thyme ct. thujanol* (*Thymus vulgaris* L. ct. thujanol) from the South of France, also with a sweeter fragrance, is dominated by c. 50% monoterpenols (incl. trans-thujanol-4 <40%, terpinene-4-ol, cis-myrcenol, linalool 10%) and monoterpenes c. 20% (incl. myrcene, γ-terpinene 15%); it contains no phenols, unlike most other thyme chemotypes

- *Thyme ct. geraniol* (*Thymus vulgaris* L. ct. geraniol) from the South of France, with its rosy-sweet, herbaceous fragrance, from its high levels of the monoterpenol geraniol (24–55%); esters (10–50%), including geranyl acetate, make up most of its remaining constituents

- *Moroccan thyme* (*Thymus satureioides* Cosson) from Northwest Africa (sometimes popularly known as Thyme ct. borneol) with its mildly acrid, herbaceous aroma, the result of a unique combination of high levels of monoterpenols (32–64%), especially borneol (28–54%) and α-terpineol (c. 10%), and only moderate amounts of thymol (c. 10%) and carvacrol (4–20%)

- **Acrid-herbaceous thyme oils with phenols dominant**

  These phenolic oils are highly irritant to the skin and mucosa. They are therefore used mainly for environmental and internal administration with the appropriate delivery method (see profiles below).

  - *Thyme ct. thymol* (*Thymus vulgaris* L. ct. thymol, *T. zygis* ct. thymol), with its more pungent-herbaceous aroma from the high content in the phenol thymol (<48%) and monoterpenes (<56%) (this profile)

  - *Thyme ct. carvacrol* (*Thymus vulgaris* L. ct. carvacrol) from the dry, rocky scrublands of southern France, with carvacrol levels <42% and thymol c. 10%

  - *Wild thyme* or Mother of thyme (*Thymus serpyllum* L.) from the Eastern Mediterranean and North Africa, with its deep sweet-herbaceous, acrid aroma, is dominant in carvacrol (15–30%) and thymol (<20%) with an assortment of mixed monoterpenes (headed by p-cymene 14%) and monoterpenols such as geraniol, linalool and borneol

  - *Capitate thyme* or Cretan thyme (*Thymus capitatus* Hoffmanns. & Link) (syn. *Coridothymus capitatus* [L.] Rchb. f.) is confusingly also called 'Wild oregano', 'Spanish oregano' or 'Headed savoury'. With its strongly acrid-pungent, warm-herbaceous aroma, this thyme from the Eastern

Mediterranean (especially Cyprus and Turkey) contains high levels of carvacrol (usually 40–50%, but occasionally up to 81%) and smaller amounts of the sesquiterpenes p-cimene (5–10%), γ-terpinene (3–9%) and β-caryophyllene (2–4%)

- **Spiked thyme** (*Thymbra spicata* L.) from the Eastern Mediterranean (Turkey, Greece), with an aroma very similar to Capitate thyme; very high in carvacrol (<80%), this herb is still used locally to treat roundworms (Ascaris) and other intestinal parasites

- **Fresh-pungent thyme oils with monoterpenes and cineole dominant**

  - **Thyme ct. cineole** (*Thymus vulgaris* L. ct. cineole) from the south of France is high in 1,8 cineole, with a marked fresh-camphor aroma

  - **Mastic thyme** or Spanish thyme (*Thymus mastichina* L.), Tomillo blanco in Spanish, from Spain and Portugal, is sometimes confusingly called 'Spanish wild marjoram' in commerce; it is dominant in 1,8 cineole (<60%), with monoterpenes (c. 15%), monoterpenols (<20%, mostly linalool), phenols (thymol <5%) and camphor (4%)

  - **Thyme ct. paracymene** (*Thymus vulgaris* L. ct. paracymene) from the south of France is high in the monoterpene p-cymene with only moderate levels of thymol

  - **Spanish sauce thyme** (*Thymus zygis* L. ct. paracymene) (syn. *Thymus tenuifolius* Mill.), with its high levels of the monoterpene p-cymene

- **Other useful Thyme oils sometimes distilled from the prolific *Thymus* genus**

  - **Caraway thyme** (*Thymus herba-barona* Loisel.), with its characteristic caraway aroma from its high content in the ketone carvone

  - **Lemon thyme** (*Thymus x citriodorus* [Pers.] Schreb.), with its fresh lemony fragrance from its high citral content; this is a garden hybrid of broad-leaf thyme, *Thymus pulegioides*, and garden thyme, *T. vulgaris*

## Therapeutic Functions and Indications

SPECIFIC SYMPTOMATOLOGY – *All applications*

Spaciness, apathy, low motivation, loss of self-confidence, physical and mental fatigue, debility, depression, low sex drive, cold hands and feet, cold skin, recurring or chronic infections, chest distension, cough with expectoration and wheezing, appetite loss, epigastric and abdominal pain, chronic diarrhoea, irregular bowel movement, undigested food in stool, chronic vaginal discharges, scanty or absent periods, painful scanty periods, muscle and joint pain, cramping and stiffness

## PSYCHOLOGICAL – *Aromatic diffusion, whole-body massage*

**Essential PNEI function and indication:** Stimulant in weakness conditions

**Possible brain dynamics:** Increases basal ganglia and prefrontal cortex functioning

**Fragrance category:** Top tone with pungent, green notes

**Indicated psychological disorders:** ADD, depression

### PROMOTES WILLPOWER, COURAGE AND SELF-CONFIDENCE

- Low willpower or strength, indecision
- Discouragement with apathy, loss of motivation, self-neglect
- Low self-confidence and self-esteem, pessimism, depression

### STIMULATES THE MIND AND PROMOTES ALERTNESS

- Lethargy, drowsiness, stupor
- Mental confusion, disorientation, poor concentration
- Mental and emotional burnout

## PHYSIOLOGICAL – *Gel cap, suppository, external applications*

**Therapeutic status:** Mild remedy with potential mild cumulative toxicity

**Topical safety status:** Moderate skin irritant and sensitizer

**Tropism:** Nervous, respiratory, digestive, reproductive systems

**Essential diagnostic function:** Stimulates and warms asthenic/cold and restores chronic hypotonic/weak terrain conditions

### PRIMARILY STIMULANT AND WARMING:

*strong systemic nervous and vascular stimulant, SNS and central arterial circulatory stimulant:* a wide range of asthenic (cold) and hypotonic (weak) conditions with circulatory deficiency, chronic physical and mental debility, fatigue and cold; incl. convalescence, neurasthenia, CFS

- *cerebral stimulant:* mental debility, depression
- *adrenal stimulant, hypertensive:* adrenal fatigue syndrome (esp. with afternoon or evening fatigue), hypotension

   – *reproductive stimulant, aphrodisiac:* sexual debility, loss of libido

   – *uterine stimulant, emmenagogue:* amenorrhoea, oligomenorrhoea

PRIMARILY STIMULANT AND RELAXANT:

*bronchial stimulant and relaxant, mucolytic expectorant, spasmolytic, bronchodilator, antitussive:* congestive and spasmodic upper respiratory conditions with cough and dyspnoea; chronic bronchitis, emphysema, asthma; croup, whooping cough

*gastrointestinal stimulant and relaxant, aperitive, stomachic, carminative, spasmolytic, analgesic, detoxicant:* asthenic (cold) digestive conditions with indigestion, appetite loss, flatulence, diarrhoea, aerophagia; enteritis, colitis, colic, IBS, abdominal pain in general, intestinal fermentation, food poisoning

*neuromuscular stimulant and relaxant, analgesic, spasmolytic, anti-inflammatory:* chronic rheumatic and arthritic conditions with pain, cramping, stiffness; rheumatoid arthritis

*mucostatic astringent:* vaginitis with leucorrhoea

*strong antioxidant*

ANTIMICROBIAL ACTIONS:

*broad-spectrum anti-infective, immunostimulant, anti-inflammatory, detoxicant, diuretic:* a wide range of acute and chronic infections, esp. respiratory, gastrointestinal, urogenital

   – *strong antibacterial:* bacterial infections both gram-negative and gram-positive, esp. respiratory, intestinal, urinary; incl. with Salmonella, E. coli, Pseudomonas aeruginosa, Haeomophilus influenzae, Staph. aureus, Strep. pneumoniae, Strep. pyogenes, incl. common cold, sinusitis, tonsillitis, laryngitis, bronchitis; intestinal microbial toxicosis, gastroenteritis, mucous colitis, food poisoning; cystitis, urethritis; MRSA

   – *strong antifungal:* fungal infections, incl. with Candida albicans, Aspergillus spp.

   – *antiviral:* misc. viral infections, incl. influenza, sinusitis, acute bronchitis; Rhinovirus, Adenovirus, Herpes zoster

   – *anthelmintic:* intestinal and other parasites, incl. hookworm, tapeworm, lice, scabies

SYNERGISTIC COMBINATIONS

All for short-term use only: see 'Therapeutic precautions' below.

- Thyme ct. thymol + Niaouli: strong broad-spectrum anti-infective, immunostimulant, lymphatic stimulant and detoxicant in a wide range of acute or chronic bacterial, viral and fungal infections of all body systems in general

- Thyme ct. thymol + Clove bud: strong broad-spectrum anti-infective and immunostimulant in a wide range of acute infections, bacterial, viral, fungal and parasitic; esp. with cold-weak terrain, debility

- Thyme ct. thymol + Black spruce: anthelmintic for intestinal parasites

COMPLEMENTARY COMBINATIONS

Generally for short-term use: see 'Therapeutic precautions' below.

- Thyme ct. thymol + Rosemary: nervous and cerebral restorative in chronic physical and mental fatigue, depression, neurasthenia, CFS

- Thyme ct. thymol + Rosemary/Black spruce: strong adrenal restorative, hypertensive for adrenal fatigue syndrome (esp. with afternoon or evening fatigue), hypotension

- Thyme ct. thymol + Ginger: reproductive restorative, aphrodisiac and emmenagogue for sexual debility, loss of libido, atonic amenorrhoea

- Thyme ct. thymol + Thyme ct. linalool: anti-bacterial and antifungal in a wide range of bacterial and fungal infections with weak or cold terrain, especially chronic (also topically), respiratory, digestive

- Thyme ct. thymol + Ravintsara/Saro: antiviral, immune and arterial circulatory stimulant for chronic or recurring viral infections, esp. with fatigue, cold extremities

- Thyme ct. thymol + Spearmint: mucolytic expectorant for chronic congestive bronchitis and dyspnoea

- Thyme ct. thymol + Hyssop: strong bronchodilator, anti-inflammatory and antitussive for acute or chronic asthma, spasmodic dyspnoea, whooping cough; esp. with chronic fatigue

- Thyme ct. thymol + Fennel: gastrointestinal stimulant-relaxant, carminative for weak and tense digestive conditions with chronic indigestion, colic, flatulence

- Thyme ct. thymol + Cajeput/Spike lavender: neuromuscular stimulant and analgesic for chronic rheumatic and arthritic conditions with cold and pain; low-back pain

## TOPICAL – *Liniment, lotion*

See 'Pharmacological precautions' below.

**Skin care:** Oily, dry or mature skin types – in low dilution only

*rubefacient, analgesic:* cold, lifeless, devitalized skin, incl. the scalp; hair loss; rheumatic and neuralgic conditions in general; cellulite

*strong antiseptic:* infected cuts and wounds, acne, eczema, psoriasis, MRSA

*antiparasitic:* skin parasites, lice, fleas, mites(?), ticks(?)

*antiviral:* verrucas, warts

**Therapeutic precautions:** Thyme ct. thymol is a strong warming stimulant to nervous, adrenal and circulatory functions, and is therefore contraindicated in hypersthenic/hot, hypertonic/tense and dry conditions; this includes high fevers, acute inflammation, hypertension, agitation, dry cough, thirst and constipation. It should be avoided in babies, infants and sensitive individuals. However, Thyme ct. thymol is able to treat both acute and chronic conditions in the context of asthenic/cold and hypotonic/weak terrain. Being a uterine stimulant, the oil is also contraindicated during pregnancy and breastfeeding.

Internal use should be limited to eight- to ten-day courses, and then usually within a formula rather than on their own, as with all high-phenol oils. Long-term internal use may cause liver damage and inhibit the healthy microflora; this should be prevented with the adjunctive use of liver restorative oils and/or herbs, and prebiotic foods, supplements or oils. Inhalation with an essential oil nebulizer is not recommended to avoid serious irritation to the mucous membrane.

**Pharmacological precautions:** Although Thyme ct. thymol is somewhat irritant to the skin and mucosa, it is essentially non-irritant to the skin when used in proper dilution. Still, care should be taken to avoid any potential long-term sensitization in some people. Internally, the phenols thymol and carvacrol may interfere with blood clotting, making Thyme ct. thymol contraindicated in bleeding disorders or in those taking anticoagulant medication.

**Preparations:**

- Diffusor: 2–4 drops

- Massage oil: 0.5–1% dilution in vegetable oil

- Liniment: 1–2% dilution in vegetable oil

- Gel cap: 1–3 drops with olive oil usually for short-term use, e.g. an eight-day course; and usually as part of a formula; the maximum daily dose is 8 drops. Like all phenolic oils, Thyme ct. thymol should always be combined with other oils to soften its intensity and enhance treatment results; especially with sweet, monoterpenol-rich oils such as Tea tree, Lavender, Palmarosa or Thyme ct. linalool.

## Chinese Medicine Functions and Indications

**Aroma energy:** Pungent, sweet, green

**Movement:** Circulating

**Warmth:** Warm to hot

**Meridian tropism:** Kidney, Lung, Spleen, Stomach

**Five-Element affinity:** Water, Metal, Earth

**Essential function:** To tonify the Yang, warm the interior and strengthen the Shen

1. **Tonifies the Yang, warms the Kidney and strengthens the Shen and libido**

   - **Yang deficiency with Shen weakness,** with physical and mental fatigue, apathy, cold hands and feet, recurrent infections:

     Rosemary/Ginger/Pimenta berry

   - **Kidney Yang deficiency** with loss of sex drive, weak loins and knees, fatigue, cold skin and extremities, apathy, spaciness:

     Black spruce/Nutmeg/Clove bud

2. **Warms the Lung, expels phlegm, circulates and descends Lung Qi, and relieves coughing and wheezing**

   - **Lung phlegm-cold with Qi accumulation,** with coughing, wheezing, sputum expectoration, chest distension, cold extremities:

     Hyssop/Grand fir/Laurel

   - **Lung Qi accumulation in other patterns,** with wheezing, chest distension, coughing:

     Siberian fir/Cypress/Basil ct. methylchavicol

3. **Warms and harmonizes the Middle Warmer, resolves damp and relieves pain**

   - **Stomach-Spleen damp-cold** with chronic diarrhoea, undigested food in stool, cold limbs, debility, poor appetite:

     Patchouli/Nutmeg/Black pepper

   - **Stomach-Spleen empty cold** (Spleen Yang deficiency with cold) with epigastric or abdominal pain, appetite loss, chronic diarrhoea, irregular bowel movement:

     Black pepper/Nutmeg/Ginger

4. <u>**Warms and activates the Lower Warmer, breaks up stagnation, promotes menstruation and stops discharge**</u>

- **Lower Warmer Blood and Qi stagnation with cold**, with scanty or absent menstrual flow, painful periods, loss of sex drive:

  Niaouli/Rosemary/Juniper berry/Pimenta berry

- **Lower Warmer damp-cold** with chronic vaginal discharge, fatigue, lethargy:

  Geranium/Atlas cedarwood/Sage/Green myrtle

REMARKS

In contrast to the commonly used linalool chemotype of Thyme oil (the yin type) (see Volume 1), the chemotype thymol is the most important yang type. In France it is produced from wild or cultivated plants on the French plateau at 300–500 metres altitude. Its chief phenolic constituent thymol was discovered by Berlin apothecary Caspar Neuman as early as 1719 and became a marker for other phenols. With the rise of coal-tar-based chemistry, synthetic thymol became a widespread ingredient in over-the-counter creams, lotions and ointments, as well as in antiseptic products such as mouth washes and temporary dental fillings.

Since the biochemist Pierre Franchomme in the 1960s was able to define the various chemotypes of *Thymus vulgaris*, the clinical uses of Thyme ct. thymol have been well explored. These are summarized below in a general overview of all Thyme oil chemotypes and species currently in common practice.

Despite its mildly acrid basenotes, the spicy, herbaceous-green fragrance of Thyme ct. thymol may work well as a psychological remedy by olfaction in some individuals. Its functions in this context are broadly the same as Oregano oil, only with greater emphasis on its mental aspect of promoting alertness.

**General summary of thyme oils:** Numerous species and chemotypes of the extremely polymorphic thyme genus are useful for the particular emphasis they are able to bring to a treatment. French practitioners value them especially and will often make fine distinctions among them, much like Chinese herbalists who make fine distinctions among several herbs that basically all have the same actions but excel at treating just one or two particular symptoms.

Grouping the thyme oils by fragrance and pharmacognosical dominance combined allows us to establish clear differentiations. The primary distinction is between the sweet thymes dominated by monoterpenols, and the acrid thymes dominated by phenols. Clinically the most commonly used sweet thyme is Thyme ct. linalool (see Volume 1), while the chief acrid thyme is Thyme ct. thymol (the above profile); it is the mildest and easiest of all the phenol-based oils to use in practice.

**Sweet-herbaceous thyme oils with monoterpenol dominance**

These are noted for being restorative in hypotonic/weak conditions or terrain, and especially when chronic. Monoterpenol thyme oils excel at supporting the individual's healthy energy (vital force, zheng qi in Chinese medicine) rather than (over)stimulating it to overcome particular pathogens (as do the phenolic thymes). Simply put, they focus on the terrain rather than the symptoms, while conversely, the phenolic thymes focus on the symptoms rather than the terrain.

Monoterpenol thyme oils all enjoy mild therapeutic status with no cumulative toxicity. Their main tropism is the nervous, respiratory, digestive and immune systems. As a group, they are also immunostimulant and anti-infective in the treatment of infections arising from weak terrain; they are especially valuable for chronic, lingering infections. Gentle and non-skin irritant by nature, these thyme oils are often chosen for treating children, the elderly and sensitive individuals; they are sometimes dubbed the 'paediatric thymes'. Their sweet fragrance is always appreciated during treatment, so they also lend themselves brilliantly to addressing the emotional component of a weak condition. Their final clinical advantage is that they carry virtually no contraindications and may be used for extended periods of time without negative effects.

**Thyme ct. linalool** (*Thymus vulgaris/zygis* L. ct. linalool), produced from wild or cultivated plants at 500–1,300 metres elevation, is the classic go-to sweet thyme oil of this group. Physiologically it is a broad restorative to nervous, cerebral, adrenal, respiratory, intestinal and immune functions. Its immunostimulant and anti-infective actions are especially useful for treating chronic upper and lower respiratory infections underpinned by a weak terrain, both physiologically and psychologically. Thyme ct. linalool is also a good detoxicant, particularly useful for bacterial infections and the aftermath of any infection in general. Psychologically, the oil aids emotional instability, conflict and stagnation with distressed feelings (see Volume 1 for a full profile).

**Thyme ct. thujanol** (*Thymus vulgaris* L. ct. thujanol) with its sweet, herbaceous, pungent fragrance is a gently warming, stimulant but non-skin irritant oil that acts as a nervous restorative and regulator in hypotonic/weak and hyposthenic/cold terrain. It is considered especially valuable for neurasthenia, autonomic nervous dysregulation, states of chronic fatigue, mood disorders, nervous breakdown, etc. Thyme ct. thujanol shares many similarities with Thyme ct. linalool as a gentle but highly effective anti-infective and immunostimulant remedy and is a particularly strong antiviral and antibacterial. In this role it will successfully treat respiratory (upper and lower), oral, gastrointestinal, urogenital and dermal infections, depending on the delivery method used. Particular infections such as vaginitis, chlamydia, cervicitis and bronchitis respond well to it. Thyme ct. thujanol is also particularly valued for its restorative, detoxicant and regenerating action on the liver, much like Rosemary ct. verbenone. It carries no cautions apart from avoiding use with babies. Standard dilutions and doses apply.

**Thyme ct. geraniol** (*Thymus vulgaris* L. ct. geraniol), uniquely rosy and herbaceous, is a pure restorative for hypotonic/weak terrain with a good tropism for the nervous system, heart and reproductive organs. As a supportive nervous and cardiac restorative, it treats nervous and heart weakness, like Palmarosa, especially in chronic conditions of all kinds, and in convalescence and postpartum. Thyme ct. geraniol is also an excellent uterine restorative for chronic dysmenorrhoea and parturient for stalled labour (uterine dystocia). It is also valued for being a broad-spectrum anti-infective with strong immunostimulant, antifungal and antiviral action. It is given especially for chronic upper and lower respiratory infections, and for reproductive and urinary infections of most kinds. The oil is also successful in treating viraemia. Topically it is an antiseptic astringent, like Geranium, and is often used for acne and dry and wet forms of eczema. It carries no precautions apart from avoiding use with babies. Standard dilutions and doses apply.

**Moroccan thyme** (*Thymus satureioides* Coss. and Bal.) belongs to the sweet thyme oils because of its borneol dominance, but also has a phenolic aspect; it could be thought of as a bridge oil in that sense, combining the gentleness of monoterpenols with the power of phenols. This oil exerts a deeply, strongly, systemically restorative, revitalizing and gently warming effect in individuals with chronic weak terrain that tends towards cold. In this respect, Moroccan thyme is usually engaged for treating severe debility or general asthenia with chronic fatigue, sexual debility, chronic uterine weakness and, with its strong analgesic effect, in chronic, cold-type arthritis. It is seen as one of the best reproductive stimulants and aphrodisiacs for sexual debility and loss of libido. For adrenal exhaustion, a good synergistic combination based on alcohol constituents would be Geranium or Thyme ct. geraniol.

Moreover, Moroccan thyme has the specific function of boosting and reorganizing immune functions. Practitioners often select it specifically for its strong immunostimulant and broad-spectrum anti-infective action when treating compromised immunity with chronic and/or recurring infections, whether viral, bacterial, fungal or parasitic. Excellent results have been obtained in chronic respiratory and urinary infections, such as chronic cystitis and lung TB, for instance. Moroccan thyme is also one of the few oils proven helpful in managing autoimmune conditions which, like the indicated infections, suggests a link to its exceptionally high content in the monoterpenol borneol (Faucon 2015). The same precautions, dilutions and doses as for Thyme ct. thymol apply.

### Acrid-herbaceous thyme oils with phenol dominance
These thyme oils are characterized by their warming, stimulating effects in hypotonic/weak and hyposthenic/cold conditions, especially when acute. Phenolic thyme oils are designed to strongly stimulate the healthy energy (vital force, zheng qi) rather than simply supporting it in order to resolve pathogens (as do the monoterpenol thymes).

As a result, they are able to focus almost exclusively on treating the symptoms rather than the terrain.

Thyme oils with phenols dominant all possess medium-strength therapeutic status with some cumulative toxicity over time. This is their strong suit, but it comes at a price. Like most thyme oils, their main tropism is the nervous, respiratory, digestive and immune systems. They are specifically strongly immunostimulant and anti-infective in the treatment of severe infections and excel at managing the acute phase of an infection. Being the most aggressive of all thyme oils, their use comes at the cost of various side effects. They are skin irritant, and their internal use always involves important precautions. Phenolic thymes are generally contraindicated in hypersthenic/hot, hypertonic/tense and dry conditions, including high fevers, acute inflammation, hypertension and agitation, as well as with pregnant and breastfeeding mothers, babies, infants and sensitive individuals. Their internal use should be limited to eight-day courses, and then always within an individualized formula rather than on their own.

From the pharmacological perspective, long-term internal absorption of phenols may cause liver damage, inhibit the healthy intestinal microflora (microbiome) and may interfere with blood clotting, making them additionally contraindicated in bleeding disorders and in those taking anticoagulant medication.

Finally, the fragrance of phenolic thyme oils is intense, acrid, 'medicinal' and not immediately pleasant – another indication that they are suited mainly to tackle the presenting symptoms or infection, and not to support the individual terrain.

Everything said here about phenolic thyme oils applies equally to the phenol-rich oils in the genera *Origanum* (Oregano), *Satureja* (Winter savoury), *Syzygium* (Clove) and *Cinnamomum* (Cinnamon). The cinnamaldehydes in Cinnamon bark oil act in virtually the same way as the phenols.

**Thyme ct. thymol** (*Thymus vulgaris/zygis* L. ct. thymol) (this profile) is the classic go-to acrid-herbaceous, phenolic thyme oil of this group with <48% thymol content. This aggressive constituent is balanced by a nice variety of other minor constituents that soften its harsh edge, making it less aggressive. Thyme ct. thymol is considered less toxic to the liver than Oregano, Winter savoury and the other thyme oils dominated by carvacrol. It thus has the advantage of being the least toxic of the phenolic oils, while still packing the punch of the phenols. In practice this means that it can be taken in repeated eight-day courses if necessary – although always combined into a formula with other oils, as all high-phenol oils.

Physiologically Thyme ct. thymol is an excellent systemic warming stimulant for chronic weak, cold and damp conditions in general. However, Thyme ct. thymol is also a premier broad-spectrum anti-infective remedy with strong immunostimulant and anti-infective/antimicrobial actions. It will treat both acute and chronic infections, esp. respiratory, gastrointestinal and urogenital ones, focusing on resolving the infection rather than supporting the terrain.

Along with Wild thyme and Winter savoury, Thyme ct. thymol contains monoterpenes in addition to phenols – unlike Clove and Oregano. As a result, Thyme ct. thymol possesses a stronger energizing effect and a better tropism for the brain than these other high-phenol oils. The additional monoterpenes also create a more complex pattern of constituents, making Thyme ct. thymol somewhat less drug-like than Clove and Oregano. This means that the body can utilize its phenols more easily and readily, resulting in a more balanced and forgiving form of stimulation.

**Thyme ct. carvacrol** (*Thymus vulgaris* L. ct. carvacrol), an acrid-pungent oil dominant in carvacrol, has the same therapeutic and topical safety status as Oregano, with potential for some cumulative toxicity and moderate to severe skin irritation and sensitization. However, carvacrol is many times more hepatotoxic than thymol, an important caution in its clinical use.

This oil's nature, functions, indications and cautions are essentially the same as for Oregano oil. Practitioners will often use Thyme ct. carvacrol for its somewhat more aggressive effect when treating acute infections. Also, the phenol carvacrol is thought to exert a better tropism for the organs in the lower trunk, making this oil an excellent choice for infections of the large intestine, urinary tract and reproductive organs.

**Wild thyme** (*Thymus serpyllum* L.), or Serpolet in French, presents an acrid, sweet-green oil dominant in both carvacrol and thymol. It has the same therapeutic and topical safety status as Thyme ct. thymol, with potential for mild cumulative toxicity and moderate skin irritation and sensitization.

Wild thyme's clinical uses as a remedy are also identical to those of Thyme ct. thymol; it is also a good nervous and cerebral restorative. However, it is more often given for its potent broad-spectrum anti-infective actions than its restorative action. Respiratory infections respond very well to it, with the same actions as Thyme ct. thymol. Wild thyme also exerts a good analgesic action, including for headaches during infections, e.g. the flu. It is considered an excellent analgesic neuromuscular sedative for muscle and tendon pain in particular, as in tendinitis, torticollis, low-back pain, sciatica and all contractions in general. The same cautions, contraindications, dilutions and doses as for Thyme ct. thymol apply.

Various varieties of this species also exist, such as Lemon-scented wild thyme (*T. serpyllum* var. *citriodorus*), which contains the pleasant-scented citral and citronellal.

**Capitate thyme** (*Thymus capitatus* Hoffmanns. & Link, syn. *Thymbra capitata* Cav.), with its strongly acrid-pungent aroma and dominant in carvacrol, has the same therapeutic and topical safety status as Thyme ct. carvacrol, with potential for some cumulative toxicity and moderate to severe skin irritation and sensitization. It belongs to the more aggressive group of phenolic oils and shares the same nature, functions, indications and cautions as Thyme ct. carvacrol and Oregano.

**Ajowan** (*Trachyspermum ammi* Sprague) from India and Afghanistan is a seed oil in the carrot (Umbelliferae) family and similar to Thyme ct. thymol in its nature and uses. Ajowan seed is an important Ayurvedic remedy and culinary spice. Like Thyme ct. thymol, it has the same therapeutic and topical safety status as Thyme ct. thymol, with potential for some cumulative toxicity and moderate skin irritation and sensitization. Thymol ranges are 40–49%, carvacrol 1–9%, with additional monoterpenes (γ-terpinene 19–36%, p-cymene 20–25%).

Ajowan is a strong stimulant, heating, phenol-rich oil useful for treating chronic hypotonic/weak and hyposthenic/cold terrain, especially with bacterial, viral or parasitic infection present. It is especially effective in cases of infectious and parasitic skin conditions such as erysipelas. Its actions, indications, precautions, dilutions and doses are essentially the same as for Thyme ct. thymol. As always with high-phenol oils, Ajowan should be suitably diluted and combined with monoterpenol-rich oils such as Palmarosa or Tea tree in a 5–10% dilution liniment.

### Fresh-pungent thyme oils with monoterpene and cineole dominance

These thyme oils are basically restorative, warming and drying by nature and are appropriate for treating hypotonic/weak and hyposthenic/cold conditions that tend to damp congestion. They resemble other similar oils such as Rosemary, Cajeput, Ravintsara and Saro, and could be seen as specialized variants of these others.

**Mastic thyme** or Spanish thyme (*Thymus mastichina* L.) is pungent fresh and somewhat green-herbaceous. It is essentially restorative in hypotonic/weak conditions with fatigue, debility, etc. It is also used conversely as a good mucolytic expectorant and anti-infective in bronchial infections with copious sputum. Upper respiratory infections with painful sinus congestion, headache and excessive mucus production respond very well to its decongestant effect and need steam inhalations as well as chest rubs (liniments). Mastic thyme has mild therapeutic and topical safety status; it is non-irritant to the skin and has no other cautions apart from avoiding use in babies and infants.

**Thyme ct. paracymene** (*Thymus vulgaris* L. ct. paracymene) is low in the phenol thymol but in contrast high in the monoterpene p-cymene, making it an excellent topical analgesic in arthritic conditions – its main clinical use. This chemotype of thyme has mild therapeutic and topical safety status; it is non-irritant to the skin and has no other cautions apart from avoiding use in babies and infants.

# Winter Savoury

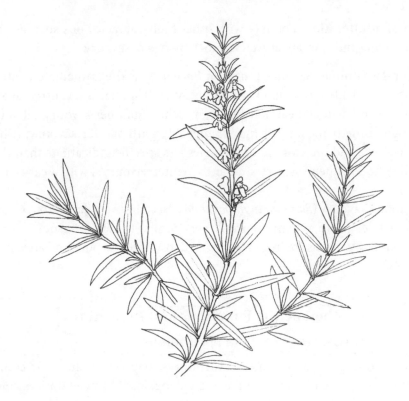

**Botanical source:** The herb of *Satureja montana* L. (Lamiaceae/Labiatae – lipflower/mint family), a herb of the warm temperate regions of southern Europe

**Other names:** Sariette des montagnes (Fr), Bohnenkraut (Ge), Satureia (It), Ajedrea (Sp)

**Appearance:** A colourless or pale yellow mobile liquid with a strong spicy-warm, herbaceous odour with somewhat acrid bottom notes

**Perfumery status:** A heart note of medium intensity and poor persistence

**Extraction:** Steam distillation from the whole herb in late summer

**1 kg oil yield from:** 300–500 kg of the fresh herb (a moderate to low yield)

**Production areas:** This Mediterranean native is produced in Spain, Morocco and several Balkan countries

**Typical constituents:** Phenols 38–76% (incl. carvacrol 37–75%, thymol 1–5%, eugenol) • monoterpenes 40–50% (incl. α and γ-terpinenes <20%, p-cymene 6–20%, limonene, terpinolene, α-thujene, α-pinenes, β-pinenes, α-phellandrene) • sesquiterpenes 6%

(incl. β-caryophyllene, α-humulene, α- and γ-cadinene, calamene, aromadendrene, β-bisabolene) • esters (incl. bornyl, linalyl, terpenyl and geranyl acetate) • oxide 1,8 cineole <1%, caryophyllene oxide • trace camphor, damascenone • carvacrol methyl-ether

**Chance of adulteration:** Possibly with other high-carvacrol oils such as Oregano, Capitate thyme and Ajowan, as well as other species of savoury

**Related oils:** Summer Savoury (*Satureja hortensis*) is the immediate relative most commonly available (see below), although over 50 species are centred around the Mediterranean basin and eastward to Iran. While Summer savoury oil is used for physiological medicine almost interchangeably with Winter savoury, it has seen less clinical use and therefore to date carries less specific indications than the latter. Its profile of constituents is very similar to Winter savoury's, with a carvacrol range of 35–40%.

Mountain savoury (*Satureja thymbra*) oil is sometimes available from Cypriot and Turkish distillers, with a chemical profile very similar to Winter savoury. The various Oregano and Thyme oils are in genuses related to Winter savoury and are equally rich in phenols.

## Therapeutic Functions and Indications

### Specific symptomatology – *All applications*

Apathy, discouragement, spaciness, listlessness, depression, low self-confidence, lethargy, chronic fatigue, poor stamina, mental fog, loss of concentration, cold hands and feet, loss of sex drive, loss of periods, urinary symptoms, poor appetite, loose stool, abdominal pains, chronic cough, wheeze, muscle and joint coldness, stiffness and pain; frequent or recurring infections

### Psychological – *Aromatic diffusion*

**Essential PNEI function and indication:** Stimulant in weakness conditions

**Possible brain dynamics:** Increases basal ganglia and prefrontal cortex functioning

**Fragrance category:** Top tone with pungent, green notes

**Indicated psychological disorders:** ADD, depression

#### Promotes courage and self-confidence

- Loss of courage with apathy, discouragement, loss of motivation, depression

- Low self-esteem and self-confidence, pessimism, self-neglect

S<small>TIMULATES THE MIND AND PROMOTES ALERTNESS</small>

- Lethargy, drowsiness, stupor

- Mental confusion, disorientation, poor concentration

## P<small>HYSIOLOGICAL</small> – *Suppository, gel cap, external applications (with caution)*

**Therapeutic status:** Medium-strength remedy with some cumulative toxicity

**Topical safety status:** Strong skin irritant and sensitizer

*vulnerary, antispetic:* insect bites, sores, abscesses

*rubefacient, analgesic:* muscle and joint pain and coldness, cramps, toothache, ear pain

*antiparasitic:* skin parasites

**Tropism:** Nervous, endocrine, respiratory, digestive, urogenital systems

**Essential diagnostic function:** Stimulates and warms asthenic/cold and restores chronic hypotonic/weak terrain conditions

P<small>RIMARILY STIMULANT AND WARMING:</small>

*strong systemic nervous and vascular stimulant, SNS and central arterial circulatory stimulant:* a wide range of asthenic (cold) and chronic hypotonic (weak) conditions with circulatory deficiency, chronic physical and mental debility, fatigue and cold; incl. convalescence, CFS

*cerebral stimulant:* mental debility, neurasthenia, depression

*adrenal stimulant, strong hypertensive:* adrenal fatigue syndrome (esp. with afternoon or evening fatigue), chronic hypotension

*strong reproductive stimulant, aphrodisiac:* sexual debility, loss of libido, impotence

*progesteronic:* progesterone deficiency syndrome

P<small>RIMARILY STIMULANT AND RELAXANT:</small>

*strong uterine stimulant and relaxant, emmenagogue, analgesic:* amenorrhoea, spasmodic dysmenorrhoea

*urinary stimulant and relaxant, diuretic:* metabolic toxicosis, anuria, dysuria *strong gastrointestinal stimulant and relaxant, aperitive, stomachic, carminative, spasmolytic, analgesic:* digestive atony with indigestion, appetite loss, flatulence, diarrhoea; enteritis, colitis, colic, abdominal pain in general

*strong musculoskeletal stimulant and relaxant, analgesic, spasmolytic, anti-inflammatory:* chronic rheumatic and arthritic conditions with pain, cramps, stiffness; rheumatoid arthritis, fibromyalgia

*bronchial stimulant and relaxant, expectorant, mucolytic, spasmolytic, antitussive:* congestive and spasmodic lower respiratory conditions with dyspnoea and cough; chronic bronchitis, emphysema, croup

*antipyretic, antimalarial:* intermittent fevers, malaria

*strong antioxidant*

ANTIMICROBIAL ACTIONS:

*broad-spectrum anti-infective, antimicrobial, immunostimulant, detoxicant:* a wide range of severe infections, acute and chronic, esp. urogenital, gastrointestinal, respiratory, lymphatic

- *strong antibacterial:* bacterial infections both gram-positive and gram-negative, incl. cystitis, nephritis, gonorrhoea, prostatitis; gastroenteritis, colitis, dysentery; microbial toxicosis, intestinal fermentation, food poisoning; bronchitis, pharyngitis, strep throat; malaria, lymphadenitis, bacteraemia

- *antifungal:* fungal infections, incl. Candida spp., fungal cystitis, lung and kidney TB

- *strong antiparasitic, anthelmintic:* amoebiasis, amoebic dysentery, roundworms (Ascaris), tapeworms (Taenia)

- *antiviral:* misc. viral infections, esp. urogenital, gastrointestinal, respiratory, neurological

SYNERGISTIC COMBINATIONS
All for short-term use only: see 'Therapeutic precautions' below.

- Winter savoury + Niaouli: strong broad-spectrum anti-infective and immunostimulant for severe acute infections, esp. urinary, genital, digestive and respiratory; esp. with debility, cold-weak terrain

- Winter savoury + Cinnamon bark + Black spruce: strong anthelmintic for intestinal parasites of most kinds; esp. with debility, cold-weak terrain

COMPLEMENTARY COMBINATIONS

All for short-term use only: see 'Therapeutic precautions' below.

- Winter savoury + Ravintsara: strong nervous, cerebral and arterial stimulant and antiviral in severe neurasthenic conditions with weak, cold terrain; with fatigue, debility, cold, depression, hypotension

- Winter savoury + Rosemary: analgesic, spasmolytic, antirheumatic, liver-protective in chronic rheumatic-arthritic conditions with pain, cramping, stiffness

- Winter savoury + Juniper berry/Sage: strong urinary antibacterial in severe chronic urinary infections

- Winter savoury + Palmarosa: broad-spectrum antifungal for fungal infections, incl. fungal cystitis

- Winter savoury + Nutmeg: antiparasitic and anthelmintic for intestinal parasites, esp. amoebic dysentery

- Winter savoury + Tea tree: antipyretic (febrifuge) for low-grade and intermittent fevers of all kinds, incl. dengue, malaria

- Winter savoury + Cardamom: strong aperitive, stomachic, nervous stimulant for severe digestive atony with appetite loss, fatigue, debility

- Winter savoury + Black pepper: strong digestive spasmolytic, analgesic, antibacterial, antidiarrhoeal for severe intestinal colic, colitis, infectious diarrhoea, incl. dysentery

TOPICAL – *Liniment, lotion*

See 'Pharmacological precautions' below.

**Therapeutic precautions:** Winter savoury oil is strongly stimulating, warming and drying; it is a strong nervous, adrenal and circulatory stimulant that should not be used in those presenting with hypersthenic/hot, hypertonic/tense and dry conditions of any kind. It is therefore contraindicated in high fevers, acute inflammation, hypertension, agitation and all symptoms of dryness (e.g. thirst, dry cough or constipation). It should also be avoided in babies, infants and sensitive individuals. Being a uterine stimulant, Winter savoury is also contraindicated during pregnancy and breastfeeding.

Internal use should be limited to a single eight-day course, and then always within a formula rather than on its own, as with all high-phenol oils (see below). Long-term internal use may cause liver damage and inhibit the healthy microflora; this should be prevented with the adjunctive use of liver restorative/protective oils and/or herbs, and prebiotic foods and supplements. Inhalation with an essential oil nebulizer is not recommended to avoid serious irritation to the mucous membrane.

**Pharmacological precautions:** Only low dilutions of this highly dermocaustic oil should be used topically. Absorbed internally, the constituents carvacrol and thymol may interfere with blood clotting, making Winter savoury contraindicated in bleeding disorders and for those taking anticoagulant medication.

**Preparations:**

- Diffusor: Not suitable

- Massage oil: Not used

- Liniment: 0.25–1% dilution in vegetable oil

- Gel cap: 1–2 drops with some olive oil for short-term use, e.g. an eight-day course; and usually as part of a formula; the maximum daily dose is 5 drops. Like all phenolic oils, Winter savoury should always be combined with other oils to soften its intensity and enhance treatment results; especially with sweet, monoterpenol-rich oils such as Palmarosa, Tea tree, Thyme ct. linalool or Lavender.

## Chinese Medicine Functions and Indications

**Aroma energy:** Pungent, green

**Movement:** Rising

**Warmth:** Warm to hot

**Meridian tropism:** Kidney, Spleen, Stomach, Lung, Bladder

**Five-Element affinity:** Water, Earth, Metal

**Essential function:** To tonify the Yang, warm the interior and strengthen the Shen

1. **Tonifies the Yang, warms the Kidney and strengthens the Shen and libido**

   - **Yang deficiency with Shen weakness**, with mental and physical fatigue, cold hands and feet, recurrent infections, apathy, depression:
   Ginger/Black spruce/Clove bud

   - **Kidney Yang deficiency** with loss of sex drive, weak loins and knees, fatigue, cold skin and extremities:
   Black spruce/Clove bud/Thyme ct. thymol

2. **Warms and harmonizes the Middle Warmer, resolves damp and relieves pain**

- **Stomach-Spleen empty cold** (Spleen Yang deficiency with cold) with epigastric or abdominal pain, appetite loss, chronic diarrhoea, irregular bowel movement:

  Juniper berry/Nutmeg/Basil

- **Stomach-Spleen damp-cold** with chronic diarrhoea, undigested food in stool, cold limbs, debility, poor appetite:

  Patchouli/Nutmeg/Black pepper

3. **Warms the Lung, expels phlegm, circulates and descends Lung Qi, and relieves coughing and wheezing**

- **Lung phlegm-cold with Qi accumulation**, with coughing, wheezing, sputum expectoration, chest distension, cold extremities:

  Hyssop/Grand fir/Green myrtle

- **Lung Qi accumulation in other patterns**, with wheezing, chest distension, coughing:

  Siberian fir/Fennel/Basil ct. methylchavicol

4. **Warms and opens the meridians, dispels wind-damp-cold, relaxes the tendons and relieves pain**

- **Internal cold with wind-damp-cold obstruction**, with muscle and joint aches, pain, coldness and cramping:

  Black pepper/Nutmeg/Ginger

5. **Warms and activates the Lower Warmer, breaks up stagnation and promotes menstruation**

- **Lower Warmer Blood and Qi stagnation with cold**, with scanty or absent menstrual flow, painful periods with cramps, loss of sex drive:

  Rosemary/Niaouli/Juniper berry

REMARKS

Like many other plants in the lipflower (mint) family, winter and summer savoury from the Eastern Mediterranean and Western Asia have a long history of culinary and medicinal use. Savoury is an important ingredient in the cuisines and herb mixtures of not only Italy and France, but also of Bulgaria, Romania, Georgia and Azerbaijan (where it is used to flavour black tea). Savoury's botanical name derives either from the Latin *saturare*, meaning 'to satiate', or from the Greek *saturos*, meaning 'satyre'. Either way, Winter savoury in Greek and Roman days certainly enjoyed a huge reputation as an aphrodisiac. The poet Ovid noted that 'its name comes from the satyres, whose amorous exploits are well known'. The herb was freely consumed at Roman orgies where it did double duty to both mitigate the unholy digestive side effects of gluttony and stimulate venery at the same time. Fast forward to the Christian Middle Ages: cultivating savoury was forbidden in monastery physick gardens, and where Monk's pepper, or chasteberry seed, was used freely to control the libido of the religious fraternity.

Still, savoury's secular reputation does not seem to have deterred the likes of Hildegard of Bingen, abbess of the St. Gallen cloister in Switzerland, from growing the herb in her physick garden. Like many of her herbalist colleagues past and future, she valued Savoury for treating digestive problems, rheumatic pain and other conditions caused by cold. In European herbal medicine, Savoury was in general as highly valued as the herbal panaceas Sage, Thyme and Angelica root.

Today, Winter savoury essential oil enjoys as much a reputation among European practitioners as the herb and tincture have always done. In contrast to other acrid, pungent phenol-rich oils such as Clove and Oregano, Winter savoury (like Thyme ct. thymol) possesses monoterpenes in addition to phenols. This creates a more complex pattern of constituents that acts in a less drug-like and more balanced manner, allowing the body to better utilize its powerful effect in general.

A systemic warming stimulant, the oil is highly effective for treating conditions stemming from weak, cold terrain, especially chronic neurasthenia, debility, nervous and mental exhaustion, and hypotension. A strong sympathetic nervous, adrenal and central circulatory stimulant, Winter savoury is Europe's answer to Asian spice stimulants such as Clove, Cinnamon and Black pepper. In general, the oil has a good tropism for the organs of the lower trunk and is often chosen whenever urinary, reproductive or intestinal stimulation is required. Chronic, cold infections of the urogenital organs are also its domain, especially bacterial and parasitic infections. In tandem, Winter savoury is a good detoxicant, both systemic and to the digestive tract: it can resolve metabolic toxicosis as much as GI tract toxins specifically, including pathogenic microflora, as well as help resolve digestive fermentation. As such, it is thought to inhibit pathogenic microflora while sparing the beneficial saprophytic flora.

Musculoskeletal pain conditions, both rheumatic and arthritic, also respond well to Winter savoury, as do menstrual cramps and painful urination. Its constituent p-cymene has been identified as analgesic in this respect.

In a few individuals not put off by its acrid basenotes, the spicy, herbaceous-green fragrance of Winter savoury may work well as a psychological remedy by gentle olfaction. Its functions in this context are broadly the same as those of Oregano oil, only with greater emphasis on its mental function of promoting alertness.

# Wintergreen

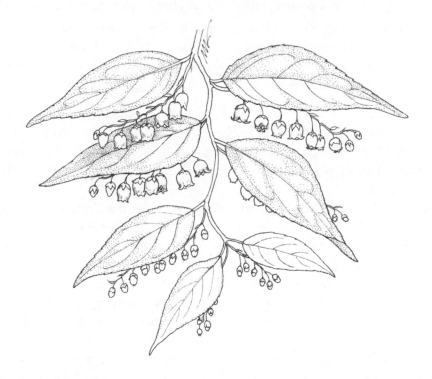

**Botanical sources:** *Gaultheria procumbens* L., *G. fragrantissima* (L.) Wallich. (Ericaceae – heather family), a widespread small evergreen shrub from temperate biomes

**Other names:** Gaultheria; Gaulthérie (Fr), Sempreverdi (It), Gaulteria (Sp)

**Appearance:** A mobile pale yellow or pinkish fluid with an intense warm, spicy, sweet, somewhat woody-balsamic odour with slightly fruity top notes

**Perfumery status:** A heart note of very high intensity and good persistence

**Extraction:** Steam distillation of the fresh herb from June to October; the leaves are first macerated in water overnight before distillation; the enzymatic fermentation ensures full extraction of the esters

**1 kg oil yield from:** 80–110 kg of the dried fermented herb (a good yield)

**Production areas:** United States (*G. procumbens*, native to the Eastern seaboard), Nepal (*G. fragrantissima*). Small-scale production of Wintergreen oil began in the 1810s in the States of New England, and soon spread to the forested hill-regions of Pennsylvania, New Jersey, New York, Maryland and Virginia. The Asian species of *G. fragrantissima* gained currency as a source of Wintergreen oil as early as the 1870s.

**Typical constituents:** Aromatic esters 99% (incl. methyl salicylate <99%, ethyl/propyl/butyl/benzyl/cis-3-hexenyl salicylates) • benzyle benzoate • cis-3-hexenyl/bornyl/menthyl/terpenyl acetates • phenol eugenol • phenolic methylether asarone • aldehydes 2 and 3-methyl-butanals, hexanal, trans-2-decan, benzaldehyde, cinnamaldehyde

**Chance of adulteration:** High. Wintergreen oil is often reconstructed from synthetic methyl salicylate and sometimes from herbal sources of methyl salicylate, including the root of *Polygala paucifolia* (fringed polygala), the stems and roots of *Filipendula ulmaria* and *F. lobata* (meadowsweet) and *Monotropa hypopitys* (Dutchman's pipe).

**Related oils:** The *Gaultheria* genus includes about 135 species of shrubs in the heather family. In addition to the main two species above, several others are often used for the production of Wintergreen oil, including *Gaultheria hispidula*, *G. leucocarpa* and *G. punctata*. They share similar properties because of their dominant constituent, methyl salicylate.

The related Birch oil is produced extremely rarely today, if at all, and for all practical purposes should be considered non-existent. All so-called Birch oil offered today is almost certainly reconstituted from either synthetic methyl salicylate and/or any of its other natural plant sources listed above.

For the record, genuine Birch bark oil in the past was distilled from the comminuted and macerated bark (and sometimes young twigs) of *Betula lenta*, the black, sweet or cherry birch, and possibly also from *Betula alleghaniensis*, the yellow birch; distillation began in 1865 in Luzerne county, Pennsylvania. This oil was closely related to Wintergreen oil in terms of its chemical and energetic properties, consisting of over 90% methyl salicylate. Because Wintergreen enjoyed such a huge reputation in those days, Birch oil used to be sold as Wintergreen oil throughout the 19th century. In those days it was also common for Birch bark to be co-distilled with Wintergreen. In terms of clinical usage, the two oils were used completely interchangeably (King *et al.* 1898; Gildemeister 1899; Arctander 1960).

## Therapeutic Functions and Indications

### SPECIFIC SYMPTOMATOLOGY – *All applications*

Loss of self-confidence and self-assertion, insecurity, discouragement, negativity, low willpower, fearfulness for no reason, paranoia, despair, addictive and compulsive behaviour, insomnia, fatigue, debility, headache, hot spells, alternating fever and chills, low-grade fever with debility, acute bladder pains, painful urination, acute menstrual cramps, chronic urinary and vaginal discharges, sexual overstimulation, chest oppression, sharp chest pains, red painful swollen or stiff joints, muscle cramping, muscle aches, nerve pains

## PSYCHOLOGICAL – *Aromatic diffusion, whole-body massage (with caution)*

**Essential PNEI function and indication:** Stimulant in weakness conditions

**Possible brain dynamics:** Increases prefrontal cortex and regulates basal ganglia functioning

**Fragrance category:** Middle tone with sweet, pungent notes

**Indicated psychological disorders:** Addictions, compulsions

PROMOTES WILLPOWER, COURAGE AND SELF-CONFIDENCE

- Loss of willpower or strength, poor personal boundaries
- Discouragement with apathy, pessimism, escapism, negativity, despair
- Loss of self-confidence with insecurity, anxiety
- Mental and emotional burnout, shock

PROMOTES EMOTIONAL STABILITY AND INTEGRATION

- Mental-emotional instability, fearfulness
- Self-neglect, self-destructive tendencies

## PHYSIOLOGICAL – *Nebulizer inhalation, gel cap, suppository, external applications*

All to be used with caution.

**Therapeutic status:** Medium-strength remedy with some cumulative toxicity

**Topical safety status:** Mild skin irritant and mildly sensitizing

**Tropism:** Musculoskeletal, urinary, reproductive, digestive systems

**Essential diagnostic function:** Cools hypersthenic/hot conditions and decongests congestive/damp terrain conditions

PRIMARILY COOLING AND RELAXANT:

*strong refrigerant, antipyretic:* hot spells, hot flushes; fevers, esp. intermittent

*strong anti-inflammatory, analgesic, spasmolytic, antirheumatic, antineuralgic:* a wide range of acute inflammatory conditions with pain and spasm, esp. musculoskeletal, urinary, reproductive, intestinal and cardiovascular; incl.:

- rheumatic, arthritic and neuralgic conditions with acute pain and cramping, incl. tendinitis, epicondylitis, sciatica, fibromyalgia, arthritis, low back pain

- – acute cystitis, interstitial cystitis, urethritis, prostatitis, nephritis; spasmodic dysuria

- – acute spasmodic and congestive dysmenorrhoea

- – colic, IBS

*cardiovascular relaxant, anti-inflammatory, analgesic, spasmolytic, vasodilator, hypotensive:* acute spasmodic coronaritis, arteritis, angina pectoris (all types), Raynaud's disease; headache, hypertension

*anticoagulant:* haematoma

*sexual sedative, anaphrodisiac:* sexual overstimulation (nymphomania, satyriasis)

PRIMARILY STIMULANT AND DECONGESTANT:

*moderate arterial circulatory and nervous stimulant:* weakness, fatigue

*uterine stimulant, emmenagogue:* amenorrhoea

*liver stimulant/decongestant:* liver congestion (esp. with headaches), liver disease

*uterine and prostatic decongestant:* congestive dysmenorrhoea, prostate congestion with dysuria

*mucostatic:* chronic mucus discharges, incl. leucorrhoea, blennuria, gonorrhoeal discharges

*diuretic:* dysuria, bladder irritation

SYNERGISTIC COMBINATIONS
None.

COMPLEMENTARY COMBINATIONS
All for short-term use only: see 'Therapeutic precautions' below.

- Wintergreen + Lemon + Tea tree: strong refrigerant, antipyretic for acute hot spells and fevers of most kinds

- Wintergreen + Lemon eucalyptus: strong anti-inflammatory, analgesic, antirheumatic for painful acute rheumatic and arthritic conditions

- Wintergreen + Tea tree/Niaouli: strong anti-inflammatory, analgesic, antirheumatic for painful chronic rheumatic, arthritic, tendonic, neuralgic and other pain conditions

- Wintergreen + Atlas cedarwood: anti-inflammatory, analgesic, diuretic, mucostatic for painful urinary and reproductive conditions with spasmodic dysuria, incl. (interstitial) cystitis, urethritis, incl. with mucus discharges

- Wintergreen + Cypress: anti-inflammatory, pelvic and prostatic decongestant for prostate congestion with hyperplasia, prostatitis, haemorrhoids

- Wintergreen + Green myrtle: mucostatic for chronic mucus discharges, esp. vaginitis with leucorrhoea

- Wintergreen + Yarrow: uterine decongestant, analgesic and emmenagogue: amenorrhoea, congestive dysmenorrhoea with dragging pelvic pains

- Wintergreen + Niaouli/Rosemary ct. verbenone: liver decongestant for chronic liver congestion with headaches

## TOPICAL – *Liniment, lotion*

see 'Pharmacological precautions' below.

**Skin care:** Not used

*anti-inflammatory:* eczema, dermatitis, pityriasis, acne

*analgesic, rubefacient, antipruritic:* headache, toothache; skin, muscle and joint pain in general; skin itching

*analgesic, antihaematomal, detumescent:* acute injuries or tissue trauma with severe bruising/contusion, haematoma, ecchymosis, swelling; tears, sprains, strains

*antiparasitic:* head lice (*Pediculus capitis*)

**Therapeutic precautions:** Wintergreen is a strong cooling and hypotensive remedy and is therefore for short-term use in acute conditions only. It is contraindicated in hyposthenic/cold and atonic/weak conditions in general; this includes debility, hypotension and chronic inflammation. The oil should only be given for acute forms of inflammation. Wintergreen is also contraindicated during pregnancy and breastfeeding by internal use as it is a uterine stimulant and teratogenic; it should also be avoided in babies, infants and sensitive individuals.

**Pharmacological precautions:** French medicine allows a maximum 2% dilution on the skin of this mildly irritating and sensitizing oil. Wintergreen is also contraindicated in individuals with salicylate sensitivity (e.g. seen in ADD and ADHD), in those taking anticoagulant medication or allergic to aspirin, and those with haemophilia or other bleeding disorders. Because of its extremely high content in methyl salicylate, Wintergreen should also be avoided in gastroesophageal reflux disease (GERD), as there is a risk of developing Reye's syndrome.

**Preparations:**

- Diffusor: Not suitable

- Massage oil: 1% dilution in vegetable oil, preferably with other oils

- Liniment: 1–2% dilution in vegetable oil

- Gel cap: 1 drop with some olive oil for short-term use, e.g. an eight-day course; and usually as part of a formula; the maximum daily dose is 4 drops. Wintergreen is best combined with other oils to soften its intensity and enhance treatment results; especially with sweet, monoterpenol-rich oils such as Lavender, Tea tree or Thyme ct. linalool. Internal use should be limited to a single maximum eight-day course.

## Chinese Medicine Functions and Indications

**Aroma energy:** Sweet, woody, pungent

**Movement:** Sinking, stabilizing

**Warmth:** Cool to cold

**Meridian tropism:** Liver, Bladder, Kidney, Heart

**Five-Element affinity:** Wood, Water

**Essential function:** To clear heat, activate Blood and Qi, harmonize the Shen and relieve pain

1. **Clears heat, calms the Liver, descends the Yang and harmonizes the Shen**

   - **Liver Yang rising (floating Yang) with heat**, with hot spells, headache, insomnia, tinnitus, irritability, apprehensiveness:

     Clary sage/Roman camomile/Spikenard

   - **Shao yang-stage and shao yin-stage heat**, with alternating fever and chills, or low-grade fever with weakness, debility:

     Lavender/Tea tree/Lemongrass

2. **Clears heat, drains damp, astringes fluids and stops discharges**

   - **Kidney-Bladder heat with Lower Warmer damp**, with acute bladder pains, painful urination, chronic urinary and vaginal discharges, fatigue:

     Lemon eucalyptus/Atlas cedarwood/Green myrtle

   - **Kidney fire** with sexual overstimulation:

     Marjoram/Cypress

3. <u>**Activates Blood and Qi, breaks up stagnation and relieves pain**</u>

- **Blood and Qi stagnation** with pain, swelling, discoloration, contusion from tissue trauma; nerve, muscle, tendon and joint pains; headaches:

  Roman camomile/Helichrysum/Spike lavender/Frankincense

- **Heart Blood and Qi stagnation** with chest pains, general tension, panicky feelings, emotional neurosis:

  Fennel/Laurel/Helichrysum

4. <u>**Activates the Lower Warmer, reduces stagnation and promotes menstruation**</u>

- **Lower Warmer Blood and Qi stagnation** with scanty or stopped periods, heavy dragging pelvic pains, pain referring to the low-back, dribbling urination:

  Yarrow/Clary sage/Niaouli/Angelica root

5. <u>**Opens the meridians, dispels wind-damp-heat, relaxes the tendons and relieves pain**</u>

- **Wind-damp-heat obstruction** with red, painful swollen joints, joint stiffness, muscle cramping, aches and pains:

  Lime/Lemon eucalyptus/Kaffir lime petitgrain

REMARKS

The scent of wintergreen is indelibly embedded in the collective North American psyche. Ever since the 1810s when the essential oil was first distilled in the forests of New England, wintergreen became irretrievably associated with syrups, pastilles, cough drops, liniments and an array of other popular preparations. Although largely replaced by synthetic methyl salicylate since the early 1900s, Wintergreen oil has long since found a place as a premier remedy for pain, inflammation and, among practitioners of energetic medicine, for clearing heat.

Named after French medical herbalist Jean-François Gaulthier of Quebec, Wintergreen was one of many herbal remedies fluent among Native American tribes of the Northeast. Like many other medicinal plants, it crossed the osmotic cultural barrier to white doctors in the late 18th century. Tonic teas were made from the leaves of this Eastern teaberry, and its tart berries were eaten freely. Among early pioneers and city dwellers alike, Wintergreen became as American a folk remedy as Birch and Sassafras.

The story of the extremely popular Swaim's Panacea, first produced in 1815 and brazenly redolent of wintergreen, is apocryphal for the stellar reputation conferred on this syrup by its analgesic essential oil. A certain Philadelphia bookbinder named Swaim found himself apparently cured of syphilis by the famous 18th-century French formula Rob de Boyveau-Laffecteur. Very impressed, Swaim became inspired to produce his own version. Somehow managing to obtain a copy of the formula, Swaim simply added Wintergreen oil to the blood-purifying Sassafras in the original formula – and voilà, a highly palatable best-seller was born. The sore throats and colicky stomachs of countless thousands of suffering individuals were mercifully soothed by its cooling, pain-relieving liquor. Its reputation sealed by the widespread fame of Swaim's Panacea, Wintergreen oil then became the defining sweetener among American druggists and pharmacists for correcting and disguising the taste of unpleasant remedies – as well as drinks such as root beer. While its sweet, fresh-woody scent had an undeniable appeal to the 19th-century nose, its cooling, pain-relieving actions were understandably, if not compassionately, beneficial in that age of burgeoning materialism, expansive geographic exploitation and modernistic industrial progress.

The paradox of Wintergreen oil is that it feels like a strong stimulant when inhaled, but is actually a cooling, pain-relieving remedy when used in practice, both topically and internally. Its general stimulant action is in reality quite moderate. Wintergreen's dominant function is to clear heat both locally and systemically. Acute painful inflammatory conditions are its prime indication, whether involving smooth or striped muscle systems. Wintergreen is most often a key ingredient in formulations for acute tendino-rheumatic, neuralgic and arthritic conditions, and for acute painful urogenital inflammation, with or without infection. It is one of the few oils with a strong tropism for the urinary and reproductive organs. Likewise, with topical applications, Wintergreen is a major oil for severe acute tissue trauma with pain, inflammation, swelling, haematoma or contusion.

Any heat rising, whether from a hot spell or a fever, the oil will also treat. Practitioners have also seen excellent results in particular with tense, spasmodic conditions of the circulatory vessels, such as coronaritis and angina pectoris. Its vasodilatant, hypotensive actions engage nicely here.

Wintergreen's secondary actions may be useful in individuals presenting a weak or damp, congestive terrain. The oil will support general weakness and fatigue, for instance, underlying a chronic fever or chronic pain and inflammation. With urogenital inflammations, Wintergreen's mucostatic and uterine stimulant actions will treat chronic vaginal discharges, congestive dysmenorrhoea and sluggish periods.

Used by gentle inhalation, Wintergreen through olfaction also makes for a unique psychological remedy if the individual can get past its somewhat 'medicinal' smell and associations with root beer. With its sweet, pungent fragrance, the oil stimulates and warms up psychic, i.e. mental-emotional, cold and weakness – essentially supporting self-affirmation, a strengthening of the ego-self. Wintergreen is for the individual who has not only lost his or her self-confidence and self-assertion, but is suffering from a deeper loss of will, their sense of power and very passion for living. Along with that, on the emotional level too, Wintergreen can help bring back to earth deep oceanic fear and paranoia.

A strong boost to the soul, Wintergreen is able to jump-start the wounded individual, powerless and exhausted from abuse – as seen in addictions, for instance, as well as from external trauma. It will support anyone intent on making a fresh start, wanting a second chance to live and thrive.

# Yarrow

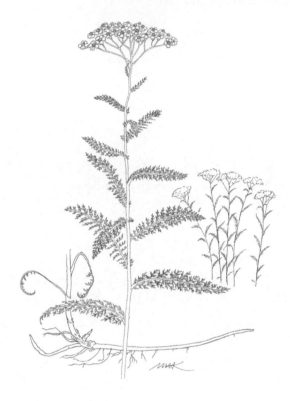

**Botanical source:** *Achillea millefolium* L. ct. chamazulene (Asteraceae/Compositae – daisy family), a widespread temperate herb

**Other names:** Milfoil; Millefeuille, Achillée (Fr), Schafgarbe (Ge), Millefoglio (It), Milenrama (Sp)

**Appearance:** A mobile cobalt to turquoise blue liquid with a sweet, herbaceous-green odour with mild to moderate fresh-camphoraceous top notes; with ageing, Yarrow oil may turn a yellowish green

**Perfumery status:** A heart note of very high intensity and good persistence

**Extraction:** Steam distillation of the fresh herb in flower during the summer

**1 kg oil yield from:** 250–1,000 kg of the herb (a highly variable field)

**Production areas:** Hungary, Austria, Bulgaria, Germany, France

**Typical constituents:** Monoterpenes 20–68% (incl. sabinene 7–41%, β-pinene 6–12%, γ-terpinene <3%, α-pinene <4%, camphene <2%, β-myrcene <2%, α-terpinene <1%, limonene <1%) • sesquiterpenes 17–52% (incl. chamazulene 5–33%, germacrene

D 9–14%, caryophyllene 2–5%) • monoterpenols 2–15% (incl. terpinen-4-ol 2-6%, borneol 1–12%, artemisia alcohol) • oxides 2–13% (incl. 1,8 cineole 2–11%, caryophyllene oxide <2%) • ketones <17% (incl. camphor 3–14%, β-thujone 0–3%) • esters <10% • bornyl acetate <2% • aromatic p-cymene <1% • sesquiterpenol cadinol <1% • lactone achilline

**Chance of adulteration:** Moderate, although increasing as the therapeutic value of this oil gains wider recognition. In addition, confusion may exist among identification of different species of *Achillea*, e.g. with *A. moschata* (used in the liqueur Iva), *A. nobilis* (Ligurian yarrow), *A. coronopifolia* and *A. ageratum*.

**Related oils:** Varieties include Ligurian yarrow (*Achillea ligustica* All.) and the Musk yarrow or Iva (*Achillea moschata*), from which essential oils are also sometimes produced. In addition, several chemotypes or type variations have been identified, including camphor, β-pinene and 1,8 cineole chemotypes (Baczek *et al.* 2015). However, more data is needed from the various countries that produce Yarrow oil before a clear picture of Yarrow chemotypes can be drawn.

## Therapeutic Functions and Indications

SPECIFIC SYMPTOMATOLOGY – *All applications*

Irritability, frustration, mood swings, negativity, shame feelings, rigidity of outlook, mental fog, confusion, loss of insight, morning lethargy, fatigue, dragging pelvic pains and distension, haemorrhoids, painful heavy periods with clots, painful, scanty late or stopped periods, ankle oedema, varicose veins, urinary incontinence, frequent scanty irritated urination, acute bladder pain, indigestion with chronic epigastric or abdominal pain, distension, flatulence, irregular bowel movement, red, itchy skin eruptions, painful swollen joints, chronic muscle aches and pains, tendency to acute inflammation and allergy

PSYCHOLOGICAL – *Aromatic diffusion, whole-body massage*

**Essential PNEI function and indication:** Regulating in dysregulation conditions

**Possible brain dynamics:** Reduces deep limbic system functioning and increases prefrontal cortex functioning

**Fragrance category:** Middle tone with sweet, green, pungent notes

**Indicated psychological disorders:** Bipolar disorder, minor depression, addiction

PROMOTES EMOTIONAL STABILITY, FLEXIBILITY AND RENEWAL

- Emotional instability with distressed feelings (including negativity, cynicism, jealousy, shame, self-deprecation, suicidal tendencies.

- Irritability, mood swings, anger management issues

- Mental/emotional conflict with rigidity, lack of flexibility

PROMOTES GOOD JUDGEMENT, INSIGHT AND ALERTNESS

- Poor judgement with loss of insight and critical thinking

- Mental fogginess, confusion, disorientation

- Loss of visualization or envisioning

## PHYSIOLOGICAL – *Nebulizer inhalation, gel cap, suppository, external applications*

**Therapeutic status:** Mild remedy with no cumulative toxicity

**Topical safety status:** Non-irritant, non-sensitizing

**Tropism:** Urinary, reproductive, digestive, respiratory systems

**Essential diagnostic function:** Stimulates congestive/damp conditions and cools hypersthenic/hot terrain conditions

PRIMARILY STIMULANT AND DECONGESTANT:

*urinary stimulant and detoxicant, diuretic, antilithic, alterative metabolic detoxicant:* anuria, kidney stones, metabolic toxicosis, gout, rheumatic-arthritic conditions; all with dysuria

*uterine stimulant and decongestant, emmenagogue:* dysmenorrhoea (esp. congestive), oligomenorrhoea, irregular cycles

*progesteronic hormonal regulator, oestrogen inhibitor:* dysmenorrhoea, oestrogen accumulation syndrome, irregular or long menstrual cycles, menopausal syndrome; repeated miscarriage, postpartum depression

*venous and lymphatic decongestant:* venous congestion with varicose veins, pelvic congestion, oedema, haemorrhoids

*hepatobiliary stimulant, cholagogue:* liver and gallbladder atony with congestion

*gastrointestinal stimulant, aperitive, stomachic, carminative:* digestive atony with appetite loss, flatulence, indigestion, constipation, mild colic

*mild respiratory stimulant, expectorant and decongestant:* head colds, sinus congestion, bronchial congestion

PRIMARILY COOLING:

*strong anti-inflammatory, analgesic:* a wide range of acute and chronic inflammatory conditions with pain:

- *urinary:* cystitis, interstitial cystitis, nephritis, kidney stone pain; all with dysuria

- *reproductive:* menstrual pain (uterine, ovarian), prostatitis, pelvic inflammatory disease

- *nervous:* headache, backache, neuritis, neuralgia (incl. sciatica), MS, Parkinson's and other neurodegenerative disorders

- *neuro-musculoskeletal:* rheumatic, arthritic and tendon pain; fibromyalgia, tendinitis

- *gastrointestinal:* gastritis, ulcerative colitis, inflammatory bowel disease (incl. Crohn's)

- *other:* phlebitis, cellulitis

*antiallergic, antihistamine, tissue-regenerative (mucosal and dermal):* atopic eczema/dermatitis, shingles, sinusitis, otitis, cystitis, intestinal hyperpermeability with food allergies

*vasodilator:* hypertension

*antipyretic (febrifuge):* fevers, esp. intermittent

*radiation protectant:* radiation exposure, radiation treatment with burns (x-ray, g-ray, 5G mobile phones.

*antiviral*(?)

SYNERGISTIC COMBINATIONS

- Yarrow + Rosemary ct. verbenone: progesteronic hormonal regulator for oestrogen accumulation, dysmenorrhoea, irregular or long cycles

- Yarrow + Cypress: strong venous and lymphatic decongestant for venous congestion with varicose veins, pelvic congestion, oedema, haemorrhoids

- Yarrow + German camomile/Roman camomile: strong anti-inflammatory, analgesic in a wide range of inflammatory conditions with pain, esp. musculoskeletal, urinary, reproductive and gastrointestinal

- Yarrow + Frankincense: analgesic, anti-inflammatory for rheumatic and arthritic conditions with pain, swelling and contraction; also for acute tissue trauma (also topically)

- Yarrow + Blue tansy: strong anti-allergic, antihistamine, analgesic in a wide range of immediate/type-I allergies with pain and inflammation, esp. dermal and mucosal; incl. atopic dermatitis, some food allergies, asthma, cystitis

- Yarrow + Patchouli: strong gastrointestinal mucosal tissue regenerative, anti-inflammatory, antiallergic for intestinal hyperpermeability with food allergies and sensitivities, gastric ulcers, ulcerative colitis, inflammatory bowel disease

COMPLEMENTARY COMBINATIONS

- Yarrow + Juniper berry/Fennel: diuretic, antilithic and detoxicant in all conditions of renal insufficiency, incl. metabolic toxicosis, kidney stones, gout, chronic rheumatic-arthritic conditions

- Yarrow + Clary sage: decongestant and analgesic uterine stimulant for congestive dysmenorrhoea, amenorrhoea

- Yarrow + Rosemary: emmenagogue and uterine stimulant for atonic amenorrhoea and dysmenorrhoea

- Yarrow + Palmarosa: strong gastrointestinal mucosal tissue regenerative, anti-inflammatory, antiallergic for intestinal hyperpermeability with food allergies and sensitivities, gastric ulcers, ulcerative colitis, inflammatory bowel disease

- Yarrow + Cardamom: gastrointestinal/digestive stimulant in a wide range of atonic digestive conditions with appetite loss, indigestion, flatulence

- Yarrow + Lemon: liver decongestant and detoxicant for hepatobiliary atony with congestion

- Yarrow + Helichrysum: strong vulnerary, antiseptic, analgesic and antihaematomal for acute and chronic tissue trauma with severe pain and haematoma, slow healing; chronic non-healing ulcers, abscesses, fissures (for topical use)

## TOPICAL – *Liniment, ointment, cream, compress and other cosmetic preparations*

**Skin care:** Sensitive and oily skin types

*vulnerary, skin regenerator, antiseptic, analgesic, antihaematomal:* acute and chronic tissue trauma with pain and bruising/haematoma; wounds (incl. chronic, non-healing), cuts, ulcers (incl. varicose ulcers, bed sores), fissures; sprains, strains, scars, cellulite; muscle aches and pains

*anti-inflammatory, antiallergic:* burns (incl. from radiation), sunburn, acne, eczema/dermatitis (incl. allergic), phlebitis, cellulitis

*antitumoural*

*mild antiviral:* warts

**Hair and scalp care:**

*hair restorative:* oily scalp, dandruff, hair loss

**Therapeutic precautions:** Yarrow is contraindicated during pregnancy as it is a uterine stimulant. Use with caution in babies, infants and children. In male patients, Yarrow is always best combined into a blend or formula if used long term as a single remedy; the oil is known to cause irritation of the seminal vesicles, resulting in headaches, irritability, vesical damage and temporary incompetent sperm (Catty 2018).

**Pharmacological precautions:** None

**Preparations:**

- Diffusor: 1–3 drops in water
- Massage oil: 2–5% dilution in vegetable oil
- Liniment: 4–10% dilution in vegetable oil
- Gel cap: 1–2 drops with olive oil

## Chinese Medicine Functions and Indications

**Aroma energy:** Sweet, green, pungent

**Movement:** Circulating

**Warmth:** Neutral to cool

**Meridian tropism:** Liver, Stomach, Bladder

**Five-Element affinity:** Wood, Earth

**Essential function:** To invigorate the Blood, reduce stagnation and resolve damp

1. <u>Activates the Lower Warmer, breaks up stagnation, promotes menstruation and relieves pain</u>

   - **Lower Warmer Blood and Qi stagnation** with painful, late scanty periods, loss of periods:

   Juniper berry/Angelica root/Fennel

2. <u>**Invigorates the Blood in the Lower Warmer and lower limbs, reduces stagnation and relieves varicosis**</u>

- **Lower Warmer Blood stagnation** with dragging pelvic pains and distension, painful clotted periods, heavy flow:

  Geranium/Clary sage/Niaouli/Yarrow

- **Blood stagnation in the lower limbs** with varicose veins, ankle oedema, fatigue:

  Cypress/Tea tree/Rosemary

3. <u>**Resolves damp and turbidity, harmonizes urination and astringes leakage**</u>

- **Lower Warmer turbid-damp** (stone, damp lin) with frequent scanty urination, incontinence, irritation:

  Juniper berry/Fennel/Lemon

4. <u>**Activates the Qi, harmonizes the Middle Warmer, regulates digestion and relieves distension**</u>

- **Stomach-Spleen Qi stagnation** with indigestion, chronic epigastric or abdominal pain, distension, irregular bowel movement:

  Lemon/Lavender/Fennel/Cardamom

5. <u>**Dispels wind-damp from the skin and meridians, and relieves pain**</u>

- **Wind-damp-heat in the skin** with red, itchy, painful eruptions:

  Lavender/Geman camomile/Blue tansy/Tea tree

- **Wind-damp-cold/heat obstruction** with painful swollen joints, chronic muscle aches and pains:

  Juniper berry/Frankincense/Wintergreen

REMARKS

Yarrow is an age-old aromatic medicinal plant that down the ages has always presented different images to different practitioners. This is no less true today, and especially if the herbal remedy is used in essential oil form. Its traditional repute as a superlative topical remedy, for example, remains intact whether used in the form of an infusion, tincture or essential oil. The apocryphal story of the celebrated Greek warrior Achilles treating his injuries with Yarrow after the battle of Troy is testimony to this perennial use. To the modern herbalist, Yarrow can be a good diaphoretic, a nice digestive relaxant and much more. Yarrow essential oil provides several other and different uses that again attest to its innate versatility.

The most important task for the modern practitioner is to separate the uses of Yarrow in infusion and tincture form from those in essential oil form. At first this may be no easy task, but the pharmacological justification is evident: the essential oil does not have the advantage of the plant's content in alkaloids and saponins, for instance. This does change its therapeutic profile.

Key to understanding Yarrow essential oil is its strong tropism for the metabolic organs below the diaphragm, and especially those in the pelvis. Working as a general stimulant and decongestant, the oil acts mainly on the level of the fluids – water, lymph and blood. Like Geranium and Juniper berry, Yarrow is a remedy for resolving damp, congestive forms of stagnation. These range from liver congestion, pelvic congestion with its collection of menstrual and venous symptoms, and venous insufficiency in the legs, to urinary atony with a range of symptoms due to urinary dysfunction and toxicosis. In all these scenarios of sluggish eliminatory transport, toxin accumulation is the net result. Yarrow clearly ends up acting here as a detoxicant alterative. The oil's ketones are also considered lipolytic and mucolytic by some in reducing levels of fats and mucus – reminding one of Helichrysum.

Yarrow oil's action on the uterus is particularly comprehensive. As a uterine stimulant, decongestant and progesteronic hormonal regulator, the oil is a versatile woman's ally for both menstrual and menopausal complaints, much in the league of Geranium and Clary sage.

The pharmacology of Yarrow is particularly well balanced and nicely expressed in its fragrance qualities. Fresh, pungent monoterpenes and oxides provide stimulation that is balanced by sweet, green, cooling, relaxant esters, sesquiterpenes and monoterpenols. Among the sesquiterpenes are the notable anti-inflammatory constituents germacrene D and chamazulene – the latter declaring itself visibly in the cobalt blue colour of the oil. Many practitioners will use Yarrow merely for the excellent, wide-ranging reduction of inflammation and pain that it provides on its target organs and tissues.

As a topical remedy with good skin-regenerating, anti-inflammatory and analgesic actions, Yarrow is a strong rival to Helichrysum. Tissue trauma involving injury and haematoma are its chief indications. Local inflammatory conditions of all kinds will also find relief. Here the oil clearly upholds Yarrow's hoary reputation as a superlative remedy for topical conditions.

When used by olfaction in the context of psychological treatment, Yarrow again engages its interesting complex of sweet, green and pungent notes. As an herbaceous-sweet blue oil, like Blue tansy, it supports a striving for balance and harmony in both the mental and emotional spheres of the psyche. Aromatic therapy with Yarrow is particularly useful during times of change and transition, whether entailing internal or external events, including menarche, menopause, work or career changes, relationships or simply surges of inner renewal. Here the oil can be a valuable ally in helping us let go of the old and in allowing us to move forward with the new with grace and poise.

Yarrow is for those who, set in their ways and habits, find it difficult to adapt to the pressure of changing circumstances and who feel unsure about being able, and perhaps confused about even wanting, to adjust to an increasingly vulnerable situation. With its gentle but persistent energy of renewal and forward impetus, the oil is especially effective in helping resolve long-held stagnant emotional patterns with their attendant distressed feelings, including suppressed anger, negativity and shame. It supports the breaking of bad habits and addictions, whether related to pathogenic emotions or drugs. Equally active on the mental plane, Yarrow can also help open us to clarity and insight into a challenging situation, helping us sort out the issues involved and envision future possibilities and potentials for resolution. It is no accident that the traditional instruments for divination using the ancient Chinese oracle, the *Yi Jing* (*I Ching*), are dried stalks of Yarrow.

# Appendix A

# The Energetic Functions of Essential Oils

| Fragrance tone | Fragrance quality | Energetic movement | Tropism | Specific fragrance quality | Typical constituents | Essential functions and indications | Essential oil examples |
|---|---|---|---|---|---|---|---|
| Top | Pungent | **Rising** to uplift and energize | Brain and chest area, lungs | **Fresh-pungent** | Monoterpenes 1,8 cineole | **Restoring, stimulating, drying**<br>• Weak, damp, congestive conditions tending to cold | Cajeput, Rosemary, Saro, Niaouli, Ravintsara, Eucalyptus, Spike lavender |
| | | | | **Spicy-pungent** | Monoterpenes eugenol | **Warming, stimulating**<br>• Cold conditions tending to weak | Ginger, Pimenta berry, Clove, Nutmeg, Black pepper |
| | | | | **Acrid-pungent** | Miscellaneous phenols | **Warming, stimulating, drying**<br>• Acute cold, weak, damp conditions | Thyme ct. thymol, Oregano, Winter savoury |
| | Lemony | **Expanding** to disperse and clarify | Brain, chest and solar plexus | **Fresh-lemony** | Monoterpenes | **Stimulating, decongesting, detoxifying**<br>• Congestive, toxicosis conditions | Lemon, Bergamot, Grapefruit, Grand fir |
| | | | | **Green-lemony** | Aldehydes | **Cooling, relaxing, decongesting**<br>• Acute hot, tense, congestive conditions | Lemongrass, May chang, Lime, Melissa, Citronella |

| | | | | | | | |
|---|---|---|---|---|---|---|---|
| **Middle** | **Sweet** | **Regulating** to harmonize and restore | Solar plexus and abdomen | **Lemony-sweet** | Esters, monoterpenols | **Regulating, restoring**<br>• Dysregulated, weak conditions | Neroli, Sweet orange, Nerolina, Mandarin, Ylang ylang |
| | | | | **Rosy-sweet** | Monoterpenols | **Regulating, restoring, decongesting**<br>• Dysregulated, weak, damp conditions | Geranium, Palmarosa, Rose, Rosewood |
| | **Green** | **Moving** to relax and calm | Solar plexus and abdomen | **Sweet-green** | Sesquiterpenes, esters | **Relaxing, calming**<br>• Tense conditions tending to heat | German/Roman camomile, Yarrow, Blue tansy |
| | | | | **Herbaceous-green** | Monoterpenols, esters | **Relaxing, restoring, regulating**<br>• Tense, weak, dysregulated conditions | Lavender, Clary sage, Marjoram, Sweet basil |
| | | | | **Pungent-green** | Monoterpenols, ketones | **Stimulating, relaxing**<br>• Energy stagnation of all types | Laurel, Spearmint, Peppermint, Green myrtle |
| **Base** | **Woody** | **Centring** to stabilize and strengthen | Lower abdomen | **Sweet-woody** | Sesquiterpenes, sesquiterpenols | **Restoring, decongesting, relaxing**<br>• Weak, damp, tense conditions | Cedarwood, Patchouli, Siam wood, Sandalwood |
| | | | | **Pungent-woody** | Monoterpenes | **Restoring, stimulating, drying**<br>• Chronic weak, damp conditions | Scotch pine, Black spruce, Cypress, Juniper berry |
| | **Rooty** | **Sinking** to ground and calm | Lower abdomen | **Rooty** | Sesquiterpenes | **Cooling, calming, regulating**<br>• Acute hot, tense conditions | Vetiver, Spikenard, Lovage root, Dong quai |

# The Six Diagnostic Conditions
# of Functional Pathology

**Nervous System**
*Tissue Tone*

### TENSE
**Hypertonic condition**
**Pulse** hard, tight, wiry
**Tongue** dusky, long with lateral lines
**Complexion** drawn, haggard

**Warmth System**
*Tissue Stimulation*

### HOT
**Hypersthenic condition**
**Pulse** rapid, slippery, flooding
**Tongue** red, yellow-orange coat
**Complexion** reddish, ruddy

**Fluid System**
*Tissue Hydration*

### DRY
**Dry condition**
**Pulse** rough, thin/small, hollow
**Tongue** thin, dry, cracked, peeled
**Complexion** thin, dry, matt

### DAMP/CONGESTION
**Damp/Congestive condition**
**Pulse** full, slippery
**Tongue** swollen, wet
**Sublingual veins** swollen
**Complexion** puffy, moist, shiny

### COLD
**Hyposthenic condition**
**Pulse** slow, knotted
**Tongue** pale, white coat
**Complexion** pale, bluish tinge

### WEAK
**Hypotonic/atonic condition**
**Pulse** soft/empty, deep, weak, thin
**Tongue** pale, scalloped, flaccid, trembling
**Complexion** flat, droopy

# Selective Bibliography

This includes titles referenced in the text and selective additional texts for further reading.

Ackerman, D. *A Natural History of the Senses*. London 1990

Aftel, M. *Essence and Alchemy*. New York 2001

Amen, D. *Change Your Brain, Change Your Life*. New York 1998

------. *Magnificent Mind at Any Age*. New York 2008

Andernach, Winther von. *De medicina veteri et nova*. Basiliae 1571

Anderson, C., Lis-Balchin, M. and Kirk-Smith, M. 'Evaluation of massage with essential oils on childhood atopic eczema', *Phytother Res*. 14, 6 2000

Anderson, E.F. *Plants and People of the Golden Triangle*. Portland 2008

Arcier, M. *Aromatherapy*. London 1990

Arctander, S. *Perfume and Flavor Materials of Natural Origin*. Elizabeth, NJ 1960

Arnould-Taylor, W.E. *Aromatherapy for the Whole Person*. Cheltenham 1981

Baczek, K. *et al.* 'Intraspecific variability of yarrow (*Achillea millefolium* L.) in respect of developmental and chemical traits', *Herba Polonica* 61, 3 2015

Baerheim, S.A. and Scheffer, J.J.C. *Essential Oils and Aromatic Plants*. The Hague, Netherlands 1989

Barille, E. *The Book of Perfume*. New York 1995

Baudoux, D. *Formulaire d'aromathérapie pratique*. Luxembourg 2004

------. *Les cahiers pratiques d'aromathérapie selon l'école francaise, Vols 1–6*. Luxembourg 2006–2011

Belaiche, P. *Traité de phytothérapie et d'aromathérapie, Vols 1–3*. Paris 1979

Bensouilah, J. and Buck, P. *Aromadermatology*. Abingdon 2006

Berendes, J. *Das Apothekerwesen*. Stuttgart 1907

Bitsas, A. *Aromathérapie, corps et âme*. Bruxelles 2009

Boiteau, P. and Allorge-Boiteau, L. *Plantes médicinales de Madagascar*. 1993

Boland, D.J., Brophy, J.J. and House, A.P.N. *Eucalyptus Leaf Oils*. Melbourne 1991

Bonneval, P. and Dubus, F. *Manuel practice d'aromathérapie*. Paris 2014

Bosson, L. *L'Aromathérapie énergetique*. Bruxelles 2004

Boullard, B. *Plantes médicinales du monde*. Paris 1999

Bowles, E.J. *The Chemistry of Aromatherapeutic Essential Oils*. Crow's Nest, Australia 2003

Brooker, M.I.H. and Kleinig, D.A. *A Field Guide to Eucalypts*. Sydney 2002

Brunschwygk, H. *Liber de Arte Distillandi Simplicibus*. Strassburg 1500

Buckle, J. *Clinical Aromatherapy*. Philadelphia, PA 2003

Burfield, T. *Natural Aromatic Materials – Odours and Origins*, Vols 1 and 2. Tampa 2000. See www.users. globalnet.co.uk/~nodice/new/magazine/october/october.htm, accessed 25 March 2019

Burkill, I.H. *A Dictionary of the Economic Products of the Malay Peninsula*, 2 vols. Kuala Lumpur 1966

Cadéac, M. and Meunier, A. *Recherches expérimentales sur l'action antiseptique des huiles essentielles*. Paris 1880

Catty, S. 'Hydrosols for the 21st century'. Talk at Aromatherapy Conference, Yixing, 2018

Chabènes. *Les grandes possibilités par les matières odoriférantes*. Paris 1838

Chamberland, M. *Les essences au point de vue de leurs propriétés antiseptiques*. Paris 1887

Chao, W-W. and Lin, B-F. 'Bioactivities of major constituents isolated from *Angelica sinensis* (Danggui)', in *Chinese Medicine* 2011. http://cmjournal.biomedcentral.com/articles/10.1186/1749-8546-6-29

Clarke, S. *Essential Chemistry for Aromatherapy*. Edinburgh 2008

Classen, C., Howes, D. and Synnott, A. *Aroma*. London 1994

Clavel, L. *Classification des huiles essentielles suivant leur valeur antiseptique*. Paris 1918

Comfort, J.W. *The Practice of Medicine on Thomsonian Principles*. Philadelphia, PA 1843

Cook, W.H. *The Science and Practice of Medicine*. Chicago, IL 1879

––––––. *A Systematic Treatise on Materia Medica and Therapeutics*. Chicago, IL 1898

Cordus, V. *Historia de Plantis*. Venezia 1554

Crenshaw, T.L. *The Alchemy of Love and Lust*. New York 1996

Culpeper, N. *London Dispensatory*. London 1659

Dugan, H. *The Ephemeral History of Perfume: Scent and Sense in Early Modern England*. Baltimore, MD 2011

Dunglison, R. *A Dictionary of Medical Science*. Philadelphia, PA 1874

Dupont, P. *Propriétés physiques et psychiques des huiles essentielles*. Le Tremblay 2002

Duraffourd, C. and Lapraz, J-C. *Traité de phytothérapie clinique*. Paris 2002

Duraffourd, C., D'Hervicourt, L. and Lapraz, J.C. *Cahiers de phytotherapie clinique*. Paris 1988

Easley, N. Physiology lecture notes, National College of Naturopathic Medicine. Portland, OR 1991

Eckman, P. *In the Footsteps of the Yellow Emperor*. San Francisco, CA 2007

Ellingwood, F. *A Systematic Treatise on Materia Medica and Therapeutics*. Chicago, IL 1898

––––––. *The Eclectic Practice of Medicine*. Chicago, IL 1910

Eysenck, H. and Eysenck, S.B.G. *Personality Structure and Measurement*. London 1969

Faucon, M. *Traité d'aromathérapie scientifique et médicale*. Paris 2015

Faure, P. *Parfums et aromates de l'antiquité*. Paris 1987

Federici, C.T., Roose, M.L. and Scora, R.W. 'RFLP analysis of the origin of *Citrus bergamia, Citrus jambhiri*, and *Citrus limonia*', *International Society for Horticultural Science. Acta Hort.* (ISHS) 535, 55–64 2000

Felter, H.W. *Eclectic Materia Medica, Pharmacology and Therapeutics*. Cincinnati, OH 1922

Fischer-Rizzi, S. *Duft und Psyche*. Munich 1991

Flückiger, F. *Documente zur Geschichte der Pharmacie*. Halle 1876

––––––. *Pharmacognosie des Planzenreiches*. Berlin 1882

Forbes, R.J. *A Short History of the Art of Distillation*. Leiden 1970

Foster, F. (ed.). *A Reference Book of Practical Therapeutics*. New York 1896

Foster, S. *Herbal Renaissance*. Layton 1997

Franchomme, P. *La science des huiles essentielles médicinales*. Paris 2015

Gallesio, G. *Traité du citrus*. Paris 1811

Gattefossé, R.M. *Propriétés bactéricides de quelques huiles essentielles*. Paris 1918

––––––. *Aromathérapie: les huiles essentielles, hormones végétales*. Paris 1937

––––––. *Gattefossé's Aromatherapy*. London 1993

Gatti, G. and Cayola, R. 'Action thérapeutique des huiles essentielles', in *Rev. Ital. Ess. Prof.* 4; 16 and 4; Milano 1922

Gildemeister, E. and Hoffmann, F. *Die Aetherischen Oele*, 4th edition, 8 vols. Berlin 1956–1966 (1st edition 1899)

Girault, M. *Traité de phytothérapie et d'aromathérapie (P. Belaiche), Tome III: Gynécologie*. Paris 1979

Grieve, M. *A Modern Herbal*. New York 1971

Guba, R. *Toxicity Myths – The Actual Risks of Essential Oil Use*. Melbourne 1999

––––––. 'Beyond Aromatherapy', in Proceedings of the AIA Conference. New Brunswick, 2017

Guenther, E. *The Essential Oils, Vols. I–VI*. Malabar, FL 1972

Halpern, G.M. and Weverka, P. *The Healing Trail: Essential Oils of Madagascar*. North Bergen 2003

Harris, B. *The Aromatherapy Data Base*. Provence 2007

Harris, B. and Harris, R. (eds). *International Journal of Clinical Aromatherapy*, Vols. 1–7, Le Martre, France 2004–2005

––––––. (eds). *International Journal of Essential Oil Therapeutics*, Vols. 1–4, Le Martre, France 2005–2010

––––––. 'Aromatic Pharmacology' seminar workbook. Toronto 2006a

------. 'Clinical Aromatherapy in Infectious Disease' seminar workbook. Calgary 2006b

Hay, R.K.M. and Waterman, P.G. *Volatile Oil Crops*. Harlow, Essex 1993

Henriette's Herbal. 'Cinnamon and Diabetes.' 2006. www.henriettes-herb.com/blog/cinnamon-and-diabetes.html, accessed 25 March 2019

Heyd, W. *Geschichte des Levantehandels im Mittelalter*. Berlin 1879

Hoblyn, R.D. *A Dictionary of Terms Used in Medicine and the Collateral Sciences*. Philadelphia, PA 1855

Holliday, I. *Melaleucas*. Sydney 1998

Holmes, P. 'Using Essential Oils in Chinese Medicine' seminar workbook. Boulder, CO 1994–2014

------. *Jade Remedies: A Chinese Herbal Reference for the West*. Boulder, CO 1999

------. *The Energetics of Western Herbs* (2 vols), 4th ed. Boulder, CO 2007

------. *Clinical Aromatherapy*. Cotati 2008

Iwata, H., Kato, T. and Ohno, S. 'Triparental origin of damask roses.' *Gene* 259(1–2), 23 2000

Iwoaka, Y., Hashimoto, R., Koizumi, H., Yu, J. and Okabe, T. 'Selective stimulation by cinnamaldehyde of progesterone secretion in human adrenal cells.' *Life Science* 86, 23–24 2010

Jellinek, P. *Die Psychologischen Grundlagen der Parfümerie*. Heidelberg 1973

Jouhanneau, D.G. *La médecine des plantes aromatiques*. Paris 1991

Jourdan, A.J.L. *Pharmacopée universelle*. Paris 1828

Juliani, H. *et al.* 'Searching for the real Ravensara essential oil. A case study for NATIORA – the Malagasy natural product label', *Perfumer and Flavorist* 30(1), 60–65 2005

Juliani, H.R., Simon, J.E., Ramboatiana, M.M.R., Behra, O., Garvey, A. and Raskin, I. 'Malagasy aromatic plants: essentials, antioxidant and antimicrobial activities.' *Acta Horticulturae* 629, 77–81 2004

Kettenkoffen, P. Ylang Ylang. Medical thesis at Bonn University. Bonn 1906

Khan, M.A., Ali, R., Parveen, R., Najmi, A.K. and Ahmad, S. 'Pharmacological evidences for cytotoxic and antitumor properties of Boswellic acids from *Boswellia serrata*.' *Journal of Ethnopharmacology* 191 2016

Kharrazian, D. 'Functional Endocrinology Assessment and Nutritional Management.' Seminar text. Los Angeles, CA 2003

King, J., Felter, H. and Lloyd, J.U. *King's American Dispensatory*. Cincinnati, OH 1898

Kirk-Smith, M. 'Possible Psychological and Physiological Processes in Aromatherapy', in Conference Proceedings, Aroma '95. Brighton 1995

Lawless, A. *Artisan Perfumery*. Stroud 2009

Lawless, J. *Aromatherapy and the Mind*. London 1994

Lawrence, B.M. Reviews of Essential Oils in *Perfumer & Flavorist*. Wheaton, IL. www.perfumerflavorist.com, accessed 25 March 2019

Le Guérer, A. *Scent*. New York 1994

Lémery, N. *Cours de chymie*. Paris 1757

------. *Pharmacopée universelle*. Paris 1761

------. *Dictionaire des drogues simples*. Paris 1798

Leopold, S. 'Saving Sandalwood', in Proceedings of the AIA Conference. New Brunswick 2017

Lis-Balchin, M. *Aromatherapy Science*. London 2006

LoBisco, S. 'Sniffing Out Pain, Parts 1 and 2.' Townsend Letter for Doctors, Nov. and Dec. 2016. Townsend 2016

Longuefosse, J.-L. *Plantes médicinales de la Caraïbe*. Fort-de-France 2008

Loughran, J.K. and Bull, R. *Aromatherapy and Subtle Energy Techniques*. Berkeley, CA 2000

Lubinic, E. *Handbuch Aromatherapie*. Heidelberg 1997

Mailhebiau, P. *Portraits in Oils*. Saffron Walden 1995

------. *La nouvelle aromathérapie*. Paris 2002

Maury, M. *Le capital jeunesse*. Paris 1961

------. *Marguerite Maury's Guide to Aromatherapy*. London 2004

McIntosh, S. *Integral Consciousness and the Future of Evolution*. St. Paul 2007

Meurisse, P. *La thérapeutique par les huiles essentielles*. Macon, GA 1919

Mills, S. and Bone, K. *Principles and Practice of Phytotherapy*. London 2000

Mojay, G. *Aromatherapy for Healing the Spirit*. London 1996

------. 'Aromatic Acupressure Course' workbook. London 2008

Morel, A. and Rochaix, A. *Contribution a l'étude de l'action microbicide de quelques essences végétales.* Paris 1925

Morita, K. *The Book of Incense.* Tokyo 1992

Morris, E.T. *Fragrance: The Story of Perfume from Cleopatra to Chanel.* New York 1983

Nabhan, G.P. *Cumin, Camels and Caravans: A Spice Odyssey.* Berkeley, CA 2014

Nadkarni, K.M. and Nadkarni, A.K. *Indian Materia Medica.* Bombay 1954

Needham, J. *Science and Civilisation in China* (Volume 4). Cambridge 1980

Oyen, L.P.A. and Dung, N.X. (eds). *Plant Resources of South-East Asia, No. 19.* Leiden 1999

Pénoel, D. and Franchomme, P. *L'Aromathérapie exactement.* Limoges 1990

Pomet, P. *Histoire générale des drogues.* Paris 1735

Powell, D. *Endocrinology & Naturopathic Therapies.* Seattle 2000

Price, S. and Price, L. *Aromatherapy for Health Professionals.* London 2007

Priest, A.W. and Priest, L.R. *Herbal Medication.* London 1981

Raimondo, F.M. and Lach, W.H. *Le Mele d'Oro.* Palermo 1998

Rasoanaivo, P. and de la Gorce, P. 'Essential oils of economic value in Madagascar', *Herbalgram* 43 1998

Rhind, J.P. *Essential Oils.* London 2012

------. *Fragrance and Wellbeing.* London 2013

------. *Listening to Scent.* London 2014

Roques, J. *Traite des plants usuelles.* Paris 1837

Rovesti, P. *Alla ricerca dei profumi perduti.* Venezia 1980

------. *Auf der Suche nach den Verlorenen Duften.* München 1995

Rubeus, H. *Liber de Destillationi.* Basiliae 1581

Ryff, W.H. *Neu Gross Destillirbuch.* Basiliae 1545

------. *Reformierte Deutsche Apotheck.* Basiliae 1573

Ryman, D. *Danièle Ryman's Aromatherapy Bible.* London 2002

------. *Danièle Ryman's Secrets of Youth and Beauty.* London 2007

Salmon, W. *Pharmacopoeia Londinensis, or, The New London Dispensatory.* London 1691

Schafer, E.H. *The Golden Peaches of Samarkand.* Berkeley, CA 1963

------. *The Vermillion Bird.* Berkeley, CA 1967

Schnaubelt, K. *Medical Aromatherapy.* Berkeley, CA 1999

------. *Aromatherapy Lifestyle.* San Rafael, CA 2004

Scudder, J.M. *Specific Medication.* 1870

------. *Specific Diagnosis.* 1874

Serafino, A. *et al.* 'Stimulatory Effect of Eucalyptus Essential Oil on Innate Cell-Mediated Immune Response', in *BMC Immunology,* April 2008

Sheil, D. *Eucalyptus – The Essence of Australia.* Melbourne 1985

Southwell, I. and Lowe, R. (eds). *Tea Tree: The Genus Melaleuca.* Amsterdam 1999

Stamelman, R. *Perfume.* New York 2006

Stansbury, J. 'Botanical Therapies for Depression and Anxiety', in *Proceedings of the AHG Symposium.* Williams Bay 2002

Thurston, J.M. *The Philosophy of Physiomedicalism.* Richmond, IN 1900

Tisserand, R. *The Art of Aromatherapy.* Rochester 1977

Tisserand, R. and Young, R. *Essential Oil Safety,* 2nd edition. London 2013

Torii, S. 'Odour mechanisms: the psychological benefits of odours', *International Journal of Aromatherapy* 8(3), 34–39 1997

Treichler, R. *Von einer Psychologie der Organe zur Organischen Behandlung Psychischer Stoerungen.* Stuttgart 1952

Tucker, A.O. 'Botanical Nomenclature of Commercial Sources of Essential Oils', in *Herbs, Spices and Medicinal Plants.* Phoenix, AZ 1987

Valnet, J. *Aromathérapie.* Paris 1975

Van Toller, S. and Dodd, G.H. (eds). *Perfumery: The Psychology and Biology of Fragrance.* London, 1988

Vanhove, M. and Devlieghere, G. *Etherische Olien.* Bruxelles 2002

Viaud, H. *Huiles essentielles, hydrolats*. Paris 1983

Vroon, P. *Smell*. New York 1997

Wabner, D. and Stefan, T. *Klinikhandbuch Aromatherapie*. Munich 2017

Walker, B. *The Woman's Encyclopedia of Myths and Secrets*. New York 1983

Walther, A.F. *De Oleis Vegetabilium Essentialibus. Dissertatio*. Leipzig 1745

Watt, M. 'Essential Oils: Their Lack of Skin Absorption but Effectiveness via Inhalation.' www.nature-helps.com/agora/skinabso.htm 2002, accessed 25 March 2019

Webb, M. *Bush Sense*. Adelaide 2000

Webster, H.T. *The Principles of Medicine as Applied to Dynamical Therapeutics*. Oakland, CA 1891

------. *Dynamical Therapeutics*. San Francisco, CA 1898

Weiss, E.A. *Essential Oil Crops*. Wallingford 1997

Weiss, R.F. *Herbal Medicine*. London 2000

Werheij, E.W.M. and Coronel, R.E. *Plant Resources of South-East Asia, No. 2*. Leiden 1999

Werner, M. *Aetherische Oele*. München 1993

Wildwood, C. *The Encyclopedia of Aromatherapy*. Rochester 1996

Williams, C. *Medicinal Plants in Australia, Vols 1 and 2*. Dural 2011

Williams, D. *The Chemistry of Essential Oils*. Weymouth 1997

Williams, M. *Only the Essentials*. Los Alamos, NM 2004

Yarnell, E. *Phytochemistry and Pharmacy for Practitioners of Botanical Medicine*. Wenatchee, WA 2003

Yilmaz, N. 'Rose Essential Oil.' In IGME Export Production Center of Turkey Report 2010

Zhu Liangfeng *et al. Aromatic Plants and Essential Constituents*. Hong Kong 1995

# Glossary of Terms

**adaptogenic:** enhances adaptation response to stress

**AIDS:** acquired immune deficiency syndrome

**alterative:** promotes systemic changes

**anaesthetic:** deadens local sensation or pain

**analeptic:** revives from shock or poisoning

**analgesic:** relieves pain internally

**anhydrotic:** reduces or stops sweating

**anodyne:** relieves pain

**antacid:** reduces gastric acid

**anthelmintic:** treats intestinal worms/parasites

**antiabortive:** prevents miscarriage

**antiageing:** retards ageing

**antiallergic:** treats allergies or hypersensitivities

**antiarthritic:** treats arthritis

**antiasthmatic:** treats asthma

**antibacterial:** inhibits bacteria

**anticatarrhal:** reduces catarrh (excessive mucus production)

**anticoagulant:** reduces blood clotting

**anticonvulsant:** treats convulsions

**antidepressant:** treats depression

**antidiarrhoeal:** treats diarrhoea

**antidyskratic:** rebalances the fluids in the presence of a fluid's dyskrasia (disharmony)

**antiemetic:** treats vomiting

**antienuretic:** treats enuresis (involuntary urination)

**antifungal:** inhibits fungus

**antigenic:** reduces antibody production

**anti-infective:** treats infection

**anti-inflammatory:** reduces inflammation

**antileucorrhoeal:** treats leucorrhoea

**antilipaemic:** lowers blood lipid levels in the presence of hyperlipaemia

**antilithic:** prevents or dissolves and flushes out stones

**antimicrobial:** inhibits microbes

**antineoplastic:** treats neoplasm or cancer

**antioxidant:** reduces oxidation

**antiparasitic:** inhibits or reduces parasites

**antipruritic:** relieves skin itching

**antipyretic:** reduces fever by lowering temperature

**antirheumatic:** treats rheumatism

**antisecretory:** reduces secretions

**antiseptic:** topically prevents or reduces infection or putrefaction

**antitumoural:** treats tumours

**antitussive:** relieves coughing

**antiviral:** inhibits viruses

**aperitive:** stimulates the appetite

**aphrodisiac:** promotes sexuality

**asthenic:** lacking stimulation; also known as 'cold'

**astriction:** a tightening effect

**astringent:** astricts or tightens tissue to reduce or stop a secretion

**atonic:** lacking tone or strength; also known as 'weak'

**BPH:** benign prostate hyperplasia

**bronchodilatant:** dilates the bronchi

**cardiac:** relating to the heart

**carminative:** relieves intestinal flatus

**CFS:** chronic fatigue syndrome

**cholagogue:** promotes bile flow

**choleretic:** enhances bile quality and quantity

**cicatrisant:** promotes tissue repair; the same as vulnerary

**CNS:** central nervous system

**CO2:** supercritical carbon dioxide (extract)

**coagulant:** promotes blood clotting

**cold:** one of the four qualities; a qualitative concept used in pharmacognosy, diagnostics and pathology to designate an effective quality; in pathology it defines a hyposthenic condition presenting insufficient objective or subjective warmth, as in hypothermia with feeling cold

**congestion:** a pathological condition involving pathological stagnation of one of the fluids, i.e. blood, mucus, phlegm, interstitial or other fluid

**constraint:** a pathological condition involving mental or emotional, and therefore nervous, tension

**contraceptive:** prevents conception

**counterirritant:** irritates to cause derivation

**CT:** chemotype or chemical type

**CTS:** carpal tunnel syndrome

**damp:** one of the four qualities; a qualitative concept used in pharmacognosy, nosology and pathology to mean an effective quality; in pathology defining a condition caused by a stagnation of one of the pure or impure fluids, and therefore often qualified, e.g. mucus damp, water damp, phlegm damp; if unqualified, then usually referring to excessive mucus secretion (catarrh)

**decongestant:** relieves fluid or blood congestion

**deficiency:** a pathological condition presenting a functional or structural insufficiency or weakness

**demulcent:** soothes and moistens the mucous membrane

**depressant:** reducing mental/cerebral functions

**derivation:** a therapeutic technique that uses counterirritation to draw blood away from an area of disease to another body part, usually through the methods of cupping or bloodletting, or the topical use of rubefacient, vesicant or pustulant remedies

**dermal:** relating to the skin

**dermatropic:** having a tropism for the skin

**detergent:** cleans and disinfects wounds

**detoxicant:** resolves and clears toxin(s)

**detumescent:** reduces swelling

**DHEA:** dehydroepiandrosterone, an adrenocortical hormone

**diaphoretic:** promotes sweating

**diathesis:** an individual tendency or predisposition for disharmony inherent in an individual's natural condition (*physis* in Greek medicine)

**digestant:** promotes digestion

**discutient:** resolves tumours

**dissolvent:** promotes solution (dissolving) of hard deposits, tissues or exudates

**diuretic:** promotes increased urination

**draining diuretic:** relieves fluid congestion (oedema) and increases urination

**dryness:** one of the four qualities; a qualitative concept used in pharmacognosy, diagnostics and pathology to denote an effective quality; in pathology designating a condition with insufficient mucus or other fluid secretion present

**Eclectic:** refers to the Eclectic medical doctors of the 19th and 20th centuries, and to the Eclectic school of medicine in North America

**effective qualities:** qualitative aspects of the nature of any substance – mineral, herbal, animal or human; applied to remedies, they consist of taste, warmth and moisture; they are effective since they produce physiological therapeutic effects (see 'four qualities' below).

**eliminant:** promotes elimination through an excretory channel

**emetic:** causes vomiting

**emmenagogue:** promotes menstrual discharge

**emollient:** soothes and moistens the skin

**excess:** a pathological condition presenting a redundancy of function or substance

**expectorant:** promotes coughing up of sputum

**febrifuge:** reduces fever

**FM:** fibromyalgia

**foetal relaxant:** relaxing/calming to the foetus and therefore reducing abnormal foetal movement

**four qualities:** energetic, dynamic effective qualities used in traditional medical systems to describe substances and processes such as remedies (pharmacognosy) and pathological conditions (pathology); hot/cold, dry/damp are the four basic qualities

**free radical inhibitor:** reduces free radicals

**GABA:** gamma-aminobutyric acid

**galactagogue:** produces milk flow

**GC:** gas chromatography

**ground:** the place where disease occurs, whether the whole person, constitution or particular tissue; also known as 'terrain'

**haemogenic:** builds blood (cells)

**haemolytic:** destroys blood (cells)

**haemostatic:** stops bleeding

**heat:** (also hot); one of the four qualities; a qualitative concept used in pharmacology, diagnostics and pathology; in pathology designating a hypersthenic condition with excessive warmth response, such as fever or inflammation, as well as subjective feelings of excessive warmth

**HIV:** human immunodeficiency virus

**HPA:** hypothalamus-pituitary-adrenal

**HPG:** hypothalamus-pituitary-gonadal

**HPV:** human papilloma virus

**HSV:** herpes simplex virus

**hydragogue:** expels water through the bowels

**hydrogenic:** retains fluids

**hypersthenic:** having excessive stimulation; also known as 'hot'

**hypertensive:** increases blood pressure

**hypertonic:** having excessive tone or strength; also known as 'tense'

**hypnotic:** calming the mind

**hypoglycaemiant:** lowers blood sugar levels

**hypotensive:** reduces blood pressure

**IBS:** irritable bowel syndrome

**immune potential:** the potential of the immune system for effective response to pathogen

**immune regulator:** regulates immunity in hypersensitivity (i.e. allergic and autoimmune) disorders

**immune restorative:** boosts immune potential

**immunostimulant:** stimulates immune functions

**interferon inducent:** produces interferon

**laxative:** promotes gentle bowel movement

**lenitive:** reduces irritation

**leukocytogenic:** increases white blood cells

**LHRH:** luteinizing hormone-releasing hormone

**litholythic:** dissolves stones

**lymphatic:** relating to lymphatic flow

**lymphocyte stimulant:** increases T-lymphocytes and lymphocyte transformation rate

**ml:** millilitre

**mucogenic:** promotes mucus production

**mucolytic:** reduces sputum production

**mucostatic:** stops mucus/catarrhal discharge

**mucus:** mucosal fluid

**nervine:** relating to the nervous system

**nutritive:** promotes nutrition or provides nourishment

**OCD:** obsessive-compulsive syndrome

**optitropic:** having a tropism for the eyes and vision

**oxytocic:** promotes labour contractions by releasing oxytocin hormone

**parasiticide:** kills parasites

**parturient:** promotes labour

**pattern of disharmony:** a syndrome, consisting of a complex of specific signs and symptoms

**phagocyte stimulant:** enhances phagocyte functions

**pharmacognosy:** the study of the nature of remedies

**pharmacology:** the study of the physiological effects of remedies

**phenomenology:** the study of empirically observed phenomena

**PMS:** premenstrual syndrome

**PNEI:** psycho-neuro-endocrine-immune

**PNS:** parasympathetic nervous system

**puerperal:** relating to childbirth

**purgative:** promotes copious bowel movement

**pustulant:** causes pustules

**Qi:** the Chinese medicine term for bioenergy or vital energy

**rash-promoting:** promoting eruptions in eruptive fever

**refrigerant:** promotes a cooling down and clears heat

**relaxant:** promotes relaxation

**resolvent:** resolves a state of toxicosis

**resorbent:** promotes catabolic resorption

**restorative:** restores and strengthens

**rubefacient:** causes hyperaemia with skin reddening

**secretory:** promotes secretions

**sedative:** reduces activity or function

**simple:** a single remedy

**SNS:** sympathetic nervous system

**spasmolytic:** reduces spasm or cramp

**spermicidal:** kills sperm

**stages of adaptation:** the theory of the three stages of adaptation to stressors, being the alarm, resistance and exhaustion stages; also known as the general adaptation syndrome

**stages of disease:** the theory of the four stages of disease according to vital activity; illness begins in the acute stage and progresses to the subacute, chronic and degenerative

**stagnation:** a pathological condition denoting a slowing down of normal processes and buildup

of injurious or toxic substances (e.g. mucus, sputum, endotoxins, fatty and mineral deposits)

**stimulant:** increases activity or function

**structive:** producing substance and form; the opposite/complementary of active

**styptic:** stops bleeding through topical application

**syndrome:** a specific complex of signs and symptoms presenting a symptom picture; synonymous with 'pattern of disharmony'

**TB:** tuberculosis

**teratogenic:** injures the foetus

**terrain:** the place where disease occurs, whether this is the whole person, the constitution or particular tissue; also known as 'ground'

**toxicosis:** (also 'toxaemia' and 'autotoxicosis'); a pathological condition involving the accumulation of endogenous or exogenous toxins

**toxins:** injurious (pathological) substances generated internally or from the environment

**tri dosas:** the three fundamental energies in Ayurvedic (Indian) medicine

**trophorestorative:** nourishes and builds tissue

**tropism:** the property of a remedy of having an affinity or bias for treating certain organs, systems, tissues or body parts

**UV:** ultraviolet

**vasoconstrictor:** constricts blood vessels

**vasodilator:** dilates blood vessels

**vermicide:** kills intestinal parasites

**vermifuge:** expels intestinal parasites

**vesicant:** causes watery blisters

**vulnerary:** treats wounds by promoting tissue healing

# Common Name Cross Index

river red gum *Eucalyptus camaldulensis*
woolly-butt *Eucalyptus macarthurii*

Female helichrysum *Helichrysum gymnocephalum*
Fennel
    bitter *Foeniculum vulgare subsp. vulgare var. vulgare*
    sweet *Foeniculum vulgare var. dulce*
Fieldmint *Mentha arvensis*
Fir
    balsam *Abies balsamea*
    Douglas *Abies menziesii/douglasii*
    grand *Abies grandis*
    Nordmann's *Abies nordmanniana*
    Siberian *Abies sibirica*
    silver *Abies alba*
Forest red gum *Eucalyptus tereticornis*
Fragonia *Agonis fragrans*
Frangipani *Plumeria spp.*
Frankincense *Boswellia sacra*
    India *Boswellia serrata*
    Saudi Arabia *Boswellia sacra*
    Somalia *Boswellia sacra*

Galangal *Alpinia officinarum*
Galbanum *Ferula galbaniflua/gummosa*
Gardenia *Gardenia spp.*
Geranium *Pelargonium cv. group Rosat*
German camomile *Matricaria recutita*
Ginger *Zingiber officinalis*
Gingergrass *Cymbopogon martini var. sofia*
Goldenrod *Solidago canadensis*
Grand fir *Abies grandis*
Grapefruit *Citrus x paradisi*
Greek oregano *Origanum heracleoticum*
Greek sage *Salvia fruticosa*
Green mallee *Eucalyptus viridis*
Green myrtle *Myrtus communis*
Grey peppermint eucalyptus *Eucalyptus radiata var. phellandra*
Guaiacum *Bulnesia sarmienti*
Guggul *Boswellia serrata*
Gully gum *Eucalyptus smithii*
Gurjun balsam *Dipterocarpus spp.*

Havozo *Ravensara aromatica*
Hazomboay *Oliganthus pseudocentauropsis*
Helichrysum *Helichrysum angustifolium*
    female *Helichrysum gymnocephalum*
    fragrant *Helichrysum odoratissimum*
    Italian *Helichrysum angustifolium*
    male *Helichrysum bracteiferum*
    splendid *Helichrysum splendidum*
Hemlock spruce *Tsuga canadensis*
Hiba *Thujopsis dolobrata*
Himalaya cedarwood *Cedrus deodora*
Hinoki *Chamaecyparis obtusa*
Ho leaf *Cinnamomum camphora ct. linalool*
Hoary basil *Ocimum canum ct. linalool*
Holy basil *Ocimum sanctum*
Hummingbird sage *Salvia spathacea*
Hyssop *Hyssopus officinalis*
    decumbent *Hyssopus var. decumbens*

Spanish *Hyssopus off. ssp. canescens*

Iary *Psidia altissima*
Indian frankincense *Boswellia serrata*
Indian spikenard *Nardostachys jatamansi*
Indian valerian *Valeriana wallichii*
Inula *Inula graveolens*

Jack pine *Pinus divaricata*
Jasmine
    royal *Jasminum grandiflorum*
    sambac *Jasminum sambac*
Jatamansi *Nardostachys jatamansi*
Juniper berry *Juniperus communis*
Juniper
    cade *Juniperus oxycedrus*
    mountain *Juniperus communis var. montana*
    Nepal *Juniperus squamata*
    Phoenicia *Juniperus phoenicea*
    savin *Juniperus sabina*

Katrafay *Cedrelopsis grevei*
Khella *Amni visnaga*
Kunzea *Kunzea ambigua*

Labdanum *Cistus ladaniferus and spp.*
Lantana *Lantana camara*
Larch *Larix decidua*
Large-leaf basil *Ocimum basilicum*
Laricio pine *Pinus laricio*
Laurel *Laurus nobilis*
Lavandin *Lavandula x fragrans*
Lavender *Lavandula angustifolia*
    Dalmatia *Lavandula x hybrida*
    Spanish *Lavandula stoechas*
    spike *Lavandula latifolia*
    true *Lavandula angustifolia*
Lavender oregano *Origanum dubium ct. linalool*
Lavender sage *Salvia lavandulifolia*
Lavender tea tree *Melaleuca ericifolia*
Ledum *Ledum groenlandicum*
Lemon *Citrus limonum*
Lemon eucalyptus *Corymbia/Eucalyptus citriodora*
Lemon myrtle *Backhousia citriodora*
Lemon tea tree *Leptospermum petersonii*
Lemon thyme *Thymus x citriodorus*
Lemon verbena *Lippia/Aloysia citriodora*
Lemon-scented ironbark *Eucalyptus staigeriana*
Lemongrass *Cymbopogon citratus*
    East India *Cymbopogon flexuosus*
    Jammu *Cymbopogon pendulus*
    West Indies *Cymbopogon citratus*
Lime *Citrus x aurantifolia*
    Italy/sweet *Citrus limetta*
    kaffir/leech/combava *Citrus hystrix*
    key *Citrus x aurantifolia*
    Persia *Citrus x latifolia*
Linaloeswood *Bursera delpechiana*
Longoza *Hedychium coronarium*
Lotus *Nelumbo nucifera*
Lovage *Ligusticum levisticum*
Lovage, Sichuan *Ligusticum wallichii*

Mace *Myristica fragrans*
Madagascar cypress *Cupressus lusitanica*

Madagascar niaouli *Melaleuca quinquenervia ct. viridiflorol*
Magnolia bud *Magnolia spp.*
Male helichrysum *Helichrysum bracteiferum*
Mandarin *Citrus reticulata*
Manuka *Leptospermum scoparium*
Marjoram *Origanum maiorana*
Massoia *Cryprocaria massoia*
Mastic *Pistacia lentiscus*
Mastic thyme *Thymus mastichina*
May chang *Litsea cubeba*
May rose *Rosa gallica*
Melissa *Melissa officinalis*
Monarda *Monarda fistulosa*
Morocco oregano *Origanum virens*
Morocco thyme *Thymus satureioides*
Morocco wild camomile *Ormenis mixta*
Mother of thyme *Thymus serpyllum*
Mountain juniper *Juniperus communis var. montana*
Mountain pine *Pinus mugo*
Mountain savoury *Satureja thymbra*
Mugwort *Artemisia vulgaris*
    California *Artemisia douglasiana*
    white *Artemisia alba, Artemisia herba-alba*
Muhuhu *Brachyleana hutchinsii*
Myrrh *Commiphora myrrha*
    bisabol *Opopanax guidotti*
    East India *Commiphora erythraea*
    guggul *Commiphora wightii*
    Yemen *Commiphora habessinica*
Myrtle *Myrtus communis*
    green *Myrtus communis*
    red *Myrtus communis*

Narrow-leaf eucalyptus *Eucalyptus radiata*
Narrow-leaf paperbark *Melaleuca alternifolia*
Narrow-leaf tea tree *Melaleuca linariifolia*
Neem *Azadirachta indica*
Nepal juniper *Juniperus squamata*
Neroli *Citrus aurantium subsp. amara*
    China *Poncirus trifoliata*
    Portugal *Citrus x sinensis*
Nerolina *Melaleuca quinquenervia ct. nerolidol/linalool*
Niaouli *Melaleuca quinquenervia ct. cineole*
    Madagascar *Melaleuca quinquenervia ct. viridiflorol*
Nordmann's fir *Abies nordmanniana*
Northern white cedar *Thuja occidentalis*
Norway spruce *Picea abies*
Nutmeg *Myristica fragrans*
Nutsedge *Cyperus rotundus*

Oakmoss *Evernia prunastri*
Oleander *Nerium oleander*
Opopanax *Opopanax chironium and spp.*
    Africa *Commiphora kataf*
Orange
    bitter *Citrus aurantium var. amara*
    sweet *Citrus aurantium var. dulcis/x sinensis*
Oregano *Origanum spp.*

common *Origanum vulgare*
compact *Origanum compactum*
Cretan *Origanum onites*
Greek *Origanum heracleoticum*
Lavender *Origanum dubium* ct. *linalool*
Moroccan *Origanum virens*
wavering *Origanum dubium*
Osmanthus *Osmanthus fragrans*

Palmarosa *Cymbopogon martini* var. *motia*
Palo santo *Bursera graveolens*
Argentine *Bulnesia sarmienti*
Parsnip *Pastinaca sativa*
Parsley seed ct. apiol *Petroselinum sativum*
Parsley seed ct. pinene *Petroselinum crispum*
Patchouli *Pogostemon cablin*
China *Microtoena insuavis*
Java *Pogostemon heyneanus*
Pepper
black *Piper nigrum*
Brazil *Schinus terebinthifolius*
cubeb *Piper cubeba*
green *Piper nigrum*
long *Piper longum*
pink/Peru *Schinus molle*
Sichuan *Zanthoxylum bungeanum*
Peppermint *Mentha x piperita*
Peppermint eucalyptus *Eucalyptus piperita*
Peru balsam *Myroxylon pereirae*
Peru pepper *Schinus molle*
Petitgrain bigarade *Citrus aurantium* subsp. *amara*
Phoenicia juniper *Juniperus phoenicea*
Pimenta berry/leaf *Pimenta racemosa*
Pine
Aleppo *Pinus halepensis*
black *Pinus nigrum*
jack *Pinus divaricata*
laricio *Pinus laricio*
mountain *Pinus mugo*
Scotch *Pinus sylvestris*
sea *Pinus pinaster*
Swiss *Pinus cembra*
white *Pinus strobus*
Pink grapefruit *Citrus x paradisi*
Plai ginger *Zingiber cassumunar*

Rambazina *Helichrysum gymnocephalum*
Ravensara *Ravensara aromatica*
Ravintsara *Cinnamomum camphora* ct. *cineole*
Red myrtle *Myrtus communis* ct. *myrtenyl acetate*
Red spruce *Picea rubens*
River red gum *Eucalyptus camaldulensis*
Roman camomile *Anthemis nobilis*
Rosalina *Melaleuca ericifolia*
Rose *Rosa damascena*
Damask *Rosa damascena*
Gallic *Rosa gallica*
Japan *Rosa rugosa*
May/cabbage *Rosa centifolia*
moonseason/China *Rosa chinensis*

musk *Rosa moschata*
white *Rosa damascena* var. *alba*
Rose geranium *Pelargonium* cv. group *Rosat*
Rosemary *Rosmarinus officinalis*
Rosewood *Aniba roseodora*

Sage *Salvia officinalis*
Algeria *Salvia algeriensis*
black *Salvia mellifera*
blue mountain *Salvia stenophella*
garden *Salvia officinalis*
Greek/Lebanese *Salvia fruticosa*
hummingbird *Salvia spathacea*
lavender *Salvia lavandulifolia*
Spanish *Salvia lavandulifolia*
white/bee *Salvia apiana*
Sambac Jasmine *Jasminum sambac*
Sandalwood
Australia *Santalum spicatum*
Hawai'i *Santalum ellipticum*
India *Santalum album*
New Caledonia *Santalum austrocaledonicum*
New Guinea *Santalum mcgregorii*
Sanna *Hedychium spicatum*
Saro *Cinnamosma fragrans*
Savin juniper *Juniperus sabina*
Savoury
garden *Satureja hortensis*
mountain *Satureja thymbra*
winter *Satureja montana*
Scotch pine *Pinus sylvestris*
Sea pine *Pinus pinaster*
Siam wood *Fokienia hodginsii*
Siberian fir *Abies sibirica*
Silver fir *Abies alba*
Sitka spruce *Abies sitchensis*
Smith's gum *Eucalyptus smithii*
Spanish lavender *Lavandula stoechas*
Spanish sage *Salvia lavandulifolia*
Spanish sauce thyme *Thymus zygis*
Spanish thyme *Thymus mastichina*
Spearmint *Mentha spicata*
curly *Mentha spicata* var. *crispa*
Moroccan *Mentha viridis* var. *nana*
Russian *Mentha verticellata*
Scotch *Mentha gracilis*
Spike lavender *Lavandula latifolia*
Spiked gingerlily *Hedychium spicatum*
Spiked thyme *Thymbra spicata*
Spikenard
China *Nardostachys chinensis*
Nepal *Nardostachys jatamansi*
Spruce
black *Picea mariana*
hemlock *Tsuga canadensis*
Norway *Picea abies*
red *Picea rubens*
sitka *Picea sitchensis*
white *Picea glauca*
Star anise *Illicium verum*
Styrax *Liquidambar styraciflua*
Sugi *Cryptomeria japonica*
Summer savoury *Satureja hortensis*
Sweet basil *Ocimum basilicum* ct. *linalool*
Sweet fennel *Foeniculum vulgare*
Sweet orange *Citrus sinensis*

Swiss pine *Pinus cembra*

Tagette *Tagetes glandulifera*
Tangerine *Citrus x tangerina*
Tarragon *Artemisia dracunculus* ct. *methylchavicol*
Russia *Artemisia dracunculus* ct. *sabinene*
Tea tree *Melaleuca alternifolia*
black *Melaleuca bracteata*
broad-leaf *Melaleuca viridiflora/ cajuputi*
citronella *Leptospermum liversidgei*
lavender *Melaleuca ericifolia*
lemon *Leptospermum petersonii*
narrow-leaf *Melaleuca linariifolia*
weeping *Melaleuca leucadendra*
Texas cedarwood *Juniperus mexicana*
Thyme *Thymus vulgaris, Thymus zygis*
capitate *Thymus capitatus*
caraway *Thymus herna-barona*
Cretan *Thymus capitatus*
garden/common *Thymus vulgaris*
lemon *Thymus x citriodorus*
mastic *Thymus mastichina*
Moroccan *Thymus satureioides*
Spanish *Thymus mastichina*
Spanish sauce *Thymus zygis*
spiked *Thymus spicata*
wild *Thymus serpyllum*
Tree basil *Ocimum gratissimum*
Tree wormwood *Artemisia arborescens*
Tropical basil *Ocimum basilicum* ct. *linalool*
Tuberose *Polianthes tuberosa*
Tulsi *Ocimum sanctum*
Turmeric *Curcuma longa*

Valerian *Valeriana officinalis*
India *Valeriana wallichii*
Vanilla *Vanilla planifolia*
Vetiver *Vetiveria zizanioides*
Virginia cedarwood *Juniperus virginiana*

Weeping tea tree *Melaleuca leucadendra*
Winter savoury *Satureia montana*
Wintergreen *Gaultheria procumbens* and spp.
White camphor *Cinnamomum camphora*
White cypress *Cupressus lusitanica*
White ginger lily *Hedychium coronarium*
White grapefruit *Citrus x paradisi*
White mugwort *Artemisia alba*
White pine *Pinus strobus*
White sage *Salvia apiana*
White sagebrush *Artemisia ludoviciana*
White spruce *Picea glauca*
White wormwood *Artemisia alba*
Wild thyme *Thymus serpyllum*
Winter savoury *Satureja montana*
Woolly-butt eucalyptus *Eucalyptus macarthurii*
Wormwood *Artemisia absinthium* ct. *thujone*
African *Artemisia afra*
annual *Artemisia annua*
tree *Artemisia arborescens*
white *Artemisia alba*

Yarrow *Achillea millefolium*
  Ligurian *Achillea ligustica*
  musk *Achillea moschata*
Yellow ginger *Hedychium flavescens*

Ylang ylang *Cananga odorata forma genuina*
Yuzu *Citrus junos*

Zdravetz *Geranium macrorrhizum*
Zedoary *Curcuma zedoaria*
Zinziba *Lippia javanica*

# Index

# Essential Oils Index

therapeutic functions/
indications, 269–72
topical uses, 272
tropism, 269
uplifting/clarifying effects, 15
*versus* Zinziba, 276
Lemon myrtle, *versus* Lemon
eucalyptus, 276–7
Lemon petitgrain, 351
Lemon verbena, *versus* Lemon
eucalyptus, 275
Lemon-scented ironbark, *versus*
Lemon eucalyptus, 276
Lemon-scented tea tree, *versus*
Lemon eucalyptus, 277
Lemongrass
for acute discouragement, 22
for ambient diffusion, 23
as insect repellent, 48
as lymphatic decongestant, 87
as neuromuscular relaxant, 83
as neuromuscular sedative, 86
psychological *vs.* physiological
effects, 22
as sedative, 86
as skin irritant, 27, 47
uplifting/clarifying effects, 15
Lilyturf root, 86
Lime, **278–86**
antiviral effects, 282
cautions, 282
chemical constituents, 279
Chinese medicine functions/
indications, 283–4
*versus* Citron, 279–80, 285–6
clarity and, 280
*versus* Combava lime, 285
complementary combinations,
282
emotional renewal and, 280
Five-Element affinity, 283
foresight and, 280
fragrance characteristics, 283
good judgment and, 280
Heart clarifying action, 283
heat clearing action, 283
insight and, 280
*versus* Italian lime/Limette, 279,
285
*versus* Kaffir lime, 279, 285
*versus* Kaffir lime petitgrain, 285
*versus* Key lime, 283
meridian tropism, 283
optimism and, 280
overview, 278–9
*versus* Persian lime, 279, 285
physiological effects, 281–2, 284
preparations, 283
psychological effects, 280, 284
Qi activating action, 283
related oils, 279–80, 285–6
Shen calming action, 283
skin care uses, 282

specific symptomatology, 280
synergistic combinations, 281
terrain, 281
therapeutic functions/
indications, 280–3
topical uses, 282
tropism, 281
Linaloeswood, *versus* Frankincense,
217
Long pepper, *versus* Black pepper,
131
Lovage root
*versus* Angelica root, 107–8
for manic elation, 21

Madagascar jasmine, 251
Madagascar niaouli, 321
Magnolia bark, 83
Mandarin
as cerebral sedative, 86
for digestive issues, 35
as digestive relaxant, 83
incongruence between olfactory/
physiological effects, 16
for travel situations, 21
Mandarin petitgrain, 351
Manuka, *versus* Niaouli, 330
Marjoram, 74
acupoint applications, 56
as cerebral sedative, 86
dilution recommendations, 52
for inflammation, 45
nervous system tropism, 69
for racing mind, 21
regulating properties, 53
as relaxant, 51
relaxant nervous restorative
properties, 54
relaxant sedative properties, 54
as sexual sedative, 86
stimulant spasmolytic properties,
54
as systemic relaxant, 75
as urinary relaxant, 83
Marshmallow root, 86
Mastic
*versus* Cistus, 166–7
as prostatic decongestant, 167
Mastic thyme, 476
May chang
for acute discouragement, 22
as neuromuscular sedative, 86
psychological *vs.* physiological
effects, 22
as sedative, 86
as skin irritant, 27, 47
uplifting/clarifying effects, 15
Melissa, **287–95**
antifungal actions, 290
antimicrobial actions, 290
antiviral actions, 290
brain dynamics, 288
cautions, 291

chemical constituents, 287–8
Chinese medicine functions/
indications, 292–3
clarity and, 288
complementary combinations,
290–1
as decongestant, 290
emotional renewal and, 288
Five-Element affinity, 292
foresight and, 289
fragrance characteristics, 288,
292
good judgment and, 289
Heart clarifying action, 292
heat clearing action, 292
historical uses, 293–4
insight and, 289
meridian tropism, 292
optimism and, 288
physiological effects, 289–91, 294
PNEI function, 288
preparations, 292
psychological effects, 288–9, 295
Qi activating action, 292
related oils, 288
as relaxant, 289–90, 294
as sedative, 86, 294
Shen calming action, 292
skin care uses, 291
specific symptomatology, 288
synergistic combinations, 290
therapeutic functions/
indications, 288–92
topical uses, 291–2
tropism, 289
Moroccan thyme, 473
Mugwort, *versus* Tarragon, 460–1
Myrrh
for acute worry, 21
antibacterial actions, 300
antifungal actions, 301
antimicrobial actions, 300–1
antiparasitic actions, 301
*versus* Benzoin, 307–9
brain dynamics, 298
as calming, 300
cautions, 302
chemical constituents, 297
Chinese medicine functions/
indications, 302–3
cognitive flexibility and, 289
cold compresses with, 50
complementary combinations,
301
*versus* Copaiba, 306–7
Damp resolving action, 303
as decongestant, 87, 299
*versus* Elemi, 307
Five-Element affinity, 303
fluid astringing action, 303
fragrance characteristics, 298,
302
haemostatic action, 303

# Repertory

*Repertory refers to Aromatica Volume 1 (Holmes, 2016) and Volume 2 (this volume).*

## A

**abdominal pain:** Angelica root; Black pepper; Cardamom; Frankincense; Myrrh; Oregano; Peppermint; Pimenta berry; Tarragon; Thyme ct. thymol; Winter savoury; Yarrow

**abscesses:** Basil ct. methylchavicol; Carrot seed; Myrrh; Pimenta berry; Saro; Winter savoury

**acne:** Atlas cedarwood; Basil ct. methylchavicol; Eucalyptus; Geranium; Grapefruit; Green myrtle; infected: Clove bud; Pimenta berry; Jasmine; Laurel; Lemon eucalyptus; Lemongrass; Mandarin; Marjoram; May chang; Niaouli; Palmarosa; Patchouli; Roman camomile; Rose; Rosemary ct. verbenone; Sandalwood; Saro; Sweet orange; Thyme ct. thymol; Vetiver; Wintergreen; Yarrow; Ylang-ylang

**ADD:** Angelica root; Basil ct. methylchavicol; Black pepper; Black spruce; Cajeput; Cistus; Clove bud; Cypress; Eucalyptus; Frankincense; Ginger; Grand fir; Green myrtle; Juniper berry; Laurel; Lemon; Lemon eucalyptus; Lemongrass; Lime; May chang; Melissa; Niaouli; Nutmeg; Oregano; Peppermint; Pimenta berry; Ravintsara; Rosemary ct. Cineole and ct. Camphor; Sage; Saro; Siberian fir; Spearmint; Tarragon; Tea tree; Thyme ct. thymol; Vetiver; Winter savoury; Ylang-ylang

**addictive behaviours:** Bergamot; Green myrtle; Helichrysum; Jasmine; Palmarosa; Rose; Wintergreen; Ylang-ylang

**ADHD:** Angelica root; Atlas cedarwood; Bergamot; Carrot seed; Clary sage; Grapefruit; Lavender; Mandarin; Marjoram; Myrrh; Neroli; Patchouli; Petitgrain bigarade; Sweet orange

**adhesions:** Geranium; Helichrysum; Palmarosa; Patchouli

**adrenal dysregulation:** Grand fir; Niaouli

**adrenal fatigue:** Black pepper; Black spruce; Clary sage; Clove bud; Coriander seed; Cypress; Geranium; Oregano; Palmarosa; Pimenta berry; Rosemary ct. Cineole and ct. Camphor; Sage; Scotch pine; Siberian fir; Thyme ct. linalool; Thyme ct. thymol; Winter savoury

**adrenocortical dysregulation:** Angelica root

**aerophagia:** Basil ct. methylchavicol

**age spots:** Carrot seed; Rosemary ct. verbenone

**agitation:** Angelica root; Blue tansy; Carrot seed; Marjoram; Myrrh; Patchouli; Roman camomile; Spikenard; Vetiver

**agoraphobia:** Nutmeg

**AIDS:** Clove bud; Sage

**allergies:** Blue tansy; Clove bud; German camomile; Helichrysum; Melissa; Niaouli; Scotch pine; skin, Spikenard; Tarragon; Vetiver

**alopecia:** Atlas cedarwood; Rosemary ct. Cineole and ct. Camphor; Ylang-ylang

**altitude sickness:** Ginger; Nutmeg

**amenorrhea:** Angelica root; Cinnamon bark; Clary sage; Clove bud; Fennel; Frankincense; Ginger; Green myrtle; Hyssop; Jasmine; Juniper berry; Laurel; Lavender; Marjoram; Myrrh; Niaouli; Nutmeg; Oregano; Pimenta berry; Rose; Rosemary ct. Cineole and ct. Camphor; Sage; Scotch pine; Spikenard; Thyme ct. linalool; Thyme ct. thymol; Vetiver; Winter savoury; Wintergreen

**anaemia:** Carrot seed; Lemon; Vetiver

**aneurism:** Tea tree

**anger:** Basil ct. methylchavicol; Mandarin; Neroli; Roman camomile; Sambac jasmine; suppressed, Helichrysum; Sweet orange; Yarrow; Ylang-ylang

**angina pectoris:** Fennel; Helichrysum; Melissa; Neroli; neurogenic: Spikenard; Tarragon; Patchouli; Rosemary ct. verbenone; Wintergreen; Ylang-ylang

**animal bites:** Cinnamon bark

**ankles, swollen:** Sandalwood

**anorexia:** Angelica root; Black pepper; Cardamom; Fennel; Ginger; Hyssop; Lemon

**anuria:** Angelica root; Winter savoury

**anxiety:** Angelica root; Atlas cedarwood; Basil ct. methylchavicol; Blue tansy; Cardamom; chronic: Cardamom; Geranium; Petitgrain bigarade; Cistus; Clary sage; Frankincense; Geranium; German camomile; Helichrysum; Lavender; Lime; Marjoram; Melissa; Myrrh; Palmarosa; Patchouli; Petitgrain bigarade; Roman camomile; Rose; Sambac jasmine; Sandalwood; Vetiver; Ylang-ylang

**apathy:** Black pepper; Black spruce; Cinnamon bark; Cistus; Clove bud; Coriander seed; Cypress; Eucalyptus; Ginger; Grand fir; Juniper berry; Niaouli; Nutmeg; Oregano; Peppermint; Pimenta berry; Ravintsara; Sage; Siberian fir; Thyme ct. thymol; Winter savoury

**aphthous sores:** Marjoram; Sage

**apnoea:** Frankincense

**appetite loss:** Angelica root; Black pepper; Cardamom; Clove bud; Coriander seed; Fennel; Grapefruit; Hyssop; Laurel; Lime; Mandarin; May chang; Melissa; Nutmeg; Oregano; Pimenta berry; Sage; Spearmint; Sweet orange; Thyme ct. thymol; Winter savoury; Yarrow

**arrhythmia:** Lemon eucalyptus; Marjoram; Melissa; Rosemary ct. verbenone; Spikenard; Ylang-ylang

**arteriosclerosis:** Basil ct. methylchavicol; Juniper berry; Laurel; Lemon; Myrrh

**arthritic pain:** Angelica root; Black spruce; Blue tansy; chronic, Cajeput; Clove bud; Coriander seed; Cypress; Eucalyptus; Frankincense; Geranium; Ginger; Grand fir; Grapefruit; Juniper berry; Laurel; Lavender; Lemon; Lemon eucalyptus; Lemongrass; Lime; May chang; Melissa; Nutmeg; Oregano; Petitgrain bigarade; Pimenta berry; Ravintsara; Roman camomile; Rosemary ct. Cineole and ct. Camphor; Sage; Saro; Scotch pine; Siberian fir; Tea tree; Vetiver; Winter savoury; Wintergreen; Yarrow

**ascites:** Juniper berry

**asthma:** Angelica root; atopic, Sandalwood; Basil ct. methylchavicol; Black spruce; Blue tansy; Cajeput; Cardamom; Clary sage; Clove bud; Eucalyptus; Fennel; Frankincense; German

camomile; Helichrysum; Lemon eucalyptus; Myrrh; Niaouli; Oregano; Petitgrain bigarade; Roman camomile; Rose; Rosemary ct. Cineole and ct. Camphor; Scotch pine; Siberian fir; spasmodic: Lavender; Siberian fir; Tarragon; Tarragon; Tea tree; Thyme ct. linalool; Thyme ct. thymol; Ylang-ylang

**atherosclerosis:** Helichrysum; Hyssop

**athlete's foot:** Carrot seed; Clove bud; Eucalyptus; Lavender; Lemon eucalyptus; Lemongrass; Myrrh; Niaouli; Palmarosa; Patchouli; Pimenta berry; Thyme ct. linalool

**atony, gastrointestinal:** Ginger; Rosemary ct. Cineole and ct. Camphor

**attention span, poor:** Lemon; Lemongrass; Lime; May chang

**autism:** Patchouli

**autonomic nervous system dysregulation:** Angelica root; Cardamom; Lemongrass; May chang; Petitgrain bigarade; Sage

# B

**bacterial infections:** Angelica root; Black pepper; Cajeput; Cinnamon bark; Cistus; Clove bud; Coriander seed; Eucalyptus; German camomile; Helichrysum; Lavender; Lemongrass; Marjoram; May chang; Niaouli; Oregano; Rosemary ct. Cineole and ct. Camphor; Sage; Sandalwood; Saro; Spearmint; Tea tree; Thyme ct. linalool; Thyme ct. thymol; Winter savoury

**bearing-down pains, premenstrual:** Basil ct. methylchavicol

**bedwetting:** Cypress; Sandalwood

**betrayal:** Helichrysum; Rose

**bile stones:** Melissa

**bipolar disorder:** Basil ct. methylchavicol; Bergamot; Blue tansy; Cardamom; Clary sage; Coriander seed; Fennel; German camomile; Grapefruit; Green myrtle; Hyssop; Laurel; Lavender; Mandarin; Marjoram; Neroli; Peppermint; Petitgrain bigarade; Roman camomile; Rose; Rosemary ct. verbenone; Sage; Sambac jasmine; Spearmint; Sweet orange; Tarragon; Ylang-ylang

**Bladder damp-heat:** Eucalyptus; Spearmint

**Bladder Qi constraint:** Marjoram; Melissa; Tarragon

**bleeding:** intermenstrual, Rose; uterine, Geranium

**bloating:** abdominal: Carrot seed; Hyssop; Peppermint; Angelica root; Basil ct. methylchavicol; Black pepper; chronic abdominal, Lemon; epigastric, Spearmint; Laurel; Sage; Spearmint; Sweet orange; Thyme ct. linalool; worse stress, Mandarin

**Blood and Qi stagnation:** Helichrysum; Wintergreen

**Blood and Yin deficiency:** Geranium

**Blood cold, with Lower Warmer Qi and Blood stagnation:** Ginger

**Blood deficiency:** Geranium; with menopausal syndrome: Sage; Vetiver; Niaouli; in perimenopause, Rose; with scanty/absent/irregular cycles: Sage; Vetiver; with Shen dysregulation, Rose; with Shen weakness, Jasmine; with stopped periods, Clary sage

**blood hyperviscosity:** Lime

**Blood stagnation:** from acute trauma, Frankincense; Helichrysum; in lower limb: Neroli; Sandalwood; Yarrow; in lower limbs: Atlas cedarwood; Basil ct. methylchavicol; Cajeput; Clary sage; Cypress; Geranium; Lemon; Patchouli; Rosemary ct. Cineole and ct. Camphor; Tea tree; in Lower Warmer, Clary sage

**boils:** Basil ct. methylchavicol; Carrot seed; Clove bud; Geranium; infected, Petitgrain bigarade; Laurel; Lemongrass; Mandarin; May chang; Myrrh; Niaouli; Pimenta berry; Roman camomile; Sandalwood; Saro; Spikenard

**boundaries, poor:** Cistus; Frankincense; Laurel; Wintergreen

**bowel movement, irregular:** Oregano

**BPH:** Basil ct. methylchavicol; Cistus; Cypress; Green myrtle; Niaouli; Sandalwood; Tarragon

**breast engorgement:** Fennel

**breathing:** irregular, Petitgrain bigarade; shallow: Green myrtle; Hyssop; Scotch pine

**bronchial spasms:** Basil ct. methylchavicol; Helichrysum

**bronchitis:** Angelica root; Atlas cedarwood; Black pepper; Black spruce; Cardamom; chronic: Cajeput; Ginger; Rosemary ct. verbenone; Thyme ct. thymol; Winter savoury; Cinnamon bark; Eucalyptus; Fennel; with foetid sputum, Sandalwood; Frankincense; Grand fir; Green myrtle; Laurel; Lavender; Lemon eucalyptus; Marjoram; Myrrh; Niaouli; Oregano; Palmarosa; Pimenta berry; Ravintsara; Rosemary ct. Cineole and ct. Camphor; Sage; Saro; Scotch pine; Spearmint; Spikenard; Sweet orange; Tarragon; Thyme ct. linalool

**brooding:** Fennel

**bruises:** Black pepper; Fennel; Geranium; Hyssop; Lemongrass; Marjoram; Wintergreen; Yarrow

**burnout:** Angelica root; Atlas cedarwood; Black pepper; Black spruce; Cistus; Clary sage; Clove bud; Cypress; Frankincense; Ginger; Juniper berry; Laurel; Marjoram; Myrrh; Nutmeg; Oregano; Palmarosa; Petitgrain bigarade; Pimenta berry; Sandalwood; Saro; Scotch pine; Siberian fir; Thyme ct. thymol; Vetiver; Wintergreen

**burns:** Bergamot; Carrot seed; German camomile; Lavender; Niaouli; from radiation, German camomile; Rosemary ct. verbenone; Yarrow

**bursitis:** Roman camomile

# C

**Callouses:** Sweet orange

**cancerous conditions:** Clove bud; Frankincense; Geranium; Lemongrass; Melissa; Rose; Sage

**candidiasis:** Angelica root; Black spruce; Carrot seed; Cistus; Fennel; Geranium; Helichrysum; Laurel; Lavender; Myrrh; Oregano; Palmarosa; Patchouli; Peppermint; Petitgrain bigarade; Pimenta berry; Rosemary ct. verbenone; Sage; Sandalwood; Thyme ct. linalool; Thyme ct. thymol

**capillaries, broken:** Geranium; Lemon; Melissa; Neroli; Palmarosa; Roman camomile; Rose; Rosemary ct. verbenone

**carbuncles:** Myrrh

**cardiac arrhythmia:** Lemongrass; Lime; May chang; Tarragon

**cardiac disorders, stress-related:** Palmarosa

**cardiac dysrhythmia:** Petitgrain bigarade

**cardiac oedema:** Black pepper

**cardiac spasms:** Neroli

**cardiac weakness:** Rosemary ct. Cineole and ct. Camphor; Sandalwood

**catatonia:** Cinnamon bark

**cellulite:** Fennel; Juniper berry; Lemongrass; Oregano; Patchouli; Sage; Sweet orange; Yarrow

**cervical dysplasia:** Niaouli; Saro

**chemotherapy:** Coriander seed

**chest congestion:** Myrrh; Scotch pine

**chest constriction:** Green myrtle

**chest discomfort:** Tarragon

**chest distention:** Hyssop; Laurel; Lemon eucalyptus; Thyme ct. thymol

**chest infections, with cough:** Eucalyptus

**chest oppression:** Wintergreen; Ylang-ylang

**chest pain:** Fennel; Lemon eucalyptus; Neroli; Wintergreen

**chickenpox:** Cistus; Lemon eucalyptus; Ravintsara

**chills:** Cardamom

**chlamydia:** Palmarosa

**cholecystitis:** Basil ct. methylchavicol; Peppermint; Roman camomile; Rose; Rosemary ct. Cineole and ct. Camphor; Scotch pine; Tarragon

**cholera:** Pimenta berry; Ravintsara; Rosemary ct. verbenone

**cholesterol, high:** Geranium; Helichrysum

**Chong and Ren mai deficiency:** Black spruce; Jasmine; Niaouli; Rose; Sage; Vetiver

**chronic fatigue syndrome:** Black pepper; Black spruce; Cajeput; Cinnamon bark; Clove bud; Frankincense; Lemon; Oregano; Petitgrain bigarade; Pimenta berry; Ravintsara; Rosemary ct. Cineole and ct. Camphor; Rosemary ct. verbenone; Sage; Scotch pine; Siberian fir; Tea tree; Thyme ct. linalool; Thyme ct. thymol; Vetiver; Winter savoury

**circulation, poor:** Black spruce; Cajeput; Ginger; Grand fir; Myrrh; Niaouli; Peppermint; Ravintsara; Rosemary ct. Cineole and ct. Camphor; Sage

**cirrhosis:** Carrot seed; Helichrysum; Rosemary ct. Cineole and ct. Camphor

**Clear Yang Qi deficiency, with Shen weakness:** Black pepper; Cajeput; Eucalyptus; Grapefruit; Laurel; Lemon; Niaouli; Nutmeg; Peppermint; Ravintsara; Rosemary ct. Cineole and ct. Camphor; Saro

**clotting disorders:** Angelica root

**codependency:** Basil ct. methylchavicol; Helichrysum; Jasmine; Palmarosa; Rose; Ylang-ylang

**cognitive impairment:** Frankincense; Peppermint; Thyme ct. linalool

**cold, internal, with wind-damp-cold obstruction:** Ginger

**cold abdomen:** Cinnamon bark

**cold hands/feet:** Black pepper; Cajeput; Cinnamon bark; Clove bud; Ginger; Grand fir; Green myrtle; Hyssop; Juniper berry; Myrrh; Niaouli; Nutmeg; Oregano; Pimenta berry; Ravintsara; Rosemary ct. Cineole and ct. Camphor; Sage; Saro; Thyme ct. thymol; Winter savoury

**cold skin:** Cinnamon bark; Ginger; Grand fir; Juniper berry; Sage; Saro; Thyme ct. thymol

**cold sores:** Bergamot; Lemongrass; May chang; Oregano; Peppermint; Ravintsara; Saro; Tea tree

**colds:** Green myrtle; Scotch pine; with sneezing, Eucalyptus

**colic,** Ylang–ylang; Angelica root; Basil ct. methylchavicol; Blue tansy; Cajeput; Cardamom; Cinnamon bark; Clary sage; Coriander seed; Fennel; Geranium; Ginger; Helichrysum; Marjoram; May chang; Neroli; Oregano; Patchouli; Petitgrain bigarade; Roman camomile; Rosemary ct. verbenone; Siberian fir; Spikenard; Tarragon; Yarrow

**colitis:** acute, Blue tansy; Angelica root; Cinnamon bark; Fennel; Helichrysum; Jasmine; Lemongrass; May chang; Melissa; mucous: Pimenta berry; Sage; Niaouli; Nutmeg; Oregano; Rosemary ct. Cineole and ct. Camphor; Siberian fir; Tarragon; Thyme ct. linalool

**colon cancer:** Geranium

**coma:** Marjoram; Peppermint; Tarragon

**compulsivity:** Carrot seed; Sandalwood; Spikenard; Wintergreen

**concentration, poor:** Black pepper; Ginger; Grand fir; Grapefruit; Melissa; Niaouli; Nutmeg; Ravintsara; Rosemary ct. Cineole and ct. Camphor; Sage; Saro; Spearmint; Winter savoury

**condyloma:** Sage

**confidence, excessive:** Rosemary ct. verbenone

**confusion:** Basil ct. methylchavicol; Bergamot; Black pepper; Clary sage; with conflict, Ylang-ylang; Eucalyptus; Frankincense; Ginger; Grand fir; Green myrtle; Hyssop; Laurel; Lavender;

Lemon; Lemongrass; May chang; with negative outlook, Marjoram; Niaouli; Oregano; Palmarosa; Peppermint; Petitgrain bigarade; Rosemary ct. verbenone; Sage; Saro; Spearmint; Tea tree; Thyme ct. linalool; Yarrow

**congestive heart failure:** Rosemary ct. Cineole and ct. Camphor

**conjunctivitis:** Helichrysum; Roman camomile

**connective tissue weakness:** Vetiver

**constipation:** alternating with diarrhoea: Angelica root; Cardamom; Neroli; Petitgrain bigarade; Black pepper; Clove bud; Fennel; Nutmeg; Palmarosa; Sweet orange; Yarrow

**convalescence:** Angelica root; Basil ct. methylchavicol; Black pepper; Cajeput; Cinnamon bark; Clove bud; Laurel; Neroli; Oregano; Petitgrain bigarade; Sage; Saro; Thyme ct. thymol; Winter savoury

**convulsions:** Marjoram; Vetiver

**cough:** Black pepper; chronic: Frankincense; Helichrysum; Rosemary ct. verbenone; Siberian fir; Winter savoury; chronic dry, Sandalwood; chronic productive: Cardamom; Laurel; with difficult expectoration: Hyssop; Niaouli; Eucalyptus; with expectoration: Cistus; Grand fir; Lemon eucalyptus; Thyme ct. thymol; with hard sputum, Black pepper; Melissa; painful, Myrrh; with productive phlegm, Angelica root; Scotch pine; severe, Marjoram; spasmodic and nervous: Angelica root; Basil ct. methylchavicol; Marjoram; Rose; Tarragon; Ylang-ylang; with sputum, Green myrtle; Thyme ct. linalool; Thyme ct. thymol; weak, Hyssop

**courage, loss of:** Sage

**critical thinking, loss of:** Grand fir; Lemon eucalyptus; Lemongrass; Lime; Yarrow

**Crohn's disease:** Cistus; Lemon eucalyptus; Nutmeg; Spikenard

**croup:** Basil ct. methylchavicol; Cypress; Fennel; Helichrysum; Hyssop; Marjoram; Melissa; Oregano; Ravintsara; Siberian fir; Tarragon; Thyme ct. thymol; Winter savoury

**cynicism:** Hyssop; Jasmine; Sambac jasmine

**cystitis:** Atlas cedarwood; Carrot seed; Eucalyptus; Fennel; Grand fir; Green myrtle; Juniper berry; Lavender; mucousy: Myrrh; Saro; Niaouli; Nutmeg; Palmarosa; Peppermint; Pimenta berry; Sage; Scotch pine; Siberian fir; Spearmint; Tarragon; Thyme ct. linalool; Wintergreen; Yarrow

# D

**dampness:** Carrot seed; Lemon; with Shen dysregulation, Grapefruit

**dandruff:** Bergamot; Eucalyptus; Juniper berry; Laurel; Lemon; Lemon eucalyptus; Patchouli; Rosemary ct. Cineole and ct. Camphor; Rosemary ct. verbenone; Yarrow; Ylang-ylang

**defensiveness:** Palmarosa

**delirium:** Vetiver

**delusion:** Angelica root; Basil ct. methylchavicol; Carrot seed; Myrrh; Patchouli; Petitgrain bigarade; Pimenta berry; Sandalwood; Spikenard; Vetiver

**dengue fever:** Basil ct. methylchavicol; Clove bud; Pimenta berry

**denial:** Palmarosa

**dental caries:** Spearmint

**depression:** acute, Ylang-ylang; with agitation: Helichrysum; Lavender; Melissa; Roman camomile; Rose; Sambac jasmine; Spikenard; with anxiety: Basil ct. methylchavicol; Blue tansy; Clary sage; Geranium; Green myrtle; Laurel; Mandarin; Neroli; Rose; Rosemary ct. verbenone; Basil ct. methylchavicol; Bergamot; Black pepper; Black spruce; Cajeput; causeless, Pimenta berry; chronic, Cardamom; Cinnamon bark; Cistus; Clary sage; Clove bud; Coriander seed; Eucalyptus; Frankincense; German camomile; Ginger; Grand fir; Grapefruit; Green myrtle; Hyssop; Jasmine; Juniper berry; Laurel; Lemon; Lemon eucalyptus; Lemongrass; Lime; Marjoram; May chang; Melissa; minor: Mandarin; Peppermint; Tea tree; Niaouli; Nutmeg; Palmarosa; postviral: Ravintsara; Saro; Ravintsara; Rosemary ct. Cineole and ct. Camphor; Sage; Saro; Siberian fir; Thyme ct. linalool; Thyme ct. thymol; Vetiver; Winter savoury; Ylang-ylang

**dermatitis:** Atlas cedarwood; Carrot seed; Helichrysum; May chang; Myrrh; Roman camomile; Sambac jasmine; Spikenard; Tarragon; Thyme ct. linalool; Wintergreen; Yarrow

**despair:** Jasmine; Melissa; Neroli; Rose; Sambac jasmine; Wintergreen

**despondency:** Eucalyptus; Frankincense; Geranium; Rosemary ct. verbenone; Sage

**diabetes:** Blue tansy; Eucalyptus; Geranium; Juniper berry; Lemon; Scotch pine; Ylang-ylang

**diabetic gangrene:** Tea tree

**diarrhoea:** alternating with constipation: Angelica root; Cardamom; Neroli; Petitgrain bigarade; Black pepper; with bloody stool, Cistus; chronic: Pimenta berry; Thyme ct. thymol; Clary sage; Fennel; Lemon; mucoid: Frankincense; Grand fir; Sandalwood; with mucousy stool; Nutmeg; Oregano; Palmarosa; Patchouli; with undigested food, Cinnamon bark; Winter savoury

**digestive problems:** acute and chronic, Cajeput; with bloating, Sage; chronic: Lemongrass; May chang; Palmarosa; Patchouli; Rosemary ct. Cineole and ct. Camphor; Thyme ct. linalool; Clove bud; Nutmeg; worse stress: Bergamot; Lime; Melissa; Sweet orange

**disappointment:** Geranium

**discharges, chronic:** Geranium; Grand fir; Green myrtle

**disconnection:** Angelica root; with fantasizing/delusion, Patchouli; Petitgrain bigarade; Pimenta berry; Rose; Vetiver

**discouragement:** Angelica root; Black pepper; Black spruce; Cardamom; Cinnamon bark; Cistus; Clove bud; Cypress; Fennel; Frankincense; Ginger; Grand fir; Jasmine; Juniper berry; Lime; Melissa; Nutmeg; Oregano; Pimenta berry; Rose; Rosemary ct. Cineole and ct. Camphor; Scotch pine; Siberian fir; Sweet orange; Thyme ct. thymol; Winter savoury; Wintergreen

**disempowerment:** Myrrh

**disorganization:** Lemongrass; Rosemary ct. Cineole and ct. Camphor

**disorientation:** Basil ct. methylchavicol; Cardamom; Grapefruit; Green myrtle; Juniper berry; Lemongrass; May chang; Ravintsara; Thyme ct. linalool; Winter savoury; Yarrow

**dissociative disorder:** Angelica root; Atlas cedarwood; Black pepper; Carrot seed; Clove bud; Cypress; Frankincense; Ginger; Jasmine; Myrrh; Patchouli; Pimenta berry; Sandalwood; Siberian fir; Spikenard; Vetiver; Ylang-ylang

**distraction:** Carrot seed; Grapefruit; Green myrtle; Hyssop; Lemon; Lemongrass; Lime; May chang; Melissa; Palmarosa; Petitgrain bigarade; Roman camomile; Rosemary ct. verbenone; Sage; Sweet orange; Tea tree; Ylang-ylang

**dizziness:** Basil ct. methylchavicol; Black pepper; Cinnamon bark; Marjoram; Nutmeg; Peppermint; Sweet orange; Tarragon

**dreams, intense:** Spikenard

**drowsiness:** Basil ct. methylchavicol; Eucalyptus; Ginger; Niaouli; Oregano; Peppermint; Ravintsara; Rosemary ct. Cineole and ct. Camphor; Sage; Saro; Tea tree; Thyme ct. linalool; Thyme ct. thymol; Winter savoury

**drug toxicosis:** Carrot seed; Grapefruit; Rosemary ct. verbenone

**dysentery:** Cinnamon bark; Cistus; Lemongrass; Nutmeg; Oregano; Pimenta berry; Ravintsara

**dyslexia:** Patchouli

**dysmenorrhea:** Angelica root; Cajeput; Cinnamon bark; Clary sage; congestive: Cypress; Niaouli; Rose; Scotch pine; Wintergreen; Cypress; Fennel; Frankincense; Geranium; Jasmine; Laurel; Myrrh; Oregano; Petitgrain bigarade; Roman camomile; Rose; Rosemary ct. verbenone; Sage; Scotch pine; severe, Marjoram; spasmodic: Angelica root; Clary sage; Cypress; German camomile; Ginger; Juniper berry; Lavender; Melissa; Roman camomile; Winter savoury; Spikenard; Tarragon; Yarrow

**dyspepsia:** atonic: Lemon; Mandarin; Cajeput; chronic, Patchouli; epigastric, Peppermint; German camomile; May chang; Siberian fir; Spearmint; Thyme ct. linalool

**dyspnoea:** Angelica root; Black pepper; congestive, Hyssop; Frankincense; Oregano; Petitgrain bigarade; Saro; spasmodic: Cardamom; Melissa; Tarragon; Thyme ct. thymol

**dysrhythmia:** Spikenard

**dysuria, spasmodic:** Fennel; Grand fir; Laurel; Sage; Tarragon

# E

**earache:** Laurel; Roman camomile; Winter savoury

**ecchymosis:** Wintergreen

**eczema:** Atlas cedarwood; atopic: Spikenard; Yarrow; Basil ct. methylchavicol; Bergamot; Black spruce; Carrot seed; Green myrtle; Helichrysum; Juniper berry; Marjoram; Melissa; Myrrh; Niaouli; Palmarosa; Roman camomile; Rosemary ct. verbenone; Thyme ct. thymol; Vetiver; Wintergreen; Yarrow

**edema:** ankles, Clary sage; Atlas cedarwood; Juniper berry; Lavender; Lemon; Lemongrass; May chang

embitterment: Rose

emotional coldness: Cinnamon bark; Clove bud; Sandalwood; Ylang-ylang

emotional deprivation: Rose

emotional inhibition: Cardamom; Coriander seed; Fennel

emotional instability: Carrot seed; Coriander seed; Fennel; Helichrysum; Hyssop; Mandarin; Neroli; Petitgrain bigarade; Pimenta berry; Rosemary ct. verbenone; Sandalwood; Spikenard; Wintergreen; Ylang-ylang

emotional outbursts: Basil ct. methylchavicol; Tarragon

emotional sensitivity: Spikenard

emotionalism: Neroli; Spearmint; Tarragon

emotions, acute: Rose; Sambac jasmine; Ylang-ylang; negative, Palmarosa; stuck: Basil ct. methylchavicol; Hyssop; Laurel; Lavender; Lemongrass; Marjoram; May chang; Peppermint; Rosemary ct. verbenone; Sage; Tarragon; Thyme ct. linalool

emphysema: Black pepper; Black spruce; Blue tansy; Eucalyptus; Frankincense; Green myrtle; Lemon eucalyptus; Niaouli; Oregano; Rosemary ct. verbenone; Saro; Thyme ct. thymol; Winter savoury

encephalitis: Basil ct. methylchavicol

endocrine deficiencies: Black spruce; Scotch pine

endurance, low: Black pepper; Ginger; Juniper berry; Siberian fir

enteritis: Clove bud; Pimenta berry; Sage; Tarragon

enuresis: Cypress; Fennel

envy: Rose

enzyme deficiency: Basil ct. methylchavicol; Cypress; Peppermint

epidemic infections: Ravintsara

epigastric fullness: Cardamom; Spearmint

epigastric pain: Mandarin; Oregano; Petitgrain bigarade; Thyme ct. thymol; Yarrow

escapism: Wintergreen

euphoria: Angelica root; Carrot seed; Myrrh; Petitgrain bigarade; Sandalwood; Spikenard; Vetiver

excitability: Neroli

external Wind-cold: Hyssop; Laurel; with Middle Warmer damp, Sage; with Qi deficiency, Sage; with Qi or Yang deficiency: Niaouli; Ravintsara; Saro

External wind-cold, with Qi or Yang deficiency: Rosemary ct. Cineole and ct. Camphor

External wind-cold/heat: Peppermint; with Qi or Yang deficiency, Cajeput

external wind-heat: Hyssop; with Qi deficiency, Tea tree; Spearmint

External wind-heat, with wind in head: Eucalyptus

eye conditions: Thyme ct. linalool

eyebrows, loss: Laurel

# F

faintness: Nutmeg; Peppermint

fancy, flights of: Spikenard

fatigue: after exercise, Sandalwood; afternoon: Oregano; Pimenta berry; Rosemary ct. Cineole and ct. Camphor; Scotch pine; alternating with restlessness, Vetiver; Cardamom; Carrot seed; chronic mental and physical: Basil ct. methylchavicol; Carrot seed; Cinnamon bark; Ravintsara; Saro; Scotch pine; Clove bud; Coriander seed; Cypress; Frankincense; Grand fir; Grapefruit; Green myrtle; Hyssop; Jasmine; Laurel; long-term, Palmarosa; Niaouli; physical, Black pepper; Ravintsara; Rosemary ct. verbenone; Sage; Scotch pine; Tea tree; Thyme ct. linalool; Thyme ct. thymol; Wintergreen; worse morning: Grapefruit; Rosemary ct. verbenone; Sweet orange; Yarrow

fear: Black pepper; Carrot seed; Nutmeg; Patchouli

fears: hidden, Sandalwood; Petitgrain bigarade; Pimenta berry; Spikenard; Wintergreen; without reason, Wintergreen

fevers: Bergamot; empty heat in late stage, Sage; German camomile; intermittent: Eucalyptus; Roman camomile; Winter savoury; Wintergreen; Lemon; low-grade, eruptive, Lavender; May chang; Myrrh; Patchouli; Rose; Sambac jasmine; Spearmint; Spikenard; tidal, Sage

fibrocystic breasts: Lemon; Lemongrass; May chang

fibromyalgia: Basil ct. methylchavicol; Blue tansy; Helichrysum; Juniper berry; Nutmeg; Ravintsara; Roman camomile; Rosemary ct. Cineole and ct.

Camphor; Tarragon; Vetiver; Winter savoury; Wintergreen; Yarrow

**Fire toxin:** Tea tree

**Fixation:** Neroli

**flank pain:** right, Carrot seed; Rosemary ct. verbenone

**flat affect:** Eucalyptus; Juniper berry; Lemon; Lemon eucalyptus; Lemongrass; May chang; Oregano; Ravintsara; Siberian fir

**flatulence:** Angelica root; Basil ct. methylchavicol; Black pepper; Fennel; Ginger; Laurel; Lemon; May chang; Nutmeg; Oregano; Petitgrain bigarade; Roman camomile; Rosemary ct. Cineole and ct. Camphor; Sweet orange; Tarragon; Winter savoury; Yarrow

**fleas:** Lemongrass; May chang; Oregano; Thyme ct. thymol

**floating Yang:** German camomile

**flu:** Eucalyptus

**fogginess, mental:** Black pepper; Frankincense; Hyssop; Laurel; Lemon; Lemongrass; Lime; May chang; Niaouli; Peppermint; Ravintsara; Rosemary ct. Cineole and ct. Camphor; Saro; Winter savoury; Yarrow

**food allergies:** Atlas cedarwood; Ginger; Helichrysum; Palmarosa; Patchouli; Sandalwood; Tea tree; Yarrow

**food poisoning:** Angelica root; fish and mushroom, Black pepper; Lemongrass; Nutmeg; Patchouli

**frigidity:** Black pepper; Black spruce; Cinnamon bark; Clary sage; Coriander seed; Jasmine; Niaouli; Nutmeg; Oregano; Sage; Sandalwood

**frustration:** Blue tansy; German camomile; Neroli; Petitgrain bigarade; Sambac jasmine; Sweet orange; Yarrow; Ylang-ylang

**fungal infections:** Angelica root; Cajeput; Cinnamon bark; Clove bud; Geranium; German camomile; Hyssop; Lavender; Lemon; Lemongrass; Oregano; Palmarosa; Patchouli; Peppermint; Pimenta berry; Rosemary ct. Cineole and ct. Camphor; Saro; Spearmint; Tea tree; Thyme ct. linalool; Vetiver

**furuncles:** Basil ct. methylchavicol; Carrot seed; Clove bud; Laurel; Niaouli; Petitgrain bigarade; Pimenta berry

# G

**gall-stones:** Lemon; Melissa; Niaouli; Peppermint; Roman camomile; Rosemary ct. Cineole and ct. Camphor; Scotch pine

**Gallbladder Qi stagnation:** Peppermint

**gangrene:** Laurel; Myrrh

**gastritis:** Basil ct. methylchavicol; Marjoram; Niaouli; Peppermint; Roman camomile; Tarragon; Thyme ct. linalool

**gastroenteritis:** Angelica root; Black pepper; chronic, Juniper berry; Coriander seed; Hyssop; Lavender; Myrrh; Nutmeg; Oregano; Palmarosa; Patchouli; Peppermint

**gastrointestinal mucus overproduction:** Patchouli

**genital discharges:** Frankincense; Grand fir

**genital herpes:** May chang; Niaouli; Ravintsara; Sage; Sandalwood; Saro

**gingivitis:** Myrrh; Rose

**glands, swollen:** Grapefruit; Laurel; Lemon; Lemongrass; May chang; Niaouli; Ravintsara; Sandalwood; Saro; Scotch pine; Tea tree

**gleet:** Frankincense; Grand fir; Green myrtle; Myrrh

**glomerulonephritis:** Frankincense

**gluten sensitivity:** Ginger; Palmarosa; Patchouli; Tea tree; Vetiver

**glycaemic disorders:** Vetiver

**gonorrhoea:** Grand fir; Myrrh; Winter savoury; Wintergreen

**gout:** Angelica root; Carrot seed; Coriander seed; Fennel; Roman camomile; Scotch pine; Yarrow

**grief:** Coriander seed; Frankincense; Geranium; Ravintsara; Rose; Saro; Siberian fir

**guilt:** Geranium; Jasmine; Mandarin; Roman camomile; Ylang-ylang

**gum inflammation:** Pimenta berry; Roman camomile; Sage

**gums:** spongy, Myrrh; swollen, Frankincense

**gynaecological spasms:** Ylang-ylang

# H

**Haemorrhage:** Rose

**haemorrhoids:** Atlas cedarwood; Basil ct. methylchavicol; bleeding: Cistus; Cypress; Cajeput; Clary sage; Cypress; Geranium; Green myrtle; Lemon; Myrrh; Niaouli; Patchouli; Sandalwood; Spikenard; Tea tree; Yarrow

**hair greying:** Spikenard

**hair growth, poor:** Frankincense; Laurel; Lemon

**hair loss:** Cypress; Fennel; Juniper berry; Pimenta berry; Rosemary ct. Cineole and ct. Camphor; Sage; Spikenard; Yarrow; Ylang-ylang

**halitosis:** Cardamom; Nutmeg

**headaches:** Angelica root; Basil ct. methylchavicol; Blue tansy; chronic: Lemongrass; May chang; Peppermint; Rosemary ct. Cineole and ct. Camphor; Rosemary ct. verbenone; Coriander seed; Eucalyptus; Fennel; Laurel; Lemon; Lemongrass; Marjoram; May chang; Melissa; Neroli; Nutmeg; Palmarosa; Patchouli; Peppermint; Pimenta berry; Rose; Rosemary ct. verbenone; Spikenard; Tarragon; tension and vascular: Helichrysum; Marjoram; Roman camomile; Wintergreen; Yarrow

**hearing loss:** Helichrysum

**heart, nervous:** Sweet orange

**Heart and Kidney Yin deficiency:** with empty heat and Shen agitation, Marjoram; with Shen agitation: Sandalwood; Spikenard; Vetiver

**Heart and Liver Blood deficiency:** Carrot seed

**Heart and Liver Qi constraint:** with Shen agitation: Basil ct. methylchavicol; Lime; Sambac jasmine; Tarragon; with Shen dysregulation: Neroli; Petitgrain bigarade; Sweet orange

**Heart and Lung Qi deficiency, with Shen weakness:** Frankincense; Rosemary ct. verbenone; Tea tree

**Heart Blood and Qi deficiency, with Shen weakness:** Palmarosa

**Heart Blood and Qi stagnation:** Helichrysum; Wintergreen

**Heart Blood and Spleen Qi deficiency, with Shen weakness:** Palmarosa

**Heart Blood deficiency:** Clary sage; with Shen disharmony: Cardamom; Petitgrain bigarade; with Shen weakness: Coriander seed; Jasmine; Neroli; Rose; Ylang-ylang

**Heart fire:** May chang; with Shen agitation: Lemon eucalyptus; Lime; Melissa; Neroli

**Heart Qi and Blood deficiency, with stagnation:** Sandalwood

**Heart Qi constraint:** with Shen dysregulation: Fennel; Rose; Rosemary ct. verbenone; Spikenard; Ylang-ylang

**Heart Qi constraint w/Shen disharmony:** Blue tansy; Geranium; Helichrysum

**Heart Qi deficiency:** Neroli

**Heart Qi/Yang deficiency:** Rosemary ct. Cineole and ct. Camphor

**heart weakness:** Fennel; Lavender; Myrrh; Nutmeg; Tea tree

**Heart Yin deficiency, with Shen agitation:** Blue tansy; German camomile; Lavender; Marjoram; Melissa; Neroli; Patchouli; Rose; Sambac jasmine

**heartburn:** Cardamom

**heavy legs:** Basil ct. methylchavicol; Spikenard

**heavy menses:** Basil ct. methylchavicol; Cistus; with clots, Yarrow; Cypress; Rose; Scotch pine

**helplessness:** Clove bud

**hematomas:** Lavender

**hepatitis:** Basil ct. methylchavicol; Carrot seed; Clove bud; Helichrysum; Peppermint; Petitgrain bigarade; Pimenta berry; Rosemary ct. Cineole and ct. Camphor; Rosemary ct. verbenone; Scotch pine; Tarragon

**herpes simplex:** Bergamot; Clove bud; Lemon eucalyptus; Lemongrass; May chang; Melissa; Peppermint; Rose; Sandalwood; Tea tree

**herpes zoster/shingles:** Bergamot; Ravintsara; Thyme ct. thymol

**hiccups:** Cajeput; Mandarin; Spearmint; Tarragon

**hidden virus syndrome, Rosemary ct. verbenone**

**HIV:** Cistus

**hoarseness:** Jasmine

**hookworm:** Black spruce; Fennel; Roman camomile; Thyme ct. thymol

**hopelessness:** Clove bud

**hormonal disorders:** Clary sage; Geranium; Jasmine; Niaouli; Palmarosa; Rose; Rosemary ct. verbenone; Sage; Scotch pine; Vetiver

**hot flashes:** Cardamom; Geranium; Lemon eucalyptus; Lime; May chang; Melissa; Petitgrain bigarade; Rose; Sage; Sambac jasmine; Spikenard; Vetiver; Wintergreen

**HPA axis deficiency:** Niaouli; Sage; Siberian fir

**HPV:** Sage; Saro

**HSDD:** Jasmine

**hyperacidity:** Basil ct. methylchavicol; Tarragon

**hyperhistamine syndrome:** Myrrh

**hyperlipidemia:** Fennel; Helichrysum; Hyssop; Nutmeg; Rosemary ct. Cineole and ct. Camphor; Rosemary ct. verbenone; Sage

**hyperpnoea:** Spikenard; Ylang-ylang

**hypertension:** Blue tansy; Clary sage; Helichrysum; Laurel; Lavender; Lemon eucalyptus; Lemongrass; Lime; Mandarin; Marjoram; May chang; Melissa; Neroli; Palmarosa; Rose; Spikenard; Sweet orange; Wintergreen; Ylang-ylang

**hyperthyroid conditions:** Marjoram; Melissa; Myrrh; Neroli; Petitgrain bigarade

**hyperviscous blood:** Lemon

**hypochlorhydria:** Juniper berry

**hypoglycaemia:** Geranium; Palmarosa; Scotch pine; Vetiver

**hypomania:** Clary sage; Lavender; Marjoram

**hypotension:** Carrot seed; Clove bud; Grand fir; Hyssop; Oregano; Palmarosa; Peppermint; Pimenta berry; Rosemary ct. Cineole and ct. Camphor; Sage; Scotch pine; Thyme ct. thymol; Winter savoury

**hypothermia:** Cinnamon bark

**hypothyroid syndrome:** Black spruce; Carrot seed; Clove bud; Pimenta berry; Sage

**hysteria:** Vetiver

# I

**IBS:** atonic, Juniper berry; Blue tansy; Cinnamon bark; Clary sage; Fennel; Geranium; German camomile; Ginger; Helichrysum; Lemongrass; Marjoram; May chang; Melissa; mucous colitis-type, Patchouli; Neroli; Oregano; Petitgrain bigarade; Roman camomile; Rosemary ct. verbenone; Siberian fir; spasmodic: Angelica root; Basil ct. methylchavicol; Clove bud; Peppermint; Pimenta berry; Tarragon; Ylang-ylang; Spikenard

**immune deficiency:** chronic, Ravintsara; Cistus; Clove bud; Frankincense; Rosemary ct. verbenone; Sage; Tea tree; Thyme ct. linalool; Vetiver

**immune stress:** Ginger

**immunodeficiency disorders:** Black spruce

**impotence:** with anxiety, Ylang-ylang; Black pepper; Black spruce; Cinnamon bark; Clove bud; Ginger; Jasmine; Niaouli; Nutmeg; Oregano; Sandalwood; Vetiver; Winter savoury

**impulsivity:** German camomile; Roman camomile; Sambac jasmine

**indecision:** Angelica root; Black spruce; Cajeput; Cypress; Green myrtle; Juniper berry; Oregano; Ravintsara; Saro; Siberian fir; Thyme ct. thymol

**indigestion:** atonic: Black pepper; Cypress; Hyssop; Nutmeg; Winter savoury; Yarrow; Black pepper; with bloating: Green myrtle; Pimenta berry; with bloating and constipation, Cinnamon bark; with bloating and flatulence: Coriander seed; Fennel; Cardamom; Carrot seed; chronic with bloating: Angelica root; Juniper berry; Hyssop; Lemon eucalyptus; Myrrh; Neroli; nervous: Basil ct. methylchavicol; Blue tansy; Cardamom; Marjoram; with pain and bloating, Basil ct. methylchavicol; Rosemary ct. verbenone; upper: Grapefruit; Lemongrass; worse stress: Laurel; Mandarin; Petitgrain bigarade; Yarrow

**infections:** chronic/recurrent: Cinnamon bark; Niaouli; Ravintsara; Saro; Tea tree; Thyme ct. thymol; Winter savoury; proneness to, Thyme ct. linalool; Tea tree

**infertility:** Clary sage; Geranium; Jasmine; Rose; Sage

**inflammatory bowel disease:** Cistus; Frankincense; Helichrysum; Lemon eucalyptus; Lemongrass; May chang; Melissa; Palmarosa; Spikenard; Tea tree; Yarrow

**influenza:** Basil ct. methylchavicol; Cajeput; Coriander seed; Melissa; Pimenta berry

**inhibition:** Patchouli; Sandalwood

**insect bites:** Atlas cedarwood; Basil ct. methylchavicol; Bergamot; Clove bud; Eucalyptus; German camomile; Lemon; Niaouli; Roman camomile; Sandalwood; Thyme ct. linalool; Winter savoury

**insecurity:** Black pepper; Cardamom; Carrot seed; Cistus; Clove bud; Frankincense; Geranium; Jasmine; Laurel; Myrrh; Nutmeg; Palmarosa; Patchouli; Pimenta berry; Ravintsara;

Rose; Sandalwood; Saro; Spikenard; Vetiver; Wintergreen; Ylang-ylang

**insight, poor emotional:** Grand fir; Lemon eucalyptus; Melissa; Neroli; Peppermint; Yarrow

**insomnia:** Angelica root; Blue tansy; Cardamom; Cistus; Clary sage; German camomile; Green myrtle; Lavender; Lemon; Lemon eucalyptus; Lime; Marjoram; Melissa; Neroli; Palmarosa; Patchouli; Petitgrain bigarade; Ravintsara; Roman camomile; Rose; Saro; Spearmint; Spikenard; stress-related, Mandarin; Sweet orange; Vetiver; Wintergreen; Ylang-ylang

**insulin resistance:** Juniper berry

**interstitial cystitis:** Lemon eucalyptus; Wintergreen; Yarrow

**intestinal dysbiosis:** Cinnamon bark; Clove bud; Coriander seed; Juniper berry; Laurel; Lemon; Lemongrass; May chang; Myrrh; Nutmeg; Palmarosa; Patchouli; Pimenta berry; Sage; Tea tree; Thyme ct. linalool

**intestinal fermentation:** Clove bud; Coriander seed; Laurel; Nutmeg; Pimenta berry; Sage

**intestinal hyperpermeability:** Helichrysum; Lemon; Palmarosa; Patchouli; Tea tree; Thyme ct. linalool; Vetiver; Yarrow

**intestinal spasms:** German camomile

**irregular menses:** Geranium; Niaouli; Rosemary ct. verbenone; Yarrow; Ylang-ylang

**irritability:** Bergamot; Blue tansy; Clary sage; Geranium; German camomile; Hyssop; Lavender; Lemon eucalyptus; Mandarin; Marjoram; Melissa; Neroli; Petitgrain bigarade; Roman camomile; Rose; Rosemary ct. verbenone; Sambac jasmine; Sweet orange; Yarrow; Ylang-ylang

**isolation:** Ylang-ylang

**itching:** German camomile; Melissa; Wintergreen

# J

**jaundice:** Carrot seed; Peppermint; Rosemary ct. Cineole and ct. Camphor

**jealousy:** Rose

**jet lag:** Geranium

**jock itch:** Lemongrass; Palmarosa; Pimenta berry

**joint aches:** acute, Lime; Cajeput; Melissa

**joint subluxations:** Vetiver

# K

**kidney colic:** Lemon; Peppermint

**kidney disorders:** Carrot seed

**Kidney Essence deficiency:** Black spruce

**Kidney fire:** Wintergreen

**Kidney Qi deficiency:** Myrrh; Sandalwood

**kidney TB:** Thyme ct. linalool

**Kidney Yang deficiency:** Black spruce; Cinnamon bark; Clove bud; Ginger; with Shen weakens, Scotch pine; with Shen weakness: Black pepper; Nutmeg; Pimenta berry; Thyme ct. thymol; Winter savoury

**Kidney Yin deficiency, with Shen agitation:** Patchouli

**Kidney-Bladder heat:** Lemon eucalyptus; with Lower Warmer damp, Wintergreen

**Kidney-Bladder Qi deficiency w/Lower Warmer damp:** Atlas cedarwood; Myrrh; Sandalwood

# L

**Labour, difficult/stalled:** Lavender; failure to progress: Angelica root; Clove bud; Fennel; Myrrh; Nutmeg; Pimenta berry; Sage

**labour pains:** Clary sage; Fennel; Jasmine; Niaouli

**lactation:** excessive: Clary sage; Geranium; Jasmine; Peppermint; Sage; Fennel; insufficient, Jasmine; scanty or absent, Lemongrass

**Large Intestine damp-cold:** Black spruce; Cistus, Myrrh

**Large Intestine damp-heat:** Cistus; Lemongrass; Lime; May chang; Melissa; Sandalwood

**laryngitis:** Bergamot; Lemon eucalyptus; Palmarosa; Peppermint; Sage; Scotch pine; Spearmint

**late menses:** Hyssop

**laughing, excessive:** Ylang-ylang

**leprosy:** Hyssop; Niaouli

**lethargy:** Basil ct. methylchavicol; Black pepper; Carrot seed; Cypress; Eucalyptus; Ginger; Grand fir; Green myrtle; Hyssop; Juniper berry; morning: Spearmint; Yarrow; Niaouli; Oregano; Ravintsara; Rosemary ct. Cineole and ct. Camphor; Rosemary ct. verbenone; Saro; Tarragon; Thyme ct. linalool; Thyme ct. thymol; Winter savoury

**letting go, difficulty:** Hyssop; Spikenard; Thyme ct. linalool; Vetiver

**leucorrhoea:** Cinnamon bark; Frankincense; Grand fir; Green myrtle; Jasmine; Juniper berry; Myrrh; Rosemary ct. verbenone; Sage; Sandalwood; Saro; Thyme ct. thymol; Wintergreen

**libido, low:** Black pepper; Cinnamon bark; Clove bud; Ginger; Jasmine; Neroli; Niaouli; Nutmeg; Oregano; Patchouli; Pimenta berry; Rose; Rosemary ct. verbenone; Sandalwood; Scotch pine; Thyme ct. thymol; Vetiver; Winter savoury; Ylang-ylang

**lice:** Black spruce; Cinnamon bark; Clove bud; Geranium; Laurel; Lemongrass; May chang; Niaouli; Oregano; Patchouli; Tea tree; Thyme ct. thymol; Wintergreen

**lichen plana:** Niaouli

**listlessness:** Cinnamon bark; Frankincense; Grapefruit; Jasmine; Lemon; Lemon eucalyptus; Neroli; Niaouli; Nutmeg; Thyme ct. linalool; Vetiver; Winter savoury

**Liver -Stomach disharmony:** Basil ct. methylchavicol; Cardamom; Fennel; German camomile; Lavender; Melissa; Neroli; Petitgrain bigarade; Sweet orange; Tarragon

**Liver -Stomach disharmony/Qi stagnation:** Bergamot; Blue tansy

**Liver and Heart Qi constraint, with Shen disharmony:** Bergamot; Mandarin; Marjoram; Melissa; Ylang-ylang

**Liver and Uterus Qi constraint:** Clary sage; Lavender; Melissa; Roman camomile; Tarragon

**Liver Blood deficiency, with Shen weakness:** Geranium; Jasmine; Rose; Ylang-ylang

**liver congestion:** Basil ct. methylchavicol; Carrot seed; Geranium; German camomile; Grapefruit; Green myrtle; Helichrysum; Lavender; Lemon; Melissa; Niaouli; Peppermint; Petitgrain bigarade; Rose; Rosemary ct. Cineole and ct. Camphor; Rosemary ct. verbenone; Wintergreen; Yarrow

**liver disease:** Basil ct. methylchavicol; Carrot seed

**Liver fire, with Shen agitation:** Lemon eucalyptus; Lime; May chang

**Liver Qi constraint:** Ylang-ylang

**Liver Qi constraint, with Shen disharmony:** Mandarin; Roman camomile; Spearmint; turning to fire, Lemongrass

**Liver Qi constraint w/Shen disharmony:** Bergamot; Helichrysum

**Liver Qi stagnation,** German camomile; turning to fire, May chang

**liver toxicosis:** Ginger

**Liver wind, internal:** Basil ct. methylchavicol; Clary sage; German camomile; Marjoram; Roman camomile; Tarragon

**Liver Yang rising:** Basil ct. methylchavicol; German camomile; with heat, Wintergreen; Marjoram; Roman camomile; with Shen agitation, Clary sage; Tarragon

**Liver Yin deficiency:** with floating Yang: Spikenard; Vetiver; with internal wind: Spikenard; Vetiver; with Shen agitation: Blue tansy; German camomile; Helichrysum; Roman camomile; Sambac jasmine; Vetiver

**Liver-Spleen disharmony:** Blue tansy; Cardamom; Cypress; Fennel; German camomile; Lavender; Lime; Marjoram; Melissa; Neroli; Petitgrain bigarade; Roman camomile; with Shen agitation, Basil ct. methylchavicol; with Shen dysregulation, Angelica root; Sweet orange; Tarragon; Ylang-ylang

**Liver-Stomach disharmony:** Mandarin; Spearmint

**lochial retention:** Ginger

**low back weakness:** Cinnamon bark; Saro

**low-back pain:** Fennel; Juniper berry; Wintergreen

**Lower Warmer Blood and Qi stagnation:** Cinnamon bark; with cold: Clove bud; Pimenta berry; Thyme ct. thymol; with internal cold, Angelica root; Juniper berry; Laurel; Lavender; Marjoram; Myrrh; Nutmeg; Oregano; Winter savoury; Wintergreen; Yarrow

**Lower Warmer Blood stagnation:** Basil ct. methylchavicol; Clary sage; Geranium; Green myrtle; Sandalwood; Yarrow

**Lower Warmer damp-cold:** Black spruce; Geranium; Sage; Thyme ct. thymol

**Lower Warmer damp-heat:** Eucalyptus; Sandalwood

**Lower Warmer turbid-damp:** Fennel; Green myrtle; Juniper berry; Yarrow

**lumbar pain:** Black pepper

**lung abscess:** Laurel

**Lung and Heart Qi deficiency, with Shen weakness:** Eucalyptus

**Lung and Kidney Yang deficiency:** Black spruce; Scotch pine

**Lung dryness:** Ravintsara

**Lung heat:** Lavender

**Lung phlegm-cold:** Angelica root; Black pepper; Cajeput; Cardamom; Frankincense; Ginger; Grand fir; Hyssop; Laurel; with Lung Qi deficiency, Green myrtle; Niaouli; with Qi accumulation: Fennel; Oregano; Thyme ct. thymol; Ravintsara; Rosemary ct. Cineole and ct. Camphor; Saro; Siberian fir; Winter savoury

**Lung phlegm-damp:** Angelica root; Atlas cedarwood; Black pepper; Cardamom; Cistus; Frankincense; Ginger; Green myrtle; Hyssop; Myrrh; Niaouli; with Qi accumulation, Sage; Rosemary ct. verbenone; Scotch pine

**Lung phlegm-dryness:** Eucalyptus; Helichrysum; Hyssop

**Lung phlegm-heat:** Eucalyptus; Hyssop; Lemon eucalyptus; Ravintsara

**Lung phlegm-heat-dryness:** Saro

**Lung phlegm-heat/damp:** Spearmint

**Lung Qi accumulation:** Basil ct. methylchavicol; Cypress; Frankincense; Helichrysum; Hyssop; Laurel; Lavender; Marjoram; Melissa; Oregano; Petitgrain bigarade; Sage; Siberian fir; Tarragon; Thyme ct. linalool; Thyme ct. thymol; with wheezing/cough, Blue tansy; Winter savoury

**Lung Qi deficiency:** Cypress; Hyssop; Scotch pine; Thyme ct. linalool

**Lung Qi deficiency w/Shen weakness:** Black spruce

**lung weakness:** Frankincense

**Lung wind-cold:** Cajeput; Grand fir; Hyssop; Laurel; Niaouli; Ravintsara; Sage; Saro; Siberian fir

**Lung wind-heat:** Eucalyptus; Helichrysum; Hyssop; Lavender

**Lung Yin deficiency:** Sandalwood; Tea tree; Thyme ct. linalool

**Lungs phlegm-cold:** Laurel

**lupus:** Frankincense

**lymph swellings:** Cypress; Lemongrass; Ravintsara

**lymphatic congestion:** Atlas cedarwood; Cypress; Grapefruit; Laurel; Lemongrass; May chang; Scotch pine

**lymphedema:** Niaouli

## M

**mania:** Melissa

**mastitis:** Fennel

**measles:** Cistus; Coriander seed

**memory problems:** Lemon; Nutmeg; Rosemary ct. Cineole and ct. Camphor; short-term: Cajeput; Eucalyptus; Grapefruit; Lemongrass; May chang; Niaouli; Peppermint; Ravintsara; Rosemary ct. Cineole and ct. Camphor; Sage; Saro

**meningitis:** Sage

**menopausal syndrome:** Black spruce; Clary sage; Cypress; Fennel; Geranium; Neroli; Niaouli; Petitgrain bigarade; Rose; Rosemary ct. verbenone; Scotch pine; Vetiver; Yarrow; Ylang-ylang

**menorrhagia:** Cistus; Cypress; Geranium; Rose; Scotch pine; Ylang-ylang

**menses, clots in:** Scotch pine

**menstrual disorders:** Black spruce; long cycles, Rosemary ct. verbenone; Niaouli; with pain, Cajeput; Rose; Sage; Scotch pine; Yarrow

**menstrual flooding:** Cistus

**mental fatigue:** Black spruce; Lemon; Lemongrass; May chang

**mental focus, loss of:** Cardamom

**mental hyperactivity:** Sandalwood

**metabolic toxicosis:** Angelica root; Black pepper; Carrot seed; Coriander seed; Cypress; Geranium; Grapefruit; Helichrysum; Juniper berry; Lemon; Lemongrass; May chang; Palmarosa; Rose; Rosemary ct. verbenone; Scotch pine; Tea tree; Thyme ct. linalool; Winter savoury; Yarrow

**metritis:** Thyme ct. linalool

**metrorrhagia:** Cinnamon bark; Cistus; Cypress

**migraine:** Angelica root; Coriander seed; Eucalyptus; Marjoram; Melissa; Roman camomile; Rose; Spikenard; Vetiver

**miscarriage, habitual:** Rosemary ct. verbenone; Yarrow

**mononucleosis:** Ravintsara

**mood swings:** Basil ct. methylchavicol; Bergamot; Cardamom; Coriander seed; Fennel; Geranium; Grapefruit; Green myrtle; Hyssop; Laurel; Lavender; Mandarin; Neroli; Palmarosa; Peppermint; Petitgrain bigarade; Roman camomile;

Rose; Sambac jasmine; Spearmint; Sweet orange; Tarragon; Thyme ct. linalool; Yarrow; Ylang-ylang

**moralizing:** Sandalwood

**morbid thoughts:** Grapefruit

**morning sickness:** Melissa; Nutmeg

**mosquito repellant:** Basil ct. methylchavicol; Cajeput; Cinnamon bark; Clove bud; Lemongrass; May chang; Pimenta berry

**motion sickness:** Cardamom; Nutmeg

**motivation, poor:** Black pepper; Carrot seed; Cinnamon bark; Clove bud; Coriander seed; Ginger; Grand fir; Juniper berry; Nutmeg; Saro; Scotch pine; Thyme ct. thymol; worse morning: Melissa; Niaouli

**mouth ulcers:** Rose; Sage; Sweet orange

**MRSA:** Niaouli; Sandalwood; Thyme ct. thymol

**mucus overproduction:** Green myrtle; Sandalwood

**multiple sclerosis:** Basil ct. methylchavicol; Clove bud; Hyssop; Laurel; Niaouli; Sage; Scotch pine; Yarrow

**muscle aches:** Angelica root; Black pepper; Black spruce; Cajeput; Cistus; Cypress; Frankincense; Ginger; Grand fir; Juniper berry; Lemon eucalyptus; Lemongrass; Marjoram; Niaouli; Pimenta berry; Roman camomile; Sage; Saro; Scotch pine; Siberian fir; Wintergreen; Yarrow

**muscle spasms:** Basil ct. methylchavicol; Cardamom; Cypress; Fennel; Juniper berry; Laurel; Rosemary ct. Cineole and ct. Camphor; Tarragon; Ylang-ylang

**muscle tension:** Clary sage

**muscle tone, poor:** Lemongrass; Sweet orange

**muscle weakness:** Ravintsara; Saro

**muscular weakness:** Ravintsara

# N

**nail fungus:** Lemongrass; Palmarosa; Pimenta berry; Saro; Thyme ct. linalool

**nappy rash:** Palmarosa

**nausea:** Basil ct. methylchavicol; Black pepper; Cardamom; Ginger; Laurel; Mandarin; Melissa; Patchouli; Spearmint; Tarragon

**neediness:** Geranium; Helichrysum

**nephritis:** Coriander seed; Grand fir; Pimenta berry; Scotch pine; Thyme ct. linalool; Wintergreen

**nerve pains, shooting:** Blue tansy; German camomile; Roman camomile; Wintergreen

**nervous breakdown:** Basil ct. methylchavicol; Cardamom; Marjoram; Neroli; Sandalwood; Vetiver

**nervous exhaustion:** Carrot seed; Coriander seed; Neroli

**nervous tension:** Angelica root; with fatigue, Clary sage; German camomile; Lavender; Mandarin; Marjoram; Neroli; Petitgrain bigarade; Sambac jasmine; Sandalwood; Spikenard; Sweet orange; Ylang-ylang

**neuralgia:** Basil ct. methylchavicol; Black pepper; Blue tansy; Coriander seed; Eucalyptus; Fennel; Helichrysum; Juniper berry; Marjoram; Palmarosa; Peppermint; Pimenta berry; Roman camomile; Sandalwood; Tarragon; Yarrow

**neurasthenia:** Angelica root; Basil ct. methylchavicol; Carrot seed; Clary sage; Clove bud; Frankincense; Grand fir; Grapefruit; Green myrtle; Hyssop; Lemon; Neroli; Niaouli; Nutmeg; Palmarosa; Ravintsara; Rose; Rosemary ct. Cineole and ct. Camphor; Scotch pine; Siberian fir; Tea tree; Thyme ct. thymol; Vetiver

**neurocardiac syndrome:** Spikenard

**neurodegenerative disorders:** Basil ct. methylchavicol; Hyssop; Laurel; Niaouli; Sage; Scotch pine; Yarrow

**neurogenic bladder:** Cypress; Marjoram; Melissa; Tarragon

**night sweats:** Sage

**nightmares:** Lemon; Rose; Spikenard

**nipple soreness:** Frankincense

**nipples, cracked:** Roman camomile

**nosebleeds:** Cistus; Geranium; Lemon

# O

**obesity, abdominal:** Grapefruit

**obsessive-compulsive disorders:** Atlas cedarwood; Carrot seed; Myrrh; Neroli; Patchouli; Sambac jasmine; Sandalwood; Spikenard; Vetiver

**oedema, ankle and leg:** Cypress; Sandalwood; Yarrow; Black pepper; Carrot seed; Fennel; Grapefruit; Scotch pine; Sweet orange; Yarrow

**oestrogen accumulation syndrome:** Clove bud; Yarrow

**oestrogen deficiency:** Clary sage; Cypress; Fennel; Niaouli; Rose; Sage; Scotch pine

**oligomenorrhoea:** Angelica root; Clove bud; Fennel; Frankincense; Ginger; Green myrtle; Hyssop; Myrrh; Niaouli; Nutmeg; Oregano; Pimenta berry; Rosemary ct. Cineole and ct. Camphor; Sage; Spikenard; Thyme ct. thymol; Vetiver; Yarrow

**oliguria:** Black pepper; Sage; Spearmint

**orchitis:** Roman camomile

**osteoarthritis:** Laurel

**otitis:** Green myrtle; Marjoram; Palmarosa; Yarrow

**otorrhoea:** Jasmine

**ovarian cysts:** Cypress; May chang

**ovarian pain:** Cajeput; Roman camomile

**oversensitivity:** Angelica root; Black pepper; Blue tansy; Carrot seed; Clove bud; German camomile; Myrrh; Patchouli; Pimenta berry; Roman camomile; Vetiver

**overstimulation:** Spearmint

**overweight:** Atlas cedarwood

**overwhelm:** Cistus; Niaouli

**ovulation pain:** Clary sage

# P

**painful conditions:** acute and chronic, Marjoram; Helichrysum; Lemon; Roman camomile

**palpitations:** with chest pains, Spikenard; Cinnamon bark; Fennel; Lavender; Lemon eucalyptus; Lemongrass; Lime; Mandarin; Marjoram; May chang; Melissa; Neroli; Palmarosa; Petitgrain bigarade; Rosemary ct. verbenone; severe, Ylang-ylang; Spikenard; Sweet orange; Tarragon

**pancreatic weakness:** Neroli; Vetiver

**pancreatitis:** Black pepper; Nutmeg; Peppermint; Roman camomile

**panic attacks:** Blue tansy; Clary sage; German camomile; Lavender; Marjoram; Roman camomile; Sambac jasmine

**paralysis:** Laurel; Marjoram; temporary, Black pepper

**paranoia:** Angelica root; Carrot seed; Myrrh; Patchouli; Pimenta berry; Spikenard; Vetiver; Wintergreen

**parasites:** Bergamot; Black spruce; Cajeput; Clove bud; Coriander seed; Eucalyptus; Fennel; Hyssop; Lavender; Lemongrass; Neroli; Nutmeg; Pimenta berry; Tarragon; Tea tree; Thyme ct. linalool; Thyme ct. thymol

**Parkinson's disease:** Yarrow

**pelvic congestion:** Basil ct. methylchavicol; Cajeput; Cistus; Geranium; Green myrtle; Lemon; Niaouli; Rose; Rosemary ct. Cineole and ct. Camphor; Yarrow

**pelvic inflammatory disease:** Lemon eucalyptus; Yarrow

**pelvic pain, dragging:** Yarrow

**pericarditis:** Lemon eucalyptus

**perineal tears:** Vetiver

**periodontal disease:** Sage

**peripheral vasoconstriction:** Helichrysum

**perseverance, poor:** Angelica root; Cistus; Cypress; Frankincense; Green myrtle; Scotch pine; Vetiver

**pessimism:** Basil ct. methylchavicol; Cardamom; Carrot seed; Eucalyptus; Fennel; Grand fir; Grapefruit; Green myrtle; Hyssop; Jasmine; Lemon; Lemon eucalyptus; Lemongrass; Lime; May chang; Melissa; Neroli; Niaouli; Oregano; Rosemary ct. Cineole and ct. Camphor; Rosemary ct. verbenone; Sambac jasmine; Sweet orange; Thyme ct. thymol

**pharyngitis:** Marjoram; Scotch pine; Spearmint

**phlebitis:** Basil ct. methylchavicol; Blue tansy; Cistus; Geranium; Helichrysum; Lavender; Lemon; Spikenard; Yarrow

**phobias:** Blue tansy; Clary sage; German camomile; Lavender; Marjoram; Melissa; Nutmeg; Palmarosa; Roman camomile; Sambac jasmine

**pinworm:** Cinnamon bark; Eucalyptus

**pityriasis:** Wintergreen

**placenta, retained:** Angelica root; Lavender; Myrrh

**plan, inability to:** Grand fir; Lemon; Lemon eucalyptus; Lemongrass; Lime; May chang

**plantar fasciitis:** Blue tansy; Marjoram; Peppermint; Roman camomile; Rosemary ct. Cineole and ct. Camphor

**pleurisy:** Basil ct. methylchavicol; Clove bud; Lemon eucalyptus; Neroli; Niaouli; Oregano; Tarragon

**PMS:** Blue tansy; Clary sage; Fennel; Geranium; German camomile; Jasmine; Neroli; Rose; Sage; Sambac jasmine; Scotch pine; Vetiver; Ylang-ylang

**pneumonia:** Eucalyptus; Hyssop; Lemon eucalyptus; Thyme ct. linalool

**poliomyelitis:** Basil ct. methylchavicol; Clove bud; Pimenta berry

**polyarthritis:** Helichrysum

**pores, enlarged:** May chang

**post-antibiotic use:** Thyme ct. linalool

**post-hysterectomy syndrome:** Rose

**post-traumatic stress disorder (PTSD):** Blue tansy; Clary sage; German camomile; Helichrysum; Jasmine; Lavender; Marjoram; Patchouli; Roman camomile; Sambac jasmine

**postpartum convalescence:** Angelica root; Coriander seed; Jasmine; Laurel; Petitgrain bigarade

**postpartum depression:** Clove bud; Neroli; Rose; Yarrow

**precordial pain:** Angelica root; Fennel; Lime; Melissa; Neroli; Tarragon; Ylang-ylang

**prediabetes:** Sage

**premature ejaculation:** Myrrh; Vetiver

**procrastination:** Angelica root; Cistus; Lemon; Lemongrass; Lime; Niaouli; Ravintsara; Rosemary ct. Cineole and ct. Camphor; Siberian fir

**progesterone deficiency:** Cinnamon bark; Coriander seed; Niaouli; Rose; Rosemary ct. verbenone; Scotch pine; Winter savoury

**prostate adenoma:** Cypress

**prostate hyperplasia:** Black spruce; Cajeput

**prostatitis:** Basil ct. methylchavicol; Black spruce; Carrot seed; Grand fir; Myrrh; Niaouli; Peppermint; Scotch pine; Tarragon; Thyme ct. linalool; Winter savoury; Wintergreen; Yarrow

**protective Qi deficiency:** Black spruce; Laurel; Niaouli; Ravintsara

**pruritis:** Helichrysum; Myrrh; Palmarosa

**psoriasis:** Carrot seed; Frankincense; Geranium; Helichrysum; Juniper berry; Myrrh; Niaouli; Spikenard; Thyme ct. linalool; Thyme ct. thymol

**psychotic conditions:** Angelica root; Black spruce; Cistus; Clove bud; Cypress; Frankincense; Ginger; Juniper berry; Marjoram; Melissa; Pimenta berry; Siberian fir; Spikenard

# Q

**Qi and Blood stagnation:** Frankincense

**Qi constraint:** with allergies, Helichrysum; with pain: Angelica root; Blue tansy; German camomile; with Shen agitation: Angelica root; Basil ct. methylchavicol; with Shen dysregulation: Sweet orange; Tarragon; turning to heat w/Shen disharmony: Blue tansy; German camomile; Lime; Marjoram; Melissa; Sambac jasmine; turning to heat with Shen dysregulation, Lavender

**Qi deficiency:** Black spruce; with Shen dysregulation, Green myrtle; with Shen weakness: Cypress; Frankincense; Grand fir; Hyssop; Laurel; Niaouli; Ravintsara; Rosemary ct. Cineole and ct. Camphor; Rosemary ct. verbenone; Sage; Saro; Scotch pine; Siberian fir; Tea tree; Thyme ct. linalool

**Qi stagnation:** Peppermint

# R

**radiation exposure:** Cajeput; Niaouli; Tea tree; Yarrow

**rage:** Blue tansy; German camomile

**rashes:** Melissa

**Raynaud's phenomenon:** Cinnamon bark; Helichrysum; Laurel; Wintergreen

**rectal prolapse:** Myrrh

**red complexion, hot spells with:** Vetiver

**resentment:** Sambac jasmine

**resignation:** Atlas cedarwood

**respiratory problems:** acute and chronic, Cajeput; Angelica root

**restlesness:** German camomile; Lavender; Marjoram; Roman camomile; Sambac jasmine; Spikenard; Ylang-ylang

**rheumatic conditions:** Angelica root; Black pepper; Black spruce; chronic, Cajeput; Clove bud; Coriander seed; Cypress; Eucalyptus; Frankincense; Geranium; Ginger; Grand fir; Grapefruit; Juniper berry; Laurel; Lavender; Lemon; Lemongrass; May chang; Melissa; Nutmeg; Oregano; Palmarosa; Petitgrain bigarade; Pimenta berry; Ravintsara; Roman camomile; Rosemary ct. Cineole and ct. Camphor; Sage; Scotch pine; Siberian fir; Tarragon; Tea tree; Thyme ct. linalool; Vetiver; Winter savoury; Wintergreen; Yarrow

**rheumatoid arthritis:** Basil ct. methylchavicol; Coriander seed; Frankincense; Ginger; Niaouli; Tarragon; Thyme ct. thymol; Winter savoury

**rhinitis:** allergic: German camomile; Helichrysum; Cajeput; Green myrtle; Hyssop; Niaouli; Rosemary ct. Cineole and ct. Camphor; Rosemary ct. verbenone; Sage; Spearmint; Tea tree

**rigidity:** Roman camomile; Rose; Sambac jasmine; Yarrow

**ringworm:** Geranium; Lemon eucalyptus; Lemongrass; Myrrh; Palmarosa; Patchouli; Peppermint; Petitgrain bigarade; Pimenta berry; Sandalwood; Spearmint; Vetiver

**rosacea:** Carrot seed; Geranium; Rosemary ct. verbenone

**roundworms:** Cajeput; Cinnamon bark; Eucalyptus; Tea tree; Winter savoury

**routine, habitual:** Niaouli

**rumination:** Hyssop

# S

**Sadness:** Green myrtle

**safety, loss of:** Myrrh

**salpingitis:** Pimenta berry; Thyme ct. linalool

**salt cravings:** Geranium; Rosemary ct. Cineole and ct. Camphor; Scotch pine; Siberian fir

**SARS:** Clove bud

**scabies:** Black spruce; Thyme ct. thymol

**scanty menses:** Clary sage; Fennel; Myrrh; painful, Angelica root

**scarlet fever:** Cistus

**scars:** Carrot seed; Cistus; Coriander seed; Frankincense; Hyssop; Jasmine; Mandarin; Myrrh; Palmarosa; Patchouli; Rosemary ct. verbenone; Sage

**scattered thinking:** Angelica root; Myrrh; Sandalwood

**schizoid conditions:** Angelica root; Black spruce; Cinnamon bark; Cistus; Clove bud; Cypress; Frankincense; Ginger; Juniper berry; Palmarosa; Pimenta berry; Spikenard

**sciatica:** Angelica root; Basil ct. methylchavicol; Black pepper; Fennel; Laurel; Marjoram; Nutmeg; Sandalwood; Scotch pine; Tarragon; Wintergreen; Yarrow

**seborrhoea:** Bergamot; Eucalyptus; Niaouli; Patchouli; Petitgrain bigarade; Rosemary ct. verbenone; Ylang-ylang

**seizures:** Basil ct. methylchavicol; in children, Clary sage; epileptic, Marjoram; German camomile; Neroli; Rose; Spikenard; Tarragon; Ylang-ylang

**self-assertion, loss of:** Wintergreen

**self-deprecation:** Yarrow

**self-destructiveness:** Jasmine; Rose; Sambac jasmine; Wintergreen; Ylang-ylang

**self-esteem, low:** Black pepper; Blue tansy; Cajeput; Cardamom; Cinnamon bark; Cistus; Clove bud; Cypress; Fennel; Geranium; Ginger; Grand fir; Green myrtle; Juniper berry; Laurel; Niaouli; Nutmeg; Oregano; Pimenta berry; Ravintsara; Rose; Rosemary ct. Cineole and ct. Camphor; Rosemary ct. verbenone; Sage; Sandalwood; Saro; Scotch pine; Siberian fir; Thyme ct. thymol; Winter savoury; Ylang-ylang

**self-esteem,low:** Atlas cedarwood; Black spruce

**self-expression, poor:** Green myrtle

**self-loathing:** Ylang-**ylang**

**self-neglect:** Black pepper; Cistus; Grand fir; Niaouli; Nutmeg; Oregano; Pimenta berry; Ravintsara; Saro; Scotch pine; Thyme ct. thymol; Winter savoury; Wintergreen

**self-sabotaging tendencies:** Sambac jasmine

**seminal emissions:** Myrrh; Sandalwood

**sensory integration disorder:** Cinnamon bark; Jasmine; Patchouli; Sandalwood; Ylang-ylang

**sensory-emotional inhibition:** Patchouli

**sepsis:** Laurel; Niaouli

**sexual anxiety:** Neroli; Patchouli; Sandalwood

**sexual disinterest:** Clary sage; Neroli; Patchouli

**sexual inhibition:** Jasmine; Sandalwood; Ylang-ylang

**sexual overstimulation:** Marjoram; Myrrh; Sage; Wintergreen

**shame:** Hyssop; Jasmine; Rose; Rosemary ct. verbenone; Sambac jasmine; Sandalwood; Yarrow

**Shaoyang stage heat:** Eucalyptus; Lemon eucalyptus; Melissa; with Shen agitation: Lavender; Lemongrass; May chang; Wintergreen

**Shaoyin-stage heat:** Wintergreen

**Shen agitation:** May chang

**shingles:** Basil ct. methylchavicol; Clove bud; Lemon eucalyptus; Lemongrass; May chang; Oregano; Peppermint; Roman camomile; Rose; Saro; Tarragon; Tea tree; Thyme ct. thymol; Yarrow

**shock, emotional:** Clary sage; Frankincense; Helichrysum; Jasmine; Lavender; Peppermint; Rose; Sambac jasmine; Wintergreen; Ylang-ylang

**shortness of breath:** Fennel; Tea tree

**shyness:** Laurel

**sinus congestion:** Eucalyptus; Green myrtle; Yarrow

**sinusitis:** Cajeput; German camomile; Green myrtle; Hyssop; Marjoram; Niaouli; Palmarosa; Peppermint; Pimenta berry; Ravintsara; Rosemary ct. Cineole and ct. Camphor; Rosemary ct. verbenone; Sage; Scotch pine; Spearmint; Tarragon; Thyme ct. linalool; Yarrow

**skin:** dry: Coriander seed; Scotch pine; Vetiver; dry with rashes, Sandalwood; flabby devitalized or congested: Lemongrass; May chang; lifeless, blue, Lavender; pale sluggish/oily, Grapefruit; rough, Patchouli

**skin cancer:** Carrot seed; Sandalwood

**skin eruptions:** Yarrow

**sleep:** disturbed, Lavender; restless, Rose

**sleep difficulties:** Basil ct. methylchavicol

**sluggish energy:** Helichrysum; morning, Rosemary ct. verbenone; Rosemary ct. Cineole and ct. Camphor; Spikenard

**somnolence:** Cinnamon bark; Green myrtle; Nutmeg; Ravintsara; Rosemary ct. Cineole and ct. Camphor

**sore throat:** Roman camomile; Scotch pine

**sores:** Grand fir; Jasmine; Lemon eucalyptus; Myrrh; non-suppurating, Frankincense; Nutmeg; Rose; Winter savoury

**sorrow:** Green myrtle; Rose

**spaciness:** Angelica root; Black pepper; Carrot seed; Clove bud; Jasmine; Juniper berry; Myrrh; Patchouli; Petitgrain bigarade; Pimenta berry; Sage; Thyme ct. thymol; Vetiver; Winter savoury

**spasmodic conditions:** Clove bud; Cypress; Ginger; Helichrysum; Laurel; Lavender; Lime; Marjoram; Patchouli; Saro; Spikenard; Tarragon; Vetiver

**speech, irrational:** Spikenard

**sperm, incompetent:** Rose

**sperm count, low:** Rose; Scotch pine

**spermatorrhoea:** Myrrh; Sage; Sandalwood

**Spirochetes infections:** Patchouli

**spleen enlargement:** Lemongrass; May chang

**Spleen Qi deficiency:** Geranium; Palmarosa; Patchouli; Thyme ct. linalool; with toxic-damp, Myrrh; Vetiver

**Spleen toxic-damp:** Black pepper; Carrot seed; Cinnamon bark; Clove bud; Geranium; Grapefruit; Green myrtle; Hyssop; Juniper berry; Laurel; Lemon; Nutmeg; Palmarosa; Patchouli; Sage; Thyme ct. linalool

**Spleen Yang deficiency:** Black pepper; Cinnamon bark

**split ends:** Ylang-ylang

**sprains:** Black pepper; Ginger; Hyssop; Laurel; Lemongrass; Marjoram; Nutmeg; Rose; Rosemary ct. Cineole and ct. Camphor; Sweet orange; Tarragon; Vetiver; Wintergreen; Yarrow

**stamina, low:** Geranium; Grand fir; Niaouli; Oregano; Sage; Scotch pine; Winter savoury

**stiffness:** Black pepper; Frankincense; Ginger; Laurel; Nutmeg; Oregano; Siberian fir; Winter savoury; Wintergreen

**Stomach cold:** Cardamom; with epigastric pain/colic, Cajeput; with food stagnation: Clove bud; Pimenta berry; with Qi rebellion: Black pepper; Cajeput; Clove bud; Fennel; Ginger; Nutmeg; with shan qi: Clove bud; Fennel; Pimenta berry

**stomach cramps:** Cajeput

**Stomach Qi and food stagnation:** Coriander seed; Fennel; Laurel; Peppermint

**Stomach Qi rebellion:** Spearmint

**Stomach Qi stagnation:** Basil ct. methylchavicol; with rebellious Stomach Qi, Peppermint

**Stomach-Spleen Blood stagnation:** Laurel; Peppermint; Rosemary ct. Cineole and ct. Camphor

**Stomach-Spleen damp-cold:** Black pepper; Cinnamon bark; Ginger; Nutmeg; Oregano; Pimenta berry; Thyme ct. thymol; Winter savoury

**Stomach-Spleen empty cold:** Angelica root; Black pepper; Cinnamon bark; Clove bud; with epigastric/abdominal pain, Cajeput; Ginger; Juniper berry; Nutmeg; Oregano; Pimenta berry; Saro; Thyme ct. thymol; Winter savoury

**Stomach-Spleen Qi stagnation:** Angelica root; Black pepper; Cardamom; Cypress; Grapefruit; Laurel; Lemon; Lemongrass; Mandarin; May chang; Peppermint; Rosemary ct. Cineole and ct. Camphor; Rosemary ct. verbenone; Siberian fir; Yarrow

**stool:** irregular: Basil ct. methylchavicol; Nutmeg; Petitgrain bigarade; Tarragon; loose, mucousy: Myrrh; Nutmeg; Winter savoury; mucus in, Carrot seed; undigested food in: Pimenta berry; Thyme ct. thymol

**strains:** Black pepper; Ginger; Hyssop; Laurel; Lemongrass; Marjoram; Nutmeg; Rose; Rosemary ct. Cineole and ct. Camphor; Sweet orange; Tarragon; Vetiver; Wintergreen; Yarrow

**strep throat:** Bergamot

**stress:** Angelica root; chronic, Clary sage; Clary sage; German camomile; Helichrysum; Marjoram; Petitgrain bigarade; Roman camomile; Sweet orange

**stretch marks:** Carrot seed; Coriander seed; Geranium; Grapefruit; Jasmine; Lemongrass; Mandarin; Rose; Sweet orange; Vetiver

**stupor:** Eucalyptus; Ginger; Niaouli; Oregano; Ravintsara; Rosemary ct. Cineole and ct. Camphor; Saro; Thyme ct. thymol; Winter savoury

**subcostal pain:** Basil ct. methylchavicol; Tarragon

**sugar cravings:** Geranium

**suicidal tendency:** Geranium; Roman camomile; Rose; Yarrow

**sunburn:** German camomile; Yarrow

**sweating:** abnormal, Cypress; excessive: Clary sage; Cypress; Geranium; May chang; Petitgrain bigarade; Sage; feet, Cypress; foot, Scotch pine; Lemongrass; nighttime, Sage

**swelling:** German camomile

# T

**tachycardia:** Marjoram; May chang; Melissa; Petitgrain bigarade; Rosemary ct. verbenone; Spikenard; Tarragon; Ylang-ylang

**tapeworms:** Cinnamon bark; Thyme ct. thymol; Winter savoury

**teething pain:** Roman camomile

**tendinitis:** Basil ct. methylchavicol; Blue tansy; Laurel; Lemon eucalyptus; Lemongrass; May chang; Melissa; Peppermint; Roman camomile; Rosemary ct. Cineole and ct. Camphor; Wintergreen

**testosterone deficiency:** Niaouli; Rosemary ct. verbenone; Scotch pine

**thinking, excessive:** Vetiver; repetitive: Carrot seed; Patchouli; Vetiver

**thrombosis:** Angelica root; Lemon; Lime; Nutmeg; Tarragon

**thrush, oral:** Lemongrass; Palmarosa

**ticks:** Cistus; Lemon eucalyptus; Lemongrass; May chang; Pimenta berry; Spikenard

**tics:** Black spruce

**timidity:** Laurel; Nutmeg; Ylang-ylang

**tinnitus:** Helichrysum

**tonsillitis:** Bergamot; Myrrh; Niaouli

**toothache:** Angelica root; Black pepper; Clove bud; Laurel; Marjoram; Nutmeg; Peppermint; Pimenta berry; Roman camomile; Sage; Scotch pine; Winter savoury; Wintergreen

**trauma:** emotional: Rose; Sambac jasmine; Jasmine; Wintergreen

**travel sickness:** Basil ct. methylchavicol; Ginger; Laurel; Nutmeg

**tremors:** German camomile; Spikenard

**tuberculosis:** Atlas cedarwood; Cypress; Hyssop; Myrrh; Neroli; Sandalwood; Thyme ct. linalool; Winter savoury

# U

**ulcerative colitis:** Cistus; Helichrysum; Palmarosa; Tea tree; Vetiver; Yarrow

**ulcers:** Basil ct. methylchavicol; Cistus; Clove bud; gastric and duodenal, German camomile; Geranium; German camomile; Grand fir; Lavender; nonhealing, Carrot seed; peptic: Angelica root; Helichrysum; Juniper berry; May chang; Palmarosa; Patchouli; Tea tree; Vetiver; Pimenta berry; Roman camomile; Rose; Sambac jasmine; Spikenard; Tarragon; varicose, Frankincense; Yarrow

**ultraviolet radiation:** Coriander seed

**unknown, fear of:** Rose

**urethritis:** Fennel; Grand fir; Green myrtle; Palmarosa; Siberian fir; Spearmint; Thyme ct. linalool; Wintergreen

**urinary dribbling:** Myrrh; Sandalwood; Tarragon

**urinary incontinence:** Cypress; Fennel; Green myrtle; Yarrow

**urinary infections:** Basil ct. methylchavicol; chronic: Sandalwood; Scotch pine; Coriander seed; recurrent, Carrot seed

**urinary pain:** Angelica root; Basil ct. methylchavicol; Coriander seed; Cypress; Marjoram; Tarragon; Wintergreen; Yarrow

**urinary stones:** Fennel; Grand fir; Hyssop; Juniper berry; Lemon; Marjoram; pain from, Geranium; Tarragon; Yarrow

**urinary strangury:** Cypress; Marjoram; Melissa; Tarragon

**urination:** difficult, Juniper berry; dribbling: Cypress; Fennel; scanty or copious: Black pepper; Sage; Vetiver

**urogenital infections, chronic:** Sandalwood

**urticaria:** Roman camomile; Tea tree; Vetiver

**uterine dystocia:** Juniper berry

**uterine spasms:** Peppermint

**Uterus Blood deficiency:** Coriander seed; Jasmine; Rose; Sage; with Shen weakness, Rosemary ct. verbenone

**UV skin damage:** Carrot seed

# V

**vaginal discharge:** Cinnamon bark; Clary sage; Green myrtle; Myrrh; Sage; Thyme ct. thymol; Wintergreen

**vaginal dryness:** Rose; Rosemary ct. verbenone

**vaginal irritation/dryness:** Rose

**vaginitis, chronic:** Atlas cedarwood; Clary sage; Rosemary ct. verbenone; Sage; Sandalwood; Saro; Thyme ct. linalool; Thyme ct. thymol

**varicose veins:** Atlas cedarwood; Basil ct. methylchavicol; Bergamot; Blue tansy; Cistus; Clary sage; Cypress; Geranium; Lemon; Neroli; Niaouli; Patchouli; Rosemary ct. Cineole and ct. Camphor; Sandalwood; Spikenard; Tea tree; Vetiver; Yarrow

**venous congestion:** Clary sage

**verrucas:** Lemon; Lime; Mandarin; Tea tree

**vertigo:** Basil ct. methylchavicol; Marjoram; Melissa; Nutmeg; Peppermint; Rosemary ct. Cineole and ct. Camphor; Tarragon

**viral infections:** Eucalyptus; Laurel; Lemon; Niaouli; Saro; Tea tree

**vision, poor:** Black pepper; Fennel; Peppermint

**vitality, low:** Cajeput; Eucalyptus; Green myrtle; Niaouli; Pimenta berry; Sage; Saro; Scotch pine; Vetiver

**vitiligo:** Mandarin

**voice loss:** Jasmine

**vomiting:** Basil ct. methylchavicol; Black pepper; Cardamom; Fennel; Laurel; Mandarin; nervous, Cajeput; Patchouli; Spearmint

**vulnerability:** Black pepper; Clove bud; masked, Sandalwood; Myrrh; Niaouli; Nutmeg; Patchouli; Pimenta berry; Sandalwood; Vetiver

# W

**waking, difficult:** Lemon

**warts:** Basil ct. methylchavicol; Cinnamon bark; Lemon; Lime; Tea tree; Yarrow

**water retention:** Black pepper; Carrot seed; Cypress; Fennel; Grapefruit; Hyssop; Juniper berry; Lemon; in lower limbs, Fennel

**water-damp accumulation:** Black pepper; Cypress; Fennel; Juniper berry

**weaning:** Peppermint; Sage; Spearmint

**weight gain:** Grapefruit; Scotch pine

**weight loss:** Palmarosa; Scotch pine; Vetiver

**wheezing:** Angelica root; Fennel; Frankincense; Hyssop; Laurel; Myrrh; Winter savoury

**whooping cough:** Basil ct. methylchavicol; Cistus; Cypress; Fennel; Grand fir; Helichrysum; Marjoram; Oregano; Ravintsara; Siberian fir; Tarragon; Thyme ct. linalool; Thyme ct. thymol

**will power, low:** Angelica root; Atlas cedarwood; Black spruce; Cistus; Clove bud; Cypress; Frankincense; Juniper berry; Oregano; Scotch pine; Siberian fir; Wintergreen

**wind-damp, in skin:** Juniper berry

**wind-damp obstruction:** Frankincense; Tarragon

**wind-damp-cold obstruction:** Black pepper; Black spruce; Cajeput; Coriander seed; Ginger; Grand fir; Juniper berry; Laurel; Niaouli; Nutmeg; Ravintsara; Rosemary ct. Cineole and ct. Camphor; Sage; Saro; Scotch pine; Siberian fir; Winter savoury; Yarrow

**wind-damp-heat, in skin:** Blue tansy; German camomile; Helichrysum; Melissa; Tea tree; Yarrow

**wind-damp-heat obstruction:** Blue tansy; German camomile; Helichrysum; Lemon eucalyptus; Lemongrass; Lime; May chang; Melissa; Ravintsara; Roman camomile; Vetiver; Wintergreen; Yarrow

**wind-heat in sinuses:** Spearmint

**wind-phlegm obstruction:** Basil ct. methylchavicol; Marjoram; Tarragon

**withdrawal:** Cinnamon bark; Geranium; Ginger; Helichrysum; Jasmine; Palmarosa; Ravintsara; Rose; Rosemary ct. Cineole and ct. Camphor; Saro

**worry:** Basil ct. methylchavicol; Carrot seed; Laurel; Myrrh; Neroli; Patchouli; Roman camomile; Sambac jasmine; Sandalwood; Spikenard; Vetiver

**wounds:** Bergamot; chronic, Carrot seed; Cistus; Eucalyptus; Geranium; German camomile; Grand fir; Hyssop; infected: Clove bud; Oregano; Pimenta berry; Sage; Thyme ct. thymol; Lavender; Lemon eucalyptus; Myrrh; Palmarosa; Patchouli; Ravintsara; Roman camomile; Rose; Sandalwood; Scotch pine; Vetiver; Yarrow

**wrinkles:** Carrot seed; Cistus; Fennel; Frankincense; Jasmine; Lemongrass; Palmarosa; Patchouli; Rose; Rosemary ct. verbenone; Sweet orange; Vetiver

# Y

**Yang deficiency, with Shen weakness:** Cinnamon bark; Clove bud; Oregano; Ravintsara; Thyme ct. thymol; Winter savoury

**Yangming-stage heat:** Lemon eucalyptus; Lime; Melissa; with Shen agitation: Lemon; Lemongrass; May chang

**Yin and Qi deficiency, in perimenopause:** Tea tree

**Yin deficiency:** with empty heat: Lavender; Sandalwood; Spikenard; Tea tree; Vetiver; with Shen agitation: Atlas cedarwood; Clary sage; Lavender; sweating from, Sage